NURSING CARE
of
CLIENTS
with
SUBSTANCE
ABUSE

NURSING CARE
of
CLIENTS
with
SUBSTANCE ABUSE

Eleanor J. Sullivan, PhD, RN, FAAN
Dean and Professor,
School of Nursing,
University of Kansas,
Kansas City, Kansas

Illustrated

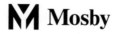 **Mosby**

St. Louis   Baltimore   Berlin   Boston   Carlsbad   Chicago   London   Madrid
Naples   New York   Philadelphia   Sydney   Tokyo   Toronto

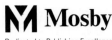

Mosby

Dedicated to Publishing Excellence

Publisher: Nancy L. Coon
Managing Editor: Jeff Burnham
Associate Developmental Editor: Linda Caldwell
Project Manager: Carol Sullivan Weis
Production Editor: Christine Carroll
Designer: Betty Schulz
Manufacturing Supervisor: Karen Lewis
Illustrations: Top Graphics

Printed in the United States of America
Composition by Village Typographers, Inc.
Printing/binding by WC Brown

Mosby–Year Book, Inc.
11830 Westline Industrial Drive
St. Louis, Missouri 63146

Library of Congress Cataloging in Publication Data

Nursing care of clients with substance abuse / Eleanor J. Sullivan.
    p. cm.
    Includes bibliographical references and index.
    ISBN 0-8016-7881-1
    1. Substance abuse—Nursing.   I. Sullivan, Eleanor J., 1938-   .
    [DNLM: 1. Substance Abuse—nursing.   WY 160 N97423 1995]
  RC564.N87   1995
  610.73'68—dc20
  DNLM/DLC
  for Library of Congress   94-30146
                                       CIP

94 95 96 97 / 9 8 7 6 5 4 3 2 1

CONTRIBUTORS

Elizabeth Bragg, RNC, MSN
Program Director of Community
   Obstetrics Outreach Program,
University of Cincinnati Hospital,
Cincinnati, Ohio

Janice Dyehouse, RN, PhD
Associate Professor,
College of Nursing and Health,
University of Cincinnati,
Cincinnati, Ohio

Dianne Felblinger, RN, EdD
Assistant Professor,
College of Nursing and Health,
University of Cincinnati,
Cincinnati, Ohio

Ann Flandermeyer, RNC, MSN
Doctoral Student,
College of Nursing and Health,
University of Cincinnati,
Cincinnati, Ohio

Michael Fleming, MD
Associate Professor, Family Medicine,
University of Wisconsin-Madison,
Madison, Wisconsin

Laina M. Gerace, RN, PhD
Assistant Professor, Psychiatric Nursing,
College of Nursing,
University of Illinois at Chicago,
Chicago, Illinois

Mary Haack, RN, PhD
Senior Research Scientist,
Center for Health Policy Research,
The George Washington University,
Washington, DC

Julia Hagemaster, PhD, RN, ARNP
Assistant Professor,
University of Kansas School of Nursing,
Kansas City, Kansas

Sandra Handley, RN, PhD, CARN
AOD Program Coordinator,
University of Kansas Medical Center,
Kansas City, Kansas

Carol Hetteberg, RN, MSN
Assistant Professor of Clinical Nursing,
College of Nursing and Health,
University of Cincinnati,
Cincinnati, Ohio

Tonda L. Hughes, RN, PhD
Assistant Professor,
Psychiatric Nursing and Post Doctoral
   Research Fellow,
School of Public Health Prevention
   Research Center,
University of Illinois at Chicago,
Chicago, Illinois

Pat Jamerson, RNC, MSN
Doctoral Student,
School of Nursing,
University of Kansas,
Kansas City, Kansas

Carole A. Kenner, RNC, DNS
Professor, Department Chair Parent Child
   Health Nursing,
University of Cincinnati,
College of Nursing and Health,
Cincinnati, Ohio

Sheila Lee, RN, MSN
Choate Health Management, Inc.,
Woburn, Massachusetts

Tona Leiker, MN, ARNP, CARN, NCACII
Director, Behavioral Health Services,
St. Francis Regional Medical Center,
Wichita, Kansas

Diana S. Look, RN, MSN, CNS, CCRN
Nurse Specialist,
Nursing Education,
Methodist Hospital,
Houston, Texas

Marianne Marcus, RN, EdD
Project Director, CSAP Faculty
    Development Grant,
Chair, Department of Nursing Systems
    and Technology,
University of Texas-Houston Health
    Science Center School of Nursing,
Houston, Texas

**Rebecca Payne McClanahan, RN, MSN,
    PhD (Candidate)**
University of Kansas School of Nursing,
Kansas City, Kansas;
Assistant Professor,
Northeast Missouri State University,
Kirksville, Missouri

Madeline A. Naegle, PhD, RN, FAAN
Associate Professor, Division of Nursing,
New York University,
New York, New York

Lynn Oswald, RN, MSN
Senior Research Nurse,
Harris County Psychiatric Center,
Houston, Texas

Ardyce Plumlee, RN, MN, CARN
Associate Professor, Retired,
University of Kansas School of Nursing,
Kansas City, Kansas

**Elizabeth A. Schenk, MSN, CRRN,
    RNCS, MDIV**
Staff Nurse,
Heather Hill, Inc.,
Chardon, Ohio

Marilyn Sawyer Sommers, PhD, RN
Associate Professor,
College of Nursing and Health,
University of Cincinnati,
Cincinnati, Ohio

Marti Stupka, RN, MS, CARN
Program Coordinator,
Chemical Dependency Services,
Evanston Hospital,
Evanston, Illinois

Eleanor J. Sullivan, RN, PhD, FAAN
Dean and Professor,
School of Nursing,
University of Kansas,
Kansas City, Kansas

Michelle Sullivan, RN, CD
Chief Psychiatric Research Nurse,
Yale University Research Unit,
New Haven, Connecticut

H. Mikel Thomas, MD
Inpatient Director of the Substance Abuse
    Treatment Unit,
Veterans Affairs Medical Center,
Kansas City, Missouri

Sandra H. Tweed, RN, PhD, CARN
Assistant Professor,
State University of New York at Buffalo,
School of Nursing,
Buffalo, New York

**Nancy M. Valentine, PhD, RN, CNAA,
    FAAN**
Assistant Chief Medical Director,
Nursing Programs,
Department of Veterans Affairs,
Washington, DC

Rothlyn Zahourek, MS, RN, CS
Assistant Clinical Professor,
University of Massachusetts School of
    Nursing-Amherst,
Amherst, Massachusetts

Douglas Ziedonis, MD
Assistant Professor/Director Dual
    Diagnosis Program,
Yale University,
New Haven, Connecticut

REVIEWERS

Jeanne A. Clement, EdD, RN, CS
Assistant Professor,
College of Nursing,
The Ohio State University,
Columbus, Ohio

Bonnie Enter-Hinrichsen, MSN, PhD
Assistant Professor,
Bradley University,
Peoria, Illinois

Pamela Billings Farley, BSN, MSN, PhD
Associate Professor,
Berea College,
Berea, Kentucky

Janice Cooke Feigenbaum, PhD, MSN, BSN
Associate Professor and Coordinator of
  Community Addictions Nursing
  Program,
D'Youville College,
Buffalo, New York

Theresa Free, PhD, MSN, BSN
Associate Professor,
College of Nursing,
University of Kentucky,
Lexington, Kentucky

Kem Louie, PhD, RN, CS, FAAN
Associate Professor,
Graduate Nursing Program,
College of Mount Saint Vincent,
Riverdale, New York

Linda Nance Marks, RN, BSN, MSN, EdD
Associate Professor,
University of Texas,
Arlington, Texas

Susan Reed, BSN, MSN
Clinical Nurse Specialist of Addictions
  Medicine and Psychiatry,
Department of Veteran Affairs,
Fort Howard, Maryland

Walter Roberson, RN, BA, MA
Assistant Patient Care Manager-Mental
  Health Services,
Deaconess Hospital,
St. Louis, Missouri

Mary Rowan, BA, MS, PhD
Assistant Professor,
College of Nursing,
The Ohio State University,
Columbus, Ohio

Joanne Sabol Stevenson, PhD, MS, BS
Professor,
College of Nursing,
The Ohio State University,
Columbus, Ohio

Antonio Suba, MD, FACS, MRO
Occupational Health Services,
St. Luke's Hospital,
St. Louis, Missouri

Arlene Thompson, RN, BSN, MS, PhD
Assistant Professor,
College of Nursing,
The Ohio State University,
Columbus, Ohio

Anita Throwe, MS, BSN, CS
Associate Professor,
College of Nursing,
Medical University of South Carolina,
Florence, South Carolina

Donna Marie Wing, RN, BSN, MS, EdD
Associate Professor and Coordinator of
  Masters Program in Nursing
  Administration,
School of Nursing,
University of Tulsa,
Tulsa, Oklahoma

DEDICATION

To my family for their continuing love and support.

Health care professionals generally skillfully manage the complications of excessive drinking, such as trauma, liver disease, and peripheral neuropathy. However, they often do not show the same skill in managing the alcohol abuse and alcoholism that cause these complications. The management of the complications is certainly important; however, the treatment of alcoholism means the modification of alcohol-seeking and alcohol-abusing behavior. If this behavior is not modified, the client experiences repeated problems caused by drinking or dies. To treat the hemorrhage or the pancreatitis and not the alcoholism is poor health care, akin to treating anemia without treating the colon cancer that causes it.

Nurses are in an excellent position to recognize the abuse of alcohol and other substances in their clients, to confront clients about their drinking, and to participate in decisions concerning referral to appropriate treatment. Nurses see clients more frequently and provide more direct, hands-on care than do other health care professionals. As a result, they form more personal, trusting relationships with those under their care. This trust may help clients accept alcoholism or other substance abuse as the cause of their medical problems and understand that the problems will continue until the underlying cause is addressed.

Nevertheless, nurses can be as negligent as physicians in identifying alcohol and other substance abuse as the basic cause of admission and readmission. Even those who wish to "do the right thing" often do not know what the right thing is. Finally, nurses who care for alcoholic or other substance-abusing clients in an alcohol or drug abuse treatment program may lack the skills necessary for successful management of their clients' problems.

The lack of adequate training in alcohol and other drug abuse by schools of nursing and other health education programs is the central reason that identifying, diagnosing, and treating or referring alcohol and other substance abusing clients has been so neglected; ultimately, increased education within the health care professions will bring a higher standard of treatment for alcoholic clients. The availability of scientifically based curricula on alcoholism and other substance abuse in health professions training is improving, but it is far from what it should be, given the number of persons who suffer from these illnesses. Thus nurses who are charged with the care of suspected or diagnosed alcohol- and other substance-abusing clients need to look beyond their current training for help.

This book, *Nursing Care of Clients with Substance Abuse* by Eleanor J. Sullivan, RN, Ph.D., FAAN, and distinguished colleagues is a primer for nurses in all clinical areas. It explains how to meet the needs of alcoholic and other substance-abusing clients. Beginning with a discussion of what alcohol and other substance abuse is, the book leads nurses through the process of identifying, diagnosing, and referring clients in all clinical settings for treatment. It also provides valuable information on the needs of alcohol- and other substance-abusing clients with special needs, such as perinatal care with multiple substance use. The payoff for those who read the various chapters is higher quality client care, improved client recovery from alcohol and other substance abuse-related complications, and savings in health care costs because of the reduction in repeat visits to the hospital or clinic for complications of drinking or substance use.

Dr. Sullivan is a distinguished leader and educator in nursing and the alcohol and substance abuse fields. Her commitment to improving the education of nurses and in turn treatment for their alcohol- and other substance-abusing clients, is no better demonstrated than in the pages of this excellent volume. I commend it to the attention and study of nurses in all settings and to any health care professional who wishes to "do the right thing."

Enoch Gordis, MD
Director,
National Institute on Alcohol Abuse and Alcoholism

The problems associated with substance abuse are complex, multidimensional, and widespread. No place are these problems more evident than in health care settings. In spite of nurses' extensive contact with clients with substance abuse problems, few educational resources are available that offer substantive, accurate information and useful techniques for dealing with this multifaceted problem. This book is designed to address such a need.

Nursing Care of Clients with Substance Abuse is based on the following three basic assumptions:

1. Substance abuse and dependence are real illnesses with both physical and psychological components.
2. Recovery from such illnesses can be realized, and return to a productive and functional life is possible.
3. Nurses play a key role in assisting clients to achieve and maintain recovery.

This book is designed to meet the growing need in both educational and clinical settings for information about nursing care of the client with substance-abuse problems. Nurses involved in caring for clients in general hospital settings, mental health units, community health settings, and alcohol and drug abuse rehabilitation programs will find this book informative and valuable in their work with clients. The book is designed as a textbook for classes in substance abuse nursing, as a reference text for specialty and advanced practice nurses working in substance abuse areas, and as an adjunct text for other courses that include substance abuse content (e.g., pediatric nursing, obstetrical nursing, community health, and mental health).

The book is arranged in three sections. Unit I, Understanding Substance Abuse, introduces the scope of the problem, describes substance abuse and diagnosis, discusses current treatment approaches, and includes an explanation of recovery and relapse. Unit II, Nursing Care of Clients with Substance Abuse, includes dimensions of substance abuse in nursing care, care of the client in the hospital, care of children and adolescents, perinatal nursing care, nursing care in community health settings, nursing care in chemical dependency treatment settings, care of clients with dual diagnoses, and nursing care of special populations, including women, minorities, and older adults. Unit III, Opportunities and Challenges in Substance Abuse, provides information about practice, education, research, and theory development; discusses financing, public policy, and legal issues; describes drug testing; and explores the variety of opportunities in substance abuse nursing practice.

A strength of the book is that many nursing and medicine experts involved in substance abuse practice and education have contributed content in their specific areas of expertise. This book brings together the best that both professions have to offer in a comprehensive, usable text. Recognizing that individuals have rights, responsibilities, and a participatory role in their own care, we have used the term *client* predominately throughout, rather than *patient*. We have attempted to use gender-inclusive language when referring to nurses and clients in this book.

For too long, society and the health care system have ignored these problems and addressed only the physical or psychological presenting problem. It is my fervent wish that this book will help nurses become sensitive, compassionate, and competent caregivers to help their clients with substance abuse problems. The health of all of us depends on it.

ACKNOWLEDGMENTS

I want to express my appreciation to the contributing authors, without whom this book would not exist. Research assistants, Marge Bott and Pat Jamerson, spent countless hours organizing and fine-tuning details. Marcia Pressly, Angela Van Buskirk, and Felicia Sappington spent significant hours typing the manuscript and taking care of other support details. Victoria Thomas, Legal Counsel, University of Kansas, provided invaluable advice regarding the legal issues in substance abuse. Finally, my research associate, Sandra Handley, oversaw the entire project. I am exceptionally grateful for her sustained commitment to this book and to providing substance abuse education for nurses.

Eleanor J. Sullivan

UNIT I   **UNDERSTANDING SUBSTANCE ABUSE**
1   Introduction to Substance Abuse   3
2   Substance Abuse and Dependency   19
3   Substance Abuse Diagnosis   47
4   Treatment for Substance Abuse   71
5   Recovery and Relapse   102

UNIT II   **NURSING CARE OF CLIENTS WITH SUBSTANCE ABUSE**
6   Dimensions of Nursing Care of Clients with Substance Abuse   117
7   Nursing Care of Clients with Substance Abuse in the Hospital   135
8   Substance Abuse in Perinatal Care   191
9   Substance Abuse in Families, Children, and Adolescents   234
10   Nursing Care of Clients with Substance Abuse in Community Settings   270
11   Nursing Care in Chemical Dependency Treatment Settings   305
12   Dual Diagnosis: A Challenge for Mental Health and Substance Abuse Caregivers   345
13   Nursing Care of Special Populations   373

UNIT III   **OPPORTUNITIES AND CHALLENGES IN SUBSTANCE ABUSE**
14   Education, Research, and Theory Development   409
15   Financing, Legal Issues, and Public Policy   422
16   Drug Testing   436
17   Challenging Practice Opportunities in Substance Abuse Nursing   444

APPENDICES
A   Diagnostic Instruments
   A-1   CAGEAID Questionnaire   463
   A-2   Michigan Alcoholism Screening Test (MAST)   464
   A-3   Alcohol Use Disorders Identification Test (AUDIT)   466
B   Organizational Resources and Services   469
C   Publications and Periodicals   471

CONTENTS

UNIT I   UNDERSTANDING SUBSTANCE ABUSE

1   Introduction to Substance Abuse   3
Eleanor J. Sullivan

Historical Perspective   4
Societal Approaches   5
   Avoidance and denial   5
   Moralistic and punitive   5
   Therapeutic approach   6
Prevalence and Incidence   6
   Prevalence   6
   Incidence   7
Definition of Terms   8
   Alcohol and drug disorder terms   8
Overview of Substances of Abuse   10
   Alcohol   10
   Sedatives and hypnotics   10
   Opiates   11
   Minor tranquilizers   11
   Stimulants   11
   Hallucinogens   11
   Inhalants   11
   Over-the-counter drugs   11
Attitudes and Myths About Substance Abuse   12
   Myths   12
   Attitudes of health care professionals   13
The Nurse's Role with Substance Abusing Clients   13
   Identification   14
   Detoxification and rehabilitation   15
   Prevention and education   15
Substance Abuse Content in Nursing Education   15
   What is needed in nursing education?   16
   Recent federal initiatives   17
Summary   17

2   Substance Abuse and Dependency   19

Michael Fleming
Janice Dyehouse
Marilyn Sawyer Sommers

Models of Illness   19
    Jellinek model   19
    Vaillant's study   21
    Chronic illness paradigm   22
Etiology and Contributing Factors   23
    Genetics   23
    Environmental factors   24
Characteristics of Substance Abuse   25
    Intoxication   25
    Tolerance   25
    Cross tolerance   26
    Dependence   26
    Loss of control   27
    Reinforcement   28
    Craving   28
    Progressive nature   28
    Common defense mechanisms   29
Categories of Substances   30
    Alcohol   30
    Amphetamines   31
    Barbiturates   33
    Benzodiazepines   34
    Opioids   34
    Cocaine   35
    Marijuana   36
    Hallucinogens   37
    Inhalants   37
    Steroids   37
    Designer drugs   38
    Nicotine   38
    Caffeine   38
    Polydrug addiction   38
Individual and Family Consequences   38
    Psychological/emotional   38
    Family   39
    Community   40
    Occupational/professional   40
    Financial   40
Societal Consequences   40
    Accidents   41
    Crime   41
    Domestic violence   41
    Child abuse   41

      Suicide   42
      Prostitution   42
      Disease   42
      Treatment costs   42
      Workplace effects   43
      Community deterioration   43
   Summary   44

3   Substance Abuse Diagnosis   47

H. Mikel Thomas
Sandra Handley

   Assessment of Substance Abuse   47
      Screening instruments for general settings   47
      Responding to positive screens   49
      Interviewing and the substance abuse history   51
      Assessment scales for clinical settings   55
      Biochemical markers   56
   Nursing Assessment and Diagnosis   57
      Nursing assessment   58
      Nursing diagnosis   59
   Medical Models of Assessment and Diagnosis   62
      DSM diagnosis   62
      Diagnostic instruments for clinical practice and research   64
   Dual Diagnosis   67
   Relationship Between Nursing and Medical Models   67
   Summary   67

4   Treatment for Substance Abuse   71

Michelle Sullivan
Douglas Ziedonis

   Substance Abuse Treatment   71
   Treatment Philosophies   72
      Disease concept   72
      Twelve step program   73
      Minnesota model   73
      Medical model   73
      Neuroscience model   73
      Psychiatric model   74
      Cognitive behavioral approach   74
      Social learning theory   74
      Sociocultural perspective   74
   Assessment and Intervention   75
   Treatment Planning and Reevaluation   76
   The Role of the Client   78
   Stages of Change   78
   Continuity of Care   78

Treatment Settings   81
    Inpatient settings   81
    Partial hospitalization   82
    Outpatient programs   83
    Halfway houses   83
    Therapeutic communities (long-term residential settings)   83
Long-Term Aftercare   84
Methadone Maintenance Programs   85
Tools of Treatment   85
    Pharmacotherapy   85
    Individual therapy   87
    Behavioral contracting   87
    Education   88
    Group therapy   88
    Family treatment   89
    Therapeutic milieu   89
    Vocational counseling   90
    Activities therapies   90
    Relapse prevention   91
    Twelve step programs   91
    Spiritual counseling   95
Effectiveness of treatment   96
    How effectiveness is determined   96
    Matching studies   97
    Does treatment work?   97
    Factors associated with improved outcomes   98
Trends in treatment   99
    Increasing outpatient treatment   99
    Changes in reimbursement   99
Summary   100

5   Recovery and Relapse   102

Laina M. Gerace
Sandra Handley
Marti Stupka

Recovery   102
Perspectives and Approaches to Recovery   103
    Spontaneous remission   103
    Harm reduction approach   104
    Twelve step approach   106
Goals of Recovery   106
    Abstinence   106
    Lifestyle change   107
    Alternative recovery goals   108
Relapse   110
    Physiological factors in relapse   110
    Models of relapse prevention   111
Summary   112

UNIT II   NURSING CARE OF CLIENTS WITH SUBSTANCE ABUSE

6   Dimensions of Nursing Care of Clients with Substance Abuse   117
Ardyce Plumlee

Using the Nursing Process   118
   Assessing the client   118
   Nursing diagnoses   123
Planning Care   124
   Intervention and referral   124
Evaluation   126
   Continuity of care   126
   Nursing care related to recovery status   127
Managing Behavior Problems in Clients with Substance Abuse   127
   Denial   127
   Manipulation   129
   Hostility   130
   Need to control   132
   Drug seeking behavior   133
   Pessimism regarding treatment success   133
Summary   134

7   Nursing Care of Clients with Substance Abuse in the Hospital   135
Marianne T. Marcus
Diana S. Look
Lynn M. Oswald

Managing Acute Withdrawal   136
   Evaluation of overall health status   137
   Physical and environmental support   137
   Psychological support   137
   Pharmacological support   137
   Alcohol   139
   Other substances of abuse   148
Care in General Medical/Surgical Units   148
   Alcohol sequelae   154
   Liver   155
   Gastrointestinal tract   161
   Cardiovascular system   167
   Musculoskeletal system   169
   Alcohol and cancer   169
   Sequelae of other substances of abuse   170
Perioperative Care for Clients with Substance Abuse   176
Pain Management   177
   Clients who admit substance abuse   178
   Clients who do not admit substance abuse   179

Nonopioid and nonpharmacological strategies   179
Emergency Care   179
General guidelines   184
Drug overdose   184
Suicide attempts   185
Other emergency care encounters   185
Discharge   188
Summary   188

8   Substance Abuse in Perinatal Care   191

Carol Hetteberg
Elizabeth Bragg
Dianne Feblinger
Ann Flandermeyer
Carole Kenner
Pat Jamerson

Alcohol   192
Placental transfer of alcohol   193
Lactation   194
Fetal Alcohol Syndrome and Fetal Alcohol Effects   194
Incidence   194
Diagnosis   195
Dysmorphic characteristics   197
Growth deficiency   198
Central nervous system dysfunction   198
Recognition and referral   200
Heroin   200
Methadone   201
Cocaine   201
Marijuana   203
Tobacco   204
Nicotine   204
Nitrosamine   204
Carbon monoxide   204
Cadmium   205
Cyanide   205
Consequences of tobacco use during pregnancy   205
Fetal effects   205
Factors associated with smoking and infancy   206
Lactation   206
Other Drugs   207
Nursing Care of the Mother   207
Prenatal care   207
Identification of substance abuse   208
Labor and delivery   209
Postnatal care   213

Substance Abuse Treatment for Pregnant Women   214
    Availability of treatment   214
    Public policy   214
The Drug Addicted Neonate   215
    Neonate abstinence syndrome   215
    Respiratory depression   218
Nursing Care of the Infant   218
    Withdrawal   218
    Fluid balance   218
    Infection control   219
    Respiratory care   220
    Developmental assessment   220
    Developmental care   222
    Parental support and education   223
Prevention   223
    Community education   223
    Warning labels   228
Summary   228

9   Substance Abuse in Families, Children, and Adolescents   234

Sandra H. Tweed
Ardyce Plumlee

Substance Abuse and the Family   234
    Dysfunctional family patterns   234
Codependency   239
    Adult children of alcoholics   248
    Family problems when the substance abuser recovers   248
    Nursing care of families with substance abusing adults   249
Effects on Children   250
    Consequences for children, adolescents, and adults   250
    Nursing care of the child from a family with substance abuse   253
Substance Abuse in Adolescents   254
    Substance use as a developmental phenomenon   254
    Patterns of adolescent substance use   254
    Influencing factors   255
    Identifying the adolescent substance abuser   260
    Current trends   260
Prevention efforts   261
Summary   266

10   Nursing Care of Clients with Substance Abuse in Community Settings   270

Elizabeth A. Schenk

Special Needs in Urban Populations   270
    Poverty   271

Unemployment   271
Homelessness   271
Unplanned pregnancies   271
HIV/AIDS   271
Violence   272
Special Needs in Rural Populations   272
Availability of Treatment Services   273
Financing treatment   273
Primary Prevention   274
Nursing role   274
Secondary Prevention   275
Adolescents   275
Minorities   275
Pregnant women   275
Mentally ill   276
Elderly   276
Families   276
Tertiary Prevention   277
Care of recovering clients   277
Nursing Care in the Home Setting   285
Individual and family assessment   285
Clues in the home   285
Abuse   286
Intervention and Referral   288
Brief intervention   288
Structured intervention   288
Intervention process   289
Follow-up   290
Nursing Care in School Settings   290
Primary prevention in schools   290
Secondary prevention in schools   291
Tertiary prevention in schools   293
Nursing Care in Occupational Settings   294
Primary prevention in the workplace   294
Secondary prevention in the workplace   296
Tertiary prevention in the workplace   297
Costs   300
Employees' rights   300
Communication with others   301
Nursing Care in Outpatient Settings   302
Prenatal and well-baby clinics   302
Surgi-centers   302
Urgent care centers   302
Primary care   303
Summary   303

11   Nursing Care in Chemical Dependency Treatment Settings   305

Sandra Handley
Tona Leiker

Factors Affecting Nursing Care in Substance Abuse Treatment   305
   Philosophy   305
   Education of nurses in a substance abuse practice   307
   Role of the nurse in the organization   308
Interdisciplinary Aspects of Substance Abuse Treatment   309
   Other professional roles in substance abuse treatment   312
Nursing Care in Detoxification   314
   Assessment of withdrawal   314
   Withdrawal patterns   315
   Management of detoxification   321
Nursing Care in Substance Abuse Treatment   330
   Dimensions of care   330
   Role modeling for clients   342
Summary   342

12   Dual Diagnosis: A Challenge for Mental Health and Substance Abuse Caregivers   345

Rothlyn Zahourek

Definition of Dual Diagnosis   345
Primary and Secondary Diagnoses   347
Treatment of the Client with Dual Diagnosis   347
   A model for treatment   348
Characteristics of Treatment for the Client with Dual Diagnosis   351
   Contingency contracts   351
   Family treatment   352
   Group treatment   352
   Educating the staff   353
The Nurse's Role in Treatment   353
   The nurse's role in inpatient treatment   354
   The nurse's role in partial hospitalization   355
   The nurse's role in residential treatment   370
   The nurse's role in outpatient, vocational, and rehabilitation
      settings   371
Summary   372

13   Nursing Care of Special Populations   373

Julia Hagemaster
Tonda L. Hughes
Rebecca Payne McClanahan

Racial and Ethnic Minorities   373
   African Americans   374

Hispanics   375
Asian Americans   377
Native Americans   378
Culturally specific treatment interventions   379
Women   381
Adolescents and young women   385
Influence of employment   386
Racial and ethnic minority women   386
Health consequences of substance abuse in women   386
Other consequences of substance abuse in women   387
Implications for treatment   387
Homosexual Men and Women   389
Implications for treatment   394
Clients with HIV and AIDS   396
Implications for treatment   397
The Homeless   397
Older Adults   398
Prescription and polydrug use   399
Problems with alcoholism   399
Psychosocial and physical complications   400
Intervention with the older adult   400
Health Care Professionals   401
Summary   403

UNIT III   OPPORTUNITIES AND CHALLENGES IN SUBSTANCE ABUSE

14   Education, Research, and Theory Development   409

Madeline A. Naegle

Curricular Change for Alcohol and Other Drug Education   410
Models for curricular change   411
Theory Development and Knowledge Building   413
Theories about addictions   416
Theoretical frameworks   417
Summary   419

15   Financing, Legal Issues, and Public Policy   422

Eleanor J. Sullivan
Mary Haack

Financing Substance Abuse Treatment   422
Evolution of financing policy   423
Reorganization of the Alcohol, Drug Abuse, and Mental Health
Administration (ADAMHA)   423
How treatment is financed today   424
Matching clients to treatment   428

Recommendations for coverage   428
A Drug-Free Workplace   429
Legal Issues in Drug Testing   429
   Civil liberty issues   430
   Due process issues   431
   Common law liability   431
Protecting Clients' Legal Rights   431
   Confidentiality of client records   431
   Protection from discrimination   433
Politics and Policy   434
Summary   434

16   Drug Testing   436

Eleanor J. Sullivan

What Is Drug Testing?   436
The Drug Testing Process   437
   Definitions   437
   Types of drug tests   437
   Elimination times   438
   Accuracy   438
Procedures for Drug Testing   440
   Collecting the specimen   440
   Chain of custody   440
   The laboratory   440
The Cost of Drug Testing   441
When Is Drug Testing Used?   441
   During treatment and follow-up   441
   To protect the public   441
   In the workplace   442
Guidelines for Testing   442
Summary   442

17   Challenging Practice Opportunities in Substance Abuse Nursing   444

Nancy M. Valentine
Sheila Lee

Context of Substance Abuse Nursing   444
The Emergence of Addictions Nursing Practice   446
Practice Opportunities   447
   Generalist roles   447
   Clinical specialists in substance abuse   453
   Consultation/liaison roles   456
   Collaborative roles   456
   Opportunities in management and administration   456
   Educational considerations   457
Summary   457

APPENDICES

A   Diagnostic Instruments

   A-1   CAGEAID Questionnaire   463

   A-2   Michigan Alcoholism Screening Test (MAST)   464

   A-3   Alcohol Use Disorders Identification Test (AUDIT)   466

B   Organizational Resources and Services   469

C   Publications and Periodicals   471

Index   475

UNIT

1

UNDERSTANDING
SUBSTANCE
ABUSE

1   **Introduction to Substance Abuse**

2   **Substance Abuse and Dependency**

3   **Substance Abuse Assessment and Diagnosis**

4   **Treatment for Substance Abuse**

5   **Recovery and Relapse**

1 Introduction to Substance Abuse

Substance abuse and addictive disorders are major health and social problems in today's society. An estimated 15.3 million Americans exhibit some symptoms of alcoholism or alcohol dependence (NIAAA, 1993). In addition, 14.5 million Americans currently use illicit drugs (NIDA, 1991). Not only are an individual's health and safety at risk when a mood-altering substance, including alcohol, is abused but the lives of family members, friends, employers, and innocent bystanders are also profoundly affected and may be irreparably damaged by resulting events such as homicides, crime, or automobile accidents. Addressing these problems is a challenge to modern health care, as well as our society.

This chapter presents the historical perspective of substance abuse and explains various approaches to the problem. Common terms are defined, and attitudes and myths explored. The nurse's role in substance abuse care is examined along with the need for this content in nursing educational programs.

The cost of alcohol and other drug abuse to individuals and society makes these disorders one of the nation's most significant and troublesome problems. It has been estimated that alcohol abuse costs impose an $85.8 billion burden on the US economy (NIAAA, 1993). Drug abuse costs are estimated at $58.3 billion (NIDA, 1991). Direct costs include health care expenses (both short- and long-term care), treatment for addictive disorders, violent crime, motor vehicle crashes, incarceration of offenders, long-term care for children born with fetal alcohol syndrome, job absenteeism, and reduced productivity. Indirect costs include the effect on individual lives, family functioning and stability, community impact, and additional job effects, including coworkers' functioning and workplace morale. The pain and suffering endured by both afflicted individuals and those around them is impossible to measure.

Substance abuse problems and addictive disorders affect people of every race, age, sex, ethnic origin, social class, income level, educational level, or occupation. They are "equal opportunity" disorders. Although family history predisposes individuals to addictive disorders, any person who consumes a psychoactive substance (or combination of substances) is at risk for substance abuse or dependency.

Because any person can suffer from addictive disorders (and millions do), all nurses care for substance-abusing clients whether they have a diagnosis of dependency or not (most do not). In addition, substance abuse disorders cause or contrib-

3

ute to a variety of other health care problems (e.g., cirrhosis, pancreatitis, cardio-vascular disease, trauma) that bring substance abusers into the health care system. The nurse is in a pivotal position to identify clients with addictive problems and work with the physician, the family, and other health care professionals to intervene and refer clients and their families to appropriate care.

HISTORICAL PERSPECTIVE

Since the beginning of the human race, the use of psychoactive substances has been part of virtually every culture. Alcohol use has been documented in ancient Greece and Egypt. Today, the use of some drugs is encouraged in one culture and forbidden in another (Mathre, 1992). For example, alcohol and caffeine are socially acceptable, legal, and widely used in most western countries while their use is prohibited in other countries (e.g., Saudi Arabia). Conversely, in the United States, "illegal" drugs (opium, mescaline, coca leaves) have ritualistic use in sacred ceremonies in other cultures (e.g., South American Indians).

Decisions to accept or prohibit a drug's use in the United States frequently have been made in the absence of knowledge or guided by misinformation. Many drugs were considered safe and not habit-forming when first introduced. Amphetamines for weight control and benzodiazepines for stress were widely prescribed and even meperidine (Demerol) was initially thought to be a non–habit-forming alternative to morphine.

When use of a specific drug becomes a problem, the usual response has been prohibition. From 1920 to 1933, alcohol use was illegal in the United States. Today, marijuana, cocaine, and heroin are prohibited substances except for medical purposes (e.g., marijuana for nausea). When a drug is designated illegal, its use goes underground and a network of crime evolves to provide illicit access to the drug. The resulting crime causes people to view the drug itself as the cause of crime rather than recognizing that *prohibiting* use of the drug is the origin of the problem.

The choice of addictive substance is based primarily on access. Access and social acceptability is why alcohol is the most widely used, and thus abused, drug in this country. Easily acquired prescription drugs are often the "drug of choice" for physicians, pharmacists, and nurses who become addicted. Access to cocaine, marijuana, and heroin encourage their use in some inner city neighborhoods.

The cause and appropriate treatment for substance abuse has been debated since the beginning of the United States. As early as 1785, Dr. Benjamin Rush, a signer of the Declaration of Independence and a physician in George Washington's army, identified "intemperance" as a disease, but controversy regarding the disease concept has continued over the years (Fingarette, 1991).

Alcoholics Anonymous (AA) was established in the early 1930s by two men suffering from alcoholism who had not been helped by medical science. They determined a method by which a person could live with the addiction but not focus on the *cause* of the problem. This organization (and its related organizations, e.g., Narcotics Anonymous, Cocaine Anonymous, Al Anon) has been successful in helping millions of people worldwide recover from addictive illnesses.

SOCIETAL APPROACHES

The United States addresses addictive disorders in one of three ways. These are (1) to ignore, avoid, or deny the problem; (2) to see the problem as a moral defect requiring punitive action; or (3) to view the problem as an illness requiring therapeutic attention and decriminalization.

Avoidance and denial

Avoidance and denial are understandable, since the difference between use, abuse, and dependence is not easy to determine. Substance use, especially alcohol, is readily accepted and even expected in many situations (e.g., wedding toasts). Indeed *excessive* use is condoned in special circumstances (e.g., New Year's Eve celebrations).

Alcohol and drug disorders are chronic and insidious problems difficult to recognize, diagnose, and treat. There is no definitive diagnostic method, laboratory test, or x-ray to identify alcohol or drug disorders. Some tests do detect organ damage (e.g., liver function) after a long progression of the illness, but these tests are unable to identify the primary illness of addiction. Adding to the confusion about these disorders, the choice of drug(s) and patterns of abuse differ between individuals. Also, alcohol and drug disorders are often accompanied by concomitant health and social problems (e.g., loss of job), thereby confounding aspects of an illness with socially unacceptable behavior. It is easy to understand why these disorders are ignored, avoided, and denied.

Moralistic and punitive

Viewing alcohol and drug abuse as a moral failing has a long and colorful history stemming from early beliefs that alcohol was the root of the "evil" of drunkenness. The Temperance Movement, begun in 1813, was founded on this belief. Fundamentalist religions, common in early American history, eschewed drinking on spiritual grounds. Both slovenliness and laziness resulting from intemperant drinking defied the inherent values of the Protestant work ethic.

In response to growing public concern about alcohol and drug abuse after the turn of the century, Congress passed the Pure Food and Drug Act of 1906, which required warning labels on prescription drugs known to be habit-forming. The Harrison Narcotic Act of 1914 further restricted sale of narcotics and provided the legal basis for intrusion of federal law enforcement agents into control of narcotics. Although the Narcotic Act expressly permitted dispensing of narcotics for "legitimate medical purposes" in the course of "professional practice only," later legal decisions based on the act limited any prescribing for an addict. The most dramatic social consequence of this approach was the association of addiction with crime, which places the emphasis on interdiction (i.e., prohibiting) rather than treatment (i.e., assisting).

The punitive approach to such moral failings has culminated most recently in the "war on drugs." Launched by the federal government in 1986, it is based on the premise that illegal drug use is morally wrong and unacceptable and users must be punished. According to the National Council of Alcohol and Drug Dependence

(NCADD), this program has reduced drug use among casual users and has led to the incarceration of large numbers of drug addicts (NCADD, 1991). It has done little, however, to reduce crime or the demand for drugs. Over 1 million people are incarcerated in the United States, more people per capita than any other country in the world. This figure represents a doubling of the prison population, including a tripling of the female prison population, since 1980 (General Accounting Office, 1991a, 1991b). This increase is due largely to incarceration of nonviolent drug addicts because of the new federal mandatory sentencing laws enforced upon this population. It is estimated that 75% of all federal and state prison and local jail inmates, probationers, and parolees need comprehensive drug treatment and aftercare services; but only 1% of federal inmates, 20% of state inmates, and less than 10% of jail inmates currently receive services (General Accounting Office, 1991a, 1991b).

Today, interdiction and law enforcement activities are the focus of this "war" rather than an equal emphasis on prevention and treatment. Over 70% of the resources spent on the drug war are utilized for interdiction and law enforcement with no evidence that these efforts have been or could be successful (NCADD, 1991). Two other factors contribute to the failure of the drug war. The target has been casual users of drugs, not those who are addicted, with indiscriminate drug screenings and punitive incarceration for drug possession. Even though the health consequences of alcohol use are far more devastating than those from illegal drugs and millions more people suffer from alcohol problems, alcohol has been excluded from the drug war.

Therapeutic approach

When addictive disorders are considered illnesses, then the appropriate approach is therapeutic. Drug and alcohol treatment has been found to be effective in breaking the cycle of addiction; returning people to productive, responsible lives; reducing health care costs; and decreasing criminal behavior (Gerstein & Harwood, 1990). Regardless, resources are woefully inadequate to meet the need. The consequences to society of nontreatment are enormous (e.g., pregnant women give birth to children with lifelong health problems, drug-dependent individuals end up in jail). Support for prevention and treatment for both alcohol and drug problems would help prevent or decrease the severe health and social problems associated with dependence.

PREVALENCE AND INCIDENCE

Prevalence

Prevalence data identify the occurrence of a disorder over a period of time (e.g., the past 12 months, lifetime). The prevalence of substance use, abuse, and dependence in the general population was estimated from a nationwide sample of more than 20,000 adults (Figure 1-1). Both lifetime and recent diagnoses were determined. Lifetime diagnosis means that the criteria for abuse or dependence was met at some time in one's life. A current problem with alcohol or other drugs is indicated when the person has met the diagnostic criteria within the past 6 months. According to this landmark study, more than 16% of the population has experienced or is experi-

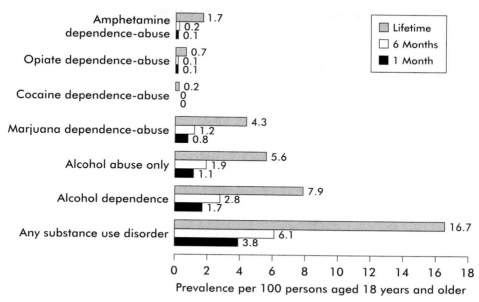

Fig. 1-1. The Epidemiological Catchment Area (ECA) study was conducted in the early 1980s on a sample of more than 20,000 adults. The data obtained from this cross-sectional study report prevalence of use, abuse, and dependence in the general population. The frequency of the problems found in this study is less than that found in ambulatory care settings. The criteria for abuse and dependence are based on DSM-III criteria. A lifetime diagnosis of alcohol dependence indicates that the subjects met criteria for dependence once in their life. Persons who met criteria in the past 6 months represent a current problem with abuse or dependence. (From Fleming, M.F. & Barry, K.L.: *Addictive disorders,* St. Louis: Mosby, 1992.)

encing a problem with alcohol or another drug (Robins & Regier, 1991).

In primary health care settings, however, higher rates of both lifetime and current use have been reported (Fleming & Barry, 1992). Lifetime alcohol disorders were estimated at 16% to 28% and drug disorders at 7% to 9%.

Incidence

Incidence measures the number of occurrences of a disorder at one point in time (sometimes expressed as "new cases") and is useful to track changes in patterns of illness (e.g., increasing breast cancer rates, decreasing rates of heart disease). Prevalence data for alcohol and drug disorders have been collected from information regarding existing cases. The incidence of these disorders, however, is more difficult to estimate because new cases are not reported to a centralized database. Thus change in the number of cases is not tracked across time as in cases such as cancer, hepatitis, or AIDS.

DEFINITION OF TERMS

Defining terms used in treating substance abuse and addiction disorders is a difficult and confusing task. The various terms used to describe addictive disorders reflect the confusion surrounding the complex processes inherent in these problems. In addition, differing philosophical perspectives guide various groups of professionals, as well as lay people, to a preference for specific terms. For example, counselors who treat clients with alcohol and drug problems often prefer the term *chemical dependents,* referring to their clients and *chemical dependency treatment,* referring to their practice. Other professionals prefer the term *substance abuse* for problems resulting from the use of alcohol or other mood-altering drugs and use *addictive disorders* when the problems have escalated to dependency. In this book, all of these terms will be used but, primarily, *substance abuse* and *addictive disorders* will be used to describe the problem and *chemical dependency* will describe a specific treatment. The Diagnostic and Statistical Manual of Mental Disorders, fourth edition (DSM-IV) will be used for diagnostic terms (American Psychiatric Association, 1994).

Following are brief explanations for common terms used to describe alcohol and drug problems and their treatment (Fleming & Barry, 1992).

Alcohol and drug disorder terms

Use.   *Light to moderate users* consume between 1 and 12 drinks per week, less than 4 drinks per occasion, and/or use other drugs 1 to 2 times per week in small quantities.

Heavy users drink more than 2 drinks per day, more than 4 drinks three or more times per week, exhibit binge patterns of use, and/or use illicit drugs more than twice per week.

Problematic users have experienced one or more alcohol- or drug-related problems, such as being arrested for driving under the influence of alcohol (DUI), medical complications, family problems, or other behavioral consequences.

Problem drinking.   *Problem drinking* is an informal term describing a pattern of drinking associated with life problems before establishing a definitive diagnosis of alcoholism.

Substance abuse.   *Substance abuse* is the harmful use of a specific psychoactive (i.e., addictive) substance(s) (e.g., alcohol or other drug(s)).

Alcoholism.   *Alcoholism* is a primary, chronic disease with genetic, psychosocial, and environmental factors influencing its development and manifestations. The disease often is progressive and fatal. It is characterized by continuous or periodic impaired control over drinking, preoccupation with the drug alcohol, use of alcohol despite adverse consequences, and distortions in thinking, most notably denial.

Addiction.   *Addiction* is the disease process characterized by continued use of a specific substance despite physical, psychological, or social harm.

Dependence.   *Physical dependence* is the physiological state of adaptation to a specific psychoactive substance, characterized by emergence of a withdrawal syndrome during abstinence, which may be relieved in total or in part by readministration of the substance.

Psychological dependence is a subjective sense of need for a specific psychoactive substance, either for its positive effects or to avoid negative effects associated with its absence. Physiological dependence is a necessary but not sufficient condition to meet the criteria for drug dependence. Psychological dependence also must occur. For example, a person receiving narcotics for pain control may experience withdrawal symptoms when the drug is discontinued but because psychological dependence has not occurred a diagnosis of drug dependence would not be accurate. Chapter 2 describes dependency in greater detail and Chapter 3 discusses diagnoses.

Recovery.   *Recovery* is a poorly understood, complex process that varies from individual to individual. Recovery refers to a chosen lifestyle without the use of addictive substances usually subsequent to treatment. Periods of abstinence may alternate with lapses (slips) of use or with full-blown relapses. (See Chapter 5 for more on the recovery process.)

Abstinence.   *Abstinence* means not using addictive psychoactive substances. It also may denote cessation of addictive or compulsive behavior (e.g., gambling, overeating).

Sobriety.   *Sobriety* is the state of complete abstinence from psychoactive substances by an addicted individual in conjunction with a satisfactory quality of life.

Relapse.   *Relapse* is the recurrence of psychoactive substance–dependent behavior in an individual who has previously achieved and maintained abstinence for a significant period of time beyond withdrawal (see Chapter 5).

Disease/illness.   Alcohol and drug disorders are often called *diseases* and those suffering from them described as *ill*. Controversy exists, however, between those who interpret disease in the narrow, biological perspective and conclude that addiction problems do not meet these criteria and those who define disease as an involuntary condition characterized by various biopsychosocial (e.g., genetic, psychological, environmental) factors.

Remission.   Since alcohol and drug disorders are regarded as lifelong problems, a recovering person is considered to be in *remission*. Individuals are not referred to as "recovered" but "in recovery" or "recovering" nor are they referred to as former alcoholics or addicts. *Partial remission* refers to some use of the substance and some symptoms of dependence that have occurred during the past 6 months. *Full remission* refers to no use of the substance and no symptoms of dependence. The remaining chapters in Unit I will describe these and other relevant terms in more detail.

OVERVIEW OF SUBSTANCES OF ABUSE

Abused substances are those that affect the central nervous system and alter an individual's perceptions. They are often called *mood-altering* because of their ability to enhance one's mood by depressing or stimulating the central nervous system. Many substances, natural and synthetic, are able to produce such effects. Substance abuse and addiction problems usually involve psychoactive drugs. Chapter 2 describes the categories of drugs in more detail.

Alcohol

Alcohol is a depressant and is the most commonly used and abused substance. It is widely available, can be legally acquired by persons over 21 (in most states), and is relatively inexpensive. Many beverages, including beer, wine, and distilled liquor, contain varying amounts (i.e., strengths) of alcohol. Figure 1-2 indicates equivalent amounts of alcohol in various drinks.

Sedatives and hypnotics

Sedatives and hypnotics depress the central nervous system and are widely prescribed for anesthesia, sleep disorders, and epilepsy. Because they produce euphoria, the potential for addiction exists. These drugs include barbiturates (Amytal,

Contents of a Standard Alcoholic Drink

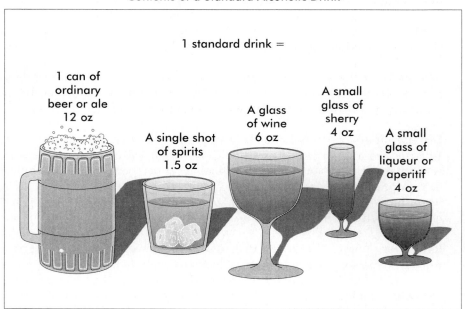

Fig. 1-2.   There is approximately 1 oz of pure alcohol in three standard drinks. A 12-oz wine cooler is equivalent in alcohol content to a 12-oz bottle of beer. (From Fleming, MF and Barry, KL: *Addictive disorders,* St. Louis: Mosby, 1992.)

Nembutal, Seconal, Luminal, Tuinal, Butisol), chloral hydrate, ethchlorvynol (Placi-dyl), glutethimide (Doriden), methyprylon (Noludar), and meprobamate (Equanil, Miltown), among others.

Opiates

Opiates also are referred to as narcotics and are effective pain-relieving drugs. The potential for addiction is great because of the euphoria they induce. Common opi-ates include morphine, heroin, methadone, meperidine (Demerol), codeine, hydro-morphone (Dilaudid), oxycodone (in Percodan), pentazocine (Talwin), and prop-oxyphene (Darvon). Because of their access in health care settings, opiates are often abused by dependent health care professionals (Sullivan, Bissell, & Williams, 1988).

Minor tranquilizers

Benzodiazepines are the most common minor tranquilizers used to treat stress and anxiety. They are readily available and commonly abused. Diazepam (Valium), chlordiazepoxide (Librium), lorazepam (Ativan), flurazepam (Dalmane), alprazo-lam (Xanax), oxazepam (Serax), chlorazepate (Tranxene, Azene), tenazepam (Res-toril), and triazolam (Halcion) are among the common benzodiazepines.

Stimulants

Stimulants excite the central nervous system and are widely used and abused. When caffeine and nicotine are included in this category (as they should be), stimu-lants are the most common group of drugs of dependence today. Stimulants in-clude cocaine, amphetamines (Benzedrine, Dexedrine, Ritalin), caffeine, and nico-tine.

Hallucinogens

Hallucinogens distort reality, produce euphoria, and are used recreationally for religious experiences in some cultures. Cannabis (marijuana), lysergic acid diethyl-amide (LSD), mescaline, peyote, and phencyclidine (PCP) are examples of hallu-cinogens.

Inhalants

Inhalants cause an altered state of mind, induce intoxication, and may produce hallucinations. Gases and solvents that can be inhaled include adhesives (e.g., rub-ber cement, airplane glue), dry cleaning substances (e.g., spot remover), solvents (e.g., paint thinner, nail polish remover), fuels (e.g., lighter fluid, camping gases), aerosols (e.g., spray paint, hair spray), amyl nitrite, and nitrous oxide. These often are used because of their potency and their fast reaction time.

Over-the-counter drugs

Over-the-counter (OTC) drugs are usually self-prescribed and administered. Many have the potential to be abused. These include analgesics, cough and cold medica-tions, appetite suppressants, and nonprescription sedatives. There is considerable controversy about whether individuals who are recovering from addictive disor-ders should use these drugs because of the potential for cross-addiction to other substances. Although this is a legitimate concern, research has not yet documented whether or to what degree these drugs are a threat to recovery.

For more information about the actions of substances of abuse, Bennett & Woolf (1991) is an excellent reference.

ATTITUDES AND MYTHS ABOUT SUBSTANCE ABUSE

In spite of the fact that millions of Americans use and enjoy the pleasurable effects of psychoactive substances (e.g., alcohol), the predominant social attitude toward the *abuse* of alcohol and the nontherapeutic use of other mood-altering drugs is negative. Historical factors, inaccurate information, stereotyping, and moralistic beliefs contribute to a generally pessimistic attitude toward alcoholics and drug abusers.

Myths

Prevailing myths perpetuate misinformation about the process of addiction, characteristics of abusers, and the outcomes of treatment. Clients, their families and friends, and health care professionals all may believe these inaccuracies, thus neglecting or delaying appropriate interventions. Myths about addictive disorders and their refuting facts follow (Sullivan, 1989).

> *Myth:* Alcoholics are skid-row bums.
> *Fact:* Only 5% of all alcoholics fit this stereotype. The majority (95%) represent a cross-section of people from all walks of life, all professions and occupations, and all socioeconomic levels.

> *Myth:* Alcoholics drink every day.
> *Fact:* There are various patterns of abuse including daily drinking (more common in later stages of the disease) and binges followed by periods of sobriety.

> *Myth:* Providing information on the dangers of alcohol and drugs will prevent addiction.
> *Fact:* Although information is essential, by itself it will not prevent addiction from occurring. Nurses, physicians, and pharmacists, who are all informed about drugs, also become addicted.

> *Myth:* People just think they're "addicted" to alcohol or other drugs. They could quit if they had more "willpower."
> *Fact:* Although initial use is under voluntary control, once a person is addicted, either physically or psychologically, it becomes nearly impossible to control one's use.

> *Myth:* Alcoholics (or addicts) must *want* to quit before anything can be done to help them.

Fact: Early treatment is beneficial as with any chronic condition. By intervening early, an individual can avoid the long-term complications and consequences that come with extensive use.

Myth: You can get addicted by using or trying a drug once.
Fact: It takes prolonged exposure to a drug to develop physiological and/or psychological dependencies. Nurses need not fear giving adequate doses of narcotics to clients in pain for fear of causing addiction.

Attitudes of health care professionals

The attitudes of health care professionals toward individuals with addictive disorders are likely to be just as pessimistic as those of others in society. In addition, health care professionals often have seen the most severe, chronic cases such as drunk drivers and drug overdoses in the emergency room or chronic alcoholics with repeated treatment failures. In one study, emergency room physicians and nurses held negative perceptions of clients with substance abuse, believed that such problems were self-caused, and expected uncooperative behavior (Biener, 1983). Health care professionals may conclude that treatment for addictive disorders is ineffective and that these cases are hopeless.

Attitudes of health care professionals correlate with the amount of knowledge they have about substance abuse and, in addition, affect the quality of care given to clients. Nurses with more knowledge about addictive disorders have more positive attitudes toward these clients (Tamlyn, 1989) and more often refer them to treatment (Reisman & Schrader, 1984). Substance abuse education and training in intervention strategies could improve attitudes, as well as provide accurate information valuable in practice.

THE NURSE'S ROLE WITH SUBSTANCE ABUSING CLIENTS

Nurses have a critical role in the successful care of clients with substance abuse in all health care settings. They play a key role in the following:
- Identifying substance abuse in their clients
- Informing other members of the health care team about their observations and findings
- Intervening and referring clients and their families to appropriate treatment
- Educating clients, families, and staff about addictive disorders
- Providing care in specialized treatment centers
- Caring for recovering clients in all clinical settings

In advanced practice roles, nurses assume greater responsibility for client care. Clinical nurse specialists, for example, may provide individual, group, and family therapy. Nurse practitioners are responsible for screening their client populations for substance abuse and, when needed, assessing the need for further intervention and/or treatment.

In hospitals, clinics, homes, schools, industry, and public health, nurses have extensive opportunities to encounter substance abuse in their clients. In the *hospi-*

tal, nurses have 24-hour responsibility for client care. This affords a unique opportunity to identify addiction problems by observing and interacting with the client and family during the hospital stay (albeit brief). The *emergency room* is especially fertile ground to identify the client admitted for alcohol or drug-related trauma or illness. Awareness of the consequences of such use often makes these clients and their families amenable to intervention. *Outpatient settings* offer opportunities for longer-term relationships with clients. Clues observed over time help the nurse identify and intervene. The *home care* nurse sees the client and family in their own environment. *School* nurses are in a pivotal position to recognize substance abuse problems in the families of children and adolescents and to aid adolescents with their own abuse problems. *Occupational health* nurses can educate, counsel, and refer employees, as well as supervise their return to work. The *public health* nurse identifies substance abuse problems, assesses community resources, and works with other health care professionals to improve substance abuse services to the community (as well as assisting law enforcement personnel and the criminal justice system in protecting community residents). The chapters in Unit II of this book discuss nursing care for clients with substance abuse in specific clinical specialties. In Unit III, the role of nurses in advanced substance abuse practice is discussed.

Identification

Just as they care for clients with a physical illness, nurses have a responsibility to identify and intervene with clients who have addictive disorders. Clients cannot always recognize diabetes or hypertension on their own; similarly, they cannot always recognize their own dependency on alcohol or drugs.

Clients with substance abuse are found in every clinical area. Clients needing emergency care, surgery, critical care, obstetric, and general medical care experience addictive disorders. Clients with other psychiatric problems also may be alcohol or drug dependent. Newborns and children may suffer the consequences of their parents' abuse, and adolescents experience substance abuse problems themselves. Even in long-term care, nurses encounter substance abuse, especially the sequelae of protracted use, in nursing home residents, persons with chronic mental illness, and clients undergoing physical rehabilitation.

Identifying the person with substance abuse requires knowledge about these disorders, recognition of the objective signs of abuse, and the interactive skills to elicit and assess subjective symptoms. There is no one indicator of substance abuse, rather a *pattern* of behavioral manifestations, life consequences, and, in some cases, physical sequelae that suggest an alcohol or drug problem. The nurse's communication skills in interviewing clients and eliciting comprehensive health histories, including alcohol and drug use histories, is essential. Also necessary is the observational skill to recognize both direct and indirect clues. Coupled with physical findings, medical diagnoses, and laboratory tests, these skills enable the nurse to participate with the health care team in identifying and intervening with individuals suffering from addictive disorders.

More about assessing a client with substance abuse is found in Chapter 6, and Chapter 3 explains substance abuse diagnoses.

Detoxification and rehabilitation

The nurse serves as a key member of the health care team in both detoxification and rehabilitation. Detoxification is the systematic withdrawal of alcohol or other drugs from the body. The process requires careful monitoring to avoid negative outcomes. Today, medication regimes properly administered have reduced the incidence of delirium tremens and death. The detoxification phase, especially when it is carried out in a chemical dependency treatment setting, is an important opportunity to begin therapeutic interventions with the client. The nurse is the major caregiver during this phase.

Detoxification also occurs inadvertently when a person whose abuse is unidentified seeks care for another illness, presents for emergency care, or requires surgery. The nurse's observational skills and quick responses are essential to protect the client in these circumstances from untoward physiological consequences.

The rehabilitation phase includes education, therapeutic treatment for substance abuse, monitoring of and treatment for concomitant physical or mental health problems, and helping the client establish lifestyle changes and support systems to maintain sobriety. The nurse serves as a member of the treatment team, which includes physicians, counselors, social workers, and psychologists, to provide care during this phase.

Prevention and education

Prevention and education are important aspects of nursing care in any setting. Because nurses are recognized as authorities on health, they can educate individuals, groups, and communities about responsible use of alcohol and the effects of substance abuse. Also, they can promote healthy alternatives to recreational drug use or to cope with stress.

The American Nurses Association *Standards of Addictions Practice* (ANA & NNSA, 1988) is a tool available to guide addictions nursing practice. Chapters 3 and 6 discuss these standards in more detail.

SUBSTANCE ABUSE CONTENT IN NURSING EDUCATION

We now know many facts about substance abuse. We know that it impacts all of society. We know that it causes long-term and sometimes irreparable physical, psychological, and social harm to millions of individuals, their families, friends, and communities. Most importantly, we know that nurses have an invaluable opportunity to make a vital contribution to the identification, intervention, and treatment of clients with substance abuse.

In spite of all this information, there is a dearth of content about substance abuse in nursing education (Hoffman & Heinemann, 1987; Murphy & Hoeffer, 1987). There are many reasons why this urgent topic receives only minimal attention in nursing curricula. Murphy (1989) suggests some of them include: (1) decreased visibility in today's integrated, nonmedical model curricula; (2) limited interest in the topic among nurse scholars; (3) agreement with current societal attitudes, which accept excessive drinking and ignore the consequences; and (4) reduced federal funding for training in substance abuse. Because substance abuse content has not been included in the educational programs of current faculty, these faculty were not exposed to this information nor to these clients except to those with poor outcomes. Thus *faculty often are unaware of their lack of knowledge.* Since few faculty are knowledgeable about substance abuse or possess clinical skills in caring for these clients, they are ill prepared to teach students. As a result, students (future nurses) are exposed to clients with substance abuse without accurate information, and they lack experience with positive clinical outcomes. Additionally, students may not have role models for competent clinical care of these clients either among the faculty or clinical staff. Add these factors to the curriculum overload with which the faculty continually contends and the status quo in nursing education continues.

What is needed in nursing education?

All programs of nursing education that prepare nurses for licensure should include basic content in substance abuse. Pharmacology and pathology of drugs is usually included, but more is needed for nurses to recognize and assist clients with substance abuse in their care. Substance abuse information is needed concerning: (1) the processes of addiction; (2) medical complications; (3) psychological complications; (4) social consequences; (5) etiology of addictions; (6) prevention; (7) public health aspects; (8) epidemiology; (9) treatment and rehabilitation; (10) the recovery process; (11) lapse and relapse; (12) relapse prevention; and, (13) self-help groups. In addition, all nursing students should have clinical exposure to clients with substance abuse *in some stage of recovery,* preferably in treatment. It is not enough that they care for a client with end-stage liver disease; they need to experience the positive aspects of treatment and recovery.

Specialist education also is needed. Clinical specialists in substance abuse are needed to work in treatment units, hospitals, clinics, industry, and schools and to manage clients with substance abuse in the community. These specialists need to be prepared at the graduate level and their program should include comprehensive content on substance abuse, intensive training in substance abuse treatment, and experience working with professionals in other health care disciplines. Only a few educational programs prepare these specialists. See Chapter 14 for more information about substance abuse in nursing education.

Also, specialists in other advanced clinical areas need to be competent in the substance abuse problems common to their area. Advanced practice nurses in maternal-child health, psychiatric nursing, community health, and adult health need to have skills in assessing and intervening with their clients. In addition, nurse practitioners, who often have front-line contact with clients, need to be especially skilled in assessing substance abuse problems. Therefore graduate programs must include sufficient and accurate substance abuse content to prepare these specialists.

Finally, doctoral programs that prepare future faculty members and nurse researchers must add substance abuse research to their areas of specialization. To do this, nurse scholars must develop programs of research on substance abuse and establish themselves as members of the alcohol and drug abuse research community. Few nurse researchers have received research funding from either the National Institute on Alcohol Abuse and Alcoholism (NIAAA) or the National Institute on Drug Abuse (NIDA) or published in the scientific journals in this field. Nursing research should target the effect that nursing care can have on identification, intervention, and recovery in clients with substance abuse. In addition, nurse researchers could participate in research on the cause, treatment, rehabilitation, and prevention of substance abuse problems for the individual, the family, and the community. Nurses also are prepared to address health policy issues related to substance abuse. There is no area of substance abuse research that nurses could not address with appropriate preparation and interest.

Recent federal initiatives

In response to the need for improvement in the education of health care professionals (physicians, nurses, social workers, psychologists), NIAAA and NIDA initiated several programs. With funding from the Office of Substance Abuse Prevention (now named the Center for Substance Abuse Prevention), the institutes offered assistance for selected schools to develop discipline-specific model curricula for teaching substance abuse content. Three schools of nursing were awarded these grants and the products of their work are now available. (See Appendix C for sources.) Grants were solicited for schools to prepare faculty from a variety of clinical areas to be experts in substance abuse. Eleven schools of nursing received grants for these 5-year training programs. Faculty on these grants develop individual training programs, serve as interns in substance abuse treatment settings, have intensive experiences as professionals in residence at renowned treatment centers (e.g., Hazelden Foundation, Betty Ford Center), and attend national meetings with faculty from other grantee schools of nursing, medicine, social work, and psychology. Collegial relationships have developed with mutual consultations occurring between and among disciplines. In addition to acquiring clinical expertise, these faculty are developing research programs in substance abuse. These programs by the federal government have the potential to impact nursing education in a positive and substantial manner. There are more than 1400 schools of nursing (diploma, associate degree, baccalaureate) in the country, however, and only eleven have grants to train faculty. Much remains to be done.

SUMMARY

Historically, society came to believe that alcoholism and drug dependence are moral problems requiring punitive, rather than therapeutic, approaches. Common use of nomenclature is elusive, and myths rather than facts contribute to pessimistic beliefs and negative attitudes regarding addiction. Nurses have a unique role to play in identifying, intervening, and caring for people with substance abuse problems. It is essential that schools of nursing include accurate, current content on the subject in educational curricula and that faculty are well informed about one of society's most complex health problems. The future care of our nation's people depends on it.

REFERENCES

American Psychiatric Association. (1994). *Diagnostic and Statistical Manual of Mental Disorders* (4th ed.). Washington, D.C.: The Association.

American Nurses Association & National Nurses on Addiction. (1988). *Standards of addictions in nursing practice.* Kansas City, MO: The Association.

Bennett, G. & Woolf, D.S. (1991). *Substance abuse: Pharmacologic, developmental and clinical perspectives.* Albany, NY: Delmar Publishers.

Biener, L. (1983). Perceptions of patients by emergency room staff: Substance-abusers versus non–substance-abusers. *Journal of Health and Social Behavior, 24,* 264-275.

Fingarette, H. (1991). Alcoholism: The mythical disease. In D.J. Pittman & H.R. White (Eds.) *Society, culture, and drinking patterns reexamined.* New Brunswick, NJ: Rutgers University Center of Alcohol Studies.

Fleming, M.F. & Barry, K.L. (1992). *Addictive disorders.* St. Louis: Mosby.

General Accounting Office. (1991a). *Drug treatment: Despite new strategy, few federal inmates receive treatment.* Report to the Committee on Government Operations, House of Representatives (GAO/HRD-91-116). Washington, D.C.: General Accounting Office.

General Accounting Office. (1991b). *Drug treatment: State persons face challenges in providing services.* Report to the Committee on Government Operations, House of Representatives (GAO/HRD-91-128). Washington, D.C.: General Accounting Office.

Gerstein, D. & Harwood, H. (Eds.) (1990). *Treating drug problems: A study of the evaluation, effectiveness, and financing of public and private drug treatments systems,* Vol. 1, Washington D.C.: National Academy Press.

Hoffman, A.L. & Heinemann, M.E. (1987). Substance abuse education in schools of nursing: A national survey. *Journal of Nursing Education, 26*(7), 282-287.

Mathre, M.L. (1992). Substance abuse in the community. In M. Stanhope & J. Lancaster, (3rd ed.). *Community health nursing: Process and practice for promoting health.* (pp 391-410). St. Louis: Mosby.

Murphy, S.A. (1989). The urgency of substance abuse education in schools of nursing. *Journal of Nursing Education, 28*(6), 247-251.

Murphy, S.A. & Hoeffer, B. (1987). The evolution of subspecialties in psychiatric and mental health nursing. *Archives of Psychiatric Nursing, 1,* 145-154.

National Council on Alcohol & Drug Dependence. (1991). *The war on drugs: Failure and fantasy.* Washington, D.C.: The Council.

National Institute on Alcohol Abuse and Alcoholism. (1993). *Eighth special report to US Congress: Alcohol and health.* (DHHS Publication No. ADM 281-88-003.) Alexandria, VA: Editorial Experts.

National Institute on Drug Abuse. (1991). *Drug abuse and drug abuse research.* The Third Triennial Report to Congress from the Secretary, Department of Health and Human Services. (DHHS Publication No. ADM 91-1704). Washington, D.C.: U.S. Government Printing Office.

Reisman, B.L. & Shrader, R.W. (1984). Effect of nurses attitudes toward alcoholism on their referral rate for treatment. *Occupational Health Nursing, 32,* 273-275.

Robins, L.N. & Regier, D.A. (1991). *Psychiatric disorders in America: The epidemiologic catchment area study.* New York: The Free Press.

Sullivan, E.J. (1989). Substance abuse. In P. Potter, (3rd ed.). *Fundamentals of nursing: Concepts, process, and practice.* (pp 1323-1343). St. Louis: Mosby.

Sullivan, E.J., Bissell, L. & Williams, E. (1988). *Chemical dependency in nursing: The deadly diversion.* Menlo Park, CA: Addison-Wesley.

Tamlyn, D.L. (1989). The effect of education on student nurses' attitudes toward alcoholics. *Canadian Journal of Nursing Research, 21*(3), 31-47.

2 | Substance Abuse and Dependency

This chapter reviews different clinical models of illness and recovery that have been observed in persons with alcohol and drug disorders. The etiology of these disorders is discussed with a focus on genetics and environmental interactions. Common clinical characteristics of substance abuse, which include symptoms of physical and psychological dependence, are described. The various categories of mood-altering substances are given and the physiological, psychological, and societal consequences associated with substance use and abuse explained.

MODELS OF ILLNESS

Until recently it was assumed that all persons with substance abuse disorders followed a progressive downhill course that resulted in only three outcomes: recovery, severe health problems, or death. Recent work suggests, however, that less than one-third of these persons actually follow this progressive course. The majority of individuals with substance abuse follow a chronic illness pattern that alternates between relapse, sobriety, controlled use, and spontaneous cessation with little or no treatment. Three models help explain this perplexing illness. They are (1) the classic model of substance dependence developed by Jellinek, (2) the natural history studies conducted by Vaillant, and (3) the chronic illness paradigm.

Jellinek model

Jellinek's model, describing four types of alcoholism (1960), was based on clinical observation and the writings of others in the field. Although his model was developed almost 50 years ago, it continues to influence the field and treatment approaches.

Alpha alcoholism is the undisciplined use of alcohol to relieve physical or emotional pain. There is no evidence of loss of control. Clients with alpha alcoholism are able to abstain without problems. Consequences are limited to family problems, interpersonal relationships, work problems, chronic absenteeism, and occasional nutritional deficiencies. There are no signs of withdrawal with abstinence or any signs of progressive disease. This species of alcoholism is usually stable and may last for decades. Although alpha alcoholism may develop into gamma alcoholism, this progression is unusual. Jellinek did not consider alpha alcoholism an illness. Current terms used for this type include *problem* and *abusive* drinking.

> Mr. V was a 55-year-old man who was evaluated for alcohol problems as part of an employee assistance program (EAP) evaluation. He reported chronic pain secondary to a previous back injury. He said he drank 8 to 12 beers a day to deal with the physical pain. His physicians refused to give him any narcotics. His family was increasingly concerned about his drinking. He missed work at least once a week because of frequent hangovers. He had long periods of abstinence but often returned to alcohol use when the back pain became intolerable. Following intensive nonpharmacological treatment of his back pain and behavioral modification therapy, Mr. V has remained abstinent for three years.

In *beta alcoholism* clients develop physical problems such as polyneuropathy, gastritis, or cirrhosis without evidence of physical or psychological dependence. The damage may be related to nutritional deficiencies. The transition from beta alcoholism to gamma alcoholism is very uncommon. There is no equivalent term used to describe this group of alcoholics in the current classification scheme.

> Mrs. X is a 42-year-old woman evaluated for end-stage liver disease. She reported a history of daily drinking for 15 years. She and her husband drank two martinis (60 grams of alcohol) each day after work. She did not meet any criteria for alcohol abuse or dependence. Two years after liver transplantation and instructions to stop drinking, the client remains abstinent.

Gamma alcoholism most closely describes persons who meet criteria for alcohol dependence. The major characteristics are an increase in acquired tolerance, withdrawal symptoms, severe craving, frequent loss of control, definite progression of disease, and marked behavioral change. There is an impairment of interpersonal relationships. Gamma alcoholism produces the most serious damage. Health, financial, and social problems are pronounced.

> Mrs. G is a 45-year-old woman with a history of daily drinking of a fifth of vodka for 12 years before becoming sober in 1989. She had been admitted to her local community hospital five times between 1986 and 1988 for treatment of pancreatitis and delirium tremens. Following her third course of treatment in an alcohol treatment program in 1989, the client became abstinent. Mrs. G remains abstinent and continues to participate in Alcoholics Anonymous (AA) and other self-recovery groups.

Delta alcoholism is similar to gamma alcoholism but instead of loss of control, persons with delta alcoholism have difficulty remaining abstinent because of physical dependence. While they develop severe symptoms of alcohol withdrawal, they do not report loss of control when drinking. They often drink throughout the day in socially acceptable settings. They do not develop social or psychological problems because of cultural norms and their ability to control their use of alcohol. Jellinek reported that this species of alcoholism is common in countries such as France where wine is part of every meal. There is no equivalent category in the current *International Classification of Diseases* or the DSM-IV.

Jellinek also discussed additional categories of alcoholism. The term *epsilon alcoholism* is used to describe persons who periodically become intoxicated. These drinking binges are associated with accidents and other health problems. In the older literature this type of alcoholism was called "dipsomania." Jellinek also recognized the presence of other species of alcoholism such as the cultural patterns of "fiesta drinking," "explosive drinking," and "excessive weekend drinking." Current terminology describes persons with these species as *abusive, hazardous,* or *harmful* drinkers. Although Jellinek's various "species" of alcoholism are no longer used to classify drinkers, his clinical descriptions of the different types of alcohol abuse have been incorporated in the current diagnostic categories.

Vaillant's study

The primary method used to determine the natural history of a chronic problem such as hypertension or alcoholism is to follow a large group of asymptomatic individuals over long periods of time and determine rates of illness and health events. For example, the Framingham study followed a large population over many decades and determined the course of untreated hypertension and the subsequent health effects such as strokes (Levy, 1990). Prospective epidemiological studies also can be used to assess the course of persons who participate in treatment activities. Such studies are particularly important to the understanding of alcohol and drug disorders, because ethical and methodological problems limit research on people in Alcoholics Anonymous (AA) and traditional treatment programs.

A long-term prospective study conducted by Vaillant (1983) has provided new insights into the natural history of alcohol disorders. The study followed three groups of males: 200 economically privileged Harvard graduates, 400 underprivileged Harvard graduates, and 100 alcoholics identified by their participation in a treatment program. The first two groups were followed for 40 years as part of a long-term study on life-span development. They were primarily asymptomatic for alcohol-related problems at the beginning of the study. The third group was followed for 8 years. Vaillant reported the following conclusions from this study.

The natural course of alcoholism can be broadly described as consisting of three stages: (1) social drinking, (2) alcohol abuse, and (3) alcohol dependence. The first stage, *social drinking,* is characterized as consumption of four to six drinks per day. As many as 30% of males report prolonged periods of heavy social drinking. It appears that about one third of heavy drinkers will continue to drink at that level with no apparent progression or development of alcohol-related consequences. A third will reduce their use to minimal levels as a result of social, peer, or family pressure. The last third will progress to the second stage of alcoholism and develop a pattern of abuse.

Abuse involves increased alcohol use, increasing loss of control over use, and the development of multiple medical, legal, social, and occupational complications. Approximately 10% to 15% of males in the general population will develop evidence of alcohol abuse. A small percentage will remain in stage two for long periods of time and not develop further problems. The rest will spontaneously become abstinent or continue to drink intermittently with no evidence of loss of control. Vaillant (1983) reports that 25% of persons who develop symptoms of abuse will progress to stage three—alcohol dependence.

Alcohol *dependence* is much less reversible than the two prior stages and usually ends in sobriety, social incapacity, or death. Vaillant (1983) estimates that 3% to 5% of adults will reach the third stage, with men outnumbering women three to one. Persons who reach this stage develop physical dependence and usually require detoxification with medical intervention. Vaillant found that the rates of spontaneous recovery in this group are lower than in the first two stages. Vaillant's work was the first long-term prospective study on the natural history of alcohol problems.

The findings presented by Vaillant suggest that further studies are needed to better define the natural course of alcohol and drug disorders. Also, a greater understanding of which clients require intensive long-term counseling and which clients would respond to brief advice therapy is needed. The high rate of spontaneous recovery found by Vaillant reinforces the importance of *treatment matching*. Treatment matching refers to applying specific treatment methods to varying client-associated characteristics.

Chronic illness paradigm

It is useful to conceptualize the clinical course and treatment of alcohol and drug problems in the context of other chronic conditions, such as hyperlipidemia and essential hypertension. Like other chronic conditions, difficulty in treating alcohol and drug disorders is due to the clinical course and behavioral manifestations of a chronic illness—not because difficulty in treatment is either the client's or the clinician's fault. The similarities among these three conditions are striking: a late onset of clinical symptoms, heterogeneity (variations in presentation), unpredictability, treatment methods, and the need for behavioral changes.

Chronic problems such as alcohol and drug disorders, hypertension and hypercholesterolemia develop slowly with few early symptoms. Many cases of hypercholesterolemia are not detected until an acute vascular event or, in the case of hypertension, the development of a hemorrhagic stroke, occurs. Cocaine-related deaths from cardiac arrhythmias, strokes, or suicide are a similar potentially preventable tragedy.

Epidemiological studies have determined the relative risk of heart disease and strokes for clients with elevated lipids and hypertension, but it is difficult to predict the clinical course for individual clients. Similarly, it is difficult for the clinician to determine which heavy drinkers are likely to develop serious consequences from their drinking. Most heavy drinkers do not develop significant end-organ damage; less than 10% develop liver failure.

Scientific studies have provided evidence that genetics is part of the etiology of these illnesses. However, these conditions also can develop as a direct result of unhealthy activities (e.g., dietary habits, lack of exercise, ineffective methods of dealing with stress, or excessive drinking). The effect of societal norms, advertising, and social pressures is a powerful environmental stimuli. It is clear that hypertension, elevated lipids, and alcohol and drug disorders develop as a result of the interaction of genetics and environmental stimuli.

Clinicians need to take a different approach to the care of clients with chronic conditions, particularly alcohol and drug disorders. Relapse is the norm rather than the exception. The primary management of chronic conditions includes changing long-term behavioral patterns. Problems with compliance are common. It may take months or years for many clients to change their behaviors and, when necessary, take medication appropriately. Many persons never make the necessary behavioral changes.

In contrast to most acute problems that can be treated and/or cured, the management of chronic conditions is dependent on the client's taking some action. No one can force a person to change eating or drinking patterns. The cause of alcoholism and other drug dependencies is unknown. Why some people can drink alcohol with no problem and others cannot continues to mystify scientists. Change often requires giving up pleasurable activities and moving against social norms. Long-term modifications in diet, exercise, or alcohol use involve a complex series of behavioral changes—often difficult to maintain.

ETIOLOGY AND CONTRIBUTING FACTORS

A number of etiological factors have been proposed as contributing to substance abuse. The primary determinants are *genetics* and *environmental influences.*

Genetics

Many studies have documented the relationship between alcoholism and *genetics.* Methods commonly used by investigators to study genetics include studies of twins, adoptees, gene identification, and other lab markers. Twin studies compare the incidence of alcoholism in identical twins with that of fraternal twins. Pickens and associates (1991) studied 169 same-sex twins and found greater agreement of alcohol dependence in identical twins than in fraternal twins. They also found higher concordance rates for male twins who met criteria for alcohol abuse. However, there was no difference between identical and fraternal female twins who met alcohol abuse criteria.

The severity of the drinking pattern also appears to have a strong genetic basis. A study of 902 Finnish twins found stronger genetic association with chronic heavy drinking than with a less severe pattern of use (Partanen et al, 1966). The primary weakness inherent in studying twins, however, is environmental influences on subjects. It is difficult to assess the impact of friends and societal effects on two different individuals, even on those raised in the same family.

Studies of adopted children have provided additional evidence of the influence of genetic factors. One method compares children raised in nonalcoholic environments, half of whom had an alcoholic biological parent. Goodwin (1974) used this method and found higher rates of alcohol dependence in children with biological parents who were alcohol-dependent. Based on these studies, Cloninger (1990) proposed Type I and Type II alcoholism. *Type I* alcoholics were described as persons who began drinking in late adolescence or early adulthood and whose drinking was influenced by social and environmental factors. *Type II* alcoholics were characterized as having early onset–drinking problems, antisocial personality traits, and male gender. Other investigators have been unable to replicate his findings, and they propose that the association of alcoholism is related more to personality disorders (Schuckit et al, 1985).

Other ongoing genetic research includes animal studies in which animals have been bred selectively to develop evidence of physiological dependence on alcohol. A number of animal studies have found strong genetic effects. These studies have found that D2 dopamine receptors are associated with reward, reinforcement, and motivation.

A number of investigators have attempted to identify a specific set of genes that may be responsible for alcoholism. Blum (1991) reported higher frequency of the A1 allele or the D2 dopamine receptor in persons with a diagnosis of alcoholism. They reported that this allele was eight times more common in alcoholics than in non-alcoholics. Other researchers, however, have been unable to replicate these findings (Gelernter et al, 1989). Difficulty in identifying the gene responsible for alcoholism may be related to the heterogeneity of alcohol disorders. The importance of the A1 allele or the D2 dopamine receptor remains to be decided. Some researchers have suggested that the D2 receptor may modulate the severity of alcoholism (Gejman et al, 1993).

Examination of the role of alcohol on neurotransmitters also is a focus of current research (Hunt & Nixon, 1993). Neurotransmitters enable neurons to transmit signals within their cells and with each other. Studies of how alcohol interrupts and distorts this communication process include effects on release of neurotransmitters, signals within the neuron, neurotransmitter binding, and studies on whether or not alcohol alters the chemical and physical structure of the cell membrane. Although this research is extremely complex, scientists have discovered a number of neurotransmitter systems (e.g., gamma-aminobutyric acid [GABA], glutamate, serotonin).

Family pedigree studies are another area of research designed to test the genetic hypothesis of alcoholism. A large, multi-site study funded by the National Institute on Alcohol Abuse and Alcoholism (NIAAA) has identified a number of family members at risk for alcohol dependence. These family members are being tested for EEG abnormalities, such as the P300 and the low voltage alpha wave, that may prove to be genetic markers. Other proposed genetic markers include the amount of body sway and platelet monamine oxidase levels. Ideally such tests could be administered to young adults to assess their level of risk if they choose to use alcohol.

Environmental factors

The relationship between *environmental factors* and the development of alcohol problems has been well described. Countries where alcohol use is discouraged (e.g., Saudi Arabia) have lower rates of alcohol-related health problems such as cirrhosis. Those countries that incorporate use of alcohol into their culture (e.g., France) have higher rates. Patterns of use also vary by culture; some Native American groups have the highest rates of alcoholism. The problem with most of the data available is in the definition of alcohol problems. Rates of cirrhosis are clearly dose-related: the greater the amount of alcohol, the greater the rate of cirrhosis. However, in countries and cultures where heavy use is the norm, the ratio of behavioral problems to alcohol use varies considerably. This variance usually depends on societal tolerance for drunkenness and even for social consequences such as family dysfunction, work performance, and accidents.

CHARACTERISTICS OF SUBSTANCE ABUSE

Intoxication

The progression from abuse to dependency evolves from excessive use with intoxication to tolerance, to dependence, and to loss of control. An individual uses a variety of defense mechanisms in an attempt (albeit unsuccessful) to control use. Intoxication is defined as the state of being poisoned by a substance. Acute alcohol intoxication can be defined legally or behaviorally. In most states, an individual is legally intoxicated when the blood alcohol concentration (BAC) is equal to 100 mg/dl (Fell, 1990). For most individuals, however, behavioral effects appear at a much lower level of alcohol ingestion. Threshold effects, such as increased reaction time, decreased fine motor control, and impaired critical thinking, occur with a BAC as low as 20 to 30 mg/dl (Rall, 1990).

Alcohol intoxication leads to depression of the inhibitory functions of the cerebral cortex and reticular-activating system. Loss of inhibition leads to behavioral signs and symptoms such as increased confidence, slurred speech, impaired judgment and memory, decreased ability to concentrate, and mood swings (Yi, 1991). Individuals are usually grossly intoxicated at a BAC of 150 mg/dl; death occurs from apnea, hypothermia, and hypotension in most people at a BAC of 400 mg/dl (Rall, 1990).

The manifestations of drug intoxication depend on the pharmacokinetics of the drug. Intoxication with central nervous system (CNS) depressants such as benzodiazepines, barbiturates, and opiates leads to inhibition of CNS neurons, sedation, and analgesia. Intoxication with CNS stimulants such as amphetamines and cocaine causes euphoria, increased alertness, and decreased need for sleep. Intoxication with hallucinogens such as those containing cannabinoids (major ingredient of marijuana and hashish) results in increased awareness of sensory input, enhanced mental activity, and sensory distortions (Hoeschen, 1991).

Tolerance

Tolerance is the adaptation of an individual or a cell to the continued presence of a foreign substance. Tolerance occurs when increased amounts of a substance are required in order to achieve intoxication or a diminished effect occurs with continued use of the same amount of a substance (Nace, 1988). Physiological tolerance is the body's adjustment to a substance that allows an individual to maintain as normal a physiological functioning as possible (Miller & Gold, 1991). Tolerance to alcohol occurs because of changes in the lipid bilayer of the cell membrane. Although several theories that explain tolerance exist, most investigators agree that receptors for neurotransmitters, such as norepinephrine and serotonin, may have altered conductance for ions such as calcium and chloride. Modification of these receptors is thought to lead to adaptation of the individual to alcohol (USDHHS, 1990).

Long-term use of alcohol leads to an increased ability to metabolize ethanol and to pharmacological tolerance. Higher blood concentrations of alcohol then are necessary to produce intoxication in chronic drinkers. With tolerance, however, there is no significant elevation of the lethal dose; severe intoxication with respiratory depression and death can occur at toxic levels, both in chronic alcoholics and in those unaccustomed to drinking regularly (Jaffe, 1990).

Tolerance to morphine is the model usually used to describe tolerance to drugs other than alcohol. Tolerance to morphine has developed when more morphine is needed than previously to produce the same expected state of intoxication (Miller & Gold, 1991). Tolerance to all of the actions of opioids does not develop uniformly; an individual may have complete tolerance to some drug actions while responses to other drug effects remain unchanged. For example, a morphine addict may have diminished intensity of pleasure and yet retain the same degree of respiratory depression at a stable dose of the drug. Manifestations of tolerance to opioids include a shortened duration and decreased intensity of analgesia, euphoria, and sedation (Jaffe, 1990).

Tolerance does not usually develop with intermittent, therapeutic use of opioids for analgesia or sedation. Opioid addicts, on the other hand, who use opioids to achieve and maintain a euphoric state, or "high," need continuous drug action at high doses (Jaffe, 1990; Miller & Gold, 1991). Jaffe (1990) notes that some persons with addiction can build up to extremely large doses of morphine (e.g., 2000 mg in a few hours) without significant changes in blood pressure, heart rate, or respiratory rate.

Cross tolerance

Cross tolerance occurs when people who drink heavily require higher-than-normal doses of other drugs to produce sedation or analgesia. Cross tolerance, or cross-reaction, occurs particularly in individuals with chronic alcohol abuse. For example, clients receiving general anesthesia may require greater doses of sedative drugs to achieve adequate analgesia. Two classes of sedative drugs that are cross tolerant with alcohol are benzodiazepines and barbiturates. Cross tolerance may occur for two reasons. First, the central nervous system may become more tolerant to other drugs that, like alcohol, cause depression. Second, cross tolerance may be due to more rapid metabolism of the drugs because the use of alcohol increases hepatic enzymatic activity. Cross tolerance only occurs in relatively sober individuals; during alcohol intoxication the depressant effects of drugs other than alcohol are additive to those of ethanol (Jaffe, 1990). Older adults are particularly susceptible to cross tolerance effects when benzodiazepines or hypnotics are prescribed.

Dependence

Dependence is defined as a set of predictable and stereotypical signs and symptoms that constitute withdrawal and occur with cessation of drug use. With resumption of drug intake, the signs and symptoms of dependence are suppressed. Dependence can be both *physical* and *psychological,* but as more is learned about dependence, the distinction between the two is blurring (Hoeschen, 1991). The relationship between tolerance, physical dependence, and psychological dependence is complex. Wide individual differences exist in people's tendency to become physically dependent and in their ability to tolerate withdrawal symptoms.

Physical dependence occurs when an individual becomes physiologically adapted to a drug because of repeated administrations. Physical dependence is primarily neuroadaptation, which necessitates continuous doses of the drug to prevent the appearance of withdrawal symptoms that are characteristic for that particular drug. In general, the degree of physical dependence is usually measured by the severity of the withdrawal syndrome that occurs when the drug is abruptly stopped (Jaffe, 1990).

Physical dependence occurs not only with ethanol, opioids, and sedatives but also with other drugs. The symptoms associated with dependence are generally explained by a rebound effect of the physiological systems that were initially modified by the drug. For example, cocaine reduces fatigue and causes euphoria, whereas cocaine withdrawal is characterized by tiredness, depression, and overeating (Jaffe, 1990).

The distinction between physiological and *psychological dependency* is less clear as our understanding of the neurochemical and neurokinetic effects of drugs increases. It is difficult to distinguish a drug's ability to reinforce drug-taking behavior from those psychological factors that influence motivation to take the drug (Miller & Gold, 1991). Alcohol dependence may be the result of an interactive process involving different psychological factors within a person with physiological vulnerability (Tarter et al, 1985).

Generally, the psychological component of drug dependency focuses on the increasing preoccupation of an individual with drug seeking, securing, and use. A behavioral pattern of compulsive drug use with overwhelming involvement emerges. The person is obsessed with the use of the drug for its pleasurable quality and, frequently, may have relapses despite efforts to stop or cut back. Drug-seeking behavior is given a sharply higher priority over other behaviors which once had significantly greater value. The faster the drug reaches the central nervous system after it is taken, the more likely the person is to maintain drug-taking behavior. Also, the magnitude of response and the unpleasant aspects of withdrawal encourage continued use. Cocaine acts quickly, is of short duration, and has a pleasurable response with minimal withdrawal symptoms. Alcohol, on the other hand, acts more slowly, and pleasurable response depends on the frequency and the amount of alcohol taken. In general, cocaine use is more difficult to discontinue than alcohol use.

Loss of control

An individual's initial experience with the substance of abuse may be pleasurable, such as in a social setting, or it may be a way to relieve stress and tension. The person then seeks to recapture this experience but finds, as time goes on, the need to increase the amount and frequency of the substance. As this behavioral pattern consumes a greater priority in thoughts and activities, the person no longer controls the substance but the need for the substance controls the person. At this point, the person has lost control. Sometimes, especially in the beginning of their drug use, substance abusers can abstain completely for some time. As a result, most individuals do not recognize that their loss of control over the substance is becoming greater. Instead, they continue to look only at the willful and voluntary aspects of their abuse patterns. There is a loss of control over the direction of one's life, with substance use gaining priority over all else: family, home, job, and, ultimately, personal health and safety.

Reinforcement

Drug self-administration is a learned behavior that is affected by the reinforcement properties of a drug. A reinforcer is defined as an event or substance that increases the probability that leads to its presentation (Roache & Meisch, 1991). In general, drugs that are known to be reinforcers in humans also can be shown to be reinforcers in laboratory animals. These drugs include CNS stimulants and depressants; dissociative anesthetics such as phencyclidine; and methylxanthines such as caffeine, nicotine, and the opioids. Cocaine is a good example of a powerful reinforcer; animals will press a lever more than 4,000 times to self-administer a single injection of cocaine (Jaffe, 1990).

The mechanism for reinforcement for many self-administered drugs involves the neurons of the central nervous system. The area of the brain most affected is the mesolimbic system, a rim of inner brain tissue that lies beneath the cerebral cortex but above the brainstem. The mesolimbic system controls feeding activities, motivation, sexual behavior, and emotions such as fear, rage, and pleasure. The neurons of the mesolimbic system are activated by electrical stimulation, a variety of drugs, or natural reinforcers such as food. The response to activation is the release of the neurotransmitter dopamine (DA) in a portion of the mesolimbic system called the nucleus accumbens. The release of DA in the nucleus accumbens results in a sense of reward or reinforcement (Jaffe, 1990).

Craving

Craving is a term that describes the intense desire to use more of a drug (Miller & Gold, 1991). Craving is such a strong drive that it often supersedes the negative aspects of intoxication and withdrawal. The physiological basis for craving depends on the pharmacokinetic properties of the substance involved. Clients who have stopped smoking frequently experience intense craving for several months. Nicotine addiction has been found to affect the acetylcholine receptor system, and it often takes long periods of time for this system to reestablish normal functioning following the cessation of the use of tobacco products. Craving for cocaine is the result of a different physiological basis: decreased availability of DA at the synapse of the nerve cell, or supersensitivity of the postsynaptic neuron. When a cocaine addict experiences these neurochemical changes, the experience is described as craving. Craving for alcohol, on the other hand, may occur because of the effects of alcohol on the cell membrane. Chronic alcohol use causes decreased DA activity because of a cell membrane that is more rigid than normal. These effects are thought to be centered primarily in the reward area of the mesolimbic system of the brain (Jaffe, 1990; Miller & Gold, 1991).

Progressive nature

When people first become involved with a drug, they are able to maintain their level of activities, but eventually preoccupation with the drug becomes more important than anything else. They begin to limit themselves to activities and friends that support the drug use. They usually will maintain relationships important to the maintenance of their self-esteem.

As dependency continues, the person begins to lie to friends and family members, which results in guilt, shame, anger, and loss of self-worth. Denial and projection are used to maintain a sense of self-respect as the individual increasingly needs to lie, hide, and become secretive. Loss of interest in others and in activities is apparent, with the resultant neglect of family, job, and personal habits. It is at this point that responsibilities interfere with substance-use behavior rather than the reverse. Wegscheider (1981) notes that there is a loss of control over the quantity of, but not the choice to, drink. For example, individuals may drink and become intoxicated for prolonged periods that continue until they either become too ill to continue drinking or deplete their stores of alcohol. Other individuals may move to a different geographical location or job to be able to maintain daily use of large quantities of alcohol.

From this point there is usually radical deterioration in family relations, loss of job, financial difficulties, and possible involvement with the law. The person is caught in a vicious circle: abusing to avoid withdrawal, abusing with reckless abandon, and abusing to despair. If intervention does not occur, the result may be death, mental illness, or irreversible debilitation.

Common defense mechanisms

With dependency, a substance pervades the individual's self-identity, cognition, and behavior and becomes the most important relationship in life. The substance becomes the major way to cope with life experiences. Whenever this relationship is threatened, the dependent person responds with a characteristic pattern of defensive strategies. These include denial, projection, and rationalization. Primitive defense mechanisms indicate that the individual has no other way of coping with overwhelming anxiety or tension. Because they are primitive, these mechanisms are resistant to intervention. It is important to understand the nature of the defenses so that the health professional can be sensitive to and supportive of the client's experience.

Denial.   Denial is a defense mechanism in which a person blocks acknowledgement of some anxiety-provoking aspects of self or reality. Denial is a hallmark of dependency. The individual does not acknowledge the effects of the drinking behavior. For this person, such an acknowledgment would mean giving up one's best friend; life would have no meaning because its meaning has been the pursuit of the next drink, smoke, snort, or line. Methods of denial include lying about use, minimizing use patterns, blaming, or rationalizing. For example, the person might comment "I drink/use every day but it does not interfere with my work" (Haber et al, 1992).

Projection.   Projection is closely related to denial because one's own unacceptable characteristics are disowned or attributed to someone else. As with denial, the individual's awareness of unacceptable characteristics is blocked. When confronted with anxiety-provoking encounters in which reality cannot be denied, a person may project the reality outside, often with some anger. Projection is apparent in such comments as "If only my wife (boss, etc.) would quit giving me such a hard time . . ." (Robak, 1991).

Rationalization. Rationalization occurs when a person tries to justify behavior by giving reasons or excuses that are not the true ones, implying that the behavior is the result of thoughtful consideration or full awareness of motives. This mechanism helps a threatened person maintain self-respect and provide socially acceptable motives for behavior. Rationalization is reflected in such comments as "I know I shouldn't drink, and I'll stop as soon as I get through this problem. Drinking keeps me calm enough to function" (Haber et al, 1992).

Delusional thinking. As an individual's self-identity becomes more and more dependent on an addictive substance, defensive strategies may take the form of delusional thinking. For example, a threatened individual may have an elaborate explanation for behavior, made up of distorted thought patterns that are not based on reality. The individual is convinced of the distortions, even though they are contradicted by logical thought and the perceptions of others.

CATEGORIES OF SUBSTANCES

Historically, individuals in every known society have used drugs to change mood, thought, and feelings (Jaffe, 1990). The types of drugs that are chosen for abuse in any society depend on the financial and technological resources of the society, the cultural history of the society, and the society's norms. The following overview summarizes the categories of substances that are of current concern in American society today.

Alcohol

Alcoholic beverages have been used since the beginning of recorded history and were considered the remedy for most diseases. The name "whiskey" means "water of life" in Gaelic (Rall, 1990). The pharmacological effects of alcoholic beverages such as wine, beer, and spirits are derived from their common ingredient, ethanol. Ethanol is the main product of the fermentation process of yeast and raw organic compounds such as grains, malt, and fruit. A colorless liquid with a bitter taste, ethanol contains small amounts of vitamins, iron, and carbohydrates but is essentially considered to have no nutritional value (Yi, 1991).

Alcohol is absorbed across mucous membranes by simple diffusion; small intestinal absorption in the duodenum and jejunum is the most rapid. Absorption is influenced by many factors. The higher the concentration of alcohol, the more rapid the absorption. The faster the rate of alcohol consumption, the higher the absorption. Dilution of alcohol by the presence of food in the stomach slows absorption. Certain foods, such as milk and food with a high fat content, also delay both gastric passage and alcohol absorption. The blood distributes alcohol to all organ systems because alcohol has a high solubility in water and a low solubility in lipids. The variation in water and lipid solubility leads to accumulation of alcohol in the organs that have the largest blood supply and the highest organ content of water, such as the brain, the gastrointestinal tract, the heart, and the liver.

More than 90% of the alcohol that an individual ingests is metabolized by the liver. Over time, the rate of oxidation of alcohol is relatively constant and does not increase as the BAC increases. Alcohol metabolism in the adult is usually 120 mg/kg/hr, or about 1 oz (30 ml) in 3 hours (Rall, 1990). A standard drink contains about one third of an ounce of alcohol. The alcohol content of a standard drink is equal in a single 12-ounce can of beer or ale, a single 1.5-ounce shot of spirits (whiskey, gin, vodka), a 6-ounce glass of wine, or a 4-ounce glass of sherry or liqueur (Brown, 1992). Therefore, it takes approximately one hour for a standard drink to be totally metabolized.

The steps in alcohol metabolism in the liver follow several pathways:

1. Hydrogen ions can be released from ethanol and accepted by nicotinamide adenine dinucleotide (NAD) under the control of a catalyst, alcohol dehydrogenase (ADH). This process results in the production of acetaldehyde.
2. Ethanol can be metabolized by microsomal oxidases from the smooth endoplasmic reticulum of the liver into acetaldehyde.
3. Ethanol can also be metabolized by catalase into acetaldehyde.

After the formation of acetaldehyde, an enzyme in the mitochondria named acetaldehyde dehydrogenase converts acetaldehyde into acetate. Acetate is then converted into acetyl-coA (the product of carbohydrate, protein, and lipid digestion), which is either oxidized or used in the synthesis of cholesterol, fatty acids, or other tissue constituents (Rall, 1990).

The metabolism of alcohol leads to several negative consequences. Increased fatty acid synthesis results in the fatty liver often associated with chronic alcohol abuse. Because of the conversion of NAD to NADP (nicotinamide adenine dinucleotide phosphate), the intracellular ratio of NAD/NADP is altered and can lead to inhibition of gluconeogenesis and hypoglycemia. The most reactive product of ethanol metabolism is probably acetaldehyde, which reacts with proteins and nucleic acids to cause massive organ damage (Murray et al, 1990). Proteins in the hepatocyte of the liver seem particularly susceptible to acetaldehyde. Chronic effects of alcohol and other drugs of abuse are described in Table 2-1.

Amphetamines

The amphetamine family is a group of drugs that are chemically similar to the catecholamines (such as epinephrine and norepinephrine) which are released in the "fight or flight" activation of the sympathetic nervous system. Amphetamines cause an increase in heart rate and blood pressure as well as pupil dilation, hyperglycemia, and bronchodilation. Amphetamines are CNS stimulants and often are abused to achieve euphoria, decrease appetite, reduce anxiety, increase self-confidence, improve alertness, and enhance energy levels. An individual who uses amphetamines appears to be hyperactive, talkative, restless, and irritable (Miller, 1991).

The CNS action of amphetamines occurs because of the release of neurotransmitters from storage sites in the neurons of the brain. Norepinephrine release leads to increased mental activity, whereas DA release probably leads to the stimulation of the central reward system, which encourages drug-seeking behaviors. Amphetamines, like cocaine, prolong the action of DA at the postsynaptic receptors; but the

Table 2-1
Chronic effects of alcohol and other drugs of abuse

Drug	Chronic effects
Alcohol	Brain damage, memory loss, sleep disturbances, psychoses, seizures Nutritional deficiencies leading to Wernicke's encephalopathy, Korsakoff's psychosis, polyneuritis Cardiomyopathy, hypertension, stroke Skeletal myopathy Diarrhea, ulcers, pancreatitis Fatty liver, liver fibrosis and necrosis Impotence, sterility, testicular atrophy, gynecomastia Depression of bone marrow, thrombocytopenia, suppression of antibody formation, suppression of white blood cell movement
Amphetamines	Mental depression, fatigue, sleep disturbances Marked weight loss Psychoses, paranoid delusions, hallucinations, drug-induced schizophrenia
Barbiturates	Thick, slurred speech, nystagmus, diplopia, strabismus Visual changes, vertigo, ataxia, decreased reflexes Liver dysfunction with altered metabolism of drugs
Benzodiazepines	Generally good toleration Sleep disturbances
Opioids	Glomerulonephritis Reduced bowel motility, severe constipation, colicky pain Hepatitis, AIDS Inflammation and infection at drug injection site Depression of the immune system
Cocaine	Venereal diseases Nasal mucosal inflammation and necrosis Nasal perforation Weight loss Seizures, perceptual changes, hallucinations, anxiety, paranoia Dysrhythmias, cardiac ischemia, myocarditis, chronic heart failure, cardiomyopathy Headaches, cerebrovascular accident, vasculitis Pulmonary hemorrhage, pulmonary infiltrates, "crack lung" Acute renal failure, rhabdomyolysis Impotence, infertility
Marijuana	Bronchitis, lung cancer, shortness of breath Chest pain, hypertension, diaphoresis Immunosuppression
Phencyclidine	Depression Lethargy, lack of ambition, lack of sexual drive Mood, sleep, and appetite variations Anhedonia

Modified from Giannini, A.J. (1991b). The volatile agents. In N.M. Miller (Ed.), *Comprehensive handbook of drug and alcohol addiction*. (pp 394-395). New York: Marcel Dekker, Inc; Rall, T.W. (1990). Hypnotics and sedatives: Ethanol. In A.G. Gilman, T.W. Rall, A.S. Nies, & P. Taylor (Eds.), *Goodman and Gilman's the pharmacological basis of therapeutics*. (pp 345-382). New York: Pergamon Press; Roselle, G.A. (1992). Alcohol and the immune system. *Alcohol Health & Research World, 16* (1), 16-22.

mechanism of action is slightly different. Amphetamines inhibit the storage of DA, whereas cocaine inhibits the removal of DA in the synapse (Cho, 1990).

Several types of amphetamines are abused in America. They are administered orally, by inhaling, or by intravenous injection. Amphetamine sulfate (Benzedrine), for example, is effective when taken orally, reaches a peak blood concentration in just over one hour, and has effects that last for several hours (Hoeschen, 1991). Methamphetamine, known as "speed," is closely related to the amphetamines but has stronger CNS effects, a longer half-life (6 to 12 hours), and fewer peripheral effects. When injected intravenously, the drug causes an immediate sense of pleasure, or "flash," that can occur even before the injection is complete. "Ice" is a pure form of methamphetamine that is viewed as more dangerous than other forms because of its purity and because it can be inhaled. When inhaled, ice causes an intense effect similar to an intravenous dose but lasts for several hours (Cho, 1990). Smoking methamphetamine (ice) compounds its effects and promotes rapid addiction (NIDA, 1991).

Tolerance to amphetamines is striking in dependent individuals. Hoffman and Lefkowitz (1990) report daily doses as high as 1700 mg per day of amphetamine (therapeutic oral dose is 5 to 10 mg daily) without apparent ill effects, and Cho (1990) reports daily doses as high as 15 grams in chronic ice abusers (therapeutic oral dose is 5 to 25 mg daily).

Barbiturates

Barbiturates are classed as *sedatives-hypnotics,* which are used to induce drowsiness and promote sleep. The earliest sedatives-hypnotics contained bromide, and during the 1800s, drugs such as chloral hydrate and paraldehyde were common. Barbital and phenobarbital, the first barbiturates, were introduced in the early 1900s. While the use of barbiturates has decreased, they remain important substances of abuse.

Barbiturates act as CNS depressants in several ways by their effect on the neuro-receptors of the postsynaptic membrane. Barbiturates increase the conductance of chloride through the gamma aminobutyric acid (GABA) receptor into the cell, making the resting membrane more negative and causing postsynaptic inhibition. In addition, barbiturates may block DA receptor stimulation and decrease calcium-dependent action potentials (Rall, 1990).

The effects of barbiturates include central nervous system depression ranging from dose-related mild sedation to general anesthesia. They may create mild euphoric effects but do not provide analgesia until the moment of unconsciousness. Barbiturates also depress the respiratory center to decrease both respiratory drive and rhythm. Other body effects include hypotension, bradycardia, decreased GI muscular tone leading to paralytic ileus and constipation, and altered liver metabolism of drugs and intrinsic substances such as steroid hormones (Rall, 1990).

Short-acting barbiturates such as pentobarbital (Nembutal, known as "reds" or "downers") and secobarbital (Seconal, known as "yellows" or "nembies") are usually preferred by abusers over longer-acting barbiturates. Abusers develop high tolerance to barbiturates and doses as high as 2.5 grams per day (therapeutic dose is 50 to 200 mg/day).

Individuals with barbiturate dependence usually fall into one of three patterns of use. Some persons, often teenagers or young adults, have episodic intoxication that creates a periodic "high." Other individuals have a pattern of chronic intoxication; often these people are middle-aged individuals who obtain a prescription from a physician for anxiety or insomnia and then develop patterns of dependency. Another pattern of use occurs in persons, often young adults, involved in the illegal drug culture. These individuals may take intravenous barbiturates, which leads to multiple areas of abscesses from repeated injections.

Acute barbiturate intoxication leads to sluggishness; slowed speech; slowed thought processes; impaired judgment, memory, and concentration; impaired motor skills; poor personal hygiene; paranoia; and suicidal tendencies. Barbiturates cause alterations in the stages of sleep that lead to a decrease in the length and density of the rapid eye movement (REM) phase of sleep. In addition, they cause several hours of drowsiness, as well as residual effects the following day (e.g., hangover).

Benzodiazepines

Benzodiazepines were first used in the 1960s. They are the drugs of choice for anxiety disorders and are generally prescribed for sedation and induction of sleep. They produce relaxation, mild motor incoordination, and drowsiness. They also can lead to impaired memory and cognition, slurred speech, and depression. Benzodiazepines are CNS depressants that lead to increased chloride conductance in brain cells. Two groups of investigators (Mohler & Okada, Squires & Braestrup) discovered benzodiazepine receptors in the brain in 1977; these receptors are part of a larger receptor complex that includes GABA receptors. The receptor complex is thought to open large chloride channels that lead to increased intracellular chloride and a hyperpolarized (more negative) cell membrane (Hoeschen, 1991).

All benzodiazepines, both short-acting and long-acting, have the potential for abuse and addiction. Benzodiazepines taken daily at several times the therapeutic dose can lead to physical dependence; abrupt cessation of the drug leads to psychosis and seizures, which produce a life-threatening withdrawal syndrome. Benzodiazepines, alcohol, and barbiturates are all cross tolerant, although the mechanism for cross tolerance is unknown. The people at most risk for benzodiazepine addiction are those who have a personal or family history of alcoholism or drug addiction. These individuals often come in contact with benzodiazepines either through treatment for various physical or psychological conditions or through misprescribing by physicians (Smith & Seymour, 1991).

Opioids

The use of opioids predates recorded history. The first written reference to opioids is found in writings from the third century B.C. (Jaffe & Martin, 1990). The term "opioids" is used to describe not only the opiate drugs derived from opium (drugs that are derived from the seeds of the poppy plant such as morphine, codeine, and heroin) but also the many semisynthetic and synthetic drugs related to morphine (such as fentanyl, meperidine, and methadone). The term "narcotic"—not a particularly useful term in a pharmacological sense—comes from a Greek word meaning "stupor" and is used to describe any drug-inducing sleep. Currently, the use of the term "narcotic" is confusing; it is often expanded to include any drug that produces tolerance, dependence, and addiction (Belkin & Gold, 1991; Jaffe & Martin, 1990).

Opioid intoxication causes CNS depression along with euphoria, a sense of well-being, analgesia, sedation, and sleepiness. Chronic abuse can lead to lethargy, apathy, anorexia, depression, and anxiety as well as constipation, hypotension, respiratory depression, nausea, vomiting, and suppression of the immune response (Belkin & Gold, 1991). Cellular action of the opioids occurs because of the interaction of the drug with a large number of opioid receptors throughout many organ systems of the body. At least three major classifications of opioid receptors have been identified. The role of these receptors, which appear on the presynaptic membrane of the nerve synapse, is to inhibit synaptic transmission by decreasing the release of excitatory neurotransmitters. In addition, opioids may affect the movement of potassium and calcium across the postsynaptic cell membrane to cause a hyperpolarized (more negative) resting membrane potential (Jaffe & Martin, 1990).

Opioid addicts usually follow two patterns: those who become addicted because of a chronic pain syndrome and those who become addicted after recreational (nonmedical) use. The incidence of opioid addiction among nurses, physicians, and other health care professionals with access to opioids is much higher than any other group with comparable educational backgrounds (Jaffe, 1990). This type of addiction is often initially associated with an injury or ailment but also is associated with on-the-job fatigue and stress.

Opioids are taken orally, intranasally, by inhalation, or intravenously. Tolerance, dependence, and addiction to opioids can occur in a few weeks, although it is not usual when the drugs are used in a therapeutic range for a short period of time. Tolerance and dependence can develop independently of addiction; individuals affected will have no preoccupation with obtaining and using a drug even if they have signs of withdrawal when drug use is discontinued. Addiction as a complication of medical treatment, therefore, is uncommon (Jaffe, 1990). The reinforcement properties of opioids probably are due to activation of the receptors in the mesolimbic system and, in particular, the receptors in the nucleus accumbens.

Cocaine

Although cocaine was first isolated from the coca plant in the 1800s, the United States is currently in the midst of a cocaine epidemic (Hoeschen, 1991; USDHHS, 1991). The number of people in this country who have used cocaine probably exceeds 20 million (Jaffe, 1990). Cocaine produces stimulating effects similar to amphetamines, which include euphoria, a feeling of well-being, increased alertness, heightened sexual awareness, talkativeness, anorexia, and wakefulness.

Cocaine's mechanism of action occurs at the nerve synapse where the drug blocks the reuptake of DA into the presynaptic terminal. The postsynaptic neuron is flooded with DA, which stimulates the postsynaptic receptors to prolong nerve stimulation and cause the cocaine "high." Cocaine is a strong reinforcer that acts by increasing concentrations of DA in the central reward system in the mesolimbic portion of the brain.

Cocaine hydrochloride ("coke"), the salt form, can be taken orally, intranasally, or intravenously; cocaine base, on the other hand, exists as a paste or a solid called "crack" or "rock." Both of these forms are of greater potency than the salt form and are inhaled (Hoeschen, 1991). Orally ingested cocaine peaks in about 60 minutes, whereas intranasal cocaine is dose-dependent and peaks in 30 to 160 minutes. The inhaled variety is the most concentrated form of the drug and provides the most effective route of administration because of the large surface area of the lungs. Inhaled cocaine has a peak level 3 minutes after inhalation (Hoeschen, 1991; Jaffe, 1990).

Cocaine toxicity can lead to increased anxiety, paranoia, and pseudohallucinations such as tactile "cocaine bugs" or visual "snow lights" (Jaffe, 1990). Tolerance, particularly to the brief "rush," occurs even after one dose of cocaine. Significant tolerance does not occur, however, to the cardiovascular effects of cocaine; even long-term users can experience major toxic cardiovascular effects such as congestive heart failure, hypertension, arrhythmias, myocardial ischemia, and cardiac arrest.

Marijuana

Although marijuana use has decreased, it is still the most widely used illicit drug in the United States (USDHHS, 1991). Marijuana is obtained from the flowering portion of the hemp plant and can be refined into either hashish or hashish oil, which is more potent. The major ingredients of both marijuana ("grass," "weed," "reefer") and hashish ("hash") are the cannabinols (particularly delta-9-tetrahydrocannabinol, [THC]), which cause euphoria, relaxation, somnolence, enhancement of the senses, distortion of time and space, and sexual arousal (Hoeschen, 1991; Jaffe, 1990). Other responses include impaired short-term memory, inability to use critical thinking, confusion, and decreased fine motor movement. Systemic involvement includes tachycardia, increased myocardial oxygen consumption, and bronchodilation.

The precise mechanism of action of THC is uncertain, but it is known that the substance can bind to a variety of neurotransmitters in the CNS. THC tends to be excitatory at low doses and inhibitory at high doses. The most serious chronic effects are damage to the lung parenchyma and destruction of nerve cells in the brain, particularly in the hippocampus (Czechowicz, 1991).

The most common route of administration of THC is by inhalation. Marijuana is usually dried and smoked either in a cigarette or in a pipe. Water pipes (called "bongs" or "hookahs") are used to humidify the smoke to allow for deeper inhalation (Gold, 1991). A marijuana joint has a concentration of 1% to 3% THC, whereas hashish usually has a concentration of at least 10% to 20%. Inhalation produces a peak plasma concentration in 3 minutes. Although the drug has a relatively long half-life (20 to 30 hours), it has subjective effects that peak in only 20 to 30 minutes and last less than three hours (Jaffe, 1990).

The long-term effects of marijuana are poorly understood. The drug has a relatively low toxicity; it rarely leads to dramatic toxic effects that occur with other drugs such as cocaine or heroin. Marijuana and hashish are moderately addictive drugs, but the greatest danger is the effect of the drugs on children and adolescents. The drugs have the potential to negatively affect learning ability and completion of developmental tasks before adulthood (Czechowicz, 1991).

Hallucinogens

Phencyclidine (PCP) is the prototype for hallucinogens, a group of substances first introduced as anesthetic agents in the 1950s. Because it led to post-anesthesia complications, after several years PCP was no longer used for humans but was reintroduced as an animal anesthetic (Giannini, 1991a). In the 1960s PCP, or "angel dust," became a street drug that caused a cluster of effects such as paradoxical sedation and stimulation, hallucinations, anesthesia, and euphoria (Jaffe, 1990). Other symptoms include rage, enlarged pupils, amnesia, excitation, ataxia, hypertension, and seizures.

PCP binds to several sites in the central nervous system and inhibits the movement of calcium and other ions into the cells. It also inhibits the uptake of DA and norepinephrine, leading to an accumulation of DA in the nucleus accumbens (Jaffe, 1990). PCP can be inhaled, injected intravenously, or taken orally. A typical "high" lasts 4 to 6 hours (Jaffe, 1990).

One of the major problems with the abuse of PCP is that the drug is associated with violent behaviors such as assaults, rapes, homicides, self-inflicted injuries, and suicides. Because PCP is an amnesiac, most individuals have no memory of committing a violent act; therefore the view of the individual's guilt is uncertain in legal terms. Verdicts in legal cases involving PCP have had a variety of outcomes (Giannini, 1991a).

Inhalants

Inhalation of volatile (easily vaporized) agents probably first occurred 2500 years ago. Today volatiles are popular for four reasons: they are readily available, they can be purchased legally, they are inexpensive, and they have a rapid onset. A variety of volatile inhalants are abused and include alcohol solvents, nitrites, gasoline, aromatics, halogenated hydrocarbons, ketones, and nitrous oxide. Usually the "high" is associated with euphoria, excitement, loss of inhibitions, increased aggressiveness, and enhanced sexual performance (Giannini, 1991b). The most significant complication is sudden death due to cardiac arrhythmias. Other important complications include respiratory depression, angina, hyperreflexia, loss of coordination, and seizures.

Steroids

Anabolic-androgenic steroids, or tissue-building steroids, refer to either the male hormone testosterone or its synthetic forms. Commonly abused agents are nandrolone, methandrostenolone, oxandrolone, and ethylestrenol. These drugs are used illegally either to increase athletic performance or enhance masculine appearance. Anabolic-androgenic steroids may increase muscle size and strength in some individuals and also may increase muscle performance (Brower, 1991). Many types of anabolic steroids exist, but they all share similar mechanisms of action: the drugs, which are lipid-soluble and can cross the cell membrane, bind with intracellular receptors to change cellular function. Complications of steroid use include myocardial infarction, cerebrovascular disease, carcinoma, and hypertension. Sterility and testicular atrophy also may occur.

Designer drugs

Since the 1970s clandestine laboratories have manufactured a number of drugs that are potent reinforcers, such as derivatives of fentanyl ("China white") or meperidine. These drugs can cause serious and even fatal side effects (e.g., a parkinson-like paralysis [Jaffe, 1990]). Another drug sometimes confused with the designer drugs is synthesized from methamphetamine—methylenedioxymethamphetamine (MDMA) or "ecstasy." MDMA is similar to mescaline, a psychedelic amphetamine, and enables individuals to talk about experiences that have been repressed. Complications include anxiety, fear, tachycardia, and hypertension.

Nicotine

Nicotine is the drug present in tobacco. Nicotine's actions in the body are unpredictable because the drug causes both stimulation and inhibition. The major results are increased mental alertness, energy, and pleasure sensation; improvement of learning; depression of appetite; and stimulation of respiration (Jaffe, 1990). It also causes nausea and vomiting, arrhythmias, coronary artery disease, and myocardial ischemia. Although not as powerful a reinforcer as cocaine, nicotine has strong reinforcement properties.

Caffeine

Caffeine is present in coffee, tea, chocolate, and soft drinks. The main effects of caffeine are bronchial dilation through smooth muscle relaxation, CNS stimulation resulting in clarity of thought, and a decrease in fatigue. Increased doses of caffeine can lead to anxiety, tremors, sleeplessness, irritability, tachycardia, hypertension, and even seizures.

Polydrug addiction

Multiple drug use is the rule rather than the exception in America. Most individuals who enter a drug treatment program in the United States admit to being multiple drug users (Chan, 1991). Many individuals have a "primary drug" that they prefer but also use a variety of other substances. Alcohol is the most frequently used drug for polydrug users. The choice of drugs depends on a multitude of variables that include drug availability, cost, and CNS effects, as well as social pressure and environmental influences.

Several reasons for multiple drug use seem to exist. First, a mixture sometimes enhances drug effects. Second, multiple drug mixtures may counteract the undesirable side effects of a primary drug. Third, an individual may use an alternative drug when the primary drug is not available (Chan, 1991). Whatever the cause, multiple drug use complicates both behavioral and pharmacological treatment.

INDIVIDUAL AND FAMILY CONSEQUENCES

Psychological/emotional

As involvement with substance abuse progresses, there is a narrowing of the individual's coping repertoire. Using the substance becomes the predominant method of dealing with all situations, especially those producing anxiety or pain. As substance use becomes the chosen method of coping, the person increasingly employs the defense mechanisms of rationalization, projection, and denial to protect a deteriorating sense of self-worth. Behavior at home and work is inconsistent; there are periods of good times and productive activity, reinforcing a self-rationalization that the substance use is still controlled.

Once a person slips into harmful dependency, any of the good feelings that accompanied substance use/abuse are replaced by a "whole catalog of painful emotions" (Wegscheider, 1981). *Anger* is expressed at those close to the person, for not understanding, for making unfair demands, for interfering—but most of all anger is turned into the self. This anger becomes hostility and resentment that alienates those closest to the person. *Fear* is experienced, including fear of being discovered and abandoned by family members and people at work; fear of deteriorating health; fear of not being able to drink, as well as not being able to stop. This fear leads to chronic tension and anxiety that lead to irritability and inability to relax or sleep. Shame, guilt, and feelings of worthlessness and remorse pervade the sense of self as the individual experiences a loss of control and is ashamed of mounting financial troubles, social rejection, and other problems. There is guilt for neglecting work and family. Shame and guilt escalate into feelings of worthlessness and remorse for a problem out of control (Wegscheider, 1981).

Preoccupation with the abused substance then may lead to impaired social relationships with families and friends, deterioration in job performance, unemployment, financial problems, violence, and criminal activities. Once there is loss of control, the person experiences a downward spiral that only intervention can halt.

Family

Substance abuse affects the entire family, its structure, functioning, and roles. The ability of the family to support growth and development of its members is distorted. Substance abuse and abusing-related behavior become the central organizing principle around which family life is structured (Steinglass et al, 1987). As the substance-abusing member, usually a parent, becomes more preoccupied with the addiction and consequently becomes isolated from the family, family members respond in a variety of ways to accommodate this behavior pattern.

Frequently the family members invest more and more energy into trying to control the abuse. They get caught up in monitoring the behavior of the abuser, trying to predict and ward off the recurrence of abusing episodes. The substance abuser becomes the center of the family's functioning. All activities are directed at responding to this behavior. Meals may be delayed, family holidays and celebrations are disrupted by the abusing behavior, social commitments are broken. The abusing parent is no longer dependable and available to the children. Family rules become unclear, and a level of chaos develops (Gerace, 1993). Family members "cover up" the substance abuser's behavior to the outside world, often isolating themselves as a result of their own shame and fear of rejection. They call to explain absence from work as well as offer excuses to friends and relatives. Because of its over-involvement with and protection of the abuser, the family does not allow the abuser to experience the consequences of the behavior. The family thereby enables the substance abuse, paradoxically maintaining the behavior they hope to stop.

Studies of the effects of parental alcoholism on children describe a pattern of behavior that is characteristic of adult children of alcoholic families (ACOA). Increasing attention, through research and treatment, is given to this population. Many of the adult children of alcoholic families find themselves caught in some form of addiction or in relationships where abuse is involved. (See Chapter 9 for more about family consequences and treatment.)

Community

Isolation from a person's community of friends and social network occurs as involvement with the substance of abuse progresses. This is an interactive process: the person who abuses substances withdraws as more time is spent in substance-abusing behavior, and as abuse continues the social network rejects the individual. Consequently the individual often develops a network of people who support the abusing behavior.

Occupational/professional

The person who abuses a substance generally experiences a series of deteriorating consequences in relation to job or occupation, which in some respects parallels the deterioration in family relationships. Initially a drug may be taken to cope with work-related problems. At first it may seem that productivity is enhanced, but as time goes on performance is inconsistent and, generally, deteriorates. Because of the inconsistency, the individual is able to rationalize the performance to oneself and to others. The abuser may be passed over for promotions and pay increases. Often decreased time is spent at work with concomitant loss of income. At work, attempts may be made to confront the individual with his or her behavior so that help may be obtained or the person may be fired. The individual then may experience a series of job failures until secure employment can no longer be found. To combat such employee turnover, most large employers now have employee assistance programs (EAPs) designed to help employees with substance abuse problems and return them to productivity.

Financial

Financial difficulties mount due to absenteeism, job loss, and unpaid bills as more financial resources are spent on the substance of abuse. Involvement with the legal system may occur because of domestic violence or charges of driving under the influence (DUI). As the abuse continues, the individual may find that all financial resources are depleted.

SOCIETAL CONSEQUENCES

The societal consequences of substance use and abuse have led to a dramatic loss of resources, both human and material; increased morbidity and mortality; reduced or lost productivity; increased crime and violence; community deterioration; and the pain and suffering of family and friends. Some of these societal effects include (1) accidents, (2) crime, (3) domestic violence, (4) child abuse, (5) suicide, (6) prostitution, (7) disease, (8) workplace consequences, and (9) community deterioration.

Accidents

Trauma is the fourth leading cause of death in the United States and the leading cause of death for children and young adults from the ages of 4 to 34 (NHTSA, 1988). Alcohol and other drugs of abuse are important cofactors in severe or fatal injuries. Alcohol is involved in more than 50% of all highway deaths and many intoxicated trauma clients are dependent on other psychoactive substances as well (Soderstrom et al, 1992). In addition, alcohol is associated with an increased severity of injury, increased frequency of operative procedures, and longer hospital stays (Sommers, in press). Alcohol is the most common substance found in work-related injuries, but other drugs such as benzodiazepines also are relatively common (Lewis & Cooper, 1989).

The cost, in both lives lost and dollars spent for traumatic injuries, is extraordinarily high. In 1987, alcohol-related motor vehicle crashes accounted for 80% of the more-than-1.5 million years of potential life lost because of alcohol (Soderstrom et al, 1992). The economic costs are staggering as well. More than 3.5 million hospital admissions each year are due to traumatic injuries, which cost the United States up to $100 billion dollars a year (Gentilello et al, 1988). The incorporation of alcohol and drug treatment programs into the management of trauma clients, therefore, is essential to decreasing these appalling outcomes.

Crime

The link between alcohol and violent crime, in particular homicide and domestic violence, has been recognized for years. While there has been an increased focus on the relationship of illicit drugs and crime, alcohol remains the primary substance implicated in violent crime (De La Rosa et al, 1990). With the advent of cocaine and crack in the 1980s, there has been an increase in the number of random or impersonal homicides; inner-city young boys and men are the most frequent victims. Most of these males are involved in the drug-distribution network either as sellers, buyers, or runners of drugs and money between sellers and buyers (De La Rosa et al, 1990). Drug involvement leads to involvement in a violent social world. Crack sellers are more likely to use violence for regulation and control. A number of studies suggest that violent crime is significantly and directly related to involvement in drugs sales, particularly for youth (De La Rosa et al, 1990). In addition, 50% to 60% of crimes against property are drug-related. These robberies are committed primarily to obtain money for drug purchase.

Domestic violence

Alcohol abuse is a greater risk factor for family violence than is illicit drug use. Family violence includes spouse abuse, child abuse, child sexual abuse, and elder abuse. Alcohol use often precedes family violence and then later is used as a means of excusing or rationalizing violent behavior (De La Rosa et al, 1990).

Child abuse

There are a few methodologically sound research studies on the relationship between alcohol and drug abuse and child abuse. It is known that the long-term effect of parental violence leads to alcohol and drug use by the child-victim as an adult.

Thus the experience of child abuse, both physical and sexual, is related to the development of alcohol problems in adulthood, especially in women. Further research is needed to ascertain the interrelationship among alcohol, drug use, and physical and sexual abuse, both from the perspective of the victim and the perpetrator (Miller, 1990).

Suicide

Suicide is the eighth leading cause of death in the United States and the third leading cause of death among adolescents (Sternberg, 1991). Although the rate of suicide has remained constant since 1950, the last 20 years have seen a rapid increase in suicide among young people, with a corresponding decline among the elderly (Sternberg, 1991).

The rate of suicide in the general population is less than 1%, but the mortality rate for suicidal persons who meet criteria for alcohol dependencies (alcoholics) is reported to be as high as 27% (Sternberg, 1991). Fifteen to twenty-five percent of suicides are committed by alcoholics, and 13% to 50% of all suicide attempts are made by alcoholics (Sternberg, 1991). In addition, the 1986 San Diego Suicide Study provided clear evidence that a sizable proportion of persons who commit suicide have had serious problems with drug addiction (Sternberg, 1991).

Prostitution

Violence and drug use are intrinsic to the world of prostitution, although there is a differential pattern of involvement for females and males. Women generally are drug users first and turn to prostitution as a means of supporting their habit. They will trade sex for money or more drugs. Men, on the other hand, are usually prostitutes first and become involved in drugs later (Sterk & Elifson, 1990). While prostitution has always been considered risky, street prostitution has become more unpredictable and dangerous with the emergence of the crack cocaine epidemic.

Disease

As a group, intravenous drug users are now the major vector of heterosexual and perinatal HIV transmission in the United States and Europe (Kravis et al, 1991). There is increased evidence that the use of alcohol accelerates the rate at which HIV-positive individuals convert to AIDS symptoms.

The use of alcohol and, in particular, cocaine increases the incidence of sexually transmitted diseases (STDs) other than AIDS. Drug use leads to increases in promiscuous behavior and prostitution, thus increasing the risk of STDs. In addition, most experts believe that syphilis, chancroid, and herpes increase the efficiency of HIV transmission by providing portals of entry for the virus at lesion sites (Kravis et al, 1991).

Treatment costs

The health care costs of alcohol abuse and alcoholism are estimated at $89.5 billion per year, and drug-related problems cost $46.9 billion per year. It is estimated that by 1995 the two combined will cost in excess of $150 billion (Kinney, 1991). Untreated alcoholics and their families have greater general health care costs than nonalcoholics by 100%. Alcoholics in the later stages of the illness can have as high as 300% times the general health care costs of nonalcoholics (USDHHS, 1990).

Individuals with alcohol dependence use approximately one and a half times more health care services, have more repeated hospitalizations for the same disease, and are hospitalized four times more often than people in the general population. Each year an estimated two million individuals are hospitalized for alcohol-related problems, and 125,000 visits with a drug abuse diagnosis are made to office-based physicians (Rice et al, 1991). Of all the clients served by health care agencies, 25% to 50% have an alcohol-related problem.

Workplace effects

Because of the tremendous impact alcohol and substance abuse has on the workplace in lost productivity, accidents, and morale, the workplace has become an area of increased focus both as a site for case finding and for treatment. More and more companies are attempting to deal with the problem with mandatory drug testing, comprehensive policies, preventive education, and treatment programs. Some are requiring mandatory drug testing at the time of employment in an attempt to avoid hiring individuals with substance abuse. Testing only identifies *recent use;* chronic abusers find many ways to thwart such tests (Sullivan et al, 1988). Written policies specify the company's expectations regarding drug or alcohol use at work and what the consequences of use will be. Also, companies are offering prevention and education programs for employees, and some employers provide on-site treatment services (e.g., employee assistance programs).

Community deterioration

Substance abuse affects communities by taxing existing resources and requiring new resources to meet the needs of the increasing population of individuals who abuse substances. Substance abusers are more likely to need medical care than nonabusers, as well as treatment for substance abuse. Communities will probably experience a deterioration in community life as domestic violence, family instability, crime, poverty, under- and unemployment, and loss of productivity increase. Greater instability of families challenges communities to support divorcing parents and children, support single-parent families, and provide for the needs of affected children.

Most larger communities have treatment programs, as well as a referral system of support services and self-help groups. Many community-based programs are offering innovative care in halfway houses, twelve-step programs, and educational programs for those convicted of DUIs. These programs provide substance abuse expertise at a much reduced cost (Fleming & Barry, 1992).

Society attempts to deal with the mammoth consequences of substance abuse primarily in one of three ways. These include (1) intervention at drug-source countries; (2) apprehension and incarceration of users and sellers of drugs; and (3) treatment for individuals dependent on alcohol or drugs. The first two efforts consume two thirds of the resources available to combat substance abuse in the "war on drugs." These costs include interdiction strategies, maintenance of the criminal justice system, legal defense and adjudication, and incarceration. Treatment receives less than one third of the money allocated for substance abuse intervention.

While exorbitant costs accrue in the health care system because of the effects of substance abuse on individuals and their families, only $15 billion is spent on treatment. The federal government provides block grants to states for prevention, education, and treatment services. Individual treatment is paid for primarily by public (Medicare, Medicaid) or private (health care insurance) third-party payers. Some reasons for the lack of support for treatment services include negative attitudes, lack of understanding about the illness of substance abuse, pessimistic beliefs about treatment outcomes, and a preference for a quick solution (e.g., regulation).

SUMMARY

Substance abuse and dependency are complex conditions. Different philosophies are used to explain these conditions. Both genetic and environmental factors contribute to the development of substance abuse problems. Substance abuse and dependency are characterized by multiple physical sequelae and psychological symptoms. Substance abuse can progress to habitual intoxication, tolerance, and, finally, loss of control. Various defense mechanisms are used to deal with the consequences of excessive use. As the disorder progresses, individual, family, and social consequences result. The community and society also suffer collectively from the substance abuse problems of its members.

REFERENCES

Belkin, B.M. & Gold, M. (1991). Opioids. In N.M. Miller (Ed.), *Comprehensive handbook of drug and alcohol addiction.* (pp 537-557). New York: Marcel Dekker, Inc.

Blum, K., Noble, E.P., Shendon, P.J., & Finley, O. (1991). Association of the A1 allele of the D-sub-2 dopamine receptor gene with severe alcoholism. *Alcohol, 8*(15), 409-416.

Brower, K.J. (1991). Anabolic-androgenic steroids. In N.M. Miller (Ed.), *Comprehensive handbook of drug and alcohol addiction.* (pp 521-536). New York: Marcel Dekker, Inc.

Brown, R.L. (1992). Identification and office management of alcohol and drug disorders. In M.F. Fleming & K.L. Barry (Eds.), *Addictive disorders.* St. Louis: Mosby.

Chan, A.W.K. (1991). Multiple drug use in drug and alcohol addiction. In N.M. Miller (Ed.), *Comprehensive handbook of drug and alcohol addiction.* (pp 87-113). New York: Marcel Dekker, Inc.

Cho, A.K. (1990). Ice: A new dosage form of an old drug. *Science, 249,* 631-634.

Cloninger, C.R. & Begluter (Eds.). (1990). *Genetics and biology of alcoholism: Banbury Report 33.* New York: Cold Spring Harbor Laboratory Press.

Czechowicz, D. (1991). Adolescent alcohol and drug addiction and its consequences: An overview. In N.M. Miller (Ed.), *Comprehensive handbook of drug and alcohol addiction.* (pp 205-210). New York: Marcel Dekker, Inc.

De La Rosa, M., Lambert, E., & Grooper, B. (1990). Introduction: Exploring the substance abuse-violence connection. In M. De La Rosa, E. Lambert, & B. Grooper (Eds.), *Drugs and violence: Causes, correlates, and consequences.* (pp 1-7). NIDA Research Monograph 103. Rockville, MD.

Fell, J.C. (1990). Drinking and driving in America: Disturbing facts-encouraging reductions. *Alcohol Health & Research World, 14*(1), 18-25.

Fleming, M. and Barry, K. (1992). *Addictive disorders.* St. Louis: Mosby.

Gejman, P.V., Ram, A., Gelernter, J., Friedman, E., Cao, Q., Picicar, D., Blum, K., Noble, E.P., Kranzler, H.R., O'Malley, S., Hamer, D.H., Whitsitt, F., Rao, P., DeLisi, L., Virkkunen, M., Linnoila, M., Goldman, D., & Gershon, E. (1993). No structural mutation in the dopamine D_2 receptor gene in alcoholism or schizophrenia. *Journal of the American Medical Association, 271*(3), 204-208.

Gelernter, J., Bunzow, J., & Grandy, D. (1989). D_2 dopamine receptor locus (hD2g1) maps close to D11s29(17) on 11q using non-CEPH families. *10th International Workshop on Human Gene Mapping: Cytogenetic Cell Genetics, 1,* 100-228.

Gentilello, L.M., Duggan, P., Drummond, E., Tonnesen, A., Degnen, E.E., Fisher, R.P., & Reed, R.L. (1988). Major injury as a unique opportunity to initiate treatment in the alcoholic. *American Journal of Surgery, 156,* 558-561.

Gerace, L. (1993). Addictive behavior. In R. Rawlins, S. William, & C. Beck (Eds.), *Mental health-psychiatric nursing: A holistic life-cycle approach,* (3rd ed). St. Louis: Mosby.

Giannini, A.J. (1991a). Phencyclidine. In N.M. Miller (Ed.), *Comprehensive handbook of drug and alcohol addiction.* (pp 383-394). New York: Marcel Dekker, Inc.

Giannini, A.J. (1991b). The volatile agents. In N.M. Miller (Ed.), *Comprehensive handbook of drug and alcohol addiction.* (pp 395-404). New York: Marcel Dekker, Inc.

Gold, M.S. (1991). Marijuana. In N.M. Miller (Ed.), *Comprehensive handbook of drug and alcohol addiction.* (pp 353-519). New York: Marcel Dekker, Inc.

Goodwin, D.W. (1974). Drinking problems in adopted and unadopted sons of alcoholics. *Archives of General Psychiatry, 31*(2), 164-169.

Haber, J., McMahon A., Price-Hoskins, P., & Sideleau, B. (1992). *Comprehensive psychiatric nursing* (4th ed.). St. Louis: Mosby.

Hoeschen, L.E. (1991). The pharmacokinetics and pharmacodynamics of alcohol and drugs of addiction. In N.M. Miller (Ed.), *Comprehensive handbook of drug and alcohol addiction.* (pp 503-519). New York: Marcel Dekker, Inc.

Hoffman, B.B. & Lefkowitz, R.J. (1990). Catecholamine and sympathomimetic drugs. In A.G. Gilman, T.W. Rall, A.S. Nies, & P. Taylor (Eds.), *Goodman and Gilman's the pharmacological basis of therapeutics.* New York: Pergamon Press.

Hunt, W.A. & Nixon, S.J. (Eds.). (1993). *Alcohol-induced brain damage.* NIAAA Research Monograph 22. Rockville, MD.

Jaffe, J. (1990). Drug addiction and drug abuse. In A.G. Gilman, T.W. Rall, A.S. Nies, & P. Taylor (Eds.), *Goodman and Gilman's the pharmacological basis of therapeutics.* (pp 522-573). New York: Pergamon Press.

Jaffe, J.H. & Martin, W.R. (1990). Opioid analgesics and antagonists. In A.G. Gilman, T.W. Rall, A.S. Nies, & P. Taylor (Eds.), *Goodman and Gilman's the pharmacological basis of therapeutics.* (pp 485-521). New York: Pergamon Press.

Jellinek, E.M. (1960). *The disease concept of alcoholism.* New Brunswick, NJ: Hillhouse Press.

Kinney, J. (1991). *Clinical manual of substance abuse.* St. Louis: Mosby.

Kravis, N.M., Weiss, C.J., & Perry, S.W. (1991). Drug and alcohol addiction and AIDS. In N.M. Miller (Ed.), *Comprehensive handbook of drug and alcohol addiction.* New York: Marcel Dekker, Inc.

Levy, D. (1990). The Framingham study. *New England Journal of Medicine, 322,* 1531-1566.

Lewis, R.J. & Cooper, S.P. (1989). Alcohol, other drugs, and fatal work-related injuries. *Journal of Occupational Medicine, 31*(1), 23-28.

Miller, B. (1990). The interrelationship between alcohol and drugs and family violence. In M. La Rosa, E. Lambert, & B. Grooper, (Eds.), *Drugs and violence: Causes, correlates, and consequences.* (pp 177-207). NIDA Research Monograph 103. Rockville, MD.

Miller, M.S. (1991). Drug and alcohol addiction as a disease. In N.M. Miller (Ed.), *Comprehensive handbook of drug and alcohol addiction.* (pp 295-310). New York: Marcel Dekker, Inc.

Miller, N.S. & Gold, M.S. (1991). A neuroanatomical and neurochemical approach to drug and alcohol addiction: Clinical and research considerations. In N.M. Miller (Ed.), *Comprehensive handbook of drug and alcohol addiction.* (pp. 729-744). New York: Marcel Dekker, Inc.

Mohler, H. & Okada, T. (1977). Benzodiazepine receptor: Demonstration in the central nervous system. *nce, 198,* 849-851.

Murray, R.K., Granner, D.K., Mayes, P.A., & Rodwell, V.W. (1990). *Harper's biochemistry.* Norwalk, Connecticut: Appleton & Lange.

Nace, E.P. (1988). Posttraumatic stress disorder and substance abuse: Clinical issues. In M. Galanter (Ed.), *Recent developments in alcoholism.* (pp 9-26). New York: Plenum Press.

National Highway Traffic Safety Administration. (1988). *Drunk driving facts.* Washington, D.C.: National Center for Statistics and Analysis.

National Institute on Drug Abuse. (1991). *Drug abuse and drug abuse research*. The Third Triennial Report to Congress from the Secretary, Department of Health and Human Services (DHHS Publication No. ADM 91-1704). Washington, D.C.: U.S. Government Printing Office.

Partanen, J., Braun, K., & Markkonen, T. (1966). *Inheritance of drinking behavior: A study on intelligence, personality and use of alcohol of adult twins* (Vol. 14). Helsinki: The Finnish Foundation for Alcohol Studies.

Pickens, R.W., Suikes, D.S., McGee, M., & Lykken, D.T. (1991). Heterogeneity in inheritance of alcoholism: A study of male and female twins. *Archives of General Psychiatry, 48*(1), 19-28.

Rall, T.W. (1990). Hypnotics and sedatives: Ethanol. In A.G. Gilman, T.W. Rall, A.S. Nies, & P. Taylor (Eds.), *Goodman and Gilman's the pharmacological basis of therapeutics.* (pp 345-382). New York: Pergamon Press.

Rice, D., Kelman, S., & Miller, L. (1991). Economic cost of drug abuse. In *Economic costs, cost-effectiveness, financing, and community based drug treatment*. NIDA Research Monograph Series 113. Washington, D.C.: U.S. Department of Health and Human Services.

Roache, J.D. & Meisch, R.A. (1991). Drug self-administration research in drug and alcohol addiction. In N.M. Miller (Ed.), *Comprehensive handbook of drug and alcohol addiction.* (pp 625-640). New York: Marcel Dekker, Inc.

Robak, R. (1991). *A primer for today's substance abuse counselor*. New York: Lexington Books.

Roselle, G.A. (1992). Alcohol and the immune system. *Alcohol Health & Research World, 16*(1), 16-22.

Schuckit, M., Li, T., Cloninger, R., & Deitrich, R. (1985). Genetics of alcoholism. *Alcohol Clinical and Experimental Research, 9*, 475-492.

Smith, D.E. & Seymour, R.B. (1991). Benzodiazepines. In N.M. Miller (Ed.), *Comprehensive handbook of drug and alcohol addiction.* (pp 405-426). New York: Marcel Dekker, Inc.

Soderstrom, C.A., Dischinger, P.C., Smith, G.S., McDuff, D.R., Hebel, J.R., & Gorelick, D.A. (1992). Psychoactive substance dependence among trauma center patients. *JAMA, 267*, 2756-2759.

Sommers, M.S. (in press). Alcohol and trauma: The critical link. *Critical Care Nurse*.

Squires, R.F. & Braestrup, C. (1977). Benzodiazepine receptors in rat brain. *Nature, 266*, 732-734.

Steinglass, P., Bennett, L., Wolin, S., & Reiss, D. (1987). *The alcoholic family*. New York: Basic Books.

Sterk, C. & Elifson, K. (1990). Drug-related violence and street prostitution. In La Rosa, M., Lambert, E., & Gropper, B. (Eds.), *Drugs and violence: Causes, correlates, and consequences.* (pp 208-221). NIDA Research Monograph 103. Rockville, MD.

Sternberg, D.E. (1991). Suicide in drug and alcohol addiction. In N.M. Miller (Ed.), *Comprehensive handbook of drug and alcohol addiction.* (pp 405-426). New York: Marcel Dekker, Inc.

Sullivan, E.J., Bissel, L., & Williams, E. (1988). *Chemical dependency in nursing: The deadly diversion.* Menlo Park, CA: Addison-Wesley.

Tarter, B.R., Alterman, I., and Edwards, K. (1985). Vulnerability to alcoholism in men: a behavior-genetic perspective. *Journal Studies on Alcohol, 46*(4), 329-356.

United States Department of Health and Human Services. (1990). *Alcohol and health.* (DHHS Publication ADM 90-1656). Rockville, MD.

United States Department of Health and Human Services. (1991). *Drug abuse and drug abuse research.* (DHHS Publication ADM 91-1704). Rockville, MD.

Vaillant, G.E. (1983). *The national history of alcoholism*. Cambridge, MS: Harvard Press.

Wegscheider, S. (1981). *Another chance: Hope and health for the alcoholic family*. Palo Alto: Science and Behavior Books, Inc.

Yi, D. (1991). Alcohol. In N.M. Miller (Ed.), *Comprehensive handbook of drug and alcohol addiction.* (pp 745-768). New York: Marcel Dekker, Inc.

3 | Substance Abuse Diagnosis

Assessment and diagnosis of substance abuse are the prerequisites of treatment. Assessment is the collection of data about a client's problem, and diagnosis is the definition of the problem based on the assessment data. Two models for assessment and diagnosis are presented: the *nursing* model and the *medical* model. Diagnostic instruments as a basis for the medical model are described. Concurrence of substance abuse and psychiatric diagnosis is discussed.

ASSESSMENT OF SUBSTANCE ABUSE

Assessment for substance abuse takes place on a continuum that includes initial screening in general health care settings, a substance use and abuse history, assessment in clinical treatment settings, and the use of biochemical markers.

Given the frequency and significance of substance abuse, assessment for substance abuse should be included in all health assessments. The type and extent depend on the setting and the goal of the assessment. In a general health care setting, a screening instrument can be used during health assessment to identify potential substance abuse problems. Screening instruments are designed to determine quickly potential problems that need further investigation. When screening is positive, additional assessment of substance abuse is necessary to better define the problem and determine if an intervention or referral is indicated. A detailed substance abuse history is often part of the additional assessment. In a clinical setting, assessment is part of the evaluation to determine appropriate substance abuse treatment. Assessment data are then used to develop nursing and medical diagnoses that guide decisions for appropriate treatment.

Data should be collected in a systematic, organized manner. The use of an assessment instrument and a data collection format is recommended. A data collection format or history increases the consistency of interview data and allows comparison with other clients or other programs. Instruments allow the data to be quantified and validated.

Screening instruments for general settings

The goal of screening is to assess a population without known substance abuse, or at high risk for substance abuse, to determine the existence of a substance abuse problem. Screening for substance abuse is important in general health care settings because abuse causes and/or complicates other physical and psychological illnesses. Screening allows early intervention either before major problems develop or early in their development.

Usually a standard instrument is used for screening. Since screening is often conducted by health care professionals with little experience in substance abuse, the instrument must be easy to use, understandable, and time-efficient. Important statistical characteristics of any instrument are *validity,* whether or not the instrument measures what it says it does, and *reliability,* whether or not the measures are consistent. Screening instruments should be sensitive and specific. *Sensitivity* refers to the instrument's ability to correctly identify persons with the illness; *specificity* is the ability to correctly identify persons without the illness. Since no instrument identifies 100% of subjects correctly, sensitivity and specificity of an instrument are determined at a precise cutoff score and users must decide acceptable levels. That is, given the characteristics of the population, is it safest to err in the direction of overidentification of potential substance abuse problems or underidentification?

Many routinely used screening instruments were developed to screen for alcohol abuse or dependence. Some of these now have newer or parallel versions that address drug abuse. Screening for alcohol abuse is much more common than screening for drug abuse, because alcohol use is legal behavior that is socially acceptable, while drug abuse is illegal and no degree of use is acceptable.

Commonly used screening instruments are the CAGE Questionnaire, the Michigan Alcoholism Screening Test (MAST), and the Alcohol Use Disorders Inventory Test (AUDIT).

CAGE Questionnaire.   The CAGE is probably the most frequently used screening instrument. The CAGE Questionnaire (Ewing, 1984) has four questions that are often answered positively by alcoholics. The term "CAGE" is an acronym for the following four questions:

1. Have you ever felt that you ought to *cut down* on your drinking?
2. Have people *annoyed* you by criticizing your drinking?
3. Have you ever felt *guilty* or bad about your drinking?
4. Have you ever had a drink first thing in the morning *(eye-opener)* to steady your nerves or to get rid of a hangover?

Two affirmative answers suggest substance abuse should be more fully investigated; this cutoff has a sensitivity of .75 and a specificity of .96, that is, it correctly identifies 75% of people with an alcohol problem and 96% of those without a problem (NIAAA, 1987). A more recent version of the test, the CAGEAID (CAGE Adapted to Include Drugs), revises the items to include drugs and is reported to have similar sensitivity and specificity (Fleming & Barry, 1992) (see Appendix A-1). The CAGE is one of the most commonly used screening tools because of its simplicity and easy recall. It is routinely included in many health examinations. It is often preceded by the introductory question "Do you drink alcohol?"

Michigan Alcoholism Screening Test (MAST).   The MAST (Seltzer, 1971) also is used extensively in screening for alcoholism. It contains 25 items describing medical, social, and behavioral events associated with excessive drinking (see Appendix A-2). Responses are differentially weighted from 0 to 4 points. A score of five points or more places the subject in a questionable category, with sensitivity and specificity in the .80s and .90s (Hedlund & Viewig, 1984).

The MAST has been widely used and validated in its original form and is now available in three other versions. The Self-Administered Alcoholism Screening Test (SAAST) has additional symptom items, includes checks on consistency of responses, and has a simplified scoring system (Swenson & Morse, 1975). Sensitivity and specificity of .95 and .96 have been reported for the SAAST (NIAAA, 1987). The Short MAST (SMAST) has 13 items and also is self-administered (Seltzer et al, 1975). The Brief MAST has 10 items (Pokorny et al, 1972). The Drug Abuse Screening Test (DAST) is a 28-item version of the MAST designed to screen for behaviors related to drug abuse and has been found to be equally valid. A score of 6 or above on the DAST indicates significant drug problems (Skinner, 1982).

Alcohol Use Disorders Identification Test (AUDIT).   The AUDIT is a 10-item questionnaire developed as part of a World Health Organization (WHO) collaborative project to identify early problem drinkers (Babor et al, 1989). The items are related to consumption, use, and consequences of drinking, and each is scored from 0 to 4. The AUDIT is easily administered and scored. A disadvantage is its focus on alcohol use only. There is an accompanying client education brochure that recommends levels of maximum safe drinking to clients. The AUDIT has been adapted to include drugs, and Appendix A-3 displays this adaptation, although this latest version has not been widely used to date (Fleming & Barry, 1992).

Responding to positive screens

The purpose of screening is to detect substance abuse in early stages so as to respond appropriately and thus prevent more serious problems. Positive screenings are not diagnostic, rather they indicate that further assessment is needed. To screen and not respond would be detrimental because it would suggest to clients that their substance use is acceptable.

It is important that the screener and the sponsoring organization plan for clients who screen positively or questionably for substance abuse. Willingness to screen carries with it the implied responsibility of appropriate follow-up. A protocol for responding to positive screenings is useful. Figure 3-1 shows one protocol based on a decision tree that incorporates the CAGE and is designed for a primary care setting (NIAAA, 1987). Variations on this model can be developed to meet the needs of a particular health care setting.

Some positive screenings clearly indicate by their magnitude the need for referral to a substance abuse professional. Referral is simple in a health care organization with an affiliating treatment program. In other settings, referral sources must be identified. Referral sources should be established when screening is initiated so that there is agreement in the organization and among personnel on the referral protocol. A resource person in the screening organization needs to develop a working knowledge of a variety of local referral sources because many factors are involved in referral, especially insurance coverage.

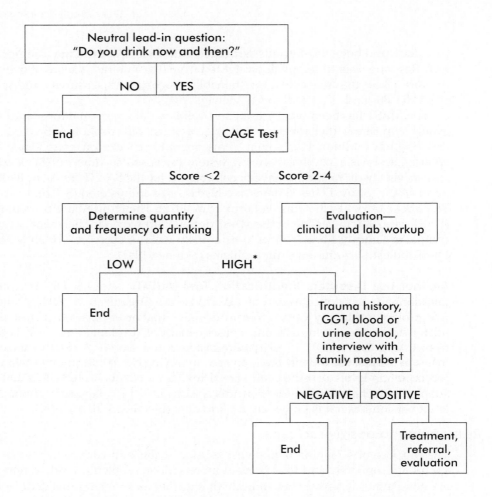

*High consumption is defined as 60 to 80 g of absolute ethanol every day.
†Significant trauma history is indicated by a score of 2 or higher on the
trauma scale designed by Israel and colleagues at the Addiction Research
Foundation. The following questions are asked: (1) Have you had any
fractures or dislocations since you were 18? (2) Have you been injured in a
traffic accident? (3) Have you injured your head? (4) Have you been injured
in an assault or fight? (5) Have you been injured after drinking?

Fig. 3-1. Decision tree for primary care alcohol screening. (From National Institute on Alcohol
Abuse and Alcoholism (1990). ADM 218-88-0002. Rockville, Maryland: United States Department of Health and Human Services.)

More difficult to assess are the questionable screenings, those that indicate some
problem but are not definitive. In health care settings where clients will be followed
for a long time, the client can be informed of the questionable screening and advised to cut back or abstain from drinking. Studies indicate that this type of response (called a brief intervention) is often quite effective in decreasing substance

use (Sanchez-Craig, 1990). Screening results also can be entered into a client's record for future follow-up and "watchful waiting."

In situations where further follow-up is doubtful or cannot be arranged easily, education or intervention must be accomplished on the spot. Brochures and other printed information are useful in giving clients more information about substance use and hints on cutting back or abstaining. Appropriate local telephone numbers should be included, such as the National Council on Alcohol and Drug Dependence (NCADD), which provides assessment, referral, and general information, and Alcoholics Anonymous (AA). Appropriate other local referral sources (e.g., treatment providers) also should be included.

Interviewing and the substance abuse history

When a screening is positive, more information about the client's actual substance use clearly is needed to determine the level and type of appropriate response. This information is most often collected by an interview, using a history form as a guide. A substance abuse history is one component of the assessment format shown in Box 3-1.

Substance abuse interviews are conducted in various situations. Taking a history could be in response to a positive screening or to further assess substance abuse and determine an appropriate response. If a client has a health problem and abuse is suspected, the interview is used to determine the degree to which abuse affects or contributes to the health problem. This information has particular implications for pain control because a client with substance abuse may have greater tolerance or sensitivity to specific medications. A history also is taken to determine the diagnosis, detoxification needs, and appropriate treatment interventions when a client enters substance abuse treatment. The degree of detail will vary according to the needs of each client and the setting.

When a client either is evasive or denies substance use, it may be useful to embed the substance abuse history within a more general social history. This allows rapport to develop before threatening questions are asked (Fleming & Barry, 1992). Since clients may underreport or inaccurately report their substance use, collateral interviews with the client's "significant others" (with the client's permission) might be needed to provide verification and additional data.

One suggested sequence of questions about drinking is as follows:
1. Do you drink now and then?
2. How many times did you drink during the last month?
3. How many times did you have six or more drinks in the last month?
4. On the occasions when you drink, how much do you usually have?

These questions can be inserted among other lifestyle questions and can be paraphrased to address other substances.

Alternatively, the following three questions from the MAST (Woodruff et al, 1976) are very sensitive to alcohol abuse:
1. Has your family ever objected to your drinking?
2. Did you ever think you drank too much in general?
3. Have others said you drink too much for your own good?

These questions too could be paraphrased to include other substances.

Whatever the introduction, a complete substance abuse history should describe

---

Box 3-1
Format For Assessment

Demographic data

Name:
Age:
Sex:
Ethnic group:
Marital status:
Religious affiliation:
Significant other:

What is the reason for coming to the hospital (e.g., symptoms of withdrawal, marital-family crisis, work problems, referred by legal source, wants help to "stop drinking" or using drugs, medical problems)?

What is the motivation for treatment?

General observations

Vital signs:	Blood pressure (hypotensive, hypertensive)
Pulse:	Rapid, regular, irregular
Temperature:	Elevated
Respirations:	Rapid, shallow, depressed
APPEARANCE	
Gait:	Unsteady, normal, weaving, shuffling
Eyes:	Conjunctival infection, bloodshot, dilated, pinpoint, normal pupils, lacrimation (tearing), vacant stare, poor eye contact, good eye contact
Skin:	Perspiration, cool, clammy, dry, bruises, needle tracks, scars, abrasions, gooseflesh, excoriations, reddened palms
Nose:	Running (rhinorrhea), congested, red
Presence of tremors:	Fine or coarse, slight to moderate or severe
Grooming:	Neat, unkempt, unshaven, odor (alcohol, foul)
BEHAVIOR	
Speech:	Slurred, incoherent, loud, soft, normal, articulates clearly, monotone, hesitant, pressured, relevant, distractive
Attitude:	Quiet, calm, demanding, agitated, irritable, impatient, vague, withdrawn, suspicious, anxious, tearful, happy, silly
Dominant mood/affect:	Euphoric, depressed, angry, sad, appropriate, inappropriate, normal
Sensorium:	Orientation to time, person, place, changes in memory
Perception:	The presence of illusions, hallucinations, delusions, hallucinosis
Potential for suicide:	Is the individual presently thinking about suicide: Is there a plan or a method to carry out that plan? A history of previous suicide attempts or gestures? Were attempts in intoxicated state or sober state? Is there a family history of suicide? Is there a recent loss or anniversary of a loss? (Assess need for emergency consultation and intervention.)

Continued.

General observations—cont'd

Potential for violence: Does behavior indicate potential for violence? Voice, manner, stance, verbal threats? Assess need for consultation, emergency intervention if necessary. Ask if individual has a history of violence when taking substances or during withdrawal period.

Present drug history

The areas that need specific assessment are the type of substance used, the amount taken, and the pattern of use.

Type: Beer, wine, whiskey, cocaine, heroin, marijuana (cannabis), sedative/hypnotics, hallucinogens; one substance only, or a combination? This may mean combination within a class (i.e., alcohol, beer, whiskey, and wine, or alcohol and sedative/hypnotics). It may be combinations in different classes (i.e., heroin and alcohol and stimulants or narcotics and sedative/hypnotics). What is the predominant substance of choice? Does the individual use "street" drugs, prescription drugs?

Amount: How much (approximate amount) does the individual drink? How many six packs, quarts, fifths? How much does individual use, bags? What route (oral, intravenous, subcutaneous)? How many pills daily? Hits?

What is the pattern of use: Daily, several times a week? Increased on weekends? Only weekends? Binge or episodic drinking? Runs? Intoxicated daily? Has the individual ever tried to control or cut down drinking or pattern of substance use? How?

When was last drink?
When was last drug dose? How taken?
What drugs currently taking?
Has individual developed tolerance? (explain)
When did it begin?
Has there been a change in tolerance?
Are withdrawal symptoms present?
Is there a previous history of withdrawal?
Is there a previous history of seizures?
Is there a history of hallucinations? (explain)
Is there a history of hallucinosis?
Was individual ever hospitalized? If yes, for what?
Are there any present medical problems?
Are there any chronic medical problems?
Is there a history of the following: liver disease? hepatitis? diabetes? heart disease? anemia? drug overdose?
Have there been any recent falls, injuries, accidents?
Is the individual taking any prescribed medication?
Has the individual any known allergies?

Past drug history

Has the individual ever stopped drinking or using drugs?
How long was the period of abstinence?

Continued.

Box 3-1
Format For Assessment—cont'd

Past drug history—cont'd

Why did the individual abstain, what was the motivation?

At what age did the individual start abusing/using substances?

At what age did the individual first begin having difficulty in life circumstances due to drug intake?

Has the individual ever been in treatment for drug abuse/dependency?

What type of treatment: detoxification, rehabilitation?

How many times in treatment for the above?

Is there a family history of alcohol abuse/dependency?

Is there a family history of other substance abuse/dependency?

Psychosocial history

Conjugal:	Married, separated, divorced, never married, widowed? What is spouse's reaction to client's abuse of substances? Does the spouse abuse substances? Is substance use causing marital conflicts?
Parenting:	Are there children? How many? What are their ages and sex? Have children had school problems, health problems, physical, emotional, sleeping problems?
Intrapersonal:	What are the individual's leisure activities, hobbies? Has there been a change in participation in these activities? Has there been a change in friends or a loss of friendships? Do the social activities center on the substance use/abuse?
Occupation/employment:	What is individual's occupation? Present employment? How long in present employment? Has the individual ever missed work due to alcohol abuse? Drug use? Has the individual abused substances while working? Is substance use jeopardizing work or business? How long has individual been employed?
Finances and living conditions:	Approximate amount spent on substances? Source of income other than employment? Family suffering from less adequate housing or food due to substance abuse or purchases? What are present living conditions? Is individual living alone, in an apartment, own house, live in a room, is there no address or no permanent living arrangement?
Legal problems:	Have there been any violations while intoxicated? Are any present legal offenses pending from substance abuse/dependency? Is present treatment court-recommended?

From Johnson, B.S. (1993). *Psychiatric-mental health nursing: Adaptation and growth.* (3rd ed.). Philadelphia: JB Lippincott.

the *frequency, quantity, duration, patterns,* and *consequences* of substance use. The history should begin with the client's drug of choice but include other substances because abuse of multiple substances is quite common. For example, almost all abusers of nonalcoholic substances also use alcohol, and many abusers of alcohol also use other substances on occasion. Prescription drug use and abuse should be included because prescription drugs—particularly pain medications, muscle relaxants, and minor tranquilizers—are often substances of abuse.

The frequency, quantity, duration, and patterns of substance use help define and categorize a client's use. Several formulas quantify alcohol intake in standard drinks so that data are comparable. At least three drinking patterns were identified in an earlier DSM (APA, 1987). These are (1) regular heavy daily drinking, (2) regular heavy drinking on weekends, and (3) long periods of sobriety with periodic heavy drinking binges lasting for weeks or months. These drinking patterns might not be apparent if quantity alone were measured.

Important information includes the consequences of use. What losses has the client experienced as a result of substance abuse (e.g., family, employment, financial, health)? Legal difficulties are common and questions about such problems should be asked. In clients with multi-drug use, specific information is necessary about each substance.

It is important to ask about the patterns of multi-drug use and if specific substances are routinely used together, which increases the potential for cross tolerance if the substances are pharmacologically related or for multiple withdrawal effects if they are not. Sequential use patterns may occur in amphetamine abuse when clients may alternate amphetamines with sedatives to "come down." Although most substance users have a drug or substance of choice, they may use other substances when their drug of choice is not available. Knowledge of the route of administration of a drug is vital for determining the degree of likely dependence and potential exposure to infectious disease such as AIDS and hepatitis B, both caused by sharing contaminated needles. All of these factors have implications for problem identification and care planning, especially for detoxification regimens.

A client's body language during the interview can indicate a problem. Frequent movements, unusual posture, avoiding eye contact, and long pauses may suggest that the client is uncomfortable with the content of the interview or is having difficulty responding truthfully (Lisanti, 1991).

The interviewer has several goals in taking a history. One is to obtain reliable and valid information. To do this, it is often necessary to meet the second goal of developing an initial level of trust and rapport with the client. Depending on the situation, a further goal may be the development of a therapeutic relationship. To meet these goals, it is necessary for the interviewer to be sensitive to the client's verbal and nonverbal cues and to present a nonjudgmental, caring attitude toward the client.

Assessment scales for clinical settings

When substance abuse or dependency is suspected, several instruments can be used to identify and quantify substance abuse problems. They are used primarily in clinical or treatment settings to determine specifics of the substance abuse problems. The purpose of these scales is case-finding rather than screening, since they yield a more precise definition of substance abuse problems within a population already identified as having the problem (Allen et al, 1988). These scales include the MacAndrew Scale, the Diagnostic Interview Schedule (DIS), and the Addiction Severity Index (ASI).

MacAndrew Scale. The MacAndrew Scale is composed of 49 selected elements from the Minnesota Multiple Personality Inventory (MMPI) that have been found to be significant in clients with alcohol abuse (MacAndrew, 1965). None of the items specifically mentions substance abuse, so this instrument is useful with clients who exhibit high levels of denial about their abuse. It is also a scale that can be extrapolated from an already existing MMPI, which is administered in many settings. The validity is not as high as other scales, however, so its main advantage is the use of an indirect approach (Preng & Clopton, 1986).

Diagnostic Interview Schedule (DIS), alcohol and drug subscales. The DIS is an interview schedule designed to determine all accepted psychiatric diagnoses. It contains two subscales related to substance abuse—alcohol abuse/dependence and drug abuse/dependence. When appropriately scored, these subscales can determine whether the criteria are met for diagnoses of alcohol or drug abuse or dependence. The interview was developed for use by nonclinical personnel (Robins et al, 1981). Self-administered computerized versions of the instrument also exist. The full interview is described later in this chapter.

Addiction Severity Index (ASI). The ASI is a semistructured interview that provides information about the client in seven spheres: drug and alcohol use, the complications of use medically, psychologically, legally, within the family and socially, and in employment (McLellan et al, 1980). These spheres represent the particular life problems manifested by the client's substance abuse. Questions in each sphere concern the number, intensity, and duration of problems. Clients rate the severity of each problem area on a 5-point scale based on events during the previous 30 days. The interviewer rates each problem area on a 10-point scale. Identifying specific life problems and their severity can direct treatment and may be useful in matching clients to treatment and in measuring outcomes.

Biochemical markers

Another source of assessment data is the measurement of biochemical markers by testing blood specimens. These blood tests are helpful as an adjunct to other assessment techniques. Common tests are liver function, mean corpuscular values, blood alcohol levels, and urine drug screens. With the exception of urine screens, laboratory tests primarily measure the physiological effects of alcohol on the body.

Liver function tests. The most common liver function tests are the gamma-glutamyl transferase (GGT), the aspartate amino transferase (AST), and the alanine amino transferase (ALT). These tests are common in laboratory screening profiles.

The GGT is the most effective biochemical test for heavy drinking because of its sensitivity to liver damage; hence it is elevated consistently in a client who has abused alcohol. Even so, an elevated GGT only corroborates a diagnosis because there are many reasons for liver damage besides alcohol abuse. The sensitivity for heavy drinking in outpatient settings is 25% to 30%, that is, the test correctly identifies that percentage of known alcohol problems (Fleming & Barry, 1992).

The AST and ALT are other liver enzymes that increase with alcohol use. A rough measure of liver function can be created by adding the AST and ALT. A normal value is two to three hundred. Elevated levels (sometimes in the hundreds or thousands) confirm the diagnosis of liver damage for which alcohol abuse is the primary, but not the only, cause.

Mean corpuscular values (MCV). Alcohol is a marrow suppressant causing a direct effect on the sternum and the femur. The levels of the MCV, an index of red blood cell size, are greatly increased in alcohol abuse. This macrocytosis often is seen early in the illness.

Blood alcohol content (BAC). A positive blood alcohol content level or the odor of alcohol on the breath is suggestive of alcohol use. Actual blood level may give little information other than the amount of recent drinking. Behavioral indicators of BAC are extremely variable.

Urine drug screens. Urine drug screening can be used to corroborate the diagnosis of substance abuse and to identify substances of abuse. Positive urine drug screens indicate prior use for some substances and vary depending on the substance and the length of time since use. For example, marijuana levels in urine may be elevated up to 30 days after use. Cocaine levels may be elevated for 5 to 7 days after use, depending on the amount used and the length of use. On the other hand, substances used very recently may not show up in the urine. (See Chapter 16 for more about drug testing.)

Because of their lack of specificity, biochemical markers are generally of less value in assessment than self-report screening instruments such as those previously described (O'Farrell & Maisto, 1987). With the exception of urine screening, markers may test positively for conditions other than alcohol or drug use. Combinations of biochemical and self-report instruments have been suggested and are currently being explored, evaluated, and tested for optimal sensitivity and cost effectiveness (Lumeng, 1986).

NURSING ASSESSMENT AND DIAGNOSIS

Screening instruments, substance abuse history, and biochemical markers are all means of assessing the client. This assessment process is not an end in itself but rather the initial step in a process of defining client problems in order to guide intervention and treatment.

Two models for assessing, defining, and subsequently intervening with, client problems are common to nursing practice: the *nursing* model and the *medical* model. While the assessment data in these models are similar, differences exist in the type of problem identified.

The medical model is based on pathophysiology and its psychological parallel, psychopathology. Substance abuse, which cannot be totally explained through pathophysiology or psychopathology, does not fit easily in the medical model.

Medical assessment focuses on data consistent with the diagnostic categories in the Diagnostic and Statistical Manual of Mental Disorders (to be described later)—the standardized psychiatric nomenclature, which includes substance abuse (APA, 1994). The medical model for assessment and diagnosis is presented in more detail later in this chapter. Although the medical model is the traditional health care model, it is somewhat reductionistic in its approach and is best used as a foundation for medical practice. The nursing model articulates with the medical model but also provides a basis for nursing practice.

Nursing practice in substance abuse is "all those nursing actions that are directed toward prevention of, and intervention with, health problems concurrent with, and consequent to, patterns of abuse and addiction" (ANA, DANA, & NNSA, 1987, p. 6). The focus on health problems is broader than a focus on disease alone. "Nursing actions" emphasizes that the nursing model is based on the independent functions of nursing practice (i.e., nursing functions that the nurse carries out independently as part of nursing care).

Both the nursing and medical models use a standardized nosology or problem list. The underlying framework for the nursing model is nursing *process,* a problem-solving format that is used to direct nursing *practice* (Potter & Perry, 1993). The components of the nursing process are (1) assessment, (2) nursing diagnosis, (3) planning care, (4) implementation, and (5) evaluation of care. Care planning, implementation, and evaluation are discussed in Chapters 6 and 11.

Nursing assessment

The goal of nursing assessment is to determine the variables necessary to develop appropriate nursing diagnoses and guide interventions. A nursing assessment of a client with substance abuse is broader than assessment of the substance abuse alone, although that abuse is included. Since nursing diagnoses may be developed in any area in which the client is experiencing real or potential problems, a broad database is necessary. The *Standards of Addictions Nursing Practice* (ANA & NNSA, 1988) recommends six basic areas for assessment: (1) past medical, psychiatric, and addictions treatment; (2) family support and family history; (3) family health history; (4) mental status; (5) spiritual health and well-being; and (6) cultural and ethnic factors. Other areas may be indicated by specific client characteristics.

An initial or baseline nursing assessment is guided by a nursing history form that collects the assessment data needed to give appropriate client care in a specific setting. For example, a screening instrument and brief substance use history would provide appropriate data in a medical-surgical environment, but a more thorough substance use history is needed in a substance abuse treatment setting. For this reason, there is no standardized nursing history form, although several models exist that can be adapted to specific settings (ANA & NNSA, 1988; NNSA, 1990). See Box 3-1 for a nursing assessment format recommended by the National Nurses Society on Addictions.

Since nurses are usually part of a multidisciplinary team, the nursing assessment uses information from the client database that includes contributions from other disciplines. Assessment of specific data may be divided among the team members; an assessment protocol is helpful in identifying which data are to be collected by whom and where the information is to be recorded in the database. Sharing assessment data increases team functioning and decreases duplicate assessment. Team meetings allow discussion of the data from a variety of disciplinary perspectives.

Data may be collected through observation, interview, examination, screening instruments, and, commonly, combinations of the above. Baseline data collection occurs with initial contact and is regularly updated based on changes in the client's condition. Elements that cannot be assessed initially are deferred for later. For example, some clients may not be able to give full histories until they complete detoxification, or a client may not share personal information until a nurse-client relationship is established. The database is continually updated as new information is obtained or as information changes.

In addictions nursing, nursing assessment data are categorized into four dimensions of human responses to addiction: (1) biological or physical responses, (2) cognitive responses, (3) psychosocial responses (including psychological-emotional and social), and (4) spiritual-belief responses (ANA & NNSA, 1988). These dimensions were developed from a survey of nurses in addictions nursing practice and collectively assess all aspects of the person.

Data analysis involves examining the data and organizing it into logically related clusters. These clusters may be further validated by acquiring additional information from the client. Data also may rule out potential problems the client is not experiencing (Little & Carnevelli, 1976).

Nursing diagnosis

A nursing diagnosis is "a clinical judgment about the client's response to actual or potential health conditions or needs" (ANA, 1991). Nursing diagnoses are developed to best describe clusters of assessment data. These clusters of data are the defining characteristics of the nursing diagnosis and can be compared for validation to the defining characteristics of standardized nursing diagnoses. Defining characteristics are, therefore, the assessment data that are typical or definitive for a particular nursing diagnosis.

Nursing diagnoses are derived from a standardized nursing diagnosis list developed by the North American Nursing Diagnosis Association (NANDA), which has identified and approved more than 100 nursing diagnoses to date in its current *Taxonomy I* (NANDA, 1992). Since standardized nursing diagnoses are relatively recent, this taxonomy is regularly revised and updated. At the 1994 NANDA conference, no new nursing diagnoses were approved. Twenty-five NANDA nursing diagnoses that are common to substance abuse nursing have been identified and described with their defining characteristics (ANA & NNSA, 1988). The 25 diagnoses are displayed in Table 3-1 with examples of their defining characteristics. Other nursing diagnoses may also be used; new diagnoses are regularly developed.

The format for a complete nursing diagnosis has three parts. The first part is the change or potential change in health. In the second part, the phrase "related to" is used to identify the cause of the change when it can be identified; this cause is the focus of nursing interventions. The last part of diagnosis uses the phrase "as evidenced by" to identify assessment data that support the diagnosis. Not all three components are used in every diagnosis or in every setting; however, use of all three creates a highly individualized nursing diagnosis. Table 3-2 offers examples of two nursing diagnoses and shows how the etiology and defining characteristics individualize the standard diagnosis. A specific nursing diagnosis may take place in

Table 3-1

Diagnoses common to addictions nursing practice

Nursing diagnosis	Examples of defining characteristics
Biological responses	
Sensory-perceptual alterations	Fluctuation in mental status, confusion, disorientation; blackouts, hallucinations
High risk for injury	Ataxia; history of flashbacks; history of seizures
Self-care deficit	Intolerance to activity; diminished self-esteem; discomfort
High risk for infection	Homeless lifestyle; practice of unsafe sex; severe withdrawal syndrome
Sleep pattern disturbance	Sleep pattern reversal; mild, fleeting nystagmus
Alteration in nutrition: less than body requirements	Report of inadequate dietary intake; change in appetite; dental caries
Alteration in comfort: pain	Distracted behavior, moaning, crying, pacing
	Guarding behavior, positioning; altered muscle tone
Altered growth and development: biological	Infants of chemically dependent mothers; newborn exhibiting drug-induced sedation; retardation of brain growth
Cognitive responses	
Knowledge deficit	Verbalization of knowledge deficit
Defensive coping	Use of denial in acknowledging addictions process
	Inaccurate perception of health status
Alteration in thought process	Mood swings, restlessness; impairment of recent memory; lack of insight; dementia
Noncompliance	Continuing pattern of addiction; verbalization of noncompliance; inability to set goals
Psychosocial responses	
Impaired communication	Inability to express feelings; slurring of speech; inappropriate speech patterns
Ineffective individual coping	Ineffective coping with feelings of defeat; replacing one chemical with another; ineffective choices and actions
Alterations in self-concept	Body image disturbance; low self-esteem: social withdrawal; role performance: role conflict
Anxiety (specific level of anxiety)	Subjective feelings of discomfort
	Affective characteristics: alarmed
	Cognitive characteristics: forgetfulness
	Behavioral characteristics: restlessness; seeking isolation from others; expressing feelings of loneliness
Social isolation	Nonverbal behaviors: staying in room; refusing to join group
Dysfunctional family process	Disturbed social communication; dependency; loss of family support system
Altered parenting	Continued substance abuse while breast-feeding; verbalization of role frustration; lack of parental attachment behavior
Altered growth and development: psychosocial	Lack of trust in adults; fear of losing control; harsh self-criticism
High risk for aggression	Threats of anger, or rage; aggressive behavior; rigid body posture

Continued.

Table 3-1

Diagnoses common to addictions nursing practice—cont'd

Nursing diagnosis	Examples of defining characteristics
Spiritual responses	
Spiritual distress	Distress in human spirit caused by guilt, shame, grief, self-blame; lack of meaning in life
Powerlessness	Passivity; a perceptual experience of loss of control Inappropriate efforts to assert control over self
Hopelessness	Diminished trust; frequent crying spells; flat affect, sadness
Grief	Potential, perceived, or actual loss of a significant object or person

Modified from: American Nurses Association. (1988). *Standards of addictions nursing practices with selected diagnoses and criteria.* Kansas City, MO: The Association.

conjunction with a variety of medical diagnoses, indicating that the nursing diagnosis is independent of medical diagnosis.

Standardized NANDA nursing diagnoses allow nurses to communicate clearly with each other and to translate the nursing diagnosis to other disciplines. In multidisciplinary settings, this sharing of discipline-specific processes adds to the total understanding of the client.

Diagnoses should be shared and validated with the client and prioritized according to the immediate health status of the client. This sets the stage for the next step of the nursing process—planning care (see Chapter 6).

Table 3-2

Nursing diagnoses with variations

Primary NANDA nursing diagnoses	Examples of complete nursing diagnoses
Sensory/perceptual alterations (visual, auditory, tactile, kinesthetic, gustatory, olfactory)	Sensory/perceptual alteration (visual) characteristic of complete alcohol dependence related to loss of job and rejection by family, evidenced by asking staff to "get rid of these bugs," while brushing at his clothing.
	Sensory/perceptual alteration (auditory) characteristic of experimentation with hallucinogens related to peer pressure, evidenced by covering ears and shouting, "Don't say those words to me," when alone in a room.
Thought processes, altered	Altered thought processes characteristic of true alcoholism related to pressures of a busy law practice and family demands, evidenced by confusion and blackouts.
	Altered thought processes characteristic of severe drug addiction to amphetamines related to desire to lose weight, evidenced by delusion that husband is having an affair with her mother.

From Stuart, G.W. & Sundeen, S.J. (1995). *Principles and practice of psychiatric nursing.* (5th ed.). St. Louis: Mosby.

MEDICAL MODELS OF ASSESSMENT AND DIAGNOSIS

DSM diagnosis

The definition of alcoholism and/or substance abuse has evolved over time to reflect recent information about the heterogeneity of the illness and the multiple factors that contribute to it. The word "alcoholism" has carried different meanings over the years, reflecting the scientific concepts and socio-political realities of the times. Such variations in usage have applied also to substance abuse. In recent studies of substance abuse terminology, there has been a lack of consensus in the addiction field, impeding communication between professionals of various disciplines, retarding deliberation of public policy, and threatening the ability of clients to get treatment. Advances are needed in the development and standardization of nomenclature to facilitate substance abuse research and to improve access to and quality of clinical care.

Historically, definitions have attempted to describe a wide spectrum of substance abuse problems. For example, Jellinek in 1960 chose to define alcoholism as "any use of alcoholic beverage that causes any damage to the individual or society or both" (Jellinek, 1960, p. 35). In 1972 a report published by the National Council on Alcoholism described *alcoholism* as a "pathological dependence on alcohol" (Criteria Committee of NCA, 1972, p. 127). Blume and others (1976) described alcoholism as a chronic, progressive, and potentially fatal disease that is characterized by tolerance and physical dependency or pathologic organ changes or both, all the direct or indirect consequence of alcohol ingestion. Also in 1976, Edwards and Gross described the alcohol dependence syndrome (ADS) for the first time. The following characteristics of alcohol dependence lie at the heart of all currently used and proposed diagnostic criteria:

- Establishment of daily drinking patterns and selective choice of alcoholic beverage
- Salience of alcohol-seeking behavior
- Increased tolerance to alcohol's effects
- Repeated withdrawal symptoms
- Drinking to relieve or avoid withdrawal symptoms
- Subjective awareness of a compulsion to drink
- Reinstatement of established drinking patterns following a period of abstinence

With these concepts in mind, the American Society of Addiction Medicine (ASAM) in 1990 defined alcoholism as "a primary, chronic disease with genetic, psychosocial, and environmental factors influencing its development and manifestations. The disease is often progressive and fatal. It is characterized by continuous or periodic impaired control over drinking, preoccupation with the drug alcohol, use of alcohol despite adverse consequences, and distortions in thinking, most notably, denial" (ASAM, 1990, p. 4). Diagnosis, then, is the first step in the treatment of the disease, and standardized nomenclature for disorders is essential for communication among clinicians and researchers. The psychiatric community in the United States historically has used the *Diagnostic and Statistical Manual of Mental Disorders* (DSM) as the diagnostic guide and source of standardized nomenclature for both mental disorders and addictive disorders. The DSM (published by the American

Psychiatric Association) first appeared in 1952. The current edition is the fourth edition (DSM-IV) (APA, 1994).

Beginning in the 1950s, DSM-I and DSM-II evolved from clinical experience and psychodynamic concepts. Both editions viewed psychiatric disorders as resulting from a person's struggle to adjust to internal and external stresses or from impaired psychological development. Thus, alcoholism and drug dependence were categorized under personality disorders (persistent, maladaptive behaviors) and other nonpsychotic mental disorders. In these DSM editions, alcoholism was a unitary or homogeneous concept defined in global terms. It designated people whose alcohol intake impaired health, personal or social functioning, or was required for daily functioning. In fact, DSM-II arbitrarily divided alcoholism into three subcategories: (1) episodic excessive drinking, in which a subject becomes intoxicated four or more times a year; (2) habitual excessive drinking, when the subject becomes intoxicated more than twelve times a year or functions under the influence of alcohol more than once a year, and (3) alcohol addiction, characterized by physical withdrawal such as a seizure or the inability to go even one day without drinking. There were no data-based explanations of the criteria or the subtypes.

In 1972, Feighner described diagnostic criteria for use in psychiatric research. His focus was on fourteen psychiatric illnesses, including alcoholism. Criteria for developing diagnoses for research were proposed, implying that these criteria have a nosological place in treatment.

Feighner recommended that descriptive studies, laboratory evaluations and family studies should be carried out whenever possible to further identify and validate these criteria. Strong emphasis was placed on objective criteria such as severe medical consequences, repeated social problems, or an inability to control use (Feighner, 1972). Concurrently, the National Council on Alcohol (NCA) was developing new criteria for alcoholism. The NCA criteria emphasized psychological problems as well as the concepts of Alcoholics Anonymous; they also defined alcoholism in more clinically relevant terms.

In general, the substance abuse field identified problems with DSM-II because of its nonspecific terminology, its view of alcoholism as a personality impairment, and the perspective of alcoholism as a unitary phenomenon. All of these factors influenced the development of DSM-III, published in 1980 (APA, 1980). Here the alcohol and other drug use disorders comprised a separate section of the manual. Although medical conditions related to substance abuse, such as withdrawal, intoxication, and organic, depressive, psychotic, and anxiety states were included as "mental disorders," abuse and dependence were not. DSM-III also renamed alcoholism as *alcohol abuse and dependence*. Alcohol dependence was defined as pathological use of alcohol impairing the client's social or occupational functioning with evidence of physical tolerance or withdrawal syndromes when the drug was stopped. Alcohol abuse included a pattern of pathological use and impaired functioning without physical tolerance or withdrawal.

DSM-III recognized the heterogeneity of alcoholism by separating abuse from dependence. However, the data to support these changes were only briefly discussed and clinician complaints resulted in a revised version, DSM-III-R. The complaints centered on the illogical and inconsistent relationships between the criteria for substance abuse and dependence (i.e., the degree of overlap between the criteria for the two concepts). Second, there were complaints that inappropriate emphasis was placed on tolerance and withdrawal as criteria for dependence. Third, clinicians felt that some key concepts, particularly tolerance, were too simplistic. Both animal and human research had demonstrated the complexities of tolerance, a phenomenon that includes learned behaviors, changes in metabolism, and alterations in brain cell sensitivity to alcohol. Moreover, due to individual variability, it is theoretically possible for clients to meet DSM-III criteria for tolerance after only limited exposure to alcohol. Fourth, the view of alcoholism was seen as simplistic. It was felt that there was not enough attention to the coexisting features of the alcohol use disorders, especially dependence. Dependence involves a broad range of behaviors, rather than simply tolerance and physical withdrawal.

The development of DSM-IV was undertaken to incorporate new research findings. It was felt that a new review of previous data and field testing was critical. In fact, DSM-IV includes tolerance as central to the diagnosis of dependence. Other changes include more clearly defined and clarified diagnostic criteria and identification of areas in which further data is needed (Woody et al, 1993). The ongoing integration of new research findings and well-established clinical practices will define DSM substance disorders in the future.

Diagnostic instruments for clinical practice and research

Instruments have been developed to objectively determine psychiatric diagnoses. This has been part of a movement to standardize psychiatric diagnosis, particularly for research and outcome studies. Currently, most of the instruments discussed develop diagnoses according to DSM-III-R criteria. New editions to accommodate DSM-IV are likely.

Alcohol disorders are part of the psychiatric nomenclature. As such, assessment of alcohol and drug use are part of psychiatric diagnosis in general. Diagnostic interviews cover the full range of psychiatric disorders, including abuse and dependence on alcohol and other substances, as well as affective, anxiety, and psychotic disorders. All the interviews include a mechanism for distinguishing between psychiatric symptoms, syndromes with organic causes, syndromes with physiological factors that mimic psychiatric symptoms, and syndromes caused by nonorganic factors. Dual diagnosis (a substance abuse disorder and a coexisting primary psychological process) and the diagnostic conundrum that surrounds these disorders are discussed later in this chapter and in more detail in Chapter 12.

The format for a diagnostic interview can be structured, semistructured, or unstructured. In a structured interview, the interviewer reads the questions to the client and records the answers exactly. Interviewers with structured interviews do not explain or reword questions or explore responses with follow-up questions. Fully structured interviews are designed to be administered by nonclinical interviewers and allow little deviation from the interview schedule. In contrast, an unstructured interview provides the interviewer with a list of conditions to evaluate but does not provide an interview schedule. The interviewer determines the questions to ascertain the appropriate information. The interviewer must have clinical training to conduct a valid unstructured interview.

Semistructured interviews fall in between. In a semistructured interview, most of the areas to be covered are in an interview schedule and the interviewer is expected to use the introductory probes. The interviewer also is expected to use clinical skills to explore responses to ensure the validity of the information. Semistructured interviews require clinically trained interviewers.

To understand the significance and the utility of the interviews, two important concepts must be discussed: reliability and validity. Reliability is the consistency of the diagnosis among different interviewers or among interview sessions with the same interviewer. Validity of an interview measures whether or not the instrument is accurately measuring the condition it is designed to measure. Validity ordinarily is demonstrated by showing that the diagnosis made by an instrument corresponds in predictable ways to patterns of conditions, traits, or behaviors. Good validity requires good reliability, because an unreliable instrument will not consistently produce accurate results. However, good reliability does not guarantee good validity, because a reliable instrument might consistently measure the wrong condition, producing good reliability without accurate diagnosis of an illness.

Several interview schedules that have both good reliability and good validity are available. The most commonly used interview schedules are the Schedule for Affective Disorders and Schizophrenia (SADS), the Diagnostic Interview Schedule (DIS), and the Structured Clinical Interview for DSM-III-R (SCID).

Schedule for Affective Disorders and Schizophrenia (SADS).

The SADS is a semistructured diagnostic interview designed to be used by interviewers with clinical training (Endicott & Spitzer, 1978). SADS was designed to evaluate symptoms using the Research Diagnostic Criteria (RDC). The SADS has standard probes for evaluating symptoms, yet the interviewer also must use clinical skills to probe responses to determine if the symptoms are consistent with the diagnostic criteria. The full SADS interview is intended for psychiatric clients. It begins with an unstructured overview of the client's condition, followed by the first section, which contains detailed questions about the severity of the subject's *current condition*. The second section of the SADS covers the subject's *history* of mental disorders including possible alcoholism. The questions are clustered according to diagnosis. These two sections of the SADS provide criteria for both current and lifetime diagnoses. After all SADS items have been rated, the interviewer makes a diagnosis using the RDC diagnostic criteria. The alcohol section of the SADS begins with unstructured questions about drinking and screening questions for alcoholism. The screening questions are criteria for alcoholism, and they cover whether or not the subject ever had a period of drinking too much, whether or not anyone ever objected to the subject's drinking, and whether or not the subject ever was unable to stop drinking. A positive response to any of these questions requires administration of the remainder of the alcohol section. This includes 15 additional questions covering withdrawal symptoms, relief drinking, blackouts, legal problems, and social and occupational problems related to drinking.

If the subject responds positively to two of the questions and also reports a period of heavy drinking that lasted at least one month, a *probable* lifetime diagnosis of alcoholism is made. If three or more responses are positive, a *definite* lifetime diagnosis is made. For example, a subject who drank heavily for several months, who thought he was drinking too much and received such feedback from others, but who had no other alcohol problems would receive a *probable* diagnosis.

Diagnostic Interview Schedule (DIS).   The DIS is a fully structured diagnostic interview designed to be administered by nonclinicians (Robins et al, 1981). The DIS was originally developed to assess lifetime diagnosis, using DSM-III-R criteria, in a large-scale epidemiological study, although it is used in clinical research as well. When administering the DIS, the interviewer reads questions exactly from the interview schedule. Exploration of the responses is neither required nor allowed. If a subject does not understand a question, the question may be repeated; however, the interviewer is discouraged from rewording the question. Like the SADS, different DIS sections cover different diagnoses. Many sections have screening questions which allow skipping if there is no evidence of disorder.

The alcohol section of the DIS begins with a few questions about alcohol consumption and drunkenness followed by a series of questions covering alcohol abuse. If responses about abuse indicate that the subject might meet criteria for alcohol dependence, additional questions are asked. All questions have a lifetime framework. No attempt is made to determine whether the symptoms cluster in time as in the SADS. Diagnosis of alcohol dependence or abuse using the DIS can result from positive responses to only two questions. DIS diagnoses can be generated using computer programs that follow the logic of the diagnostic criteria. The programs are straightforward and comprehensible to users.

Structured Clinical Interview for DSM-III-R (SCID).   The SCID is a semistructured interview designed for use by clinical interviewers (Spitzer et al, in press). The SCID was originally intended for use with DSM-III criteria, but it has been revised to DSM-III-R criteria (APA, 1987). The SCID is currently undergoing revision to make it consistent with DSM-IV.

The developers of the SCID wanted a diagnostic instrument with shorter time for administration than the SADS, one that would provide a diagnosis during the interview and would require simple training. SCID interviewers should be experienced clinicians because interviewers must ask follow-up questions to determine whether the client's symptoms actually meet the diagnostic criteria. The SCID includes directions on making DSM-III-R diagnoses during the interview. At the end of the section pertaining to each disorder, the interviewer develops a severity score based on the level of symptomatology and impairment of function.

The alcohol section of the SCID begins with an unstructured probe about drinking habits, inquiring whether the subject ever felt that his or her drinking was excessive or problematic and whether other people ever objected to the drinking. If no suggestion of alcohol problems emerges at this point, the alcoholic diagnostic is skipped.

Before proceeding with the alcohol section of the SCID, the interviewer determines the period when the subject experienced the most problematic or the heaviest drinking and orients the remaining questions to that time. Subsequent questions cover the DSM-III-R criteria, which are based on the ADS symptoms (APA 1987, p.

22). Clinical judgment determines if the experiences occurred at the diagnostic level. If the subject fails to meet criteria for dependence, then alcohol abuse may be indicated. A diagnosis of abuse or dependence is clarified as current or past based on whether the criteria were met in the month before the interview or earlier.

DUAL DIAGNOSIS

In some cases, assessment and diagnosis uncover two primary diagnoses, that is, two diagnoses of equal significance. The concurrence of substance abuse with psychiatric illness, referred to as *dual diagnosis,* is quite high. The difficulty of making an accurate psychiatric diagnosis in the face of ongoing alcohol or drug use cannot be overemphasized. It is important to keep in mind that true dual diagnosis clients have poorer prognoses, poorer compliance with medications, and much more troubled therapeutic drug treatment than clients with only substance abuse problems. Chapter 12 describes care of the client with a dual diagnosis.

RELATIONSHIP BETWEEN NURSING AND MEDICAL MODELS

The differences between the nursing and medical models have only recently been described because the nursing profession has only recently established a separate classification system as a basis for nursing practice. Clear distinctions between the two models do exist. For example, a medical diagnosis generalizes symptoms to a diagnostic category whereas a nursing diagnosis specifies the individual dimensions of a problem. Another comparison is that "the medical diagnosis describes the client's disease and a nursing diagnosis describes the client's current health responses" (Stuart & Sundeen, 1995). "The goal of a nursing diagnosis is to identify actual and potential client responses, whereas the goals of a medical diagnosis are to identify and design a treatment plan for curing the disease or the pathological process" (Potter & Perry, 1993, p. 128). These definitions all concentrate on the differing perspectives between nursing and medicine that are at the core of the different systems.

While a client usually has only one primary medical diagnosis, numerous nursing diagnoses are possible for the same client. Nursing diagnoses are similar to problem lists in problem-oriented medical records (POMR), only they are standardized. Box 3-2 shows the nursing and medical diagnoses of a particular client and exemplifies the differences between them.

The nursing and medical diagnostic models together describe the categorical and the individual needs of a client. Both are used to thoroughly identify the health care needs of the client and guide treatment interventions. Both are required in the accreditation of hospitals by the Joint Commission on Accreditation of Health Care Organizations.

SUMMARY

Substance abuse assessment includes screening individuals in a general setting, more comprehensive assessments when indications of possible problems exist, and

Box 3-2
DSM-IV and NANDA Diagnoses Related to Substance Abuse

DSM-IV*

Alcohol abuse
Alcohol dependence
Alcohol intoxication
Alcohol withdrawal
Amphetamine (or related substance) dependence
Amphetamine (or related substance) abuse
Amphetamine (or related substance) intoxication
Amphetamine (or related substance) withdrawal
Cannabis dependence
Cannabis abuse
Cannabis intoxication
Cocaine dependence
Cocaine abuse
Cocaine intoxication
Cocaine withdrawal
Hallucinogen dependence
Hallucinogen abuse
Hallucinogen intoxication
Posthallucinogen perception disorder
Inhalant dependence
Inhalant abuse
Inhalant intoxication
Nicotine dependence
Nicotine withdrawal
Opioid dependence
Opioid abuse
Opioid intoxication
Opioid withdrawal
Phencyclidine (or related substance) dependence
Phencyclidine (or related substance) abuse
Phencyclidine (or related substance) intoxication
Sedative, hypnotic, or anxiolytic dependence
Sedative, hypnotic, or anxiolytic abuse
Sedative, hypnotic, or anxiolytic intoxication
Sedative, hypnotic, or anxiolytic withdrawal
Polysubstance dependence
Other (or unknown) substance dependence
Other (or unknown) substance abuse
Other (or unknown) substance intoxication
Other (or unknown) substance withdrawal

NANDA†

Anxiety
Communication, impaired verbal
Coping, ineffective individual
Family processes, altered
Fear
Growth and development, altered
Grieving, dysfunctional
Hopelessness
Infection, potential for
Injury, potential for
Knowledge deficit
Noncompliance
Nutrition, altered
Pain
Parenting, altered
Powerlessness
Self-care deficit
Self-esteem disturbance
Sensory-perceptual alteration
Sexual dysfunction
Sleep pattern disturbance
Social isolation
Spiritual distress
Thought processes, altered
Violence, potential for

*From American Psychiatric Association. (1994). *Diagnostic and statistical manual of mental disorders.* (4th ed.). Washington, D.C.: The Association.
†From North American Nursing Diagnosis Association. (1992). *NANDA nursing diagnoses: Definitions and classifications 1992-1993.* Philadelphia: NANDA.

complete clinical assessments for individuals in substance abuse treatment. A number of instruments can be used for initial screening (e.g., CAGE, MAST, AUDIT) as well as for more comprehensive diagnoses (e.g., MacAndrew, DIS, ASI). Blood tests are used to determine biochemical markers that indicate physiological sequelae of substance use. Nursing assessment and diagnoses are directed toward the amelioration of health problems related to substance abuse and dependency. Medical assessment and diagnosis are used to determine a substance abuse or dependency diagnosis consistent with the criteria specified by the *Diagnostic and Statistical Manual of Mental Disorders* of the American Psychiatric Association. The nursing and medical models are complementary, and both are needed to develop comprehensive treatment plans.

REFERENCES

Allen, J.P., Eckartdt, M.J., & Wallen, J. (1988). Screening for alcoholism: Techniques and issues. *Public Health Reports, 103,* 586.

American Nurses Association. (1991). *Standards of clinical nursing practice.* Kansas City, MO: The Association.

American Nurses Association, Drug and Alcohol Nurses Association, & National Nurses Society on Addictions. (1987). *The care of clients with addictions: Dimensions of nursing practice.* Kansas City, MO: ANA.

American Nurses Association & National Nurses Society on Addictions (1988). *Standards of addictions nursing practice.* Kansas City, MO: ANA.

American Psychiatric Association. (1994). *Diagnostic and statistical manual of mental disorders.* (4th ed.). Washington, D.C.: The Association.

American Psychiatric Association. (1987). *Diagnostic and statistical manual of mental disorders.* (3rd ed. rev.). Washington, D.C.: The Association.

American Psychiatric Association. (1980). *Diagnostic and statistical manual of mental disorders.* (3rd ed.). Washington, D.C.: The Association.

American Society of Addiction Medicine. (1990). Disease definition of alcoholism revised. *Addiction Review, 2,* 3.

Babor, T.F., de la Fluente, J.R., Saunders, J., & Grant, M. (1989). *AUDIT: The Alcohol Use Disorders Identification Test: guidelines for use in primary health care.* Geneva: World Health Organization.

Blume, S., Cloud, S.A., & Liever, C.S. (1976). The definition of alcoholism. *Annals of Internal Medicine, 85,* 764.

Criteria Committee of the National Council on Alcoholism. (1972). Criteria for the diagnosis of alcoholism. *American Journal of Psychiatry, 129,* 127.

Edwards, G. & Gross, M. (1976). Alcohol dependence: Provisional description of a clinical syndrome. *British Medical Journal, 1,* 1058.

Endicott, J. & Spitzer, R.L. (1978). A diagnostic interview: The schedule for affective disorders and schizophrenia. *Archives of General Psychiatry, 43,* 13.

Ewing, J.A. (1984). Detecting alcoholism, the CAGE questionnaire. *Journal of the American Medical Association, 252,* 1905.

Feighner, J.P. (1972). Diagnostic criteria for use in psychiatric research. *Archives of General Psychiatry, 26*(1), 57.

Fleming, M.F. & Barry, K.L. (1992). *Addictive Disorders.* St. Louis: Mosby.

Hedlund, J.L. & Viewig, B.W. (1984). The Michigan Alcoholism Screening Test: A comprehensive review. *Journal of Operational Psychology, 15,* 55.

Jellinek, E.M. (1960). *The disease concept of alcoholism.* New Haven, CT: College and University Press.

Lisanti, P. (1991). Assessment of the adult client for drug and alcohol use. In M. Naegle (Ed.), *Substance Abuse Education in Nursing.* New York: National League for Nursing.

Little, D. & Carnevelli, D. (1976). *Nursing care planning.* Philadelphia: Lippincott.

Lumeng, L. (1986). New diagnostic markers of alcohol abuse. *Hepatology, 6*(4), 742.

MacAndrew, C. (1965). The differentiation of male alcoholic outpatients from nonalcoholic psychiatric outpatients by means of the MMPI. *Journal of Studies on Alcohol, 37,* 1215.

McLellan, A.T., Luborsky, L., Woody, G.E., & O'Brien, C.P. (1980). An improved diagnostic evaluation instrument for substance abuse patients: The Addiction Severity Index. *Journal of Nervous and Mental Diseases, 168,* 26.

National Institute on Alcohol Abuse and Alcoholism. (1987). *Screening for alcoholism in primary care settings.* Rockville, MD: USDHHS.

National Nurses Society on Addictions. (1990). *Core curriculum of addictions nursing.* Skokie, IL: The Society.

North American Nursing Diagnosis Association. (1992). *NANDA nursing diagnoses: Definitions and classifications, 1992-1993.* Philadelphia: The Association.

O'Farrell, T.J. & Maisto, S.A. (1987). The utility of self-report and biological measures of alcohol consumption in alcoholism treatment outcome studies. *Advanced Behavioral Research Therapy, 9,* 91.

Pokorny, A.D., Miller, B.A., & Kaplan, H.G. (1972). The brief MAST: A shortened version of the Michigan Alcoholism Screening Test. *American Journal of Psychiatry, 129,* 342.

Potter, P.A. & Perry, A.G. (1993). *Fundamentals of Nursing.* (3rd ed.). St. Louis: Mosby.

Preng, K.W. & Clopton, J.R. (1986). The MacAndrew Scale: Clinical application and theoretical issues. *Quarterly Journal of Studies on Alcohol, 47,* 228.

Robins, L.N., Helzer, J.E., Croughan, J., & Ratcliff, K.S. (1981). National Institute of Mental Health Diagnostic Interview Schedule: Its history, characteristics, and validity. *Archives of General Psychiatry, 38,* 381.

Sanchez-Craig, M. (1990). Brief didactic treatment for alcohol and drug-related problems: An approach based on client choice. *British Journal of Addictions, 85,* 169.

Seltzer, M.L. (1971). The Michigan Alcohol Screening Test: The quest for a new diagnostic instrument. *American Journal of Psychiatry, 127,* 1653.

Seltzer, M.L., Vinokur, A., & van Rooijen, L.A. (1975). A self-administered short Michigan Alcoholism Screening Test. *Journal of Studies on Alcohol, 36,* 117.

Skinner, H.A. (1982). The drug abuse screening test. *Addictive Behaviors, 7,* 363.

Spitzer, R.L., Williams, J.B.W., Gibbon, M., & First, M. (in press). The structured clinical interview for DSM-III-R. *Archives of General Psychiatry.*

Stuart, G.W. & Sundeen, S.J. (1995). *Principles and practice of psychiatric nursing.* (5th ed.). St. Louis: Mosby.

Swenson, W.M. & Morse, R.M. (1975). The use of self-administered screening test (SAAST) in a medical center. *Mayo Clinic Proceedings, 50,* 204.

Woodruff, R.A., Clayton, P.J., Cloninger, C.R., & Guze, S.B. (1976). A brief method of screening for alcoholism. *Diseases of the Nervous System, 37,* 434-435.

Woody, G., Schuckit, M., Weinrieb, R., & Yu, E. (1993). A review of the substance use disorders section of the DSM-IV. *Psychiatric Clinics of North America, 16,* 21.

4 Treatment for Substance Abuse

Treatment of substance use disorders can be effective, and individuals with these problems can return to being productive, contributing members of society. This chapter presents various approaches and "tools" of substance abuse treatment, including "twelve-step" programs such as Alcoholics Anonymous, individual and family psychotherapy, cognitive-behavioral therapy, contingency contracting, and medication. Combinations of different treatment approaches are determined by the needs of individuals. Individuals vary in the severity and consequences of their substance abuse problems; therefore, treatment approaches should be matched to each person's needs, problems, and assets.

Nurses must learn different approaches to substance abuse treatment. They must develop abilities in assessing, detoxifying, making appropriate referrals for, and monitoring recovery in clients. Before describing specific treatment programs and services, this chapter briefly reviews the history of substance abuse treatment and important perspectives of addictive disorders. Being knowledgeable about different treatment approaches will help nurses improve communication with a wide variety of substance abuse treatment providers.

SUBSTANCE ABUSE TREATMENT

The character of substance abuse treatment programs continues to evolve (Musto, 1992). There are many different approaches to treating individuals with addictive disorders, which include the "twelve-steps," psychiatric, medical, social, and behavioral perspectives. Each of these approaches has a particular historical bias and vocabulary. The modern addictions specialist has become fluent in all different approaches and uses eclectically the strengths of each approach. Future treatment-outcome studies will be able to determine which treatment approaches will be effective for specific problems. Although the nature of addictions has remained the same, the complexity has increased. More clients are younger and poorer, are poly-drug addicted, or have concurrent psychiatric illnesses.

Many factors have influenced the evolution of treatment programs, including social, economic, and legal issues and increased understanding of addiction treatment. During the last 15 years there has been an explosion of scientific information on the nature and treatment of addictive disorders. New research has focused on evaluating existing treatment approaches and developing new approaches. Important advances have been made using biological, psychological, social, and spiritual perspectives. In the past thirty years, research related to addictions has pioneered new technology and interest in the central nervous system. Increased understanding of neurotransmitters and receptor sites for opiates, alcohol, benzodiazepines, and other substances has resulted in the discovery and testing of new treatment approaches. In recent years, treatment-outcome studies have attempted to determine the most effective ingredients of treatment.

In 1935, Alcoholics Anonymous started the twelve-step movement, which has become an international organization with more than 1.5 million members and 73,000 groups (Alcoholics Anonymous World Services, Inc., 1987). Today there are literally hundreds of self-help programs based on this model. Widespread availability of treatment programs first appeared during the 1960s.

In the past 40 years, the most influential substance abuse treatment approach has been the Minnesota model. This approach emphasizes chemical dependency as the primary problem and other diagnoses and problems as secondary. The goal of treatment is total abstinence. Education has an important role in the recovery process. The Minnesota model is closely linked to and supportive of the twelve-step approach. The Minnesota model originated in inpatient programs that treated individuals for 28 days. In recent years, however, third-party payers are more reluctant to reimburse for inpatient care. Treatment programs have responded by adapting the Minnesota model to other less-intensive levels of care. An important part of aftercare has always been the community twelve-step programs.

TREATMENT PHILOSOPHIES

Substance abuse treatment professionals are beginning to understand and appreciate the range of treatment approaches in the addiction field. No one philosophy fully or adequately explains the range of addiction problems, and no one philosophy suggests the correct treatment approach. While some professionals may be fundamentally supportive of one particular approach, most approaches to treatment can be integrated in a comprehensive treatment program, adding unique pieces to the addiction puzzle.

Disease concept

The *disease concept* links many of the different treatment approaches, including twelve-step, medical, and current psychiatric models. This perspective considers substance abuse disorders diseases. Benjamin Rush, a physician and signer of the Declaration of Independence, described "drunkenness" as a disease. He listed the acute and chronic manifestations of the disease and observed both hereditary and nongenetic influences. Historically, the disease-concept explanation of alcoholism contrasts with the *moral defect concept*. (The assumption of this belief is that substance abuse is a moral weakness which can be overcome by willpower [Marlatt et al, 1988].) A proponent of the disease concept, E.M. Jellinek (1960), defined five subtypes of alcoholics (alpha, beta, gamma, delta, and epsilon) based on factors including possible etiology, severity of alcohol-related problems, and damage to self and situation (see Chapter 2). Subtypes of alcoholics and substance abusers have been proposed. Cloninger and Begluter (1990) defined two types of alcoholics based on family history, temperament, and age of onset of the disorder. Individuals with substance abuse problems are heterogeneous, so subtyping substance abusers may have important implications for treatment.

Twelve step program

The *twelve step program* is a self-help approach to treating addictions and has roots in medicine, religion, and psychoanalysis. The approach was begun as Alcoholics Anonymous (AA) in 1935 by two men who struggled with their own alcoholism and had not benefited from known treatments. The twelve step approach has proven to be one of the most effective methods for maintaining long-term abstinence and sobriety (Vaillant, 1983; Chappel, 1992). The twelve step program is outlined in *Alcoholics Anonymous,* (1976) known as the "Big Book," and is designed to help people with alcoholism become abstinent and then grow and develop. With the success and growth of AA, many other twelve step programs emerged to help individuals with other addictions (e.g., Cocaine Anonymous, Narcotics Anonymous, and Overeaters Anonymous). In addition, twelve step programs also have been established for family and friends of substance abusers (e.g., Al-Anon, Cocanon, and Narcanon). The specific aspects of the twelve step program are described later.

Minnesota model

The development and growth of twelve step programs were linked to professional treatment through the *Minnesota model.* This model was developed in 1948 at Pioneer House in Minnesota and quickly replicated at the Hazelden program in 1949 (Anderson, 1981). For many years, the Minnesota model of care was the leading model of treatment, and it continues to provide an important framework for program development.

Medical model

The *medical model* framework considers addictions from a public health, chronic disease, and acute infectious disease perspective. From this perspective, diseases are conducted to a host by a vector. The goal of treatment is to intervene somewhere in the chain of events. When diseases are medicalized, they become part of the domain of the health-care system. The *biopsychosocial* perspective is one medical model which proposes that etiologies are best understood by the interaction of biological, psychological, and sociocultural risk factors (Lewis, 1991).

Neuroscience model

Since the 1960s there has been an explosion of new knowledge about the brain. Much has been learned about how the brain operates by studying drugs such as LSD and opiates. The *neuroscience model* focuses on biological, genetic, and neurochemical risk factors. Modern understanding of neurotransmitters and receptors in the brain has led neuroscientists to pursue the development of medications to treat addictions.

Psychiatric model

The *psychiatric model* of addictions is represented by the American Psychiatric Association *Diagnostic and Statistical Manual of Mental Disorders (DSM)*, first published in 1952 as detailed in Chapter 3. In 1952, addictive problems were viewed as an expression of underlying psychopathology or neurotic conflict, and addictions were classified as part of the sociopathic personality syndrome. This philosophy was in direct contradiction to the disease-concept proponents, who believed addiction was the primary disease. This theoretical conflict was resolved in 1980, when addictions were classified as diseases. Psychiatrists and other mental health specialists have played an important role in understanding drug abusers with concurrent psychiatric disorders or dual diagnosis. Some clients have two disorders; for example, an alcoholic with bipolar affective disorder requires both substance abuse treatment and treatment with lithium. Some clients will be told by peers at twelve step meetings to avoid all medications and, unfortunately, some will stop their lithium. This phenomenon is decreasing because both non–mental health addictions specialists and twelve step participants are being better educated about dual diagnosis. The evolution of psychiatry and substance abuse counseling is an example of how both ideologies can benefit from mutual respect and openness to different perspectives. This process should continue to improve the treatment of addictive disorders.

Cognitive behavioral approach

The *cognitive-behavioral approach* starts with the premise that maladaptive behavior is learned and is based on a set of faulty thoughts (cognitions). Individuals can be taught to change their faulty thinking and correct dysfunctional behaviors. Cognitive and behavioral therapists explain addictions as being "caused by a composite of innate, biological, developmental, and environmental factors interacting with each other" (Beck, 1989, p. 1542). The goal of cognitive therapy is to assist individuals to identify "automatic thoughts" and learn cognitive restructuring. Learning to change their thoughts will lead to a change in behaviors and feelings. *Relapse-prevention training* developed from this theoretical base and is a useful tool in treatment. Relapse-prevention training is described later in this chapter.

Social learning theory

The *social learning theory* explains addictions as deficits in general coping skills that make an individual vulnerable to the use of alcohol or other drugs as an artificial method to modulate everyday functioning. The cause of poor coping skills is the interaction of biological factors and psychosocial determinants (Abrams & Niaura, 1987). Substance abuse treatment includes social-skills training and coping-skills development.

Sociocultural perspective

The *sociocultural perspective* suggests that substance abuse disorders can be treated by changing the social environment and/or developing new learned responses to the current social environment. The belief of the proponents of this perspective is that people can heal themselves with reassurance, reality testing, and the support of other recovering alcoholics or addicts. In the 1960s the Synanon organization was a leading example of this approach, with long-term (approximately one year or longer) inpatient programs. Residents were confronted by peers and recovering addict-counselors concerning changing their attitudes and behaviors. Residents were expected to change in recovery by increasing their responsibilities in the residential program, developing job skills, and finding independent living. These programs were criticized for the harshness of their confrontation and demands. During the past 30 years, however, proponents of this philosophy have modified their approach and incorporated other treatment strategies, including the addition of professional services (O'Brien & Biase, 1992).

Various approaches to treatment have developed and evolved over the past 50 years. There is significant overlap in perspectives, but philosophical differences still exist. Specialists must be familiar with different approaches and understand the specific vocabulary and skills required to use each approach. Addiction is a heterogeneous disorder that requires individualized treatment plans. While fundamental philosophical differences clearly drive different treatment programs, an important goal is the integration of the different approaches in the care of individual patients.

ASSESSMENT AND INTERVENTION

Chapter 3 explains the assessment and diagnosis of persons who may be in need of substance abuse treatment. There is no typical person with a substance use disorder. People vary in their motivation and readiness for treatment. In addition, they vary according to age, sex, socioeconomic status, substance abuse problem severity and duration, type of substance abused, need for detoxification, history of previous treatment efforts, goals and expectations, social skills and supports, legal problems, and medical condition. A careful and thorough evaluation marks the beginning of the treatment process. Establishing and presenting a diagnosis is the first step in treatment. The likelihood of a person's seeking referral to treatment is determined by his or her readiness for change, external forces brought to bear (e.g., threat of job loss), and the primary clinician's skills.

Many persons are initially resistant to admitting they have a problem which requires professional treatment. Treatment is most likely to be effective when a person with substance abuse admits a problem and is willing to make changes in behavior.

Denial is a paramount symptom and the classic defense mechanism seen in addiction. The client denies the problem to everyone, as well as himself. Often individuals with addictive disorders view their problems as moral weaknesses or defects in character. This explanation of the problem affects the individual's self-esteem and can lead to profound shame and guilt. Denial interferes with a client's acceptance of a diagnosis and active participation in treatment. The experienced clinician assesses the client's readiness for acceptance and change and adapts the treatment approach accordingly.

As with any disorder, a caring and empathic approach to individuals who suffer with a substance use disorder is critical. Nurses, like all other clinicians, are influenced by the attitudes of the general society and must carefully consider their attitudes toward clients with alcohol and drug abuse to improve interactions with them. Healthy and helpful attitudes can be developed by learning more about substance abuse and effective treatment approaches (Boxes 4-1 and 4-2). Chemically dependent clients often anticipate a negative attitude when they enter treatment and are pleasantly surprised and relieved when treatment staff members approach them with kindness and respect.

After assessment is completed and an initial diagnosis determined, a referral can be made to the appropriate type of treatment setting and services. The treatment plan and options should be presented to the patient for approval. If the client is extremely resistant to entering treatment, the nurse or other staff person might suggest some initial steps at further assessment or attendance at some twelve-step meetings on a trial basis.

TREATMENT PLANNING AND REEVALUATION

The treatment planning process for addictive disorders parallels the development of nursing care plans for other disorders. Perhaps the major difference in treatment

---

Box 4-1
Helpful Attitudes and Understandings in Treating Alcoholics

1. Recognize that alcoholism is a chronic, relapsing illness.
2. Recognize that alcoholism is a treatable disease.
3. Realize that alcoholism has definite signs and stages of progression.
4. Understand that treatment of alcoholism is often successful.
5. Know that help is readily available in most communities.
6. Understand that alcoholism could happen to anyone.
7. Understand that a recognition of the alcoholic's self-loathing, isolation, depression, and guilt feelings while he is drinking is essential to a successful treatment.
8. Recognize that AA, Al-Anon, and Alateen can be effective self-help groups in treating alcoholism.
9. Realize that standard psychiatric treatment methods are generally ineffective in treating alcoholism per se; they can be used by the alcoholic, in fact, to avoid dealing with the alcoholism.
10. Recognize that the alcoholic's spouse cannot cause the problem, although the spouse may aggravate it.
11. Recognize that members of the alcoholic's family need treatment as much as the alcoholic.
12. Acknowledge that—for all practical purposes—an alcoholic cannot return to normal controlled drinking.
13. Understand that to the alcoholic, following through on a referral presents an extreme life crisis: a decision to not drink. For the alcoholic, this is akin to the heroin addict's giving up heroin. In the alcoholic's view, alcohol is the only means of survival.
14. Understand that a recovery process is a frightening, difficult, lifelong task. It requires a complete reordering of social aspects of the alcoholic's life; to accomplish this, the individual will need lifelong support.

From Norris, J.L. (1978). Prevention of chronicity. *Psychiatric Annals, 8*(11), 48-53.

Box 4-2
Unhelpful Attitudes in Treating Alcoholics

1. Alcoholism is a self-inflicted illness.
2. Alcoholism is hopeless.
3. Recovering from alcoholism is simply a matter of will power.
4. Drinking in any amount is dangerous and can lead to alcoholism.
5. Let the poor, sick, unemployed, lonely, or old people with alcoholism continue to drink. They are better off that way.
6. Abstinence for an alcoholic is a primitive expectation. No one can live that way.
7. It is so hard for an alcoholic to abstain, one should merely expect the alcoholic to limit the amount.
8. Alcoholics are simply people who will not accept life's responsibilities as most people must do.

From Norris, J.L. (1978). Prevention of chronicity. *Psychiatric Annals, 8*(11), 48-53.

planning for chemical dependency is the variety of disciplines potentially involved in the care. The clinical team working with a client should review all the pertinent data and develop a plan to address and establish priority for the identified problems.

Two examples of initial treatment plans for the same client with alcohol abuse are described. In the first example, the treatment plan indicates a standard protocol with no individualized elements.

EXAMPLE 1
Problem 1   Alcohol Dependence
  Short-term goal
  • The client will detoxify safely in an outpatient setting within two weeks, as evidenced by continued compliance with facility protocol and by negative blood alcohol level
  Long-term goals
  • Client will enter rehabilitation treatment within 2 weeks
  • Client will follow up with aftercare after completion of rehabilitation treatment
  Interventions
  • Medication as ordered
  • Education
  • Referral

In Example 2, a plan has been developed to address the patient's specific problems (e.g., lack of commitment to treatment).

EXAMPLE 2
Problem 1   Alcohol Dependence
Problem 2   Noncommitment to Treatment
  Short-term goals
  • Client will state personal goals for treatment within 1 week
  • Client will engage in treatment within one week as evidenced by attending groups without prompting and actively participating in group sessions

Long-term goals
- Client will state personal problems that inhibit sobriety by the time of discharge
- Client will state personal treatment options by the time of discharge
- Client will enter continuing treatment for ongoing problems within 1 week after discharge from alcohol treatment program

Interventions
- Help patient identify why he sought assessment and treatment
- Help patient clarify whether or not the problems are still present and visualize present and future reality should he decline treatment now
- Assist patient in feeling empowered to make his own decision, while conveying respect for his choice
- Be certain patient understands the likely scenario following treatment or dropping out of treatment

The second example is a comprehensive treatment plan focused on the patient's specific problems, providing more details. Both the primary clinician and other team members now have a clearer sense of how to address the problem of alcohol dependence for the patient. To ensure active participation, the client should be involved in the process of creating the plan.

This treatment-planning process is dynamic and should be reevaluated regularly to reflect the client's progress and be adjusted as necessary (e.g., during acute detoxification the plan might be adjusted daily; but after 6 months of stable progress, the plan might need changing only every few months). Treatment planning is important and time-consuming work that provides the primary clinician and the team with a special tool to guide the therapeutic process.

THE ROLE OF THE CLIENT

The role of clients in substance abuse treatment differs from the role nurses commonly expect from their patients. The nurse usually provides care *to* the client. In substance abuse treatment, clients are expected to assume more responsibility for care. Instead of receiving medications at their bedsides, for example, clients in treatment are expected to go to the nurses' station at the time medications are needed. In other words, clients are expected to recognize their needs and to follow through with actions necessary for their care.

STAGES OF CHANGE

Clients entering treatment should be assessed for their stage of readiness for change, their motivation for change, and for the appropriate level of treatment needed. Individuals who need substance abuse treatment cover a spectrum of desire and motivation for treatment. During an initial evaluation, a clinician should investigate a person's motivation to seek treatment by asking, "Why are you coming for treatment now?" Examples of reasons given by clients include a spouse's or family members' encouragement, employment pressure, or legal problems. External pressures, such as the threat of divorce, disciplinary action at work, or legal problems, are common reasons. One short-term goal of treatment is for clients' motivation for treatment to be for themselves and not for others. Some individuals screened for substance abuse problems may be in complete denial of their problems and resistant to treatment.

One treatment model describes five stages of readiness for changing addictive behaviors (Prochaska et al, 1992): *precontemplation, contemplation, preparation, action,* and *maintenance.* In the *precontemplation* stage the individual is in complete denial of an addiction problem. Individuals in the *contemplation* stage admit that they would like to change their behavior but they do not make any attempts to make changes. During the *preparation* stage, individuals begin to make feeble attempts at change which are unsuccessful. In the *action* stage, individuals make overt behavioral changes. This stage often is seen as change itself without respect for the other stages. *Maintenance* is dedicated to the continuation of change through relapse prevention. Each one of these stages represents a level of motivation and activity in making changes in past behaviors. A continuous goal of treatment is to advance an individual to the next level of change. Clinicians improve treatment effectiveness by using specific approaches for each different stage of change.

Progression through these stages is not usually a linear process. Most individuals have relapses to substance use and regress to an earlier stage of change. The efforts of individuals who do well in recovery ought to be recognized and appreciated by addiction treatment providers. Major life improvements can occur. Unfortunately, many clinicians who work with clients who have little or no motivation do not see the later stages of progression. For example, emergency room staff often encounter intoxicated clients who are irrational and poorly motivated for treatment.

Substance abuse treatment and recovery is a process and not an event. Repeated efforts and setbacks are the natural course of the disorder. Substance abuse is a chronic, progressive, and often fatal disease; and functional periods alternate with exacerbation of the illness. Treatment plans need to be adjusted over time to match changes in the individual.

CONTINUITY OF CARE

Substance abuse treatment takes place along a continuum of different intensity levels of care and services. Clients should be assessed for the appropriate level of care required, including outpatient treatment, partial hospitalization, inpatient treatment, and residential care. In order to determine the appropriate level of care, the clinician must consider the severity of the substance abuse problem, other related problems, need for inpatient detoxification, level of motivation, previous treatment efforts, and available social supports.

Several models for matching severity of illness with characteristics of treatment have been created to help clinicians determine the appropriate level of care. Two examples include the Cleveland Criteria and the American Society of Addiction Medicine (ASAM) criteria. These models can be used in deciding if a client is being treated in the most appropriate treatment setting.

The Cleveland Criteria was first published in 1987 and defined six levels of care determined by assessment of functioning in each individual's life. The ASAM criteria refined the Cleveland Criteria to the following four levels:

Level 1   Outpatient treatment
Level 2   Intensive outpatient–partial hospitalization treatment
Level 3   Medically monitored intensive inpatient treatment
Level 4   Medically managed intensive inpatient treatment

For each level of care there are three aspects to be considered. These are (1) an overview of the intensity and frequency of services available; (2) a description of the settings, staff, and services expected at that level; and (3) a description of the criteria for admission, continued stay, and discharge (Hoffman et al, 1991).

Determination of treatment levels is made by evaluating six dimensions, which are:

1. Acute intoxication and/or withdrawal potential
2. Biomedical conditions and complications
3. Emotional/behavioral conditions or complications
   a. Psychiatric conditions
   b. Psychological or emotional/behavioral complications of known or unknown origin (e.g., poor impulse control, changes in mental status)
   c. Transient neuropsychiatric complications
4. Treatment acceptance/resistance
5. Relapse potential
6. Recovery environment

The Cleveland and ASAM criteria also help to standardize treatment approaches in the addictions field. Each patient's treatment plan is developed to meet the individual client's needs and includes the appropriate level of care. The following examples illustrate application of these criteria:

Ⅲ➤ Clinical Example

John is a 36-year-old divorced male who is currently estranged from his family. He has gastritis and, despite many efforts, has been unable to stop drinking a pint of vodka daily. Although John still has a job, he has received several warnings about his absenteeism. John knows he should stop drinking but has ambivalence about wanting to stop. His network of friends includes other heavy drinkers at the local bar. He lives alone and has no sober support system.

Clinical discussion: Using the ASAM criteria to determine the level of care needed, clinicians ascertain that inpatient treatment is appropriate for John. Reasons include the need for a close observation of detoxification, given his history of heavy drinking and medical problems; the lack of a sober support system (poor recovery environment); and his limited motivation for treatment.

Ⅲ➤ Clinical Example

Janet is a 30-year-old married mother of two small children. She drinks mostly on weekends. She has embarrassed herself and her husband on numerous occasions after drinking more than she planned and becoming intoxicated. This pattern is causing marital strife, and Janet is unable to carry out her responsibilities on weekends. Neither Janet nor her husband recognizes the problem as alcohol dependence, but they are willing to seek professional help.

Clinical discussion: In contrast to the previous case, Janet can be appropriately treated in outpatient care because she has a history of mild withdrawal, has no other medical or psychiatric complications, and her family is somewhat supportive and willing to participate in treatment. Both of these clients need treatment for alcohol dependence, but the intensity of the treatment will vary.

During treatment, clients are reassessed for the appropriate level of care. Clients can move to a less-intensive level of care; however, some clients require a higher intensity of treatment. Sometimes the decision of care level is determined by pragmatic, nonclinical conditions such as amount of insurance coverage or available openings in treatment programs.

TREATMENT SETTINGS

There are advantages and disadvantages in the various treatment settings along the continuum of care. In each setting there can be a variety of services available. Individual clinicians have a choice of "tools" to use in providing services.

There is no typical flow as a client moves from one level of care to another. The flow is determined by many factors, including severity of the problem, social supports, type of health care insurance, availability of different levels of treatment, and availability of treatment slots. Some patients initially will be treated in an inpatient unit and then transferred to a lower level of care (e.g., partial hospitalization, standard outpatient care, or community twelve step programs). Some patients will be seen at first in an outpatient setting and later will require a higher level of care such as partial hospitalization, inpatient treatment, a halfway house, or residential treatment.

Inpatient settings

Inpatient programs vary according to philosophical emphasis, available services, and setting (hospital-based or freestanding). Advantages and disadvantages for use of an inpatient setting are shown in Box 4-3.

Some treatment programs are located in psychiatric units, some are independent substance abuse units within a hospital, and others are separate hospitals devoted only to substance abuse care. In spite of these differences, most offer similar services. Patients requiring inpatient detoxification are usually treated for 2 to 5 days in an inpatient setting. Patients in a substance abuse rehabilitation program are treated as inpatients for about 14 to 28 days. Patients may need medical management of acute or chronic health problems during this phase.

The rehabilitation phase is comprised of group psychotherapy and educational lectures about chemical dependency and related issues such as health, family, living sober, and time management. The twelve step component is integrated into treatment, including the use of twelve step literature, written assignments based on the first few steps, and attendance at twelve step meetings. The staff typically includes physicians, nurses, occupational and rehabilitation therapists, psychologists, substance abuse counselors, recovering volunteers, and social workers. Often, some of

---

Box 4-3

Advantages and Disadvantages of Inpatient Treatment

Advantages

1. More intense treatment
2. Minimal access to drugs and alcohol
3. Highly structured environment
4. Minimal outside distractions
5. More integrated health care
6. Impression on client and family of seriousness of illness

Disadvantages

1. Higher cost
2. Absence from home
3. Absence from employment

---

the substance abuse counseling staff also are recovering. The therapeutic milieu provides an opportunity to assess how the client interacts and identifies with staff members and other patients. An active process of eliciting input and feedback from clients is used. This process is invaluable in reinforcing positive behavior and in providing corrective feedback on the individual's interactions and behavior. Often, the client is able to receive corrective feedback more easily from peers.

The typical inpatient day is long and structured. An example of an inpatient program schedule follows:

6:00-8:00 AM	Wake up, breakfast, and walk
8:00-9:00 AM	Daily community meeting followed by morning meditation
9:00-9:30 AM	Free time to work on assignments
9:30-11:00 AM	Group psychotherapy
11:00 AM-12:00 M	Occupational therapy
12:00 M-1:00 PM	Lunch and free time
1:00-2:00 PM	Step group and/or recovery-oriented group
2:00-3:00 PM	Individual psychotherapy or free time
3:00-4:00 PM	Psychoeducation group
4:00-5:00 PM	Free time/assignments
5:00-6:00 PM	Supper and free time
6:00-7:30 PM	Patient and family education group
7:30-8:00 PM	Visiting (approved visitors only)
8:00-9:00 PM	Twelve step meeting

Partial hospitalization

Partial hospitalization provides intensive outpatient treatment (usually 4 to 5 hours per day, 2 to 5 days per week). The typical program activities include group therapy, educational seminars, family education and counseling, and introduction to twelve step programs, as well as attendance at twelve step meetings. The advantages and disadvantages of partial hospitalization are shown in Box 4-4.

Box 4-4
Advantages and Disadvantages of Partial Hospitalization

Advantages

1. Less disruptive to patient's life
2. Less costly
3. Patient can continue to live at home
4. Patient can continue employment

Disadvantages

1. More access to drugs and alcohol
2. Less intense treatment
3. Less integrated health care
4. Difficulty in patient's managing work and treatment schedule

---

Outpatient programs

Outpatient programs generally consist of 1 to 4 hours of weekly participation in individual and/or group therapy. Behavioral contracting is also important and is generally targeted towards issues related to abstinence, important behavioral changes, and twelve step meeting attendance. If a client is unable to maintain an agreed upon contract, he or she is often referred to a more intensive level of care.

Halfway houses

Halfway houses are transitional living facilities that provide both a supportive environment and rehabilitative services for people who do not have adequate resources or are not ready to reenter the community (Geller, 1992). The typical length of stay in halfway houses ranges from several months to a year. Residents are expected to participate in the treatment offered, assist in housekeeping chores, and prepare for independent living. Many individuals will need help from community vocational rehabilitative services in order to find work, learn new job skills, or complete their education.

Therapeutic communities (long-term residential settings)

Long-term residential programs treat individuals who have an extensive history of substance abuse, multiple treatment failures in less-structured settings, significant psychosocial deficits, or histories of antisocial and criminal behavior. The model for therapeutic communities, Synanon, was founded in 1958 by Charles Dederick, who used AA principles with drug addicts. Because of the belief that an addict is never cured, Dederick advocated long-term (sometimes lifetime) residence at Synanon. Controversy regarding financial dealings related to Synanon businesses (used to provide employment for residents) emerged in the 1980s. Although the Synanon image has suffered, it still exists. The typical length of stay is 6 months to 2 years. Daytop, Phoenix House, Odyssey House and Gateway Foundation are examples of therapeutic communities, which number in the hundreds today. These therapeutic communities differ from Synanon in that they recommend returning an addict to the community. The critical elements of therapeutic communities include the following:

1. Drug-free supervised abstinence
2. Emphasis on peer self-help, with appropriate inclusion of professional staff
3. Active participation of residents
4. Active use of role modeling
5. Emphasis on accountability and socially responsible behavior
6. Strong belief in emphasizing socialization in treatment
7. Mutual support to peers and commitment to treatment environment
8. Feedback and confrontation of behavior and attitudes; self disclosure
9. Focus on present behaviors, recognition of motivations, and acknowledgment of a statement of O.H. Mowrer, an internationally known humanistic psychologist and supporter of therapeutic communities, "Only you can do it, but you can't do it alone" (O'Brien & Biase, 1992).

The therapeutic community serves as a more healthy family system for many of its residents. In this environment the individual has the opportunity to grow, mature, and develop new skills in the context of a supportive drug-free milieu.

LONG-TERM AFTERCARE

Aftercare is the term used by proponents of the Minnesota model for the long-term outpatient treatment which follows inpatient or partial hospitalization treatment. The term is used to emphasize the ongoing nature of substance abuse treatment. Aftercare programs can be quite variable in duration, site, type of treatment delivered, and type of staff delivering the treatment (Geller, 1992). The purpose of aftercare is to consolidate and maintain gains made in inpatient treatment while the individual makes the transition back to his or her normal routine. The early weeks and months after inpatient treatment are associated with the highest relapse period (Gorski & Miller, 1982). Although clients leaving an intensive treatment program may feel optimistic and determined about remaining abstinent, they are often unprepared for and unrealistic about the difficulties they will encounter in their daily routines. Some common themes dealt with during aftercare include commitment to treatment, maintaining healthier behaviors, relapse prevention, and dealing with unresolved losses and traumas. Exploration of emotionally charged issues from the individual's childhood is usually delayed until healthy coping skills are developed. Aftercare can include individual, group, or family therapy. Clients are almost always encouraged to attend twelve step meetings. Clients also may address medical and/or psychiatric problems, identify time management strategies, participate in new leisure activities, or seek employment.

METHADONE MAINTENANCE PROGRAMS

A unique type of substance abuse treatment program is the methadone maintenance program (MMP). MMPs were started in the 1960s in response to poor treatment outcomes for intravenous heroin addicts. MMPs are the only form of substance abuse treatment in which a patient is maintained on a medication which causes physical dependence and can be abused. This treatment philosophy has led some to criticize the MMP approach in spite of the numerous research studies which have proven its efficacy. Some programs offer minimal counseling or therapy, some provide a low level of outpatient group and individual counseling, and other programs provide a variety of enhanced services like family therapy, psychiatric assessment and treatment, medical care, vocational training, and social services. Methadone maintenance allows an opiate addict the opportunity to be stabilized on a once-daily medication. However, the addict remains dependent on an addictive substance, and difficulty in ultimately detoxifying from methadone is viewed as a major drawback. In some MMPs the likelihood of patients switching chemicals of abuse is another major problem (see also Chapter 5).

TOOLS OF TREATMENT

The specific approaches used in substance abuse treatment can be conceptualized as the "tools" of treatment. Knowing when to use the most appropriate one is important. Not every tool needs to be used with every patient, but proper usage can increase the effectiveness of treatment. Which tool to use and when depends on the following: the patient's drug(s) of choice, phase of the addiction, level of motivation, support system, level of premorbid functioning (e.g., education, job skills, legal problems, social skills), comorbid psychiatric or medical conditions, and level of care required. Helping a client understand the value of using "tools" in his or her own work in recovery is important. Furthermore, when a patient relapses, approaches can be reviewed to help the patient and the staff identify tools needed.

Pharmacotherapy

Pharmacotherapy is used in substance abuse treatment for: (1) detoxification, (2) treating comorbid psychiatric and medical disorders, (3) reducing drug cravings or the euphoria from drug usage, (4) substitution, (5) aversive therapy, and (6) symptomatic treatment of withdrawal effects. Medications are not "magic bullets" which will cure addictive disorders but rather are one tool in the "toolbox" of treatment. Medications are used adjunctively with the other elements of psychosocial treatment.

Nurses must know what medications are used in treatment and when their use is appropriate. Also, they must know both the indications and the limitations of medications, including interactions with other medications and potential side effects. Some treatment programs make limited use of pharmacotherapies because of philosophical bias, limited experience or skills in this area, and lack of medically trained staff (Thomas et al, in press).

Detoxification.   Detoxification is the process of helping clients withdraw from an abused drug. Physical dependence on most substances requires medical detoxification. Also, individuals may require pharmacological detoxification to facilitate their transition into rehabilitation treatment. Pharmacological detoxification is accomplished by administering progressively decreasing dosages to depress withdrawal signs and symptoms in the initial phase of treatment. There are individual variations in the intensity of medications needed and in the optimal setting (outpatient versus inpatient) for administering medications. Important considerations include the client's detoxification history, type of drug abused, social supports, medical problems, psychiatric problems, and relapse history.

Also, some patients admitted to hospitals for nonaddiction medical problems develop withdrawal symptoms. Nurses should be alert for the signs and symptoms of alcohol and other drug withdrawal. Withdrawal symptoms from depressants (including alcohol) include tremors, agitation, anxiety, diaphoresis, nausea, vomiting, and diarrhea (see Table 11-2). Withdrawal from CNS stimulants (amphetamines, cocaine) can cause fatigue, lethargy, anxiety, irritability, and depression.

In addition to monitoring the symptoms of withdrawal, nurses have an important role in helping patients through the detoxification process and in providing education about recovery. The detoxification time period can be crucial in getting patients ready for the next phase of treatment, rehabilitation.

Comorbid disorders.   Medications may be used for treating comorbid psychiatric and medical disorders. There are high rates of concurrent anxiety and depressive disorders among substance abuse treatment seekers. Many individuals with a substance use disorder will come to a primary care clinic or a psychiatric clinic for evaluation of stress and psychiatric complaints. The appropriate selection of medications for this sample of clients requires skills and knowledge in both addictions and psychiatric problems. Chapter 12 discusses care of the client with dual diagnosis, or two primary psychiatric diagnoses.

Reducing effects of drugs.   Medications may be used to reduce the reinforcing effects of a substance. For example, naltrexone is used for treatment of heroin addiction. Naltrexone (Trexan) is an opiate antagonist which acts as a blocker of the euphoric effects of opiates such as heroin. After individuals are detoxified from opiates, they can be started on naltrexone. This medication has been useful in treating impaired health professionals, who often have been addicted to opiates.

Other drugs used to reduce the effects of an abused drug include bromocriptine for cocaine withdrawal and clonidine for heroin, cocaine, and nicotine addictions. Using medications to reduce craving is to prevent the high dropout rates typical for cocaine and narcotic users in the early days of treatment.

Recent research has focused on the use of medications for reducing drug cravings. Interest in developing new, and using established, pharmacotherapies has increased because of the growing number of substance dependent clients seeking treatment, the relatively high relapse rates with nonpharmacological treatment approaches alone, the growing recognition of high rates of psychiatric comorbidity, and the increasing neurobiological and pharmacological understanding of drug abuse.

Experimental drugs that reduce craving for cocaine are being tested. These include carbamazepine, fluoxetine, mazindol, and bromocriptine. Buprenorphine is being tested for opiate detoxification as well as maintenance. Both the National

Institute on Drug Abuse and the National Institute on Alcohol Abuse and Alcoholism have initiatives to encourage research on medications to treat substance abuse.

Substitution.   Drug substitution is treatment with a medication having similar pharmacological action as the abused drug. Most short-term substitution is for withdrawal only. Maintenance therapy also may be used, such as methadone for heroin addiction (see previous section on methadone maintenance). Another example of drug substitution is nicotine gum, which is given to patients with addiction to tobacco.

Aversion therapy.   Another form of pharmacotherapy is use of agents designed to produce an aversive response. The classic example of this type of medication is disulfiram (Antabuse). Disulfiram is an antidipsotropic agent that causes an extremely unpleasant reaction when combined with alcohol. It interferes with the metabolism of alcohol and results in a buildup of acetaldehyde in the body. The result is an intense, throbbing headache, severe flushing, extreme nausea, vomiting, palpitations, low blood pressure, labored breathing, and blurred vision. Few patients drink while taking this medication.

Symptomatic treatment.   Patients sometimes require symptomatic treatment to help reduce the discomfort of withdrawal from drugs and enable them to remain in treatment. Insomnia and anxiety are two such symptoms that may be treated with benzodiazepines. Antidepressant drugs have been shown to be useful in treating the depression often experienced during cocaine withdrawal (Barnes, 1988). Desipramine (Norpramin) is commonly used.

Individual therapy

Individual psychotherapy has a role in most treatment settings. Psychotherapy is an interpersonal process designed to bring about modifications of feelings (thoughts), attitudes, and behaviors that have caused problems for persons seeking help. Historically, psychoanalytically oriented psychotherapy was viewed as a failure when used with alcoholics. This led to a bad reputation for psychotherapy in general. It is widely recognized today, however, that psychotherapy can be helpful if certain guiding principles are used (Nace, 1992). In fact, Rounsaville and Carroll (1992) identify several situations, based on their clinical experience, in which psychotherapy may be the primary mode of care. They suggest that individual psychotherapy may be useful in the following circumstances: (1) to introduce drug abusers into treatment; (2) to treat clients with low levels of drug dependence; (3) to treat failures of other modalities; (4) to complement other ongoing treatments for selected patients; and (5) to help clients solidify gains following achievement of stable abstinence.

Behavioral contracting

Behavioral contracting is an agreement between a treatment provider or team and a client about expected behaviors, with a contingency plan if the client is unable to abide by the defined behaviors. This tool serves patients who are stuck or struggling in treatment or who disagree with a recommended plan of action. For example, an assessing clinician may identify a patient's need for inpatient hospitalization. The patient agrees to treatment but does not want to go to inpatient treatment. In this case, the outpatient treatment provider can develop a contract with this client. The contract might specify total abstinence, attendance at a specified number of AA or NA meetings, and attendance at therapy sessions. The client agrees that failure to maintain the behaviors designated in this predetermined contract will require inpatient treatment.

Another example is a client who is late in turning in expected assignments. After the clinician reviews the issue with the client, always seeking to clarify the underlying resistance, the clinician could place a contingency on completion of the assignment. For example, a client might lose privileges to go outside unescorted or for a weekend pass. This tool is not meant as a punishment; rather, it is a very effective means of helping clients reflect on and explore certain resistances that they need to overcome to progress in treatment. When making contracts with clients, this goal should be clearly explained.

Education

Education is an invaluable tool. Most often, clients and family members are uninformed about alcoholism and chemical dependency. Informal education begins when the client and family first encounter the treatment system. Typically the screening clinician is doing some teaching while assessing the client and obtaining a history. This helps decrease inevitable anxiety and other negative emotional states in the client—and the family, if they are involved at this stage. A formal program of education typically is built into program schedules and takes place in group and individual forums. The format includes didactic lectures, videos, reading assignments, and discussion groups. Educational programs often occur in the context of support groups. Topics reviewed usually include the *disease* concept of chemical dependency, introductory information about twelve step programs, medical effects of the disease, family issues as they relate to the disease, recovery-related concepts, and dealing with emotional states.

Education serves to demystify what both the client and the family have been experiencing. Often clients appear defensive and ashamed and families are frustrated and angry. The educational tool serves to diffuse some of this intense effect, instills hope for the possibility of recovery, and involves the whole family in treatment.

A vast library of recovery-related reading materials exists for both chemically dependent individuals and their families. These tools can be used while the client is in treatment and can be recommended for ongoing reading after the treatment encounter is over.

Group therapy

If there is a mainstay in substance abuse treatment besides the twelve step programs, it is the use of group therapy in all types of treatment settings. It would be highly unlikely to find an inpatient, residential, or partial-hospitalization program that failed to use group therapy. Additionally, many outpatient and aftercare programs include, or sometimes rely exclusively on, this intervention. The philosophy and methods used to conduct a group vary depending on the clinician's training and philosophical background, as well as the philosophy of the treatment environment. While it is commonly believed that group therapy is effective in work with substance abusers, there are a limited number of research studies that document this. People with substance abuse have difficulty tolerating intense emotional states; therefore, too much exposure to these states often leads to relapse. The skilled therapist will recognize individual problems and guide the group accordingly.

Family treatment

There are a variety of family treatments available in substance abuse intervention. For approximately 25 years, experts in the field have recognized the value of involving the whole family in the treatment process. The family is defined as the client's immediate network, regardless of blood relationship. Originally, families were engaged in the treatment process to enhance understanding of the problem and to increase support for the newly recovering person. Today, with an appreciation of social networks and family systems, the goals have become more sophisticated. Family members of substance abusers have their own special set of problems for which they can benefit from professional help. The goal is to assist the whole family in attaining a healthier and more functional way of relating and communicating.

The types of family treatment offered vary from participation in Al-Anon to a period (usually one week) of intensive inpatient work for family members. Besides the educational component noted above, there are typically a number of family counseling sessions. The goals of these sessions are to identify and clarify issues and communication styles, to assess each family's need for ongoing family therapy, and to facilitate referrals if they are indicated. The therapist also seeks to clarify the family's position about the client's need for treatment and helps to define what support and limits they are willing to implement with this client. For example, if the client called and said, "I want to leave this place now," which frequently occurs, would the family say, "We'll be right there," or "We love you, but cannot accept you back home before you are really in recovery"? Understanding the family's posture guides the treatment staff members in using their input in the recovery process. Typically the therapist working with family members is a clinical social worker or another professional with specialized training in family work. (For more about the family, see Chapter 9.)

Therapeutic milieu

A therapeutic milieu is an environment that contributes to the therapy, healing, and learning the recovering person must do to achieve sobriety. Therapeutic milieu is of particular interest and value to nurses, because it is the nursing staff that defines and maintains the milieu 24 hours a day. Nurses and other staff members managing the milieu are always keenly tuned to tone, energy, relationships between clients, and every nuance of the environment. The milieu is the stage or backdrop for much of what is occurring in treatment. Knowledgeable clinicians are aware of the environment and take steps to influence it. For example, a staff member may hear lots of rowdy noise coming from a patient area. On closer examination it may become apparent that clients are reminiscing about their drug-use days and, by doing that, stirring up cravings for drugs or alcohol in themselves and others. The experienced clinician learns to deflect the atmosphere and redirect the group's discussion in an obvious way. A nurse may sit in the patients' areas, so as to be easily available to patients, or may engage the patients in a game of cards or Ping-Pong—using that unstructured, relaxed time to learn more about the clients and how they interact with each other. This information is useful in various client treatment plans.

Staff members also are attuned to an escalating tone in the environment and wisely intervene early to learn its source and address the excitement. Often an increased intensity in the milieu could mean that a patient or group of patients is craving and/or using drugs on the unit. Perhaps other patients sense or know this before the staff does and feel threatened, frightened, and vulnerable. When patients are encouraged to identify openly their struggles and the emotional pain contributing to their struggles, they often are able to overcome the crisis and learn much from it. The more staff members are attuned to their clients' histories, current treatment issues, and significant developments, the better they are able to successfully intervene with them. Staff members seek to *be* tools, as well as *teach* tools to clients. The use of the therapeutic milieu is indeed a very powerful one.

Vocational counseling

Although many patients admitted to private treatment settings are employed (therefore insured), approximately 62% of patients entering federally funded programs are unemployed at admission (Schottenfeld et al, 1992). To appreciate the crucial role vocational counseling plays in the rehabilitation process, one need only listen to clients. For many, a paramount concern is securing employment, not only for the income but also for the structure it will add to their lives. Patients who are successfully engaged in rehabilitation recognize unstructured time as a major relapse trigger, drawing them back to their former lifestyle.

The important components of a comprehensive vocational services program include: (1) vocational assessment and treatment planning, (2) vocational counseling, (3) work adjustment programs, (4) job seeking–skill training, and (5) job development programs. These components ideally are coordinated with or included in the treatment program. Furthermore, a vocational program identifies or matches clients to the aspects of the vocational program they most need (Schottenfeld et al, 1992).

Nationally, there is a lack of vocational programs available to and included in rehabilitation programs. Vocational programs should be considered fundamental for a select group of clients because they maximize the opportunity for a positive outcome for those clients.

Activities therapies

Activities therapies include a wide array of tools usually delivered by a psychiatric occupational therapist. One of the goals of these therapies is to teach patients social skills to use when interacting with others while sober. An activity therapist also teaches time management, leisure planning, and daily living skills. Some of the forums used for activities therapies are group settings, planned recreation, and art or expressive therapies.

Many clients with substance abuse have never learned to enjoy leisure without drugs or alcohol. In fact, it is not unusual for clients to be unable to identify one fun or leisure activity they have participated in without drugs or alcohol. Activities therapies have significant implications for overall time management and for clients' learning to enjoy life sober.

Relapse prevention

A number of relapse prevention strategies have been developed during the 1980s. Relapse prevention is a cognitive/behavioral approach that assists patients in identifying high-risk situations and behaviors, developing alternative strategies for coping, and identifying, recognizing, and intervening in relapse thinking before actually using a substance. These procedures often are used with patients who have had prior relapses, but they have utility for all substance abusers because of the relapsing nature of the illness (Marlatt & Gordon, 1984). A national training center has been established for substance abuse practitioners to become experts in relapse prevention (Gorski & Miller, 1982).

Patients respond favorably to relapse prevention. It helps them identify concrete strategies that can be rehearsed and practiced under supervision. It teaches them to visualize the full cycle of their illness should they be contemplating a return to drug use (e.g., addicts and alcoholics are known for their use of the phenomenon called euphoric recall, that is, idealizing drug use and recalling all the pleasant states associated with it). When contemplating a return to active use, rarely do these individuals meditate on the whole cycle of their use, with all the negative consequences such as physical withdrawal, legal consequences, family problems, job losses, or homelessness. When they are assisted to visualize these realities, their cravings frequently abate and they are grateful for guidance in seeing the full, real picture. Relapse prevention also helps patients recognize that they are not "bad" if they relapse but rather in need of more tools or better utilization of those tools. (See chapter 5 for more about relapse.)

Twelve step programs

There are many different types of twelve step programs, designated by type of drug abused, for addicted persons and their spouses, families, and children. Each type of program offers a wide variety of meetings.

Alcoholics Anonymous (AA).   Alcoholics Anonymous defines itself as "a fellowship of men and women who share their experience, strength, and hope with each other that they may solve their common problem and help others to recover from alcoholism" (Alcoholics Anonymous, 1976). The only requirement for membership is a desire to stop drinking. There are no dues or fees for AA membership. AA is not allied with any sect, denomination, political organization, or institution.

The AA program is defined and guided by the "Twelve Steps" (Box 4-5) and "Twelve Traditions" (Box 4-6). The twelve steps offer a prescription for recovery from alcoholism, and individuals are presented with this program when they attend AA meetings. The twelve traditions guide the structure and function of the group.

Three types of meetings are offered—speaker, discussion, and step. In *speaker* meetings, prearranged members tell their "stories" about their lives with alcohol, how they found the road to recovery, and the changes in their lives. Many attendees find these stories validating, as well as inspiring. In *discussion* meetings, an AA member relates some aspect of his or her story to a recovery topic or theme, and a discussion ensues relevant to that topic. *Step* meetings are typically closed meetings in which members systematically work on Steps 1 through 12. Meetings are usually 1 hour in length and are preceded and followed by socializing.

Many sayings and slogans are used in AA. These are simple statements valued as pearls of wisdom. Slogans are memorized and recalled as needed to reinforce positive sobriety. Some of the more common slogans are "Easy does it," "Live and let live," "It works if you work it," and "One day at a time." The "it works if you work it" slogan refers to the AA program itself. The fundamental way to "work the program" is to attend and participate in AA meetings and to acquire and relate to a

---

Box 4-5
The Twelve Steps of Alcoholics Anonymous*

1. We admitted we were powerless over alcohol—that our lives had become unmanageable.
2. Came to believe that a Power greater than ourselves could restore us to sanity.
3. Made a decision to turn our will and our lives over to the care of God as we understood Him.
4. Made a searching and fearless moral inventory of ourselves.
5. Admitted to God, to ourselves, and to another human being the exact nature of our wrongs.
6. Were entirely ready to have God remove all these defects of character.
7. Humbly asked Him to remove our shortcomings.
8. Made a list of all persons we had harmed, and became willing to make amends to them all.
9. Made direct amends to such people wherever possible, except when to do so would injure them or others.
10. Continued to take personal inventory and when we were wrong promptly admitted it.
11. Sought through prayer and meditation to improve our conscious contact with God, *as we understood Him,* praying only for knowledge of His will for us and the power to carry that out.
12. Having had a spiritual awakening as the result of these steps, we tried to carry this message to alcoholics and to practice these principles in all our affairs.

From *Alcoholics Anonymous*. (1976). (3rd ed.). New York: Alcoholics Anonymous World Services, Inc.
*Permission to reprint this material does not mean that AA has reviewed or approved the contents of this publication. AA is a program of recovery from alcoholism *only*. Use of the Twelve Steps in connection with programs and activities that are patterned after AA but address other problems does not imply otherwise.

sponsor—a more senior member (in length of time in AA)—who advises and helps direct members in maintaining sobriety.

A sponsor is another recovering person who has attained some significant degree of sobriety. The role of the sponsor is to assist in acquainting a member with the program, serve as a guide through the step work, and be available to talk during times a less-experienced member is feeling vulnerable. Many recovering people look to their sponsors as mentors who remain important figures in their lives. Sponsorship is considered one type of service members can offer as they mature in sobriety.

Another basic premise in the AA program is the concept that you "keep it" (i.e., sobriety and serenity) by "giving it away"—hence the concept of service. Service can be accomplished in many ways. AA volunteers often are ready to assist in hospital emergency areas and/or in social services departments. Others volunteer by going to schools to offer information about the twelve step meetings and sub-

---

Box 4-6
The Twelve Traditions of Alcoholics Anonymous*

1. Our common welfare should come first; personal recovery depends on AA unity.
2. For our group purpose there is but one ultimate authority—a loving God as He may express Himself in our group conscience. Our leaders are but trusted servants; they do not govern.
3. The only requirement for AA membership is a desire to stop drinking.
4. Each group should be autonomous except in matters affecting other groups or AA as a whole.
5. Each group has but one primary purpose—to carry its message to the alcoholic who still suffers.
6. An AA group ought never endorse, finance, or lend the AA name to any related facility or outside enterprise, lest problems of money, property, and prestige divert us from our primary purpose.
7. Every AA group ought to be fully self-supporting, declining outside contributions.
8. Alcoholics Anonymous should remain forever non-professional, but our service centers may employ special workers.
9. AA, as such, ought never be organized; but we may create service boards or committees directly responsible to those they serve.
10. Alcoholics Anonymous has no opinion on outside issues; hence the AA name ought never be drawn into public controversy.
11. Our public relations policy is based on attraction rather than promotion; we need always maintain personal anonymity at the level of press, radio, and films.
12. Anonymity is the spiritual foundation of all our traditions, ever reminding us to place principles before personalities.

From *Alcoholics Anonymous*. (1976). (3rd ed.). New York: Alcoholics Anonymous World Services, Inc.
*Permission to reprint this material does not mean that AA has reviewed or approved the contents of this publication. AA is a program of recovery from alcoholism *only.* Use of the Twelve Traditions in connection with programs and activities that are patterned after AA but address other problems does not imply otherwise.

stance abuse programs in their communities. Other members volunteer by going to hospitals and treatment centers to run institutional meetings. Many begin their service to the fellowship by offering to be the coffee maker at home meetings. The home meeting is each member's base meeting; many AA members attend 2 to 7 meetings weekly but view one specific meeting as their "home-base" meeting.

AA members recognize what is perhaps the most difficult reality in leaving a life of drinking and drugging behind (i.e., leaving a whole lifestyle, which usually includes leaving one's circle of friends behind as well). This is very often the single most difficult task newly recovering people face. They wonder how they will fill the huge void in their lives. AA deals with this in several ways. Meetings are available every day of the week, often several times daily in larger communities. A sponsor helps to bridge the gap from old friends to new ones. AA also sponsors many nondrinking social activities. These include dances, picnics, and meeting anniversary celebrations. During the very difficult Christmas holiday season, AA and its counterparts run "Alkathons," which are 24-hour, continuous meetings throughout the Christmas and New Year holidays.

What is the success and membership of AA? There are many in the substance abuse field who acknowledge that what works best for most people are the twelve step programs. Why, one may ask, is that so? Many theories can be postulated. The "Twelve Steps" and "Twelve Traditions" are fundamental, solid principles that can have only positive influence in anyone's life. The "Big Book's" chapter "How it works" states, "Rarely have we seen a person fail who has thoroughly followed our path" (Alcoholics Anonymous, 1976).

Another important consideration is the group process function of AA (Nace, 1992). The elements of group therapy are apparent:

1. Hope is provided by associating with other alcoholics who are not drinking and who are apparently happy, satisfied, or indeed grateful not to be drinking.
2. Universality is formed through sharing stories and experiences involving alcohol. The newcomer is struck by the value of his or her experience as AA members identify with it and express thanks and gratitude to the newcomer for sharing the story. Instead of feeling condemned, the newcomer feels bonded to these other alcoholics by virtue of his or her experience.
3. Information is provided informally through conversations, literature published by AA, and the content of the meetings themselves.
4. Imitation is a very prominent aspect of the group process. Phrases are repeated and rituals followed.
5. Learning occurs at multiple levels and includes how sober alcoholics view their disease, how they relate to others, and what to do to stay sober. The member also learns that the problem is alcohol (not a spouse, a job, or a lack of willpower). It is learned that one has a disease and alcoholism is cunning, powerful, and baffling.
6. Catharsis can occur. The opportunity is provided (but not demanded) through discussion, speaker, and step-study meetings. Again, one's experiences are appreciated and not subject to condemnation or judgment.

7. Cohesiveness follows the ability to identify, usually quickly, with the viewpoints and experiences of fellow members. Cohesiveness is also facilitated by participating in the informal socializing of AA meetings. One feels at home by helping to make coffee, set up chairs, and eventually greet newcomers (Yalom, 1975).

Although these factors offer significant healing potential, they cannot account for the entire success of AA, or all group therapy treatments would have the same results. Nevertheless, one need attend a meeting only once to recognize powerful forces at work. Students in the health professions should be encouraged to attend several meetings to experience the process firsthand. The investment will be invaluable for future practice.

The fact that AA has been so helpful in addressing issues of the struggling alcoholic has led to an explosion of self-help programs. A few of these programs include: Al-Anon for family and friends affected by the alcohol abuse; Alateen for adolescent children of alcoholics; Adult Children of Alcoholics (ACOA), which addresses problems of individuals who grew up with alcoholism; Codependents Anonymous (CODA), which addresses issues for individuals who have difficulty in relationships specifically related to sacrificing their own needs to attempt to please others; Mentally Ill Chemical Abusers (MICA), which seeks to offer special help to those who suffer from both mental illness and substance abuse. As the list of twelve step programs has grown, some clinicians have criticized the overuse of the philosophy. Despite this criticism, many value highly the support network that the twelve step programs provide.

There are individuals, however, who do not do well with these programs. It is important to discern whether the difficulty involves legitimate issues or resistance to treatment. At times that assessment is complex, so the clinician must evaluate all areas of the patient's treatment and life functioning. Some common complaints are "AA is too spiritual, I just don't relate," or "I get worse (or triggered to use) when hearing the stories repeated." It is known that some individuals have great difficulty connecting with AA, and there will be people who, for a number of reasons, may not be able to get their needs met in the twelve step programs. The level of difficulty should be carefully assessed to determine whether it is resistance and denial or sincerely legitimate, and an appropriate treatment plan should follow.

Spiritual counseling

The term "spiritual counseling" often causes discomfort in staff members (especially in the psychiatric arena), because they believe they are breaching a sacred boundary in personal belief systems. Nurses working in health care, particularly acute care, regularly offer help with or referral to pastoral counseling. In chemical dependency treatment, spirituality is conceptualized as much more than, and sometimes altogether different from, one's faith. It relates more to the persons themselves—what and who they love, how they can develop their strengths, talents, and gifts, and how they can develop and use what is referred to as positive energy. Again the goal is aimed towards finding serenity in their lives and being at peace with themselves and the world around them. For some, if not many, this includes a new connection or a reconnection with a religious belief system. The goal of spiritual counseling is to help individuals identify their spiritual needs and how these can best be met.

It is important to explore spirituality because problems in this area can make it difficult for patients to be comfortable in twelve step programs. While the AA "Big Book" specifically identifies that AA has no religious affiliation, the Lord's Prayer is sometimes repeated at meetings. Some individuals respond favorably to that while others, particularly people who are not Christians, are very uncomfortable. It is important for treatment providers to recognize these variations and be prepared to encourage patients to find meetings that meet their needs.

EFFECTIVENESS OF TREATMENT

How effectiveness is determined

To determine treatment effectiveness, studies are designed to carefully evaluate outcomes based on predetermined goals in various aspects of the client's life in the months and years following the treatment encounter. Key areas of functioning include reduction or elimination of alcohol and illicit drug use; concomitant reduction of the signs, symptoms, and consequences of the alcohol or drug use; resolution of recurring medical, psychiatric, or social problems; and modification in attitude toward drinking and drugging behavior, leading to a commitment to its amelioration in the future (Institute of Medicine, 1990).

The fundamental question is, "Did the patient get better?" Clinicians, consumers, and family members all want to know the answer to this question. Health insurance providers and government payers also need to determine effectiveness of treatment. For many years the substance abuse field was inconsistent in its attention to this important question. This omission has contributed to a reluctance of both public and private insurers to pay for treatment services.

Therefore, a major initiative is under way to obtain and provide accurate data which answer these questions. Some states have begun to mandate a management information system relevant to outcomes for programs receiving public funds. The private sector also has become involved in outcome studies, particularly since the advent of utilization review and managed care by private insurers. The Chemical Abuse/Addiction Treatment Outcome Registry (CATOR) is a private corporation specializing in providing treatment outcome data to individual treatment programs for a set fee per patient. While the registry's primary task is to provide reports for its subscribers, the data also can be employed to explore general issues in the treatment of alcohol and drug problems (Hoffman & Harrison, 1988). The utility of this information has already proven invaluable to the understanding of outcomes and also is useful in giving accurate information regarding outcomes to clients in treatment.

Fundamentally, it is known that treatment is helpful in attaining change in clients' lives. Yet a careful examination reveals that there is still much to learn about the specifics of treatment outcomes. Some studies conclude that outpatient treatment is as effective as inpatient treatment (Miller & Hester, 1986), while others have demonstrated that an inpatient modality produces a better outcome for a certain type of patient (Walsh et al, 1991). No one treatment works best for everyone, but a carefully thought-out plan relevant to each individual helps define the most cost-effective treatment likely to produce positive results. Although a good database exists for beginning to describe the treatment-outcome phenomenon, much more specific research has begun and must continue to provide answers to remaining questions.

Furthermore, effectiveness is defined in many different ways. For example, one treatment provider may define effectiveness as total abstinence with improved functioning in all life areas, the ideal and the gold standard. Another may define effectiveness as a decrease in use of substance(s). These are the two ends of the spectrum. Most researchers and providers define effectiveness as somewhere in the middle. What is important is for nurses to recognize, thoughtfully evaluate, and question information. The point to be remembered is that proper patient matching will assure effectiveness with all correctly used treatments.

Matching studies

It follows then that the answers to many of the questions regarding outcomes lie in understanding and refining treatment matching. Which kinds of individuals, with what kinds of alcohol (or drug) problems, are likely to respond to what kinds of treatments by achieving what kinds of goals when delivered by what kinds of practitioners (Institute of Medicine, 1990)?

There have been a number of matching studies to date and many more are currently under way to provide specific information regarding treatment matching. Important contributions to this area of understanding have been made by McLellan and others (1983) and a number of other researchers. A quick review of some of this work can be found in the Institute of Medicine's book, *Broadening the Base of Treatment for Alcohol Problems* (1990).

To produce valid outcome results, the process of matching must accurately represent both the assessment and treatment processes. It must be grounded in clearly documented and defined guidelines that can be understood and used by every provider.

Does treatment work?

Success commonly is measured by the number of patients treated who remain abstinent. The literature indicates that abstinence rates vary from 10% to 90%, depending on the study. Obviously this range of rates does not provide the necessary information. The Institute of Medicine summarizes the salient principles from current outcome studies. These conclusions are as follows:

1. There is no single treatment approach that is effective for all persons with alcohol problems. (This includes drugs as well.)
2. The provision of appropriate, specific treatment modalities can substantially improve outcome.
3. Brief interventions can be quite effective compared with no treatment and they can be quite cost-effective compared with more intensive treatment.
4. Treatment of other life problems related to drinking can improve outcome in persons with alcohol problems.

5. Therapist characteristics are determinants of outcome.

6. Outcomes are determined in part by treatment factors, post-treatment adjustment factors, characteristics of individuals seeking treatment, characteristics of their problems, and interactions among these factors.

7. People who are treated for alcohol problems achieve differing degrees of success with respect to drinking behavior, and alcohol problems follow different courses of outcome.

8. Those who significantly reduce their level of alcohol consumption, or who become totally abstinent, usually enjoy improvement in other areas of life, particularly as the period of reduced consumption becomes longer (Institute of Medicine, 1990).

Considering the aforementioned principles as fundamental, the reader also is referred to several large or classic bodies of outcome studies. Besides the previously mentioned CATOR research, see the *Treatment Outcome Prospective Study* (TOPS) (Craddock et al, 1985).

Factors associated with improved outcomes

The critical factor in determining outcome is the matching of the patient to the best treatment. One clinical problem commonly found in substance abuse care is a lack of medical treatment for depression. Although it is sensible to wait a prescribed period of time for the toxic effects of alcohol (a depressant) or other drugs to abate, there are frequent instances when both providers and patients resist any use of antidepressant medication. Some of these clients are able to make good progress, but others either relapse or are hindered by depressive symptoms. Often patients do not recognize their symptoms as depression but think these symptoms are normal for them. It then depends on treatment staff to identify the problem and designate appropriate treatment strategies. An example of this follows:

Ⅲ➡ Clinical Example

John was a 30-year-old divorced male with two children. He had a 10-year history of stable employment, but currently he was threatened with job loss if he continued his drug use and work performance problems. He had successfully recovered from alcoholism approximately 8 years earlier and later had become heroin dependent. He had been through approximately three inpatient programs and generally followed through on his prescribed aftercare plans. John's nurse was struck by his constricted range of affect, his anhedonia, and his inability to be comfortable in social situations, including AA and NA meetings. He stated that this feeling state left him vulnerable to relapse, but he did not identify this state as depression. In fact, he resisted the notion of depression as well as suggested treatment with antidepressant medicines. His treatment plan included weekly group psychotherapy sessions, weekly individual sessions, weekly contact with his employee assistance representative, and three to five twelve step meetings weekly. Despite this vigorous treatment plan, John slipped back into drug use. After his relapse, however, he was referred to an inpatient dual diagnosis treatment unit where his addiction and mood disturbance were addressed. He responded well to antidepressant medication, reporting he felt the best he had in his entire life. At 1 year follow-up, John was clean and sober, maintained his job, and reported an improvement in his overall quality of life.

Besides the obvious issues related to treatment matching, there are a number of other identified factors associated with more positive outcomes. These factors are related to the patient's overall state of health. An individual who is medically well, has intact support systems including family, friends, and employment, and does not have another psychiatric illness generally fares better than an otherwise similar individual who lacks these strengths.

The patient who has added social burdens such as poverty, homelessness, or unemployment to cope with will obviously have more difficulty sustaining the hope and energy necessary for recovery. If one adds the further burden of AIDS or schizophrenia, recovery is even more difficult. Nevertheless, these patients too have a chance to improve their lives if their treatment plans address the full scope of their medical, psychiatric, and social problems. It also is important to recognize that treatment expectations and goals will vary for different clients just as they would vary for patients with different types of cancers.

TRENDS IN TREATMENT

Increasing outpatient treatment

Outpatient treatment services have an important role for many patients. In fact, making outpatient services more widely available serves a number of patients whose disease severity is mild to moderate. Again, this can be compared to a patient receiving outpatient radiation or chemotherapy for cancer. Some patients' illnesses are amenable to outpatient treatment, while other clients are so ill they need all the resources an acute care hospital can provide. Although the inpatient Minnesota model was the most widely used method for the delivery of chemical dependency treatment for many years, treatment has been changing dramatically during the past ten years. Many factors have contributed to these changes (e.g., evidence that less intensive treatment is effective), but the major factor limiting inpatient use has been the necessity for cost containment in health care.

Changes in reimbursement

Because of the rapidly escalating cost of health care, government (both federal and state) and other third-party payers have attempted to reduce costs by using the least expensive methods of treatment. Retrospective reimbursement (DRGs) was a major effort begun in the mid-1980s to contain costs. Private payers soon followed the government's guidelines for reimbursement. Reimbursement for substance abuse treatment was reduced. Intensive (and expensive) inpatient treatment was replaced by less intensive outpatient treatment. The rationale for this change was based on the research that had shown outpatient treatment to be effective (e.g., Miller & Hester, 1986). What often is not considered when deciding the level of care to be reimbursed are the patient's specific problems and circumstances that may or may not be amenable to outpatient treatment. For example, some third-party payers insist that a patient fail in outpatient therapy before they will pay for inpatient treatment. There are hopes that in a reformed health care system, specific criteria can be used to determine the least-intensive treatment likely to be successful.

The development of the Cleveland Criteria in 1987, followed by the ASAM criteria in 1991, began the effort to establish a system that allows providers of chemical dependency services and payers to mutually agree on delivery of services to patients. Refinement of these guidelines, coupled with mutual agreement to use and abide by them, would be a major leap forward in delivering quality, cost-effective care most likely to produce the desired results. (See Chapter 15 for a thorough discussion of funding for treatment.)

SUMMARY

Treating patients with substance abuse can be an extremely rich experience for the clinician. It is gratifying to help clients regain their lives and to see family members do the same. In the last 25 years, great strides have been made in recognizing chemical dependency as a disease and developing treatment strategies accordingly. The challenge in the 90s and beyond is to continue to refine understanding of substance abuse and dependency and its treatment. The more this generation can assist in successfully preventing these disorders, the less expertise in intervention will be needed for the next.

REFERENCES

Abrams, D.B. & Niaura, R.S. (1987). Social learning theory. In H.T. Blane & K.E. Leonard (Eds.), *Psychological theories of drinking and alcoholism* (pp 131-178). New York: Guilford Press.

Alcoholics Anonymous. (1976). *Alcoholics Anonymous* (3rd ed.). New York: Alcoholics Anonymous World Services, Inc.

Alcoholics Anonymous World Services, Inc. (1987). A.A. surveys its membership: A demographic report. *About AA: A newsletter for professional men and women.* Fall, 1-2.

American Psychiatric Association. (1952). *Diagnostic and statistical manual of mental disorders* (1st ed.). Washington, D.C.: The Association.

Anderson, D.J. (1981). *Perspectives on treatment: The Minnesota experience.* Center City, MN: Hazelden Foundation.

Barnes, D.M. (1988). Breaking the cycle of addiction. *Science, 241,* 1029.

Beck, A. (1989). Cognitive therapy. In H.I. Kaplan & B.J. Sadock (Eds.), *Comprehensive textbook of psychiatry* (4th ed.). (pp 1432-1438). Baltimore: Williams & Wilkins.

Chappel, J.N. (1992). Effective use of Alcoholics Anonymous and Narcotics Anonymous in treating patients. *Psychiatric Annals, 22*(8), 409-418.

Cloninger, C.R. & Begluter, H. (Eds.). (1990). *Genetics and biology of alcoholism: Banbury Report 33.* New York: Cold Spring Harbor Laboratory Press.

Craddock, S.G., Bray, R.M., & Hubbard, R.L. (1985). *Drug use before and during drug abuse treatment: 1979-1981 TOPS and Mission Cohorts.* Rockville, MD: National Institute on Drug Abuse.

Geller, A. (1992). Rehabilitation programs and halfway houses. In J. Lowinson, P. Ruiz, R. Millman, & J. Langrod (Eds.), *Substance abuse: A comprehensive textbook* (p. 460). Baltimore: Williams & Wilkins.

Gorski, T.T. & Miller, M. (1982). *Counseling for relapse prevention.* Independence, MO: Herald House Independence Press.

Hoffman, N.G., Halikas, J.A., Mee-Lee, D., & Weedman, R.D. (1991). American society of addiction medicine: Patient placement criteria for the treatment of psychoactive substance use disorders. Washington, D.C.: The Society.

Hoffman, N.G. & Harrison, P.A. (1988). *Treatment outcome: Adult inpatients two years later.* Saint Paul, MN: Chemical Abuse/Addiction Treatment Outcome Registry.

Institute of Medicine. (1990). *Broadening the base of treatment for alcohol problems.* Washington, D.C.: National Academy Press.

Jellinek, E.M. (1960). *The disease concept of alcoholism.* New Haven, CT: College and University Press.

Lewis, D.C. (1991). Comparison of alcoholism and other medical diseases: An internist's view. *Psychiatric Annals, 21*(5), 256-265.

Marlatt, G.A. & Gordon, J.R. (1984). *Relapse prevention: Maintenance strategies in addictive behavior change.* New York: Guilford Press.

Marlatt, G.A., Baer, J.S., Donovan, D.M., & Kivlahan, D.R. (1988). Addictive behaviors: Etiology and treatment. *Ann Review Psychology, 39,* 223-252.

McLellan, A.T., Luborsky, L., Woody, G.E., O'Brien, C.P., & Druley, K.A. (1983b). Predicting response to alcohol and drug abuse treatments. *Archives of General Psychiatry, 40,* 620-625.

Miller, W.R. & Hester, R.K. (1986). Inpatient alcoholism treatment: Who benefits? *American Psychologist, 41,* 794.

Musto, D. (1992). Historical perspectives on alcohol and drug abuse. In J. Lowinson, P. Ruiz, R. Millman, & J. Langrod (Eds.), *Substance abuse: A comprehensive textbook* (pp 7-8). Baltimore: Williams & Wilkins.

Nace, E.P. (1992). Alcoholics anonymous. In J. Lowinson, P. Ruiz, R. Millman, & J. Langrod (Eds.), *Substance abuse: A comprehensive textbook* (pp 486-495). Baltimore: Williams & Wilkins.

Norris, J.L. (1978). Prevention of chronicity. *Psychiatric Annals, 8*(11), 48-53.

O'Brien, W. & Biase, D.V. (1992). Therapeutic community: A coming of age. In J. Lowinson, P. Ruiz, R. Millman, & J. Langrod (Eds.), *Substance abuse: A comprehensive textbook* (p 456). Baltimore: Williams & Wilkins.

Prochaska, J.O., DiClemente, C.C., & Norcross, J.C. (1992). In search of how people change: Applications to addictive behaviors. *American Psychologist, 47*(9), 1102-1114.

Rounsaville, B.J. & Carroll, K.M. (1992). Individual psychotherapy for drug abusers. In J. Lowinson, P. Ruiz, R. Millman, & J. Langrod (Eds.), *Substance abuse: A comprehensive textbook* (pp 496-506). Baltimore: Williams & Wilkins.

Schottenfeld, R., Pascale, R., & Sokolowski, S. (1992). Matching services to needs, vocational services for substance abusers. *Journal of Substance Abuse Treatment, 9,* 3-8.

Thomas, H.M., Ziedonis, D., & Kosten, T.R. (in press). *Pharmacotherapeutic approaches for drug abuse.* NIDA Monograph Series: Drug Abuse Services and Treatment Issues. Washington, D.C.

Vaillant, G.E. (1983). *The natural history of alcoholism: Causes, patterns, and paths to recovery.* Cambridge, MA: Harvard University Press.

Walsh, D.C., Hingson, R.W., Merrigan, D.M., Levenson, S.M., Cupples, L.A., Heeren, T., Coffman, G., Becker, C.A., Barker, T.A., Hamilton, S.K., McGuire, T.G., & Kelly, C.A. (1991). A randomized trial of treatment options for alcohol-abusing workers. *New England Journal of Medicine, 325,* 775.

Yalom, I. (1975). *The theory and practice of group psychotherapy* (2nd ed.). New York: Basic Books.

5 Recovery and Relapse

Recovery is a complex process and somewhat difficult to define. Nursing addictions organizations have defined recovery as "Regaining health; returning to a normal state in which the individual no longer engages in problematic behavior, can feel good about himself or herself, and is able to accomplish established goals" (ANA, 1987, p. 30). Recovery usually begins with formal treatment and continues throughout an individual's life.

This chapter describes the intricate processes of recovery and relapse according to current research and theoretical approaches. The process of change that occurs during recovery is discussed. Several approaches to recovery are described and the goals of recovery are explained. Factors related to relapse are considered and a model of relapse prevention is presented.

RECOVERY

The term "recover," when applied to diseases in general, means "to restore health or regain a normal or usual state." A person who has a disease "recovers" when the agent causing the disease is modified, alleviated, or removed. In substance abuse, substances are "removed" when a person is detoxified. Early treatment methods ended with detoxification and admonishing the client to abstain from further substance use. This approach was not effective because it did not deal with what is increasingly seen as an addictive process. That is, substance abuse is more than use of the substance itself; it involves a whole range of behavioral and physiological manifestations. Whether these behaviors are antecedents or consequences of the substance abuse is not clearly understood, but the need to change the behaviors is clear.

As understanding of substance abuse increases, it is apparent that just as addiction is more than the presence of the substance, recovery is more than the absence of the substance. Addiction is now understood as a chronic illness characterized by relapse. Maintaining recovery entails a major departure from old habits, dysfunctional behaviors and relationships that were part of the addictive lifestyle, and replacement with healthier options.

A model of behavioral change, introduced in Chapter 4, was developed (Prochaska & DiClemente, 1984) and refined (Prochaska, DiClemente, & Norcross, 1992) as a model for phases of change including maintenance or recovery. The model emerged from a comparative analysis of psychological and behavioral change-theories and is based on the assumption that any behavioral change involves a common sequence of events. Therefore, the model transcends individual theories to address change itself. Each stage of change is best facilitated by a specific type of response.

According to this model, in the first stage of change the individual does not recognize substance abuse as a problem and fails to see that change is needed. This first phase is called *precontemplation* and is essentially one of denial. What the person needs at this phase is feedback and information about the problem. The individual enters the second phase, *contemplation,* when recognition of the need for change is acknowledged. In this stage, the individual thinks about changing. Helpful at this point is information about how to begin to change. The next stage is *preparation,* in which some minor actions are taken toward change and the individual prepares for definitive action. In the fourth phase of change, *action,* change is initiated. For example, the individual makes a commitment to abstinence, enters a treatment program, or attends Alcoholics Anonymous (AA) meetings. The last phase of change is *maintenance.* The maintenance phase is concerned with the long-term efforts needed to sustain the changes begun during the action phase. Increasingly, it is recognized that maintenance is a distinctly separate phase and requires a new set of skills. Clearly, more emphasis needs to be placed on this phase of recovery. Although recovery begins with treatment, it is more fully implemented and tested when clients leave the treatment environment and return to their everyday lives.

PERSPECTIVES AND APPROACHES TO RECOVERY

There are several theoretical perspectives to recovery. Selected perspectives and specific approaches to recovery addressed in this chapter are (1) spontaneous remission, (2) harm reduction, and (3) twelve step programs.

Spontaneous remission

Some people attain recovery from alcohol and/or drug dependence without treatment. This is referred to as spontaneous remission or natural recovery. One estimate is that as many as 40% of alcoholics recover spontaneously. Very little is known about this population since they do not enter the substance abuse treatment system. Often recovery is attributed to a positive life change such as marriage, more meaningful work, or a profound religious experience (Grinspoon, 1987).

Studies of spontaneous remission in alcoholics have identified personal illness or accidents, religious experiences, alcohol-related financial problems, and extraordinary events (usually negative) as reasons subjects gave for giving up alcohol use (Tuchfield, 1981). Similarly, Ludwig (1985) found "hitting bottom," psychologically or physically, or a religious experience were precursors to a change in drinking behavior.

The results of a more recent, controlled study of spontaneous remission found that 57% of subjects attributed their recovery to a cognitive evaluation or an appraisal process rather than to a specific event, although frequently the appraisal was triggered by a buildup of negative events. To be included in the study, these subjects had achieved resolution of relatively severe drinking problems for a minimum of three years (Sobell et al, 1993). Not all subjects remained abstinent; however, those who were still drinking were not experiencing drinking-related problems. The data from these studies suggest that spontaneous remission may be more common than previously thought and deserves more study.

A concern about spontaneous remission is that the individual and family may fail to resolve the destructive behavioral patterns that develop as a result of substance abuse, creating higher risk for relapse. More research is needed to determine long-term results.

Harm reduction approach

Rather than focusing on individual lifestyle, the harm or risk reduction approach takes a broader, public health perspective. The goal of this approach is to reduce risky behaviors and harmful effects of substance use problems. Many harm reduction interventions can be classified in the *precontemplation* phase of change, because dealing with harmful effects of substance abuse helps raise individuals' awareness of their substance abuse.

Developed in the 1980s in response to the spread of the AIDS virus among intravenous drug users, the harm reduction approach holds that abstinence should not be the only objective of health care services to substance abusers. Rather, recovery should be the final goal in a series of harm-reduction objectives that seek to reduce the harm substance abuse causes.

The underlying philosophy of harm reduction is that some people are going to abuse substances regardless of prevention or treatment. Some people may never enter recovery; others will enter recovery at their own pace. From a public health perspective, health care professionals are concerned with the harmful effects of substance abuse, including infections caused by unclean needles, health problems compounded by poor nutrition, and—most important—the spread of AIDS through risky behaviors such as unprotected sex with IV drug users. In this framework, user-friendly services need to be provided so that individuals who abuse substances will receive health care. "User-friendly" means having clinics with easy access and minimal red tape within high-abuse areas, (e.g., a storefront clinic located in a high-use area). Health care workers in these settings need to have a nonjudgmental approach to drug use and provide services such as needle exchange programs, instruction on proper injection techniques, nutrition education, and hepatitis B vaccinations. Methadone maintenance may be suggested when clients are ready to move toward abstinence; however, abstinence should not be actively promoted by the health care providers (Springer, 1991).

ⅢⅢ➡ Clinical Example

Tina is a known intravenous drug user who comes to the Wheels Clinic, which is actually a van equipped to provide preventive health care to known drug users in a specific urban neighborhood. Tina seeks treatment for an abscess at an injection site on her arm. During her treatment, the nurse practitioner asks Tina about her sexual practices and drug habits.

She discusses with Tina some details about cleaning her "works" and then asks her if she has considered alternate (i.e., safer) routes of administration.

Clinical discussion: This case exemplifies how a harm-reduction program for individuals with drug addiction is implemented. The Wheels Clinic is part of a specially funded outreach health care program targeting drug users. The nurse practitioner deals with Tina in a nonjudgmental manner and expresses concern about her health and safety by discussing her drug use and sexual practices.

With alcohol abuse, the harm reduction approach seeks to promote moderate, responsible drinking and decrease problems such as drunk driving, medical complications, and alcohol-related work accidents. Moderate drinking limits are defined as no more than two standard drinks per day, no more than five days per week for women and no more than three standard drinks per day, no more than five days per week for men. In addition, drinking should not take place in potentially hazardous situations such as when operating machinery, when driving, or during pregnancy. The rationale is that since drinking is legal and normative in our society, an important part of prevention is to educate people about safe limits and harmful effects of drinking.

Ⅲ➡ Clinical Example

Derek, age 35, is brought into the emergency room with a broken arm due to falling off a ladder while painting his home. His breath smells like alcohol and his blood alcohol level is just below the legal limit of intoxication. Once his arm is set and put into a cast and he is in a sober state, a nurse who is also a certified addictions counselor meets with him to discuss his alcohol and drug use. He admits to daily drinking of "four or five beers." He has had no previous alcohol-related incidents or accidents, although his wife sometimes complains about his "television watching and drinking." He has no family history of alcoholism and drug abuse.

Based on these assessment data, the nurse counsels Derek in three areas: (1) the limits of sensible drinking, (2) the concept of standard drinks, and (3) the difference between sensible drinking, problem drinking, and dependent drinking. She closes this brief counseling session by saying, "There is some concern about the problems your drinking has created. You have just broken your arm while drinking and your wife seems concerned about your drinking. I think you need to cut down. If you are unable to cut down to sensible drinking, you may need professional help."

Derek is surprised at the feedback. He considers himself a responsible husband and father and thinks of himself as "just a beer drinker." The information about standard drinks is new to him. The nurse hands him an educational brochure about sensible drinking limits and information about Alcoholics Anonymous. She plans to telephone him in a few days to follow up.

Clinical discussion: Derek is classified as a heavy drinker. Using a harm reduction approach, the nurse seeks to raise the client's awareness about the problems created by his drinking. Rather than pushing for abstinence, she educates him about types of drinking patterns and counsels him to cut down. Cutting down should reduce potential for harm to himself, his family, and others. The rationale behind the nurse's intervention is: Drinking is normal and common in our society. Derek's drinking is creating some problems which could be minimized if he cuts down on amount and frequency. If he is not able to cut down, he may need further help.

Harm reduction is an important concept in relation to recovery because often a substance abuse related accident or illness provides impetus for change. Nurses need to use these crisis points as "teachable moments" in which to help penetrate the client's denial system. Providing feedback in a professional, nonjudgmental manner can help move an individual out of the precontemplation stage toward recovery.

Twelve step approach

Another approach to recovery is the twelve step model of which AA is the prototype. In meetings of recovering individuals, participants share their experiences and work through the twelve steps of the program that begins with admitting a powerlessness over substances. For some, this approach evokes a powerful spiritual awakening; for others, the group experiences and relationships with other recovering individuals promote recovery. This approach produces for many people a dramatic, subjective shift in experience. Life is viewed and experienced differently. Individuals are awakened to new possibilities and to a higher level of thinking and feeling. Spiritual awakening involves a belief in a power greater than oneself. Individuals may define this higher power as God, the power of the self-help group as a whole, or a power awakened within themselves. The support received in twelve step groups is itself likened to a spiritual bonding. The twelve steps provide clear and comprehensive guidelines for recovery. (See Box 4-5 for the Twelve Steps of Alcoholics Anonymous.) The twelve steps were developed empirically through group experience; so they do not have a clear theoretical framework, although beliefs about substance abuse as a disease are clearly present. Confidentiality makes research difficult, although the organization itself maintains some statistics. Most treatment programs in the United States include AA principles or are actively organized around the AA principles and steps.

GOALS OF RECOVERY

The goals of recovery are the desired outcome(s) related to the approaches mentioned above (e.g., abstinence with the AA approach, fewer negative consequences with the harm reduction approach). In recent years, there has been a broadening of the goals of recovery beyond abstinence alone, to include the lifestyle changes necessary to maintain recovery. Alternatives to abstinence as an absolute goal are the goals of controlled drinking and drug substitution.

Abstinence

Imagine giving up your favorite food (e.g., chocolate chip cookies, ice cream, or fresh bakery rolls). The food is readily available and offered to you in social settings by your friends. Furthermore, this food has been a source of great enjoyment to you because its use is part of a family ritual (e.g., donuts on Sunday mornings). Giving it up seems impossible and, quite frankly, you don't want to do so.

This example gives some sense of how difficult an abstinence goal is. Drugs, tobacco, and alcohol are readily available in our society. Alcohol especially is socially acceptable and a normal part of many events. Once initial detoxification and treatment have occurred, the individual with an addiction must learn to maintain abstinence in a world full of opportunities to resume using. Murphy (1993) found that remaining abstinent required a multidimensional approach including good coping skills, social support, and environmental control.

Lifestyle change

The addicted individual has focused much of his or her life around the substance of addiction. As a result, dysfunctional patterns of behaving and relating have developed and other more functional behaviors have dropped out. This individual's social circle revolves around substance use. A crucial goal for recovery is to make changes in self and social functioning, family relations, and employment that will support recovery. This lifestyle rehabilitation has been termed a second recovery track following psychological or inner change. This track stresses the importance of learning new pleasures (usually with social support for the process), social integration, and the creation of new goals (Sackon, 1986).

Life without the addictive substance requires a major shift for an individual (Murphy, 1993). Especially during early recovery, the individual may experience feelings of loss, psychological discomfort, or depression. Old relationships may have to be abandoned and, since so much of life was focused on acquiring, using, and withdrawing from the substance of abuse, a whole new social life needs to be developed. A period of grieving for the "lost substance" and previous lifestyle is normal.

New interests, relationships, and healthy activities such as exercise or a hobby are needed. Attendance at AA or Narcotics Anonymous may meet some of these needs. Family relations and employment are two very important components that need to be addressed in recovery.

Family relations are important because the family can be a major support for recovery. Family members may have developed dysfunctional coping strategies with the addicted individual. Often some family members have facilitated the abuse. Addiction affects the entire family system; and for optimal recovery, family members, as well as the client, may need assistance. Research indicates that recovery is more effective when a stable family environment supports it (Finney & Moos, 1992).

Addiction severely affects family subsystems and boundaries. For example, a mother addicted to benzodiazepines and alcohol is less available as a parent; and other family members, often children, may try to fill the mother role. Common roles have been observed in children from families with substance-dependent members.

When the substance-abusing individual begins recovery, the whole family needs to change to accommodate changes in the recovering family member. The family may have patterns of codependence, that is, behaviors of excessive concern and preoccupation with the dependent member that deny and enable the dependence to continue. Family members may have angry feelings about the pain and disruption substance abuse has caused. As the recovering family member assumes more family responsibility, other members may need guidance to reorganize family roles and responsibilities. Families need education on addiction and recovery so they can effectively participate in recovery. Chapter 9 discusses family systems and dysfunctional roles in families in more depth.

Employment also must be considered. If the client is employed and on a leave of absence, details may need to be worked out with the employer concerning job reentry. When an employee assistance program (EAP) is available, an EAP counselor may facilitate job reentry and help with earlier recovery.

If a client is unemployed or has been fired because of substance abuse, vocational counseling may be an important component of recovery. Vocational choices need to allow the individual to actively participate in a program of recovery. When work or the individual's particular vocational skills make this participation problematic, a better short-term choice may be one that will promote recovery.

⫸ Clinical Example

Hyram Johnson, age 33, is enrolled in an outpatient recovery program for his cocaine and alcohol addiction. He was referred to treatment through the EAP at the company where he is a factory supervisor. His job hinges on his cooperation in a treatment program.

Hyram has been divorced for several years and has a five-year-old son whom he rarely sees. Hyram spends off-work time and weekends with other single people who enjoy drinking and using cocaine. To support his cocaine habit, Hyram performs as a "male stripper" at bars and private parties. When his addiction began to interfere with his job as factory supervisor, Hyram realized that his drug and alcohol habits were out of control. He also began to feel that he could not continue his "fast track" lifestyle indefinitely.

Clinical discussion: In order for Hyram to be successful in his recovery, the lifestyle patterns he has developed need to be interrupted and other patterns need to be put in their place. For example, it would be nearly impossible for Hyram to remain substance free while continuing relationships with his partying friends. His current lifestyle, in addition to his loss of family ties, is not conducive to remaining substance free.

A recovery program for Hyram needs to include leisure counseling and explore avenues to provide structure. Boredom is often a key issue in early recovery, because previously so much time and energy were placed on obtaining and using substances. Furthermore, it is important to help Hyram explore family issues, particularly those surrounding his divorce and his role as a divorced parent. Learning to assume parental responsibility for his son is an important facet of Hyram's recovery.

Alternative recovery goals

Controlled drinking. Must an individual addicted to alcohol remain completely abstinent, or is it possible for a recovering individual to resume moderate, controlled drinking? Controlled use as a feasible goal of recovery is very controversial (Wallace, 1990). Even defining controlled drinking is problematic. Heather and Talbott (1989) define controlled drinking as drinking in the absence of intoxication or drinking-related problems. As a practical matter, controlled drinking means a pattern of light or moderate drinking that excludes daily drinking, heavy drinking, or drinking under hazardous conditions such as driving.

Some studies show that controlled drinking may be a suitable goal for selected clients, especially those who are younger, have fewer alcohol-related problems, and are able to select their treatment goals (Miller et al, 1992; McMurran, 1991; Barber, 1991). However, the follow-up for most subjects in these studies was only six months to one year. That length of time is not adequate to determine whether or not controlled drinking is consistent with long-term recovery. Therefore, controlled drinking as a treatment goal must be viewed with caution.

Substance substitution.   Another alternative to abstinence is the use of a substitute for the substance of abuse. Substitution can be a short-term, intermediate, or long-term goal of recovery. The use of benzodiazepines for withdrawal from alcohol is an example of short-term substance substitution. Methadone maintenance for heroin dependence is an example of intermediate and long-term use. In a methadone maintenance program, oral methadone is administered daily. Controversy about methadone programs concerns whether the methadone is part of a prolonged withdrawal (such as one to two years) with the eventual goal of abstinence, or whether the methadone is part of a harm reduction approach in which methadone maintenance is prescribed indefinitely in order to prevent the health risks and criminal activity associated with acquisition and use of heroin. Methadone is given in liquid form and suppresses opiate withdrawal symptoms without providing the euphoria associated with heroin. Because methadone has a longer half-life than heroin (1 to 1.5 days), methadone is only needed once a day to avoid withdrawal symptoms. The individual comes to a clinic daily and is given one dose of methadone. This method of administration brings the client into daily contact with a clinic staff member, often a nurse, and allows regular urine monitoring to determine if other drugs are being used. Because clients are no longer engaged in drug-seeking behavior and are not experiencing a euphoric high from heroin, they may be more amenable to counseling and social rehabilitation (Chenitz, 1989).

Methadone is also addicting, and withdrawal from methadone can be as problematic as withdrawal from heroin. However, methadone withdrawal can be accomplished gradually under controlled, therapeutic circumstances.

Methadone maintenance programs are not problem free. Some clients use methadone in conjunction with other illicit drugs. Others may disseminate or sell methadone. A reputable methadone maintenance program must provide counseling and monitoring of clients, using urine drug screening and frequent clinic visits (Madden, 1991).

⇒ Clinical Example

Meg, age 44, has been addicted to heroin for a number of years. She supports her heroin habit with prostitution. Numerous inpatient treatments have been tried, but Meg always reverts to her addiction and accompanying lifestyle. Despite these treatment failures, Meg persists in trying to gain control over her life. Now enrolled in an outpatient program, Meg tested HIV-positive. This news devastated Meg and she feels more strongly than ever that she wants to stop her addiction. The nurse in the outpatient treatment program develops a positive working relationship with Meg, and together they decide that the best approach for beginning her recovery is a methadone program.

Clinical discussion: This patient has made numerous attempts to discontinue her drug use. A methadone maintenance program is a good option at this point, both from a harm reduction perspective and to assist with long-term withdrawal by gradually tapering dosages. Enrolling her in such a program will reduce her need to continue prostitution, thus reducing the risk of Meg's spreading the AIDS virus. Because Meg is able to establish a working relationship with a nurse, she has the ability to develop an alliance with a methadone clinic worker as well. Through monitoring and counseling, Meg may be able to gradually withdraw from methadone and adopt a drug free lifestyle.

RELAPSE

The most challenging aspect of recovery is preventing relapse. While relapse has been defined as a return to substance abuse, current thinking expands the definition of relapse (and recovery) more broadly. In addition to a return to actual substance abuse, relapse may include a return to the psychological state or mindset that promoted substance abuse initially. Such states often precede the actual abuse.

As with other chronic illnesses, relapse is often considered an aspect of the illness. Seeing relapse as part of the process of the illness, rather than a failure of the client or the treatment system, reverses unwarranted pessimism about recovery. In actuality, relapse is the nature of the illness itself and sometimes part of the individual's testing of whether abstinence is truly required. Substance use following treatment may consist of stretches of abstinence punctuated by slips, periods of intermittent use, brief periods of daily use and/or true long-term relapse (McAuliffe et al, 1991).

Research on relapse has led to a definition of the physiological factors in relapse and to the development of relapse prevention programs that incorporate both physiological and psychological factors. These programs are currently being developed and tested but represent organized programs that anticipate, manage, and/or prevent relapse. The two frameworks for relapse prevention that follow are those of Marlatt and Gorski.

Physiological factors in relapse

Recovery is a physiological phenomenon as well as a psychological and social one. Physical withdrawal from alcohol may last for a number of weeks. Central nervous system excitability such as respiratory irregularity, unstable blood pressure, anxiety, insomnia, and depression may persist long after initial detoxification. This protracted withdrawal syndrome may produce intense craving for alcohol, leading to the desire to drink again. Individuals experiencing these symptoms may not be able to fully benefit from treatment until the symptoms abate. It is important to teach clients about these physiological phenomena. Drug withdrawal, particularly from cocaine, may produce similar symptoms. Craving for cocaine and painful anhedonia may occur for months after treatment. In client education about protracted withdrawal syndrome, the client learns to expect craving, to identify situations that may trigger craving, and to plan coping strategies.

Gorski (1986) described the "post–acute withdrawal syndrome" (PAW) symptoms that begin 7 to 14 days after cessation of drinking. Six symptom clusters were identified: mind-racing, lack of conceptual thought; emotional overreaction; memory problems, both short-term and long-term; psychomotor coordination problems; sleep impairment; and stress-management disorder. He suggested that this syndrome is related to central nervous system damage, which peaks 3 to 6 months after abstinence and requires 6 to 24 months for recovery.

Gorski incorporated this information into an exercise workbook for relapse prevention (1988). Daily study and exercises help clients assess and evaluate potential problems and obstacles to recovery. The emphasis is on diet, physical exercise, rest supplemented by vitamins, and meditation or relaxation.

Models of relapse prevention

Significant research has contributed to understanding relapse and developing relapse prevention techniques using a cognitive-social learning model. In the past, relapse was equated with treatment failure or recidivism and treated as an all-or-none phenomenon. Marlatt suggested a distinction between lapse and relapse. A lapse is a single act of "falling back: a single mistake, an error, a slip" (Marlatt, 1985, p. 32). A lapse can be compared to a fall by an ice skater who quickly recovers and continues to perform. Later, the athlete examines the reason for the slip and how to avoid it in the future. This perception is opposed to interpreting the lapse as a full-blown return to substance use. The goal is to prevent lapse, and, further, to prevent a lapse from becoming a relapse (Marlatt, 1985).

Initial lapse can be seen as a transition phase in the transtheoretical model and may mean the individual is reconsidering the commitment to abstinence. Relapse proneness is related to a combination of predisposing factors such as background and social skills and to actual precipitating factors, such as peer pressure, negative emotional states, and/or anger and resentments. Both the predisposing and precipitating factors are unique to individuals and their backgrounds. The precipitating factors may provoke cues that elicit craving, which may further provoke relapse. The lapses frequently begin with "apparently irrelevant decisions," which lead to high-risk behaviors that may lead to relapse.

The first step in relapse prevention is a thorough assessment of the client's coping skills, including behavioral techniques and cognitive strategies. Intervention builds on developing the skills lacking and strengthening those skills present. These skills include learning warning signs of high-risk behaviors, problem-solving, cognitive self-statements, and restructuring (Mackay et al, 1991).

Gorski's work on relapse prevention developed simultaneously with Marlatt's but within a treatment setting and with the ideological framework of substance abuse as a disease. Gorski worked with clients with multiple relapses. He began investigating relapse episodes using extensive relapse histories and developed a list of 37 common warning signs of relapse. He used this list to develop three categories: *recovery prone,* or those clients likely to recover, 40%; *transitionally relapse prone,* or those clients with some initial relapse characteristics but of a temporary nature, 20%; and *relapse prone,* or those who appeared likely to relapse, 40%. The relapse prone category was further subdivided into *motivated* and *unmotivated* to differentiate clients who appeared to sincerely want recovery from those who didn't. Characteristics that were associated with relapse were high-stress personality or lifestyle, social conflict or instability, poor health maintenance, multiple diagnoses, and an inadequate recovery program.

Gorski linked phases of recovery (Brown, 1985) with specific relapse prevention techniques for each phase (1986). Early-recovery clients needed social structure because early relapse is often due to direct social pressure, absence of coping skills, and chronic stress. Middle-recovery clients needed a balanced lifestyle because relapse during that time is often due to the stress of life changes. Late recovery involved clients' working on personal functioning and childhood issues because relapse then was often due to the inability to cope with unresolved childhood issues.

Some of the strategies assessed and taught throughout relapse prevention include:

1. Identifying high-risk situations
2. Developing specific ways to cope in high-risk situations
3. Identifying signs of craving
4. Modifying environmental situations
5. Practicing coping strategies in real-life situations

Both models suggest that relapse prevention should begin in the treatment setting and that some clients may be at higher risk for relapse than others. Teaching specific relapse information and helping individuals identify their specific warning signs are important components of both programs. An active posttreatment program is crucial in implementing relapse prevention.

⟫ Clinical Example

Pat is a 40-year-old business woman who has completed an intensive outpatient program for treatment of her alcoholism. Pat is continuing in a weekly aftercare group, led by a nurse, for ongoing support in the early recovery period. Pat admits to the group that she has been craving a drink after work the past two nights. The nurse-leader helps the group focus on what situations may have triggered the craving. The nurse explains protracted withdrawal and its relationship to craving. The nurse also emphasizes that craving is normal in early recovery. Group members make several suggestions to Pat about how to deal with these experiences, including restructuring her time after work so that no opportunity for drinking arises. Pat decides that attending AA right after work twice a week (rather than after dinner) is a good suggestion. In addition, she plans to join an exercise class several afternoons a week.

Clinical discussion: Because the nurse helped the group identify high-risk situations and develop ways to cope with these situations, Pat recognized that her drinking time had always been immediately after work and that this time of the day was a specific trigger for her. With the group's help she developed a plan for after-work hours that included activities where alcohol was not accessible. Over time, Pat may become "addicted" to a more positive activity: exercise.

SUMMARY

Recovery involves development of a balanced lifestyle without substances. Individuals need to learn internal controls in order to anticipate and cope effectively with the external pressures imposed by a society where alcohol and drugs are readily available. Systematic relapse prevention work is coupled with intensive involvement in self-help groups that provide the individual with the necessary skills and cognitive strategies needed to maintain sobriety.

REFERENCES

American Nurses Association, Drug and Alcohol Nursing Association, & National Nurses Society on Addictions. (1987). *The care of clients with addictions: Dimensions of nursing practice.* Kansas City, MO: ANA.

Barber, J.G. (1991). Microcomputers and prevention of drug abuse. *MD Computer, 8*(3), 150-155.

Brown, S. (1985). *Treating the alcoholic: A developmental model of recovery.* New York: Wiley.

Chenitz, W.C. (1989). Managing vulnerability: Nursing treatment for heroin addicts. *Image: Journal of Nursing Scholarship, 21*(4), 210-214.

Finney, J.W. & Moos, R.H. (1992). The long-term course of treated alcoholism. *Journal of Studies on Alcohol, 53,* 142.

Gorski, T.T. (1986). Relapse prevention planning. *Alcohol Health and Research World, 11,* 6.

Gorski, T.T. (1988). *The staying sober workbook exercise manual.* Independence, MO: Independence Press.

Grinspoon, L. (Ed.) (1987). Treatment of alcoholism, Part II. *The Harvard Medical School Mental Health Letter, 4*(1), 1-3.

Heather, N. & Talbott, J. (1989). Definitions of non-abstinent and abstinent categories in alcoholism treatment outcome classifications: A review and proposal. *Drug and Alcohol Dependence, 24*(2), 83-93.

Ludwig, A. (1985). Cognitive processes associated with "spontaneous" recovery from alcoholism. *Journal of Studies on Alcohol, 46,* 53.

Mackay, P.W., Donovan, D.M., & Marlatt, G.A. (1991). Cognitive and behavioral approaches to alcohol abuse. In R.J. Frances & S.I. Miller (Eds.), *Clinical textbook of addictive disorders.* New York: Guilford.

Madden, J.S. (1991). Detoxification, pharmacotherapy and maintenance: Drugs. In Ilana Bell Glass (Ed.), *The international handbook of addiction behavior.* (pp 216-224). New York: Tavistock/Routledge.

Marlatt, G.A. (1985). Relapse prevention: Theoretical rationale and overview of the model. In G. Alan Marlatt & Judith R. Gordon (Eds.), *Relapse prevention: Maintenance strategies in the treatment of addictive behaviors.* New York: The Guilford Press.

McAuliffe, W.E., Albert, J., Cordill-London, G., & McGarraghy, T.K. (1991). Contributions to a social conditioning model of cocaine recovery. *International Journal of Addictions, 25* (9A-10A), 1141-77.

McMurran, M. (1991). Young offenders and alcohol-related crime: What interventions will address the issues? *Journal of Adolescence, 14*(3), 245-253.

Miller, W.R., Leckman, A.L., Delaney, H.D., & Tinkcom, M. (1992). Long-term follow-up of behavioral self-control training. *Journal of Studies in Alcohol, 53*(3), 249-261.

Murphy, S.A. (1993). Coping strategies of abstainers from alcohol up to three years post-treatment. *Image: Journal of Nursing Scholarship, 25*(1), 29-35.

Prochaska, J.O. & DiClemente, C.C. (1984). *The transtheoretical approach: Crossing traditional boundaries of therapy.* Homework: Dow Jones Irwin.

Prochaska, J.O., DiClemente, C.C., & Norcross, J.C. (1992). In search of how people change: Applications to addictive behaviors. *American Psychologist, 47,* 1102.

Sackon, F.N. (1986). Lifestyle rehabilitation. *Alcohol Health and Research World, 11,* 18.

Sobell, L.C., Sobell, M.B., Toneatto, T., & Leo, G.I. (1993). What triggers the resolution of alcohol problems without treatment? *Alcoholism: Clinical and Experimental Research, 17,* 217.

Springer, E. (1991). Effective AIDS prevention with active drug users: The harm reduction model. In M. Shernoff (Ed.), *Counseling chemically dependent people with HIV illness.* New York: The Haworth Press, Inc.

Tuchfield, B.S. (1981). Spontaneous remission in alcoholics: Empirical observations and theoretical implications. *Journal of Studies on Alcohol, 42,* 626.

Wallace, J. (1990). Controlled drinking, treatment, effectiveness, and the disease model of addiction: A commentary on the ideological wishes of Stanton Peele. *Journal of Psychoactive Drugs, 22*(3), 261-284.

UNIT

II

NURSING CARE OF CLIENTS WITH SUBSTANCE ABUSE

6   Dimensions of Nursing Care of Clients with Substance Abuse

7   Nursing Care of Clients with Substance Abuse in the Hospital

8   Substance Abuse in Perinatal Care

9   Substance Abuse in Families, Children, and Adolescents

10 Nursing Care of Clients with Substance Abuse in Community Settings

11 Nursing Care in Chemical Dependency Treatment Settings

12 Dual Diagnosis: A Challenge for Mental Health and Substance Abuse Caregivers

13 Nursing Care of Special Populations

6

Dimensions of Nursing Care of Clients with Substance Abuse

Nurses are in a unique position to identify substance abuse and intervene with clients. Any client may be affected by substances, either directly from use or indirectly through a significant other's use. To provide competent care to these clients, nurses need to examine their own attitudes about substance abuse and acquire specialized knowledge about addictions and required care. This chapter describes the basic steps of using the nursing process with clients who abuse substances, the standards of addictions nursing practice, and nursing care for six troublesome behaviors frequently encountered by nurses.

Nurses' attitudes and feelings about substance use and abuse that accumulate from their own experiences can affect the quality of nursing care. Reisman and Schrader (1984) correlated positive attitudes and knowledge with referral rates for treatment. As knowledge and self-awareness of personal attitudes and feelings increased, nurses' capacity for empathetic care for clients increased.

First, nurses must understand the disease of addiction, its risk factors, how it develops, and its expected progression and subsequent symptoms. Hope for treatment success follows an understanding of the disease process. Second, nurses must be familiar with the options for treatment, and for whom each option might be successful. Third, the nursing process must be individualized for each client and appropriately applied. Last, available support and treatment options in the community must be identified.

Nurses need competent assessment skills to identify a person with substance abuse difficulties. Typically, changes occur in the psychosocial, biological, cognitive/perceptual, and spiritual dimensions of such a person's life (ANA, 1987). These changes are usually evident in physical or behavioral signs and symptoms.

Excellent interpersonal skills are necessary and important in the nursing care of a client with substance abuse. An accepting, nonjudgmental, caring attitude is essential. Even a hostile or uncooperative client responds to a caring, nonthreatening nurse. Most substance abusers are extremely sensitive to caregivers who are rejecting or judgmental. Nurses must be able to listen, be supportive, and use measures

117

to establish rapport with clients. Since clients may be defensive for several reasons, it is important to be nonthreatening. Both denial about substance use and cognitive impairment from intoxication, withdrawal, or long-term use may predispose clients to defensiveness.

Several considerations help nurses deal with defensiveness. In general, nurses should explain their purpose in being there and any procedures to be done, and they should provide clients with an opportunity to have questions answered. Responding with empathy toward any emotions expressed is especially important. It is common for nurses to feel anger or disgust at clients who are foul-smelling, combative, or yelling abusive language. It is helpful to be aware that this behavior is part of the disorder and usually can be managed. If clients are angry, reflecting the feeling expressed or implied helps them know the nurse understands. It may be necessary to reorient clients frequently if they are intoxicated or withdrawing from alcohol or drugs. Often, inappropriate behavior is a response to misperceptions of the environment.

After rapport is established, nurses must use skill to elicit pertinent information for assessment and subsequent care. A particularly difficult aspect of the interpersonal relationship with a client with substance abuse is the extensive use of denial. Denial is defined as refusal to accept or acknowledge the reality or validity of a thing or idea (Gove, 1971). This denial is pervasive and involves aspects of the addiction and other parts of the client's life. Nurses need skill in recognizing denial when it occurs and how to intervene.

Nurses need the courage and ability to communicate successfully with the family and to keep other health care professionals informed. This is not always as easy as it might seem. Many health professionals may demonstrate the same denial that the client does. In fact, denial of alcohol and drug problems is typical throughout modern society. Nurses serve as liaisons between the health care system and family and between the client and others—while functioning as team members in planning and carrying out care.

USING THE NURSING PROCESS

The nursing process provides a framework for planning and intervention with clients with substance abuse. These clients need careful assessment, appropriate nursing diagnoses, individualized plans of care, and steps for identifying outcomes, intervening, and evaluating care. Standards have been developed by the American Nurses Association to guide nursing practice with addicted clients (ANA, 1988). These standards provide criteria for providing care to addicted clients whether a nurse is on a medical unit, a psychiatric unit, or is a specialist nurse on an addictions treatment unit (Box 6-1).

Assessing the client

Assessment of drug and alcohol history is accomplished as a normal part of the complete history and physical examination. It is extremely important to obtain an accurate history of drug or alcohol use. Identification is crucial in helping the client

Box 6-1
Standards of Addictions Nursing Practice

Standard I. Theory

The nurse uses appropriate knowledge from nursing theory and related disciplines in the practice of addictions nursing.

Standard II. Data collection

Data collection is continual and systematic and is communicated effectively to the treatment team throughout each phase of the nursing process.

Standard III. Diagnosis

The nurse uses nursing diagnoses congruent with accepted nursing and interprofessional classification systems of addictions and associated physiological and psychological disorders to express conclusions supported by data obtained through the nursing process.

Standard IV. Planning

The nurse establishes a plan of care for the client that is based upon nursing diagnoses, addresses specific goals, defines expected outcomes, and delineates nursing actions unique to each client's needs.

Standard V. Intervention

The nurse implements actions independently and/or in collaboration with peers, members of other disciplines, and clients in prevention, intervention, and rehabilitation phases of the care of clients with health problems related to patterns of abuse and addiction.

Standard V-A. Intervention: therapeutic alliance

The nurse uses the "Therapeutic Self" to establish a relationship with clients and to structure nursing interventions to help clients develop the awareness, coping skills, and behavior changes that promote health.

Standard V-B. Intervention: education

The nurse educates clients and communities to help them prevent and/or correct actual or potential health problems related to patterns of abuse and addiction.

Standard V-C. Intervention: self-help groups

The nurse uses the knowledge and philosophy of self-help groups to assist clients in learning new ways to address stress, maintain self-control, or sobriety, and integrate healthy coping behaviors into their life-style.

Standard V-D. Intervention: pharmacological therapies

The nurse applies knowledge of pharmacological principles in the nursing process.

Standard V-E. Intervention: therapeutic environment

The nurse provides, structures, and maintains a therapeutic environment in collaboration with the individual, family, and other professionals.

Continued.

Box 6-1
Standards of Addictions Nursing Practice—cont'd

Standard V-F. Intervention: counseling

The nurse uses therapeutic communication in interactions with the client to address issues related to patterns of abuse and addiction.

Standard VI. Evaluation

The nurse evaluates the responses of the client and revises nursing diagnoses, interventions, and the treatment plan accordingly.

Standard VII. Ethical care

The nurse's decisions and activities on behalf of clients are in keeping with personal and professional codes of ethics and in accord with legal statues.

Standard VIII. Quality assurance

The nurse participates in peer review and other staff evaluation and quality assurance processes to ensure that clients with abuse and addiction problems receive quality care.

Standard IX. Continuing education

The nurse assumes responsibility for his or her continuing education and professional development and contributes to the professional growth of others who work with or are learning about persons with abuse and addiction problems.

Standard X. Interdisciplinary collaboration

The nurse collaborates with the interdisciplinary treatment team and consults with other health care providers in planning, implementing, and evaluating programs and other activities related to addictions nursing.

Standard XI. Use of community health systems

The nurse participates with other members of the community in planning, implementing, and evaluating community health services that attend to primary, secondary, and tertiary prevention of addictions.

Standard XII. Research

The nurse contributes to the nursing care of clients with addictions and to the addictions area of practice through innovations in theory and practice and participation in research, and communicates these contributions.

From American Nurses Association. (1988). *Standards of addiction nursing practice with selected diagnoses and criteria.* Kansas City, MO: The Association.

---

obtain treatment for the disorder. Substance use may be evident in the presenting symptoms, or it may be hidden. In either case potential withdrawal symptoms must be identified.

The first step is to determine the type of substance used and whether one substance only or a combination of several substances was used. Questions to elicit this information might include: What is the predominant substance of choice? Are these substances "street drugs" or prescription drugs? (Street drugs may contain a variety of unwanted contaminants in addition to the substance of choice.)

Next, determine how much of and when each substance was last taken. For the last episode of use, determine the amount used, asking about each substance separately. How long did this episode last? Try to determine the pattern of use. How much does the client use or drink in a usual episode? How many drinks (first determine size of drink), how many pills, or how many "hits" (a user term for each snort, injection, etc.)? Through what route are these substances taken (e.g., by mouth, smoked, injection)? How often does this occur (daily, several times a week, weekly, or in binges)? How often do binges occur?

Also, find out the history of past use. Is there a history of seizures or hallucinations during drug or alcohol withdrawal? Does the client have a history of liver disease, anemia, or overdoses? Has there been any history of falls, injuries, or accidents, especially related to use? (for a detailed use-history tool, see Box 3-1). It is important for the nurse to realize that the information given is probably at least *somewhat* inaccurate because of the client's denial. If possible, verify information with family or other persons who have observed the client's use.

Assessment questions need to be given to women as well as men. Frequently, women substance abusers, whose use may be more hidden than men's, are not assessed for substance problems. One study found that alcoholism was higher among unemployed women than those employed and among women 30 years of age or older (Kress, 1989). In addition, significantly more alcoholic women than nonalcoholic women were "homemakers."

Women who are addicted to substances may appear for health care services with nonspecific symptoms, such as anxiety, depression, or inability to sleep, and may be seeking tranquilizer medication. These women are more likely than men to have low self-esteem, to suffer from depression, self-blame, anxiety, and agoraphobia (Kress, 1989), and to experience body-image distortions such as those associated with anorexia and bulimia.

Physical assessment.   A careful physical assessment is necessary for the client with substance abuse (see Box 3-1). There may be acute alterations in physical state or alterations that are long-term and chronic. This assessment begins with taking the client's vital signs and looking for symptoms of possible substance overdose, followed by evaluation of the stage of physical withdrawal and a system-by-system assessment of complications. A urine specimen is obtained for a drug screen. (If an order has not yet been written, the specimen can be frozen until it is obtained.) A blood alcohol concentration is necessary for anyone suspected of drinking. Evaluate also the client's overall level of hygiene, fluid balance, and nutritional status.

The head, neck, and musculoskeletal and integumentary systems are assessed for presence of trauma. Broken bones, bruises, alterations in hydration status, edema, or general skin discoloration may be found. The breast and axilla examination may reveal gynecomastia, lesions, or masses.

The respiratory system is assessed for breathing pattern and signs of respiratory distress. Use of alcohol or drugs may result in or exacerbate such disorders as asthma, emphysema, chronic bronchitis, or chronic obstructive pulmonary disease. Because alcohol decreases respirations, pneumonia is common in those who drink excessively.

Many abused substances have a profound effect upon the cardiovascular system. Assessment may reveal an arrhythmia or any of a number of chronic cardiovascular difficulties. Use of alcohol or drugs also may result in a variety of gastrointestinal disorders. Anorexia and cachectic presentation are common. Alcoholics frequently have ascites and edema. Ruptured esophageal varices and pancreatitis are emergency conditions and are most frequently secondary results of alcohol use. Liver enlargement is common. A neurological examination may reveal a number of problems, ranging from hyperreflexia to peripheral neuropathy. Sleep disorders also are common.

Psychological assessment.   A mental-status examination gives the nurse information about the status of the client's cognitive processes, feeling states, and general level of functioning (see Box 3-1). The first evaluations in psychological status are for alertness and the level of consciousness. Next, what is the client's general appearance and behavior? How appropriate are the client's dress, grooming, and responses? What are the client's general posture, level of activity, and general facial expression? Are they compatible with the current situation? Is the client cooperative and responding appropriately to stimuli, or combative or nonresponsive? Does the client's behavior, such as a raised voice, threatening manner or stance, or verbal threats, suggest that the person might become violent?

What is the client's general mood? Is it congruent with the topic of conversation or the client's current situation? Does the mood change appropriately with changes in conversation? What is the intensity of the mood? Many substance users explain that they use substances because of feeling anxious or depressed.

What are the characteristics of the client's speech? Is speech slurred or clear? Does the client talk softly or loudly, rapidly or slowly? Is he or she coherent? Are answers to questions relevant to the questions asked? Are thoughts organized, is the speech pattern logical or rambling? Are there evidences of maladaptive speech patterns?

What are the client's thoughts and perceptions? Is the client in touch with reality? Hallucinating? Is there evidence of anxiety or phobias?

Alcoholics and drug users are at increased risk for suicide. While 1% of the general population is at risk for suicide, 15% of alcoholics have this risk (Trenk, 1986). Nurses must ask if clients have any thoughts of suicide. If the answer is "yes," follow up with questions determining the proposed method and whether or not the person has access to the method. If the method is lethal, and the client's ideation is serious, the suicide risk is extreme; steps must be taken to protect him or her.

Cognitive function is often disrupted in the chemically dependent client. First, the client must be assessed for orientation: person, place, time, and knowledge of the current situation. Then, how intact is the client's memory? Can the client remember the content of the last meal (recent memory)? Can the client remember family birthdates, or personal health history (long-term memory)? Attention can be measured by determining how attentive the client is to the current conversation. Do questions need to be repeated often? Concentration can be evaluated by requesting sequential subtractions such as by seven's from 100 or by three's from 25, depending on the expected competence of the client. A good measure for insight and judgment is the client's thoughts about the current situation. Does the client consider the use and abuse of substances a problem? Does the client recognize a chemical dependency? If so, is the client willing to seek treatment?

Is there evidence of mental illness? Anxiety and depressive disorders are highly correlated with substance abuse (NIAAA, 1991). The client who has bipolar affective disorder frequently may overindulge in chemical use (NIAAA, 1991). The use of cocaine and marijuana has been associated with an increase in psychotic disorders. The client with substance abuse may have an underlying mental disorder that also may need attention (see Chapter 12).

Social assessment.   A genogram is helpful in obtaining a family assessment. A genogram is a format for drawing a family tree that records information about family members and their relationships for at least three generations. Genograms provide a quick and visual means to identify the complex relationships within a family. All family members need to be identified and the relationships between significant family members described. Health status, family history of alcoholism, eating disorders, sexual or physical abuse, or other disruptions in the family (e.g., moves, desertions, divorces, accidents) are obtained (see Box 3-1).

What are the client's current living arrangements? Is there a stable family? How stable are these arrangements? Is there a support network, and what is the stability of this network?

What is the client's current economic condition? Is the client employed? What is the length of employment? Is the client able to live within his or her income?

Is there a history of legal problems? Is the client currently charged with a crime? Is it a felony or a misdemeanor? Is the client on probation? From what? Is the client being sued by anyone?

Spiritual assessment.   The client with substance abuse frequently experiences spiritual distress. Spirituality is sometimes a difficult area for nurses to assess, partially because of the wide interpretations of the term. It is useful to ask the client to state his source of hope. Does the client have a source of strength? Does the client believe in God? Does the client pray? Is that helpful? Have current circumstances affected the client's spiritual beliefs? What is meaningful or frightening right now?

Nursing diagnoses

Since the use of drugs or alcohol results in a variety of effects, almost any nursing diagnosis approved by the North American Nursing Diagnosis Association (NANDA) may be appropriate for a particular client. Twenty-five nursing diagnoses, however, have been identified as those most frequently encountered in the addicted client (ANA, 1988). (See Table 3-1.)

PLANNING CARE

Because of the wide-ranging effects of ingestion of alcohol or drugs over time, the client needs care in all aspects of life. There are, however, four main goals in the care of the addicted client. First, the client's safety must be maintained and care provided humanely. Second, a therapeutic relationship is developed so that the nurse can provide safe and caring support for the client. Third, the nurse helps the client recognize abuse of substances. Last, the nurse needs to know where and how to refer the client and family for subsequent care (Plumlee, in press).

Nursing interventions need to be directed toward the presenting problems of the client with substance abuse just as with any other client. Physical or psychological illness is often the crisis that may provide impetus for the client to recognize difficulties with substance use. During a time of crisis, the wall of denial often crumbles momentarily. It is very important to intervene by presenting reality and getting the client to accept treatment before the denial again becomes solid.

Often nurses have a closer relationship with a client than other caregivers and are with the client around the clock. This proximity and relationship form the foundation for gentle confrontation about the use of substances. It is critically important for the nurse to consistently connect the problems and consequences of abuse to the abuse and to avoid any response that might enable the client to continue denying problems with use of chemicals. Since a main goal for this client is for him or her to acknowledge that the use of chemicals is the source of problems, the nurse must be consistent in allowing the client to experience and face pain. It often is easy to try to soften the blows and rescue the client from this reality.

It may not be possible for the nurse to motivate the client to go into treatment. It is realistic, however, to expect these interventions to push the client gently toward facing reality sometime in the future. The goal is to obtain acceptance of the need for treatment and to begin treatment. A client who accepts the need for treatment has a good chance of recovering from illness.

Intervention and referral

Close cooperation among the health care team is essential when working with addicted clients. The nurse can facilitate this coordination. These clients often manipulate staff members against one another in order to maintain denial. Such maneuvers may involve pitting nurse against nurse, nurse against aide, or nurse against physician or facility administrators. It is essential to have agreement among team members that these clients do have a substance abuse problem and to sustain a consistent approach without enabling clients' denial or allowing manipulation. A defined protocol with such clients benefits all parties involved—assisting clients into treatment and team members into collaboration with one another.

Addictive disease is a family disease. All members of the family have been affected by it. It is important to include the family in the plan of care as much as possible. In the first place, families are often the most accurate source of information about clients' use of chemicals, behaviors, and current circumstances. Addicted clients frequently describe their circumstances more positively than is true.

The family of a substance abuser is usually experiencing extreme stress and subsequent pain. The members need empathy and emotional support badly and usually appreciate them when given. Often family members' denial of the problem presents an obstacle to their participation in breaking the denial of the client and moving him or her toward treatment. It is common for the family of the substance abuser to be extremely dysfunctional. If the marriage has stayed intact, members may be severely enmeshed and overinvolved with the substance abuser. These members need to be helped to meet their own needs. Typically a female spouse may stay with the addict, while the male spouse may leave his addicted wife. If the family has remained intact, the prognosis for treatment is enhanced. This support system can become increasingly functional with family therapy, either through a substance abuse treatment facility or through other counseling.

Education about addictive disease—how it develops and progresses, its symptoms, and the most frequently demonstrated behaviors—potentially provides perspective to family members. As family members learn that the disease is predictable and treatable, hope may be restored and they may be willing to take whatever steps are needed to help the client receive treatment and to obtain help for themselves.

Because the opportunity for receiving the client's agreement to treatment is often very limited, the nurse needs a repertoire of available resources. A list of treatment service alternatives may be obtained from several sources. Ideally, there is a certified addictions nurse or other substance abuse expert available, but this may not be the case. Other sources for obtaining information are the National Council on Alcohol and Drug Dependence and state or local community departments for alcohol and drug abuse.

It is important for the nurse to inquire about treatment facilities for women, whether a given facility takes women, and especially where there are women-only facilities. There are far fewer treatment facilities for women than for men, but women have a greater chance at recovery if treated where women's issues are addressed. Other important resources for women include arrangements for child care, specialized care for pregnancy, and services for women victimized by abuse or other forms of violence. From 60% to 75% of women in alcohol and drug treatment facilities have experienced sexual abuse (Kress, 1989). These women need groups for women only in which to deal with painful memories.

Often, the family and the health care team are in agreement that the client does need help for addiction. It may be decided that he or she probably will not willingly seek treatment. At this time, it is often helpful to call in an addictions professional to carry out a formal "intervention," in which the professional coordinates a carefully orchestrated group confrontation. The group may involve the nurse, family members, friends, colleagues, or work supervisor of the client. Each member is asked to write a letter to the client describing how the addiction has affected him or her. Then, they all meet with the client under the direction of the professional and read the letters to the client. Usually this heavy dose of reality given by persons who care about the client breaks the denial, at least momentarily, and the individual will agree to go for evaluation.

Before the intervention, an appointment is made with the substance abuse counselor for evaluation of the client, and a treatment setting with an opening is chosen. Identification of a third-party payer is made if one is available. Without this assistance, treatment alternatives may be limited. Immediately upon completion of the intervention, the client is taken for evaluation before the client changes his or her mind. (See Chapter 10 for more information about interventions.)

Even if the nurse does not participate in a formal intervention process, there is often opportunity to intervene briefly with the client by presenting reality that contradicts the client's view of the world. With enough of these small interventions, eventually the client may acknowledge the problem. If he or she continues to deny the problem, it is important for the nurse to accept this decision and yet provide an opening for the client to change his or her mind. It is important to make clear that if the client changes his or her mind, the nurse will be available to discuss the topic further.

The nurse, using information obtained through the assessment, can intervene by informing the client of the seriousness of drinking or drug use. Then an attempt can be made to get the client to reduce use. The lone realization that it is impossible to reduce use for a prolonged period of time can convince the client of his or her need for treatment.

EVALUATION

The major criteria for evaluation of nursing care for a client using substances are:
1. The client safely undergoes detoxification and withdrawal.
2. The client recognizes the use of substances as detrimental. Since the likelihood of reaching this goal in one short-term hospital stay may be dim, a small advance can be measured for evaluation.
3. The client connects use of substances to the problems and consequences encountered. An appropriate evaluation criterion would be a concrete, specific, and realistic step toward making this connection.
4. The client and the family agree to continued treatment for the substance abuse (Plumlee, in press).

Outcome criteria should be stated in terms that can be measured by the client's or family's response to nursing care. In addition to the above major criteria for evaluation, each client will have individualized nursing diagnoses. Outcome criteria for each diagnosis should reflect progress toward resolution of the diagnosis.

Continuity of care

Any client identified with substance abuse needs follow-up upon discharge. Even if the client has refused to acknowledge problems with substance use or abuse, follow-up is necessary. The client or the family needs telephone numbers of persons or organizations from whom they may receive help. The National Council on Alcoholism and Drug Dependence has a collection of literature that may be given to clients or their families. This organization has a variety of services, from referral resources to information about the disease, to client evaluation, and classes for family members.

Any client or family member who is receptive should be referred to support groups such as Alcoholics Anonymous or Al-Anon (the organization for family members), or any of the other related twelve step support groups (see Chapter 4).

Other groups that usually are listed in the telephone directory are Adult Children of Alcoholics, Codependents Anonymous, or Overeaters Anonymous.

Some families will need assistance from social services for any number of complications resulting from the substance abuse of a member. This may be anything from financial assistance to difficulties with parenting or need for legal assistance.

Nursing care related to recovery status

Nursing care for the client with substance abuse varies with the person's recovery status. An acknowledged and diagnosed addict who is in recovery requires special assistance to maintain that recovery. A health care crisis can trigger relapse in a recovering client. This client needs understanding and support in his efforts to maintain sobriety. The client usually is aware of what is needed and is willing to discuss this with the health care team. Since many pain and sleep medications are addictive, use of these medications may trigger relapse. It is imperative for the physician and other care providers to be educated about relapse potential and the client's need for additional support during a health crisis. In addition, family members may need assistance and support at this time. The health care crisis may have triggered their fears of a relapse, and assurance that the team is collaborating to assist the client may relieve some fears. They also may need education about relapse and defenses against it.

Some clients have problems with drugs and alcohol but do not recover. Many clients are admitted to health care facilities with medical diagnoses other than substance abuse but may have an unidentified and undiagnosed substance abuse disorder. Others may have been diagnosed but have refused treatment. The nurse will encounter all of these types of clients in various clinical settings. (Information about nursing care in clinical specialties is found in Chapters 7 through 13.)

MANAGING BEHAVIOR PROBLEMS IN CLIENTS WITH SUBSTANCE ABUSE

Frequently addicted clients demonstrate behaviors that can interfere with the nurse's ability to provide care. These behaviors include (1) excessive use of denial, (2) use of manipulation, (3) hostility, (4) need to control, (5) drug-seeking behavior while in a treatment setting, and (6) pessimism regarding treatment success. The nurse will be able to provide better care and will be comfortable in working with these clients by learning how to deal with such behaviors.

Denial

Denial is a core component of the disease of chemical dependency. As the disease develops, so does the denial system. It protects people against the consequences of the disease but also locks them into repeated patterns of self-destruction. Denial may develop as a result of the person's ego defense mechanisms, or as defense against the painful realities of the consequences of substance abuse. Organic changes in the brain from substance use further augment the denial system. Blackouts develop early in the disease of alcoholism. During blackouts, the person appears to be functioning normally but remembers nothing of these periods when sober. The person genuinely may not recall events that occurred during intoxication. Later in the disease, organic brain damage further keeps the person from being aware of what is happening. The end result is a deeply entrenched delusional system. This delusional system revolves around the belief that the person is in control of his or her life and that the substance enhances moods and causes little damage.

Many times the health professional inadvertently reinforces or enables the denial by either directly or indirectly allowing the person's view of the world to stand without challenge. In order for persons to obtain help for their disease, they must at least question whether or not they have a problem.

A variety of defenses protects the denial system. First is simple denial, the belief that something is not so. Next is minimizing or downplaying the significance of a situation or an event although acknowledging it exists. Frequently, the client reinforces the denial system by blaming painful circumstances on something or someone outside the self (e.g., "I just lost my job" or "My wife left me"). Another way of reinforcing denial is to rationalize or explain away difficulties (although the explanation is inaccurate). In addition, many of these explanations are in theoretical terms, thus the client withdraws from the emotional impact of problems. A common method of reinforcing denial is to divert attention away from the painful subject. Often nurses will find themselves discussing unrelated subjects with the client and wonder how this occurred. Last, the client's hostility is very effective in reinforcing denial when uncomfortable topics are approached. Hostility usually causes a nurse to retreat and change the subject because of the discomfort encountered.

In order for a person to receive help for substance abuse, that person must first acknowledge that there is a problem. Next, the person must be convinced of the nature of the problem. Last, the person must be convinced that something must be done about the problem.

The person with a substance abuse disorder must be helped to face the reality of the situation. The term "confrontation" often erroneously conjures up thoughts of aggressive verbal assault in the nurse. Haber (1987) explains that confrontation can be constructive as well as destructive. She describes constructive confrontation thus:

> [It] . . . means responsible unmasking of discrepancies, evasions, distortions, games, and smoke screens the client uses to hide from both self-understanding and behavioral change. It calls attention to discrepancies between what the client says (verbal communication) and what the client does (nonverbal communication). It involves challenging clients' undeveloped, underdeveloped, unused, and misused skills and resources. It also helps clients examine the consequences of behavior. Constructive confrontation is not attacking or blaming clients "for their own good." Destructive or punitive confrontation may relieve the aggressor of a burden, but it does not help the other person learn to live more effectively.

Confrontation takes place within a caring, trusting relationship. It is important to be nonjudgmental, matter of fact, and accepting of the person. A firm approach is needed, with patience and persistence. It is not likely that the person will immediately acknowledge substance abuse difficulties. Each time a person uses any of the variations of denial, the nurse must resist allowing these mechanisms to terminate the discussion. Return to the discussion at hand and attempt to establish a significant connection between the drinking or drugging and the repeated harmful consequences. Point out inconsistencies as they occur and give the person feedback about his or her diagnostic conclusion, citing specific examples as evidence for this conclusion (Box 6-2).

Forchuk and Westwell (1987) point out that denial is a defense for excessive anxiety. They suggest that the nurse can feel more successful with clients in denial if the level of confrontation is tailored to the anxiety level of the client. They believe that excessive anxiety strengthens the denial, so reality orientation must be gradual and gentle. Sometimes, all that can be accomplished is for the nurse to agree only with the portion of the client's view that is true. Often, other recovering persons are the most successful in breaking into a client's denial system.

Manipulation

Manipulation is defined as an enduring use of patterns of behavior aimed at immediately satisfying one's needs while disregarding the rights and needs of others. Typically, manipulation triggers powerful emotions in others. Therefore, it is common for the nurse to feel anger, frustration, or indifference toward the manipulative client.

The client using substances frequently has difficulty delaying gratification of needs or desires. In addition, an attempt to control others and the surrounding environment is used to protect the denial system and to prevent others from dis-

---

Box 6-2
Confronting Denial

Have a caring attitude.
Use a matter-of-fact approach.
Focus on the present.
State feedback in objective terms.
Give feedback after detoxification.
Give feedback privately.
Reflect back feelings—both expressed and implied.
Avoid labeling terms.
Use open-ended, specific, factual questions.
Insistently probe for details.
Return to main task after any diversions.
Never discuss inaccurate explanations of problems with client.
If unsuccessful, do not push, but try again later.

Modified from Kinney, J. (1991). *Clinical manual of substance abuse.* St. Louis: Mosby; Chappel, J.N. (1980). Confronting the alcohol and drug abusing patient. *Seminars in Family Medicine, 1*(4), 249-254; *Dealing with denial.* (1975). Center City, MN: Hazelden Educational Materials.

cussing any results of substance use. Manipulation may provide a sense of security and control when the client's life may be very much out of control. The end result for the client is distance and superficiality in interpersonal relationships and a lowering of self-esteem each time this kind of interaction occurs.

The first rule in managing manipulative behavior is for the nurse to set firm and clearly defined limits on behavior. Consistency is essential! It is useless for one nurse to set limits while others who deal with this client allow manipulation to occur. Therefore, all nursing staff members must be in agreement on how to manage the client and carry out plans consistently. One's own feelings are a significant clue that the client is trying to manipulate. If a nurse begins to feel very angry, depressed, or confused, it may be an indication that he or she is being manipulated. If the feelings are too intense, it may be therapeutic to break away from the client for a short time and return later.

It is important for the manipulator to realize how the behavior affects others. The nurse can help the client analyze behaviors that distance the client from others. A helpful comment is, "When you manipulate me, I feel angry with you and feel like leaving you alone. Is that what you want to happen?" It is helpful to try to get the manipulator to express feelings verbally by asking a question such as "What are you feeling right now?" If the client refuses to recognize the inappropriateness of the behavior, the nurse should refuse to "play the game" (e.g., interact in this fashion). The subject should be changed or the nurse should leave the situation.

There are several useful evaluation criteria for measuring progress in the manipulative client:

1. The client recognizes and verbalizes the manipulative behavior that is demonstrated.
2. The client asks directly for what he wants or needs.
3. The client demonstrates alternative ways to meet needs.
4. The client demonstrates learning from past experiences.

Box 6-3 lists limit-setting nursing actions.

Hostility

The client with a substance abuse disorder uses hostility for many reasons. First, it serves to cause others to back off when anything related to the use of substances is mentioned. Besides defending the denial system, hostility may result from a client's low frustration tolerance and difficulty in delaying gratification. Substance abusers generally have an external referencing system. That is, these individuals usually attribute any causes for their circumstances to something or someone outside of themselves. As a result, they do not take responsibility for their own actions but blame others for their problems.

When the client expresses hostility, the nursing goals are, first, to manage the hostility so that it will not escalate into acting-out or violence. In addition, hostility must not be allowed to divert confrontation and connection of substance use with adverse consequences. Last, it is hoped the client will be helped to acquire self-knowledge and learn how to cope with frustration in more appropriate ways.

The nurse's first step in dealing with hostility is to let the client know that the anger is heard. A statement such as "You seem very angry about this" will some-

---

Box 6-3
Limit Setting

Expectations

Make expectations clear to client and other staff members.

Client-centered limits

Be sure limits are in the best interest of the client and not punitive.

Communication

Avoid using personal statements, such as "I don't want you to drink alcohol while I'm on duty." Offer the true rationale: "Alcohol is not allowed in the hospital."

Consequences

When consequences are needed, avoid those that are absurd or cannot be enforced, such as "Put the alcohol away or I won't come into your room." Offer only enforceable consequences, such as "If you don't dispose of the alcohol, I will call security to dispose of it."

Testing

Remain firm and consistent as the client tests the limits that have been set.

Venting

Allow the client to vent feelings about limits, but do not become engaged in power struggles or attempt to rationalize (e.g., "The hospital policy was written because things would get out of control if all clients could drink alcohol. . . ."). Instead, verify the client's feelings and repeat the limit as necessary: "I hear that you are angry about this, but alcohol is not allowed."

Positive reinforcement

Return to the client's room when the affect has subsided to demonstrate that you are not angry and have not withdrawn from the client. Offer positive reinforcement for strengths.

Clarifications for staff

Explain the expectations, limits, and consequences discussed with the client to all staff members to provide consistency and avoid confusion.

From Ellis N.K. (1993). Manipulation. In R.P. Rawlins & S.R. Williams, *Mental health-psychiatric nursing: A holistic life-cycle approach.* St. Louis: Mosby.

times achieve this end. Then ascertain whether or not the client is aware of the anger. The next step is to try to connect the hostility to what happened just before the feelings. This might have been reference to the chemical dependency problem or something else. In the case of hostility in response to discussion of chemical dependency, connecting the anger to the discussion of this topic is helpful. If the client connects the hostility with the previous event, then it is appropriate to help him or her reexamine the response. What was the meaning to the client of the event or conversation? How did the client experience this as a threat? This process is thought-provoking and has the potential to increase self-awareness.

Hostility can escalate into violence, so it is important for the nurse to be alert for clues that such escalation might be taking place. Early indications of escalation are signs of excessive anxiety: shouting, pacing, clenched fist or jaw, flushed face or pallor, or talking to himself or herself through clenched teeth. When the nurse reflects back the perceived anger and the client hears sufficiently, he or she will usually shout back something like "Of course I'm angry." It is acceptable for the client to vent anger verbally through complaining about the source of anger. It is not acceptable for the client to act out the anger, so it is important for the nurse to set limits on behavior.

On the rare occasion that a client who is angry appears to be continuing to escalate, it is important for the nurse to remain calm. Any violent act such as throwing something or slamming a door is an indication of impending violence. It is important to not corner the client. The nurse must not remain alone with the client but get help with assisting the client to regain control.

Need to control

It has been said that an addictive disease is a disease of the will. Inherent in the substance abuse itself is the need to control when, where, and how much of the substance is ingested. Acknowledgment of lack of control itself breaks the denial system; therefore, addicted clients will contend that they can control their use of the substance. This delusion of control will exhibit itself in many other aspects of life also. Clients will go to extreme ends to convince themselves that they are in control and will attempt to control family members and the nurse as well. Whether in the hospital for medical care or in a substance abuse facility, these clients will attempt to control care, often becoming very difficult for those attempting to provide care. This is an especially difficult problem with health care professionals who have a substance abuse problem (see Chapter 13).

The best way to handle this need to control is to recognize that it exists and to use it in the care of clients. The nurse may have to give up a little control in some areas. Clients need to be involved in their treatment plans. The nurse needs to allow clients to have some control over daily activities—in such small ways as asking if they want their baths before or after breakfast. Clients with substance abuse usually have very low self-esteem. Helping identify strengths and using these strengths in any way possible in care will assist in increasing this self-esteem. Clients can contribute to their plan of care by sharing their needs and ideas. On a psychiatric unit, a client with leadership abilities can organize client activities. It is important to try to channel clients' talents in a socially acceptable way.

Growth takes place when clients learn self-control and acceptance of responsibility. Hospitalized clients who have regularly used alcohol or drugs are likely to be craving them. This craving and increasing awareness of emotions often lead to excessive anxiety and difficulty sleeping. The nurse can teach relaxation skills to deal with the excessive anxiety (Dodge, 1991). There is also a need for teaching problem-solving skills and assertiveness. The nurse must avoid power struggles and be supportive, honest, and very specific in responding to newly developed behaviors (Chitty & Maynard, 1986). Such clients usually will respond to extra attention when anxiety arises. The nurse can help them identify the feeling and name the emotion. Explain that substance use has been the previous mode of coping and that anxiety results because alternative coping skills have not been learned. Initially clients may need simple instructions on how to cope with specific situations. When the strategy succeeds, the nurse can point out the connection between reduced anxiety and the coping skill used. When behavior is inappropriate, it is important to point out the behavior and its connection to the consequences. The goal is for clients to learn that their own behavior is significant in meeting or not meeting needs.

Drug seeking behavior

Often addicted persons, especially those addicted to narcotics or sedatives/hypnotics, will seek health care in order to obtain the drug of choice. A thorough drug and alcohol history and assessment may uncover this addiction. A drug screen may demonstrate traces of the drug. It is important not to feed people's addictions.

Other clients will be in the hospital for medical or psychological reasons and will be unable to obtain drugs or alcohol. It is important to know that there is cross tolerance between most of the abused drugs, including alcohol and those drugs used to relieve pain, reduce anxiety, or induce sleep. An alcoholic may need increased pain medication to ease real pain. This problem requires close observation because tolerance may develop to pain relief but not to respiratory depression. For the surgical client or one with severe pain, narcotics must be given frequently and in strong enough doses to control the pain. It is inhumane to expect any person to endure excruciating pain. For the client with less severe pain, however, it is preferable to give nonsteroidal antiinflammatory medications if needed.

Also because of cross tolerance, sleep medications in therapeutic dosages will either maintain the addiction or be inadequate to initiate sleep. Withdrawal from most addictive drugs involves some sleep disturbance and it is common for a person abusing drugs or alcohol to have difficulty sleeping. Sleep medications for these clients should be avoided if at all possible. They do need assistance to rest as much as possible. Warm milk, relaxation techniques, and reduction in caffeine consumption all are options.

It is common for these clients to attempt to obtain any drug to ease anxious feelings, even though it is not the drug of choice. They sometimes will use manipulation or subterfuge to obtain medications. They will complain of severe pain to obtain narcotics or difficulty sleeping to obtain sedatives, with or without pain or insomnia. Sleeping medications are inappropriate in all but a small percentage of cases. Needs for pain medication must be carefully assessed and only given when extent of injury or other evidence of pain exists. Nonaddicting medications can be given for all other pain.

Pessimism regarding treatment success

The addicted client may feel hopeless about treatment success for several reasons, whether the treatment is for physical disease or for the addiction itself. Clients withdrawing from alcohol, sedatives/hypnotics, or cocaine frequently experience depression. For some clients, this lifts within a week or two; for others, it lingers much longer. In addition, with chronic substance use interpersonal relationships, finances, interests, and most areas of life are impaired. As the drug leaves the brain, awareness of the shambles of things increases. All of this is likely to produce a sense of hopelessness and to induce the client to return to drugs or alcohol for relief from the pain.

These clients need assurances that it is common to feel this way. There is hope—others have succeeded in undergoing treatment and now enjoy a full life, and the client can too. Teaching the client about addictive disease, the symptoms to be expected, and hoped for outcomes helps. Point out how the client's feelings are similar to those of others going through the same process. Having a member of Alcoholics Anonymous or Narcotics Anonymous come to talk with the client can provide hope. Again, including the client in planning treatment, pointing out strengths, and using these strengths in treatment as much as possible will increase hope.

SUMMARY

The use of the nursing process with addicted clients is very similar to that used with any other client. Inclusion of a careful drug and alcohol history in any assessment helps to identify the substance abuse. Nurses are in a key position to identify substance abusers and can contribute a great deal to their care. Nurses can help clients recognize the illness, help maintain their safety during intoxication or withdrawal, and assist with the special problems encountered by these clients. The nurse can teach clients new coping skills so they can cope with life without chemicals.

Several behaviors demonstrated by clients with substance abuse can be problematic for the nurse. These include denial, manipulation, hostility, need to control, drug-seeking behavior, and pessimism regarding treatment. The skillful nurse who has learned well can recognize and manage these behaviors appropriately.

REFERENCES

American Nurses Association. (1987). *The care of clients with addictions: Dimensions of nursing practice.* Kansas City, MO: The Association.

American Nurses Association. (1988). *Standards of addictions nursing practice with selected diagnoses and criteria.* Kansas City, MO: The Association.

Chitty, K.K. & Maynard, C.K. (1986). Managing manipulation. *Journal of Psychosocial Nursing, 24*(6), 9-13.

Dodge, V.H. (1991). Relaxation training: A nursing intervention for substance abusers. *Archives of Psychiatric Nursing, 5*(2), 99-104.

Forchuk, C. & Westwell, J. (1987). Denial. *Journal of Psychosocial Nursing, 25*(6), 9-13.

Gove, P.B. (Ed.), (1971). *Webster's third new international dictionary.* Springfield, MA: G. & C. Merriam.

Haber, J. (1987). *Comprehensive psychiatric nursing* (3rd ed.). New York: McGraw-Hill.

Kress, M.K. (1989). Alcoholism: A women's issue, a disability issue. *Journal of Applied Rehabilitation Counseling, 20*(2), 47-51.

National Institute on Alcohol Abuse and Alcoholism (NIAAD). (1991). Alcoholism and co-occurring disorders. *Alcohol Alert, 14,* PH302.

Plumlee, A. (in press). The client using mind altering substances. In D. Antai-Otong (Ed.), *Psychiatric nursing.* Orlando, FL: W.B. Saunders.

Reisman, B.L. & Schrader, R.W. (1984). Effect of nurses' attitudes toward alcoholism on their referral rate for treatment. *Occupational Health Nursing, 32*(5), 273-5.

Trenk, B. (1986). Biochemical abnormalities can be linked to suicide. *American Medical News, 17*(11).

7

Nursing Care of Clients with Substance Abuse in the Hospital

The nurse in a hospital setting may care for a client with substance abuse whether or not the disorder is recognized or diagnosed. This chapter describes the nursing care of the client withdrawing from alcohol or drugs, the care of the client on a general medical-surgical unit who has an acute or chronic disorder in addition to substance abuse, the surgical client with substance abuse, and the client with substance abuse in need of emergency care. Alterations in physiological function from alcohol and each group of abused drugs are described. Case examples and nursing care are provided throughout the chapter.

Clients who have alcoholism and other drug abuse as primary diagnoses may be referred to inpatient settings for detoxification or safe management of withdrawal (see Chapter 11). More commonly, substance abuse causes, complicates, or coexists with other illnesses that require admission to general hospital units. In those instances the signs and symptoms of substance abuse may not be recognized among the more obvious indicators of the admitting diagnoses. Tweed (1989) notes that although alcoholism is seldom part of the admitting diagnosis, an estimated one third of hospital clients have alcohol-related illnesses. Robin and Michelson (1988) estimate that 40% of the hospitalized client population may have underlying alcoholism or other drug abuse. Despite an apparent drop in substance use, it is predicted that high levels of substance abuse will continue, causing health problems especially in the elderly, women, minorities, and clients with dual diagnoses (Westermeyer, 1992).

There are several mechanisms whereby abuse of psychoactive substances can cause health problems and subsequent admission to the general hospital. In some cases the toxic effect of the substance directly damages body organs (e.g., alcohol's effect on the liver). Second, the route or technique of administration may pose risks to health such as occur when pathogens enter the body during parenteral drug abuse. Third, lifestyle factors associated with substance abuse cause illness. For example, malnutrition and poor hygiene challenge the immune system and threaten health. Finally, increased risk-taking or impairment while under the influence of psychoactive substances may result in life-threatening situations that can require hospitalization, such as motor vehicle accidents, fires, falls, and suicide attempts. Sometimes, clients hospitalized with diagnoses unrelated to alcohol or other drug abuse manifest unexpected responses to routine care (e.g., seizures); such responses may signal the presence of substance abuse. Hence clients with substance abuse, recognized as such or not, are admitted to the full range of hospital units, including general medicine, surgery, post anesthesia, intensive care, orthopedics, obstetrics, and emergency areas.

Because the problems associated with substance abuse span multiple hospital settings, nurses should be prepared to deal with those problems. The nursing role in caring for acutely ill individuals with illnesses compounded by addiction is multifaceted and challenging. In addition to meeting the immediate needs of the admitting diagnosis the nurse must engage in case finding, referral, and education related to the substance abuse.

To be effective in this complex role, nurses must first examine their own beliefs about substance abuse. Too often, health professionals, like the lay public, stigmatize abusers as individuals who lack willpower. While the use of substances such as alcohol may be socially sanctioned, their abuse is considered an avoidable frailty. In the hospital setting, negative attitudes may be compounded by frustration when clients return to previous abusive behaviors as soon as the immediate crisis is resolved. Clients whose diagnoses are related to substance abuse are often unwelcome in the hospital because they have ignored advice to change addictive behaviors. When a sense of defeatism occurs among health professionals confronting these clients, accurate assessment and optimistic referral are impeded (Dans, 1987).

The nurse must view the substance abuser as an individual with a legitimate health problem or disease. The approach should be a nonjudgmental attempt to understand the impetus for the behavior while offering hope for a substance-free future. The nursing response should be realistic, positive, caring, and based on the knowledge that recovery is possible. This is the only way open communication with client and family can be initiated and maintained.

One of the most difficult tasks associated with caring for clients with substance abuse in the hospital is identification of the problem. The signs and symptoms of alcoholism and other drug abuse can be subtle, masked by other more obvious physical or emotional problems, and accompanied by denial. Substance abusers are often adept at deception. Hence the nurse should understand the addiction process, be alert to its subtle signs and symptoms, and be able to gather pertinent data sensitively.

MANAGING ACUTE WITHDRAWAL

The body adapts to or becomes physically dependent on certain chemicals when they are used chronically. *Withdrawal* or *abstinence syndrome* is the set of symptoms that occurs when drugs are removed from the physically dependent individual too quickly (Schuckit, 1989; Woolf, 1991a). Withdrawal symptoms vary depending on the drug in question, and they tend to be the opposite of the drug's initial effect. For example, individuals who are physically dependent on central nervous system (CNS) depressants may develop anxiety and increased pulse and respiratory rates when the drug is withdrawn. The duration and severity of withdrawal symptoms vary with the half-life of the drug, the usual dose, and the length of time the drug was used. Clinically significant withdrawal syndromes are seen following physical dependence on CNS depressants, opiates, and stimulants (Schuckit, 1989).

Detoxification and withdrawal can be the primary focus, or can occur when clients admitted for other diagnoses no longer have access to psychoactive substances. Clients with a primary request for detoxification have three main reasons for doing so: a sincere desire to cure the habit, a desire to reduce the habit to a less expensive level, or a desire to supplement the habit with purer or cheaper drugs (Turrell et al, 1988). Because of the possibility of the third motivation, it is important to be objective with treatment regimens by providing clients with written protocols and informed consents that specify expectations for remaining in the program. Clients are informed in advance that they will have some discomfort, their blood and urine will be screened, and they may be dropped from treatment for failure to comply. The written documents are signed and witnessed, and they become a contract between the client and the treatment unit. Figure 7-1 is an example of an informed consent form for an inpatient detoxification program. The form can include clinic attendance requirements when used in an outpatient setting.

Detoxification requires knowledge of the drug in question. Protocols and nursing care for each major withdrawal syndrome are addressed. However, some general components of care should be considered in all clients experiencing withdrawal.

Evaluation of overall health status

Clients beginning detoxification need a thorough history, physical examination, and routine laboratory tests to detect the presence of any other disorders that might complicate withdrawal. Drugs of abuse and associated lifestyle factors pose major risks to health. In some instances, withdrawal itself is a significant physiological stress if the individual is already debilitated.

Physical and environmental support

Clients in withdrawal need a quiet environment and adequate monitoring to assure safety. Although withdrawal from some substances is described by clients as a serious case of flu, withdrawal from alcohol can be life-threatening and result in irreversible damage to the cerebral cortex. Prompt intervention is required. Rest and nutritional support are also appropriate.

Psychological support

Clients in withdrawal need reassurance that successful recovery is possible. Staff and peer support should be a part of detoxification. Turrell and associates (1988) note that underlying emotional disorders such as depression, anxiety, and schizophrenia may emerge as drugs are withdrawn. While treatment of these disorders will aid eventual success in recovery, the researchers caution against the use of anxiolytics, pain medications, or CNS depressants.

Pharmacological support

Withdrawal symptoms may be treated by administering the substance or another of the same class in decreasing amounts for periods varying from a few to several weeks depending on the half-life of the drug (Schuckit, 1989). The general rule is

Informed Consent for Drug Withdrawal

I, _____ (name of patient), am addicted to
_____ (name of drugs and/or alcohol) and
willingly enter treatment for withdrawal from physical dependence on this (these) substance(s).
I understand that I will receive a copy of the standardized program used for withdrawal in cases
such as mine.

I further understand that all of my symptoms of withdrawal cannot be alleviated without
simply continuing my addiction or addicting me to another drug. I therefore expect and am willing to endure a certain amount of discomfort in this withdrawal process. I agree to adhere to
the written drug reduction schedule given to me. I will not request that the time period for withdrawal be lengthened.

I agree to submit to initial and regular urine tests. I understand that I may be asked to submit to regular blood tests. If I have difficulty in cooperating and fail to demonstrate an appropriate decrease in the blood level of my drug(s) of abuse or the presence of other drugs in my
blood or urine, there will be sufficient reason for me to be dropped from the program. I would
not then be able to reapply for treatment for at least 30 days.

I further agree to participate in individual, group, or other therapeutic programs, including
a period of aftercare, as are prescribed for me. I understand that failure to do so will result in
my being dropped from the program and that I cannot then reapply for at least 30 days.

_____   _____
Signed   Witnessed

_____
Date

Fig. 7-1. Informed consent for drug withdrawal form. (Modified from Turrell, E.S., Schmetzer,
A.D., Wright, J.J., & Scherl, E.K. (1988). Drug and alcohol withdrawal: Methods for patient
management. *Indiana Medicine, 81*(5), 401-407.)

that the withdrawal process should be slow enough that symptoms are not excessively painful but rapid enough that the client will not become discouraged. Some discomfort is to be expected. Clients should be made aware of this possibility and told that such discomfort is self-limiting.

Alcohol

Alcohol causes CNS depression. The effect is dose-dependent and, in high enough concentrations, may produce anesthesia and death. In low doses a behavioral stimulant effect is produced (Schuckit, 1989). Alcohol is readily absorbed by the stomach and intestine; 5% to 15% is excreted through the lungs, in the urine, and in perspiration. The remainder is metabolized by the liver at the approximate rate of one drink per hour. The rate of alcohol metabolism is influenced by the weight and tolerance of the individual drinker.

Intoxication.   Intoxication is most frequently seen in the emergency department. Alcoholic intoxication occurs when more alcohol is consumed than can be metabolized. This condition is determined by the blood alcohol level. In most states the legal limit for intoxication ranges from 80 mg to 100 mg of alcohol per 100 ml of blood. The nontolerant individual will exhibit behavioral signs of intoxication at levels of 100 mg to 150 mg of alcohol per 100 ml of blood; however, the alcoholic may have a blood alcohol level between 200 mg and 300 mg and appear normal (Woolf, 1991b). Alcoholism should be considered when a seemingly unimpaired individual presents with a high blood alcohol level. Behavioral manifestations of intoxication include slurred speech, lack of coordination, decreased attention span, and poor memory. The physical signs of acute intoxication are those of CNS depression, including bradycardia, decreased pulse rate, and decreased blood pressure. Signs and symptoms of intoxication related to alcohol ingestion and blood alcohol are summarized in Table 7-1.

Clients with a blood alcohol level of 300 mg or more must be closely monitored. Treatment for respiratory depression or hypotension may be required. Immediate aspiration of gastric contents is recommended to prevent further absorption of any residual ethanol in the acutely intoxicated client. When initial blood alcohol levels exceed 500 mg and acidosis is present, hemodialysis may be indicated (Li, 1992).

Alcohol withdrawal syndrome.   A physiological dependence on alcohol and tolerance for increasing amounts occurs with continued use. When alcohol is withdrawn, signs and symptoms of alcohol withdrawal syndrome (AWS) may occur. Early manifestations include anxiety, restlessness, mild disorientation, insomnia, tachycardia, hypertension, and diaphoresis. The presence of these signs and symptoms can alert nurses to intervene quickly to prevent more serious consequences including tremors, hallucinations, seizures, and delirium. Most clients do not develop the full syndrome; those who have experienced previous seizures or delirium, and those who are older or have coexisting acute illnesses are more likely to develop severe symptoms (Schenk, 1991). This clinical picture should alert nurses in any hospital setting to the possibility of underlying alcoholism.

Tremors, initially involving the hands, may begin within 6 to 48 hours after alco-

Table 7-1

Intoxicating levels of alcohol

Amount (80 proof whiskey)	Blood alcohol level (per 100 ml of blood)	Signs and symptoms
2 oz = 30 ml— 1½ shot glasses	50-75 mg	Not under influence; no apparent effect
4 oz = 60 ml— 3 shot glasses	80-100 mg	Usual legal limit for operating a motor vehicle; emotional response is erratic, may have increased aggressiveness, talkativeness, muscle incoordination, slowed reaction time; decreased inhibition
6 oz = 90 ml— 4½ shot glasses	100-200 mg	Confused, staggering gait, rapid pulse, vertigo, slurred speech, diaphoresis
8 oz = 120 ml— ½ pint	200-400 mg	Marked depression in stimulus response; nausea, vomiting, drowsiness, muscle incoordination, emotional lability
16 oz = 240 ml— 1 pint	400-500 mg	Stupor, coma, hypotension, tachycardia, labored respiration, seizures, absent reflexes
24 oz = 360 ml— 1½ pints	More than 500 mg	Death caused by cardiac or respiratory arrest or aspiration of gastric contents

Based on an average 160-pound adult 30 to 45 minutes after ingestion. (Level will be higher in women due to fat/muscle ratio.)

hol is withdrawn and may persist for 3 to 5 days (Schenk, 1991). *Hallucinations* occur in 10% to 20% of clients with severe withdrawal. This manifestation ranges from nightmares to tactile, olfactory, mixed visual, and auditory hallucinations that usually recede within a few days. A small percentage of clients have *seizures* that occur within 48 hours of abstinence (Li, 1992). *Delirium tremens* (DTs) is the most serious complication of alcohol withdrawal and should be treated as an emergency. The onset of DTs is often sudden and dramatic and generally occurs 3 to 4 days after abstinence and lasts for 2 to 4 days. Occasionally, this condition persists for as long as 5 weeks (Li, 1992). Characteristic manifestations of DTs include disorientation, hallucinations, tremors, agitation, and increased autonomic nervous system (ANS) activity (diaphoresis, tachycardia, dilated pupils, fever). There is a 5% mortality rate associated with delirium tremens.

Components of care for alcohol withdrawal. Safe management of withdrawal from alcohol in the hospital setting includes the following: (1) pharmacological treatment or detoxification with decreasing doses of cross-tolerant drugs such as the benzodiazepines, (2) metabolic interventions to correct possible alterations in glucose, phosphate, magnesium, electrolytes, and water, (3) nutritional supplementation to include calories, folic acid, thiamine, B-complex vitamins, and vitamin K when prothrombin time is decreased, (4) attention to coexisting physical disorders, and (5) provision of a quiet, safe environment (Casteneda & Cushman, 1989).

Pharmacological treatment.   Alcohol withdrawal is generally accomplished with benzodiazepines. Longer-acting preparations (chlordiazepoxide [Librium]) are preferred, but shorter-acting drugs (lorazepam [Ativan]) are used when clients have concomitant liver disease (Li, 1992). A loading dose of the drug of choice is usually given. A typical protocol for the pharmacological management of alcohol withdrawal is presented in Box 7-1. Withdrawal seizures may require anticonvulsant therapy (magnesium sulfate, 2 ml of 50% solution every 8 to 12 hours, or phenytoin [Dilantin] if seizure activity persists). According to Schuckit (1989) the optimum treatment for delirium tremens has not been determined. Li (1992) notes that chlordiazepoxide (50 to 100 mg given parenterally every 4 to 6 hours to a maximum of 300 mg a day) is usually effective, but some clinicians prefer diazepam (Valium) because it is shorter-acting.

Nutritional support.   Nutrition is particularly important for the recovering alcoholic. Lifestyle factors include inadequate intake of nutrients; the majority of calories are derived from alcohol. Clients may be nutritionally depleted at entry to treatment and may experience anorexia as a consequence of withdrawal. Diet as tolerated, with liberal fluids and snacks, is encouraged. Often, coexisting conditions such as cirrhosis, hypertension, or coronary artery disease demand limitations of protein, salt, and fats. In such cases, diets will need modification and clients must be given every encouragement to eat properly. A complete nutritional assessment and appropriate education are recommended.

Providing a quiet, safe environment.   This is important for clients experiencing alcohol withdrawal because anxiety, agitation, seizures, and disturbed thought processes are common manifestations. Clients must be monitored closely to protect them and others from erratic behavior. Safety measures such as padded side rails and occasionally restraints may be indicated. Potentially harmful objects should be removed from the environment and every effort should be made to reduce stimuli

---

Box 7-1
Alcohol Withdrawal Protocol

Day 1: Chlordiazepoxide	50 mg PO QID
Day 2: Chlordiazepoxide	50 mg PO TID
Day 3: Chlordiazepoxide	25 mg PO QID
Day 4: Chlordiazepoxide	25 mg PO TID
Day 5: Chlordiazepoxide	25 mg PO BID
Day 6: Chlordiazepoxide	25 mg PO HS
Multivitamins	1 PO QD ×2 wks
Thiamine	50 mg PO QD ×2 wks
B-complex vitamins	1 PO QD ×2 wks

Table 7-2

Modified Selective Severity Assessment (MSSA)

Signs and symptoms	Quantification of signs and symptoms
1. Eating disturbances	Based on meal before exam: 0 = Ate and enjoyed all of it 3+ to 4+ = Ate about half of what was given 7+ = Ate none at all
2. Tremor	1+ = Tremor not visibly apparent, but can be felt by the examiner's fingertips when placed lightly against the patient's fingertips 3+ to 4+ = Tremor is moderate with arms extended 7+ = Marked tremor even when arms are not extended
3. Sleep disturbances	1+ = Patient gets up once 4+ = Awake half the night 7+ = Completely sleepless
4. Clouding of sensorium	0 = No evidence of clouding of sensorium 1+ = Cannot do serial 7 subtractions, or knows correct date but is uncertain 2+ = Disoriented for time by no more than two calendar days 3+ = Disoriented for time by more than two calendar days
5. Hallucinations (Record frequency, content, intensity, and patient's insight into hallucination.)	0 = None 1+ = Auditory 2+ = Visual 3+ = Nonfused auditory and visual 4+ = Fused auditory and visual
6. Quality of contact	Awareness of examiner and people around patient: 1+ = Drifts off slightly 2+ = Appears to be in contact with examiner, but is unaware of or oblivious to the surroundings or other people 3+ or 4+ = Periodically appears to become detached 7+ = Makes no contact with examiner
7. Agitation	Based on amount of movement (not anxiety or tremor): 1+ = Somewhat more than normal activity 3+ to 4+ = Moderately fidgety and restless 7+ = Paces back and forth during most of the interview
8. Paroxysmal sweats	1+ = Barely perceptible sweating 3+ to 4+ = Beads of sweat obvious 7+ = Drenching sweats

From Benzer, D.G. (1990). Quantification of the alcohol withdrawal syndrome in 487 alcoholic patients. *Journal of Substance Abuse Treatment, 7,* 117-123.

Continued.

Table 7-2

Modified Selective Severity Assessment (MSSA)—cont'd

Signs and symptoms		Quantification of signs and symptoms
9. Temperature	1	= 99.5 or below
	2	= 99.6 to 99.9
	3	= 100 to 100.4
	4	= 100.5 to 100.9
	5	= 101 to 101.4
	6	= 101.5 to 101.9
	7	= 102 to 102.4
	8	= 102.5 to 102.9
	9	= 103 and above
10. Pulse	1	= 70 to 79
	2	= 80 to 89
	3	= 90 to 99
	4	= 100 to 109
	5	= 110 to 119
	6	= 120 to 129
	7	= 130 to 139
	8	= 140 to 149
	9	= 150 and above

that might trigger agitation. The nurse contributes by offering calm reassurance, orientation to reality, and support.

Other dimensions of treatment, such as individual and group therapy, are initiated once detoxification is complete (see Chapter 4).

Assessment of alcohol withdrawal.   Effective management of withdrawal requires an efficient system for monitoring and quantifying the manifestations. Objective rating scales or standardized clinical assessments score signs and symptoms numerically to produce an index of severity (Foy et al, 1988). The Modified Selective Severity Assessment (MSSA) (Benzer, 1990) and the Clinical Institute Withdrawal Assessment (CIWA) (Shaw et al, 1981) were developed for this purpose (see Chapter 11). Benzer recommends use of the Modified Selective Severity Assessment (MSSA) for any client with a history of daily use of alcohol or other sedative hypnotics. The MSSA, presented in Table 7-2, illustrates that scores are used as one criterion for determining which clients should receive pharmacological intervention.

Withdrawal scales are useful in medical, surgical, or psychiatric units. The scales assist staff in focusing on an evolving withdrawal syndrome that might otherwise be missed among other health problems. Early recognition and intervention of alcohol withdrawal syndrome may prevent the development of the more serious complications of seizures and DTs. Care Plan 7-1 presents a typical pattern for alcohol withdrawal.

Text continued on p. 148.

Alcohol Dependence and Withdrawal

Susan, a 30-year-old Caucasian female, was brought to the hospital by her husband, Danny, for treatment of alcohol dependency. Danny stated that Susan had been drinking vodka daily for 13 years. Both informants reported that Susan's alcohol intake had increased over the last 3 years, following the death of their second child. Susan reported prior unsuccessful attempts to abstain and a current intake of a fifth of vodka daily. Her last drink was on the morning of admission.

ASSESSMENT

Relevant Subjective Information

Health history: Hepatitis 14 years ago; no history of DTs or withdrawal seizures; smokes a pack of cigarettes daily; reported crying spells, somnolence, and unprovoked irritability; recent 10-pound weight loss.

Psychosocial history: Alcoholic grandparents and parents; sexually abused at age 11; married at age 15; one child, age 11; occupation, homemaker.

Relevant Objective Information

Clinical picture: Unsteady gait; poor hygiene; odor of alcohol on breath; appeared older than stated age; some facial features characteristic of fetal alcohol syndrome; height, 5'2"; weight, 98 lb; vital signs: T—97.6°F, P—110, R—20, BP—132/100; no hepatomegaly.

Relevant Laboratory Findings

Elevated values		Low values	
Blood alcohol level	233 mg/dl	K+	2.8 mg/dl
Alkaline phosphate	210	Uric acid	1.9
SGOT	133	Ca+	8.3
SGPT	50	RBC	2.9
LDH	418	HGB	10.7
GGTP	471	HCT	32
LDL	145	Lymphocytes	14
MCV	109		
MCH	37		
Neutrophils	81		

Admitting Medication Orders

Initial dose of chlordiazepoxide 75 mg on admission; chlordiazepoxide 50 mg every 2 hours PRN for p > 110, tremors, anxiety, or agitation.

Decreasing doses of chlordiazepoxide as follows:

Day 01	Chlordiazepoxide	50 mg QID
Day 02	Chlordiazepoxide	50 mg TID
Day 03	Chlordiazepoxide	25 mg QID
Day 04	Chlordiazepoxide	25 mg TID
Day 05	Chlordiazepoxide	25 mg BID
Day 06	Chlordiazepoxide	25 mg HS

Nutritional supplements Folate, Thiamine, B complex and multiple vitamins daily.

Modified from Jack, L. (1990). *Nursing care planning with the addicted client,* Skokie, IL: National Nurse's Society on Addictions.

NURSING DIAGNOSES

Potential for injury related to the effects of alcohol withdrawal

Alteration in nutrition: less than body requirements related to long-term alcohol use, self-neglect, and inadequate diet

Sensory-perceptual alteration: visual, auditory, kinesthetic, gustatory, tactile, and olfactory related to withdrawal from alcohol

Outcome identification	Nursing interventions	Rationale	Evaluation
Nursing diagnosis: Potential for injury related to the effects of alcohol withdrawal			
1. Client will detoxify in a controlled hospital environment within 2 weeks.	1a. Assess level of consciousness, orientation, and presence of hallucinations and delusions.	1a. Important assessment to determine course of detoxification.	1. Susan experienced a difficult detoxification complicated by acute alcoholic hepatitis, toxic encephalopathy, and the large doses of chlordiazepoxide required to manage withdrawal symptoms. She experienced profound cognitive impairment, delusions, confusion, disorientation, and auditory and visual hallucinations. She required 1:1 observation and seizure precautions. She did detoxify within 2 weeks, however. Goal met.
	1b. Position the client to prevent aspiration if needed.	1b. Altered level of consciousness leaves the client at risk for aspiration.	
	1c. Provide safe, protective environment and reduction of stimuli.	1c. The client's CNS is hyperactive, and reduction of stimuli is needed.	
	1d. Assess for suicidal ideation and acting-out behavior.	1d. This client will feel distressed and will be at risk for such behaviors.	
	1e. Monitor the client's response to medication, including vital signs, degree of discomfort, and the amount of withdrawal symptoms.	1e. Changes in response to medication, VS, and other withdrawal symptoms will dictate frequency of medication administration.	
	1f. Use bedrails and supervise ADL's.	1f. When a confused client is in bed, she may fall out. In addition, she may not be able to complete own ADL's.	

Continued.

Alcohol Dependence and Withdrawal—cont'd

Outcome identification	Nursing interventions	Rationale	Evaluation
Nursing diagnosis: Alteration in nutrition: less than body requirements related to long-term alcohol use, self-neglect, and inadequate diet			
1. Client will eat well-balanced, nutritional meals by the end of 3 days.	1a. Document intake and output of fluids and calorie count of food.	1a. This is to determine quantity and adequacy of fluid and calorie intake.	1. Susan was unable to eat meals by the end of three days. She had pedal edema and an elevated ammonia level. She was placed on a low protein diet. Goal met within 7 days, however.
	1b. Assist client with eating if her tremulousness interferes with the necessary motor abilities.	1b. The withdrawing client is likely to have tremors.	
	1c. Collaborate with the client to include food preferences if possible.	1c. The client will be more likely to eat something that she likes.	
	1d. Encourage frequent, smaller feedings rather than three large meals per day.	1d. Smaller meals will be tolerated better because her stomach likely is irritated.	
	1e. Administer vitamin and mineral supplements as ordered by the physician.	1e. Chronic alcohol intake interferes with many vitamins; supplements prevent deficiency syndromes.	
2. Recognize the effect of alcohol on nutritional status within 1 week.	2a. Teach the client measures to promote good nutrition such as recognition of basic food groups, abstinence from alcohol and drugs, and avoidance of behavior patterns of addictions.	2a. Knowledge of good nutrition will assist the client to make appropriate decisions about intake of food and chemicals.	2. Susan was not able to discuss the effect of alcohol on her nutritional status within 2 weeks. Goal not met. *Revision:* She will complete goal by discharge.
	2b. Caution the client against high caffeine intake. Limit coffee, tea, cola, and chocolate. Encourage other fluid intake as desired.	2b. Caffeine will stimulate an already overactive CNS.	

Outcome identification	Nursing interventions	Rationale	Evaluation
Nursing diagnosis: Sensory-perceptual alteration: visual, auditory, kinesthetic, gustatory, tactile, and olfactory related to withdrawal from alcohol			
1. Client will become oriented and be able to perform own ADL's by 1 week.	1a. Establish rapport and confidence by use of competent bedside care and warm, positive regard. Call the client by name.	1a. Persons respond positively when they feel respected and cared for.	1. By 1 week, Susan could follow simple commands and sustain periods of orientation. It was two weeks, however, before she could attend her own ADL's and converse with staff. Goal met with longer time frame.
	1b. Monitor the client's vital signs and degree of tremor and medicate for withdrawal as ordered.	1b. Level of tremors are an indicator of severity of withdrawal.	
	1c. Assess and record mental status, especially orientation, presence of hallucinations or delusions, and coherence of speech patterns.	1c. Monitor course of withdrawal. Deterioration in orientation is a sign of impending delirium tremens.	
	1d. Reorient the client regularly.	1d. Even the client who is fairly oriented can become somewhat confused.	
	1e. Reduce stimuli in the environment.	1e. Helps calm overactive CNS.	
	1f. Reinforce behaviors that are reality-oriented.	1f. Helps the client stay in touch with reality.	
	1g. Institute measures to help the client sleep, such as relaxation techniques.	1g. Sleep will likely be disrupted in the withdrawing client.	

Other substances of abuse

As was noted with alcohol abuse, acute, life-threatening physiological and psychological complications of abuse of other drugs occur in overdose, withdrawal, and toxicity. Anticipated effects and appropriate crisis interventions for the acute phase of each category of abusive substance are summarized in Table 7-3.

Recognizing and managing withdrawal.   Withdrawal often produces significant signs and symptoms, ranging from life-threatening to mildly uncomfortable. Clients must be observed for characteristic signs and symptoms, monitored for alterations in vital signs, provided with a safe, comfortable environment, and reassured that they will be supported. Specific clinical manifestations of withdrawal and suggested pharmacological management are outlined in Table 7-4.

Multidrug withdrawal.   Many individuals abuse multiple psychoactive substances. Dependence on more than one drug and complicated patterns of withdrawal are potential problems in hospital settings. The most common patterns of multidrug withdrawal follow concomitant abuse of multiple depressants, depressants and stimulants, or opiates and depressants (Schuckit, 1989).

The clinical picture for withdrawal from multiple depressants is similar to withdrawal from CNS depressants (Table 7-4); however, a higher incidence of seizures is seen with benzodiazepines or barbiturates than with alcohol. The length of withdrawal is based on the half-life of the drugs abused and is less predictable with more than one drug (Schuckit, 1989).

Treatment is aimed at the longer-acting drug and includes (1) gradually decreasing doses of the CNS depressant used for withdrawal and (2) close observation for serious or unusual symptoms of withdrawal. Simultaneous withdrawal from depressants and stimulants produces a clinical picture close to the CNS depressant pattern described in Table 7-3, with the added features of lethargy, sadness, and paranoid thinking. Treatment follows the plan for CNS depressant withdrawal.

When opiates and depressants are abused together, the clinical manifestations of opiate withdrawal predominate and are compounded by insomnia, anxiety, and increased risk of confusion and seizures. Treatment follows the following sequence: (1) stabilization with the opiate, (2) gradual withdrawal of the CNS depressant, and (3) opiate withdrawal once CNS depressant withdrawal is accomplished. The following case illustrates withdrawal from multidrug dependence (see Care Plan 7-2).

CARE IN GENERAL MEDICAL/SURGICAL UNITS

The toxic effects of alcohol, tobacco, and other drugs are associated with significant alterations in normal physiological function. Clients who abuse these substances risk developing characteristic clinical manifestations and well-defined acute and chronic diseases. When hospitalization is required for medical management or surgical intervention, the contribution of substance abuse to the clinical picture may be overlooked because of the urgency of the admitting diagnosis. Hence nurses should be familiar with the classic consequences of abuse and prepared to assess and care for abuse or dependence.

Text continued on p. 154.

Table 7-3
Clinical manifestations and interventions for major classifications of psychoactive substances

Substance	Street names	Clinical manifestations	Acute intoxication/overdose	Interventions
CNS depressants				
Hypnotics				
Barbiturates	Barbs, Downers, Goof Balls	Initial euphoria and decreased inhibitions, drowsiness, lack of coordination, impaired judgment, slurred speech, hypotension, bradycardia, bradypnea	Respiratory depression, pupillary constriction (progressing to dilation if hypoxia occurs), shock, hyporeflexia, coma, death	Establish and maintain airway, assist ventilation, provide oxygen; evaluate cardiovascular status, monitor vital signs every 15 to 30 minutes; treat shock; monitor intake and output; monitor reflexes; lavage if recent oral ingestion; position patient on side or prone; hemodialysis may be required
Secobarbital (Seconal)	Red Devil, Seggy			
Phenobarbital (Luminal)	Phennie			
Pentobarbital (Nembutal)	Yellow Jacket, Nembies			
Amobarbital (Amytal)	Blue Devil, Blue Bird, Blue Velvet, Blue Heaven			
Barbiturate-like drugs				
Methaqualone (Quaalude)	Ludes, Wallbangers, Quads			
Glutethimide (Doriden)				
Ethchlorvynol (Placidyl)				
Others				
Chloral hydrate (Noctec)	Peter, Mickey Finn			
Temazepam (Restoril)				
Antianxiety drugs				
Carbamates				
Meprobamate (Miltown, Equanil)				
Tybamate (Salacen, Tybatran)				
Benzodiazepines				
Diazepam (Valium)				
Flurazepam (Dalmane)				
Lorazepam (Ativan)				
Chlordiazepoxide (Librium)	Roaches, Tranqs			

Continued.

Table 7-3
Clinical manifestations and interventions for major classifications of psychoactive substances—cont'd

Substance	Street names	Clinical manifestations	Acute intoxication/ overdose	Interventions
CNS stimulants				
Amphetamine (Benzedrine) Chlorphentermine (Pre-sate) Dextroamphetamine (Dexedrine) Methamphetamine (Desoxyn) Methylphenidate (Ritalin) Phenmetrazine (Preludin)	Bennies, Uppers Dexies, Speed Crystal, Meth	Euphoria, hyperactivity, hyperalertness, insomnia, anorexia, tremor, restlessness, tachycardia, hypertension, dysrhythmias, sexual arousal	Rapid respiration, tremor, restlessness, confusion, assaultiveness, hallucination (Cocaine overdose can cause convulsions, respiratory paralysis, and death.)	Establish and maintain airway; evaluate cardiovascular status; monitor vital signs until stable; provide quiet, safe environment; haloperidol or chlorpromazine may be ordered but must be used with extreme caution; cooling blankets for hyperpyrexia
Cocaine	Coke, Snow, Flake, Rock, Superblow, Topot			
Caffeine			Flushing or pallor, tachycardia, hyperpyrexia	
Other analgesics/narcotics				
Heroin	Horse, Junk, H. Brown, Scat M, Microdots Poppy, Tar, Black Smack	Analgesia, drowsiness, relaxation, detachment, pupillary constriction, nausea, constipation, slurred speech, impaired judgment	Decreased respirations, bradycardia, hypotension, pinpoint pupils, unconsciousness, coma, death	Establish airway, assist ventilation, provide oxygen; evaluate cardiovascular status, monitor vital signs every 15 to 30 minutes; treat shock; administer narcotic antagonist as ordered: Naloxone (Narcan) 0.4 mg IV; repeat as ordered (duration of naloxone is 30 to 45 minutes)
Morphine Opium Codeine Meperidine (Demerol)				
Hydromorphone (Dilaudid) Propoxyphene (Darvon) Pentazocine (Talwin) Oxycodone (Percodan)	Pinks and Grays			
Methadone (Dolophine)	Dollies			

Cannabinols

Marijuana	Pot, Reefer, Grass, Weed	Relaxation, euphoria, decreased motivation, sexual arousal, increased appetite, decreased social interaction	Intoxication: tremors, poor motor coordination, bloodshot eyes, dry mouth, decreased body temperature, nausea, headache, nystagmus, hypotension	Maintain calm environment and support
Hashish	Hash, Rope		Overdose: psychosis, anxiety, confusion, hallucinations; as ordered: Chlordiazepoxide (Librium) 10-50 mg PO	Administer antianxiety medications

Hallucinogens

Lysergic acid diethylamide (LSD)	Acid, Cube D, Window Pane Sugar, Sunshine, Blue Dots, Barrels	Perceptual distortions, hallucinations, depersonalization, heightened sensory perception, euphoria, impaired judgment, increase of body temperature, hypertension, flushed face, mydriasis, tremor	Panic, psychosis, agitation, anxiety, self-destructive behavior caused by perceptual distortion. Flashbacks are possible	Maintain calm, safe environment; reassure that total recovery will occur; antianxiety agents such as diazepam (Valium) 10 to 30 mg; PO may be ordered
Psilocybin (mushrooms)	Shroom, Magic Mushroom, Exotic Mushroom			
Dimethyltryptamine (DMT) Diethyltryptamine (DET)				
3,4-Methylendioxyamphetamine (MDA)	Love Drug, Mellow Drug of America			
Mescaline (peyote)	Cactus, Mescal, Button			

Continued.

Table 7-3

Clinical manifestations and interventions for major classifications of psychoactive substances—cont'd

Substance	Street names	Clinical manifestations	Acute intoxication/ overdose	Interventions
Phencyclidine (PCP)	Angel Dust, Hog, Peace Pill, Rocket Fuel, Embalming Fluid, Shermans	Perceptual distortion, euphoria, agitation, delusions, violence, hypertension, increased salivation, diaphoresis, hyperreflexia, nystagmus, ataxia, decreased response to painful stimuli, pupillary constriction	Hyperthermia, stupor, coma, seizures, death	Establish airway, assist ventilation; monitor cardiovascular status, IV antihypertensives may be ordered; oral suction if excess salivation occurs; gastric lavage may be indicated if drug was taken orally; provide quiet, safe environment; Benzodiazepines (Diazepam) 5 to 10 mg every 4 hours may be ordered to reduce risk of seizures; mechanical cooling may be indicated

Inhalants

Aerosol propellants		Euphoria, "high" similar to alcohol, decreased inhibitions, slurred speech, giddiness, clouded sensorium, illusions, drowsiness	Blurred vision, excessive tearing and nasal secretions, nausea, vomiting, diarrhea, anorexia, bradycardia, chest pain, dysrhythmias, bradypnea, decreased brain wave activity, seizures, altered state of consciousness, death due to cardiac dysrhythmias or suffocation	Establish and maintain airway, assist ventilation, provide oxygen, evaluate cardiovascular status, moitor vital signs every 15 to 30 minutes; treat shock; provide supportive care and reality orientation
Fluorinated hydrocarbons				
Nitrous oxide				
found in:				
Deodorants				
Hair spray				
Pesticide				
Cookware coating products				
Whipped cream spray				
Spray paint				
Solvents	"Hitting Rags" (refers to sniffing the substance from a rag)			
Gasoline				
Kerosene				
Nail polish remover (Acetone)				
Typewriter correction fluid				
Cleaning solutions (carbon tetrachloride)				
Lighter fluid				
Paint and paint thinners (ethanol, toluene, methanol)	Tolly			
Glue (toluene, naphtha, benzene)				
Anesthetic agents				
Chloroform				
Nitrous oxide				

Table 7-4

Clinical manifestations of withdrawal with suggested pharmacological treatment

Substances	Clinical manifestations	Medications
CNS depressants (other than alcohol)	Anorexia, anxiety, insomnia, tremors, tachycardia, fever, seizures, dehydration	Pentobarbital—Test dose: 200 mg (challenge) If patient falls asleep, no treatment needed; if no reaction, repeat dose every 2 hours; determine dose for 24 hours; divide QID, stabilize for 2 days; decrease by 100 mg/day (Schuckit, 1989)
CNS stimulants	Depression, lack of energy, inability to concentrate, irritability, somnolence, paranoid thinking, intense craving, agitation	Symptom management Chlordiazepoxide (Librium) for agitation Haloperidol (Haldol) for paranoid thinking Bromocriptine (Parlodel) for craving
Opiate analgesics/narcotics	*Early:* Tearing, rhinorrhea, yawning, diaphoresis, desire to sleep, drug craving, dilated pupils, anorexia, gooseflesh, back pain, tremor *Later:* Insomnia, yawning, nausea, vomiting, abdominal cramping, chills, flushing, diarrhea, myalgia	*Opiate approach* Methadone—Test dose: 20 mg PO Establish minimum daily dose to control symptoms; decrease by 10% to 20% of first day's dose according to symptoms *Nonopiate approach* Clonidine (Catapres)—0.2 to 0.3 mg to start, then 0.1-0.4 mg TID *or* Guanabenz (Wytensin) dose regulated according to systolic BP Other drugs for temporary symptom management of nausea, diarrhea, indigestion, cramps, myalgia
Nicotine	Irritability, anxiety, craving, difficulty concentrating, restlessness, drowsiness, insomnia, tremor	Nicotine transdermal patch Nicorette gum (nicotine polacrilex) Clonidine (Catapres) may suppress craving: 0.1 mg TID (investigational) (Lee & D'Alonzo, 1993)

From Lee, E.W. & D'Alonzo, G.E. (1993). Cigarette smoking, nicotine addiction, and its pharmacologic treatment. *Annals of Internal Medicine. 153,* 34-48.

Alcohol sequelae

When alcohol is ingested in moderation by healthy, nonalcoholic individuals, pathological changes are reversible (Schuckit, 1989). The potential benefits of moderate alcohol consumption (no more than two drinks a day) for such individuals include increased socialization, increased appetite, and decreased risk of cardiovascular disease (Schuckit, 1989). If moderate use gives way to alcoholism or the person has other medical problems, the consequences can be life-threatening. A brief review of classic changes in body systems secondary to excessive alcohol ingestion follows. Case examples are included to illustrate the hospital courses of several such individuals.

Liver

The liver participates in the following functions: (1) drainage of blood from the gastrointestinal tract, (2) metabolism of carbohydrates, fats, and protein, (3) detoxification of endogenous and exogenous substances, (4) metabolism and storage of vitamins and minerals, (5) bile production and excretions, and (6) bilirubin metabolism (Cassmeyer, 1995). Alcohol is particularly damaging to the liver. Even in low doses, alcohol disturbs the ability of the liver to produce sugar (gluconeogenesis) for carbohydrate metabolism and increases fatty acid and triglyceride synthesis, resulting in fatty infiltration. Hence alcohol is a direct hepatotoxic that can injure this vital organ even when nutrition is adequate. Three distinct diseases of the liver result from chronic abuse (Woolf, 1991b). They are *fatty liver* (a reversible disorder), *alcoholic hepatitis* (an acute disease with a 10% to 30% mortality), and *cirrhosis*. In cirrhosis, scar tissue replaces normal liver cells, liver function is lost, portal blood flow is obstructed, and total liver failure can occur. A liver biopsy is necessary to differentiate fatty liver, alcoholic hepatitis, and cirrhosis reliably, but abnormal bleeding and prothrombin times and ascites may preclude this procedure (Crabb & Lumeng, 1992).

The clinical progression from fatty liver to liver failure in cirrhosis includes signs and symptoms ranging from mild indigestion to coma and death. Nursing care is directed toward encouraging sobriety, improving nutritional status, managing signs and symptoms, and monitoring for major complications such as portal hypertension, ascites, esophageal varices and hemorrhage, and portal-systemic encephalopathy.

Portal hypertension. This condition results when liver necrosis obstructs portal circulation and causes a rise in portal venous pressure. Obstructed portal blood flow can cause venous congestion in the spleen and splenomegaly. This obstruction contributes to ascites because albumin and fluid from the liver leak into the peritoneal cavity. Collateral circulation develops to bypass the obstruction (Cassmeyer, 1995).

Ascites. Ascites, an abnormal collection of fluid in the intraperitoneal cavity, results from portal hypertension, decreased hepatic synthesis of albumin, increased levels of aldosterone, and obstruction of hepatic lymph flow. Sodium restriction and diuretics are conservative measures to treat ascites. Chronic, persistent ascites may be treated by insertion of a peritoneal venous shunt that allows continuous reinfusion of ascitic fluid back into the venous system (Cassmeyer, 1995).

Esophageal varices. This condition is a complex of enlarged, swollen, and tortuous veins at the lower end of the esophagus; these veins are susceptible to ulceration and hemorrhage. Bleeding is frequently painless and abrupt. Bleeding may be caused by the mechanical trauma of coarse foods, acid erosion, or increased ab-

Text continued on p. 161.

Care Plan 7-2

Multidrug Withdrawal

Jerry, a 30-year-old Caucasian male, was admitted to the hospital for treatment of multidrug dependence and withdrawal. He stated that he was currently supporting his addictions by doing odd jobs and dealing drugs; he wanted to be treated so that he could hold down a regular job. Jerry reported daily use of 30 to 80 mg of methadone, 10 to 12 beers, unspecified amounts of marijuana, and two packs of cigarettes. In addition, he reported approximate use of diazepam (Valium) 10 times a month, heroin twice a month, and IV cocaine once a month.

ASSESSMENT
Relevant Subjective Information
Health history: Needle sharing; medical detoxification twice; participated in two methadone programs in the past; no prior rehabilitation for dependence.

Psychosocial history: Physically abused by father as a child; parents divorced when he was age 4; little contact with father, whom he deeply resents; served in Marines where he received GED; previously worked as iron worker; currently unemployed; separated for 1 year from wife of 6 years; lives alone in old trailer; no contact with family.

Relevant Objective Information
Clinical picture: Untidy, unshaven appearance; no obvious physical distress; thought process logical and goal-directed; speech pattern slow and deliberate; appeared "unconcerned," depressed with blunt affect; denied suicidal or homicidal ideations.

Relevant Laboratory Findings
Urine screen positive for methadone, cocaine, and marijuana; all other lab values, including liver function tests, were normal; HIV negative.

NURSING DIAGNOSES
Alteration in comfort related to withdrawal from methadone
Potential for injury related to withdrawal
Sensory-perceptual alterations related to withdrawal from multiple chemicals
Anxiety related to the distress of withdrawal

Outcome identification	Nursing interventions	Rationale	Evaluation
Nursing diagnosis: Alteration in comfort related to withdrawal from methadone			
1. Client will state he has minimal discomfort while withdrawing from drugs and alcohol during the next 7 days.	1a. Take BP 5 times a day and monitor all vital signs.	1a. Blood pressure is a useful index of severity of opioid withdrawal symptoms. Vital signs are a good indicator of progress of alcohol withdrawal.	1. Jerry was friendly and cooperating with peers and staff during his first few days on the unit. He appeared to be experiencing minimal physical discomfort. Because of this, no Chlordiazepoxide was given. By day 3 he became increasingly irritable, noncompliant, and angry. Guanabenz was increased on day 5. The worst part of the withdrawal was on days 6 and 7. At that time he complained of abdominal cramps and bone aches. His major complaints consisted of bone aches, which responded well to naproxen. Use of other PRN medication for withdrawal symptoms was very limited. Jerry did not state minimal discomfort until day 9. Goal met, with longer time frame.
	1b. Give medication as ordered: • Chlordiazepoxide, decreased schedule • Guanabenz for high BP • Naproxen for joint pain • Dicyclomine for abdominal cramps • Acetaminophen for headache • Hydroxyzine for nausea • Prochlorperazine for vomiting • Magnesium hydroxide for indigestion • Diphenhydramine for sleep × 3 days.	1b. Chlordiazepoxide is given for alcohol withdrawal. Antihypertensive drugs have been shown to relieve withdrawal symptoms. Bone pain, abdominal cramps, nausea, and vomiting are common. Sleep disturbances are common as well.	

Continued.

Care Plan 7-2

Multidrug Withdrawal—cont'd

Outcome identification	Nursing interventions	Rationale	Evaluation
Nursing diagnosis: Alteration in comfort related to withdrawal from methadone—cont'd			
2. Client will implement a regular sleep schedule by the end of 3 weeks.	2a. Assist the client in determining and stating the severity of pain and general discomfort.	2a. Only the client can determine the extent of his discomfort.	2. Jerry slept well for two nights but began to have difficulties on the third night. This continued until the next week when his sleep began to normalize. By 3 weeks he went to bed and arose at the same time as other clients and verbalized that he slept fairly well. Goal met.
	2b. Institute and teach measures to promote sleep, such as managing dietary intake, avoiding caffeine, maintaining consistent times to go to bed and arise, manipulating the environment, and using relaxation techniques.	2b. Measures that strengthen the body's natural biological rhythms and naturally induce sleep will provide the maximum probability that client may sleep.	
Nursing diagnosis: Potential for injury related to withdrawal			
1. Client will achieve withdrawal without injury while hospitalized.	1a. Monitor frequently for clinical manifestations of withdrawal, i.e., seizures, combative behavior, confusion, impaired judgment, perceptual distortions.	1a. Withdrawal patterns may be unpredictable in a given client. Prompt response to clinical manifestations reduces risk of escalation.	1. Jerry was not injured during his hospitalization. Goal met.
	1b. Medicate as ordered and PRN as needed.	1b. Adequate, appropriate pharmacological treatment reduces risk of increased clinical manifestations.	
	1c. Provide safety measures, i.e., side rails, quiet environment.	1c. Client experiences inability to care for self related to effects of withdrawal.	

Outcome identification	Nursing interventions	Rationale	Evaluation
Nursing diagnosis: Sensory-perceptual alterations related to withdrawal from multiple chemicals			
1. Client will maintain contact with reality throughout withdrawal.	1a. Assess degree of intoxication and stage of withdrawal.	1a. Assists in planning intervention.	1. By day 6 of hospitalization, Jerry was isolative, oppositional, resistive, and hostile. He was preoccupied with his medications and spent most of his time in bed. By day 8 he was less irritable. He maintained orientation throughout withdrawal. Goal met.
	1b. Provide safe environment.	1b. Prevents injury.	
	1c. Orient client to reality: • Make eye contact • Call by name • Provide information about environment • Identify self	1c. Assists in maintaining contact with environment.	
	1d. Assess hourly or more often for orientation, safety, response to medications, behavior.	1d. Decreases or prevents injury.	
2. Client will demonstrate trust in staff by cooperating with treatment during withdrawal.	2a. Reassure client of staff support.	2a. Decreases discomfort related to sensory/perceptual distortions.	2. Even though Jerry was hostile and isolative, he complied with staff requests. By day 9, he again began attending group activities and interacting appropriately with peers and staff. Goal met.
	2b. Educate client about withdrawal process.	2b. Reduces fear related to unknown or unexpected consequences of abstinence.	

Continued.

Care Plan 7-2

Multidrug Withdrawal—cont'd

Outcome identification	Nursing interventions	Rationale	Evaluation
Nursing diagnosis: Anxiety related to the distress of withdrawal			
1. Client will identify feelings as they occur during hospitalization.	1a. Assess level of anxiety: whether mild, moderate, severe, or panic. 1b. Provide comfort measures such as quiet atmosphere or warm bath.	1a. Assists to determine appropriate interventions. 1b. Showing concern by providing comfort measures has calming effect. Reassures client of support.	1. Psychological testing during the acute phase of withdrawal revealed that he was experiencing high levels of emotional distress and anxiety, as well as trouble thinking and concentrating. Jerry stated, however, that he was too uncomfortable to talk about feelings. Goal not met.
2. Client will state that his anxiety is caused by withdrawal by 1 week.	2a. Observe and document anxiety-producing situations. 2b. Assist client to identify anxiety triggers. 2c. Give rationale for anxiety during withdrawal.	2a. Early identification will prevent escalation of anxiety. 2b. Assists client to resume control of situation. 2c. Assists client to understand and accept anxiety as related to withdrawal.	2. Even though Jerry refused to talk about feelings, he was able to connect his discomfort to his withdrawal process. Goal met.
3. Client will demonstrate adaptive coping strategies to deal with anxiety by participation in the treatment program by 1 week.	3a. Assess client's coping skills. 3b. Promote participation in treatment program to increase coping, i.e., stress management, seminars, and leisure-time activities.	3a. Assists to determine appropriate intervention. 3b. Facilitates learning of adaptive coping strategies.	3. Jerry began attending groups and participating in the treatment program on day 9. Goal met with longer time frame.

dominal venous pressure such as occurs in coughing, sneezing, vomiting, and straining at stool (Cassmeyer, 1995). Severe bleeding can lead to shock. Depending on the severity, treatment may involve gastric lavage, vasopressin to induce splanchnic vasoconstriction and lower portal pressure, balloon tamponade to exert direct pressure on the vessels, use of a sclerosing agent on the varices, and as a last resort surgical shunt. Careful estimate of blood loss and replacement of blood volume are essential. Nursing care demands close surveillance to monitor cardiac output, vascular volume, tissue perfusion, hemostasis, fluid and electrolytes, and the status of renal, respiratory, and neurological systems (Cassmeyer, 1995). Clients are often frightened by the massive hematemesis, and they need calm attention to the physiological crisis.

Portal-systemic encephalopathy.   This is an abnormal function of the brain secondary to liver disease and is another major sequelae of cirrhosis. Metabolic derangements result in the build-up of toxic substances, particularly ammonia, in the blood, and reduced liver function limits detoxification. Hypoxia and increased CNS sensitivity to depressants can also precipitate portal-systemic encephalopathy. This phenomenon may occur quickly or gradually, and it is manifested by alterations in level of consciousness, intellectual function, behavior and personality, and neuromuscular function. Other characteristic signs include asterixis (liver flap), a sweet breath odor (fetor hepaticus), EEG changes, hyperventilation, tachycardia, and temperature elevation. An elevated serum ammonia provides definitive diagnosis but is not always present in these clients (Cassmeyer, 1995; Crabb & Lumeng, 1992). Treatment includes prompt correction of known precipitating events such as constipation, infection, or ingestion of sedative-hypnotics (Crabb & Lumeng, 1992) and specific therapies are aimed at reducing serum ammonia levels. Dietary protein is restricted, and antibiotics are administered to reduce the bacterial flora that degrade protein into ammonia. Oral cathartics or enemas are given to relieve constipation and subsequent luminal protein concentrations. Lactulose, a hyperosmotic cathartic, is used because it stimulates fecal excretion of ammonia.

Clients with portal-systemic encephalopathy require close observation and care to support ventilation, cardiovascular status, and nutrition. Narcotics and sedatives are contraindicated because of the limited hepatic function. *Chlordiazepoxide,* which is excreted by the kidneys, may be ordered as a sedative on a limited basis (Cassmeyer, 1995). The following case illustrates hepatic failure in a hospitalized client (Care Plan 7-3).

Gastrointestinal tract

Alcohol is a direct irritant to gastrointestinal mucosa and promotes secretion of gastric acid. These factors contribute to erosion in the lining of the gastrointestinal tract and cause *esophagitis, gastritis,* and *duodenitis.* Complaints range from mild gastric pain to severe nausea and vomiting and may cause the alcoholic to seek medical attention. Such conditions should alert the nurse to the possibility of alcohol abuse. Alcohol is also associated with ulcer disease, and alcohol abuse should be considered in clients presenting with *gastric or duodenal ulcers* (Schuckit, 1989).

The pancreas, a fish-shaped gland that functions in digestion, is located behind

Text continued on p. 167.

Care Plan 7-3

Hepatic Failure/Alcoholism

Raymond, a 30-year-old Caucasian male with a 15-year history of alcoholism, was admitted to the hospital for increasing icterus, agitation, confusion, and one episode of hematemesis. History revealed that he had consumed more than a liter of whiskey and smoked a pack of cigarettes every day for the past 15 years. The family reported that Raymond had also abused IV drugs (substance and amount unknown).

ASSESSMENT

On admission Raymond was endoscoped, and the findings included grade 1 esophageal varices, distal erosive esophagitis, and gastritis. Abnormal laboratory studies included: Hgb/Hct = 8.4 g/dl/22.6% (started on 3 units of packed RBCs); creatinine = 2.6 mg/dl; BUN = 67 mg/dl; alkaline phosphatase = 292 U/L; bilirubin = 29 mg/dl; and WBCs = 18,430 mm³. The client was HIV negative. Vital signs: BP 120/70, P 108, T 98.2.

Other early diagnostic findings included: hepatic encephalopathy (treated with lactulose and improved nutritional status); an elevated temperature of 100.5 (blood cultures showed gram negative cocci); abdominal ultrasound showed cirrhosis, small amount of ascites, and no biliary dilatation. A paracentesis was done, and the fluid aspirated had 300 WBC, 2% polymorphs, amylase 22, and albumin 0.6, findings compatible with portal hypertension). Chest X-ray on admission was clear. Physical examination revealed hepatomegaly.

Significant laboratory studies done on the day following admission included: phosphate = 6.4 mg/dl; SGPT = 48 IU/ml; SGOT = 115 U/L; alkaline phosphatase = 316 U/L; bilirubin = 30.4 mg/dl; prothrombin time (PT) = 13 seconds; and partial thromboplastin time (PTT) = 34 seconds.

Five days after admission Raymond's chest X-ray showed bilateral pulmonary infiltrates probably caused by aspiration pneumonia, resulting from his reduced level of consciousness. Eight days after admission, Raymond lapsed into unconsciousness.

NURSING DIAGNOSES

Impaired gas exchange related to reduced hemoglobin and reduced lung function from aspiration

Altered nutritional status related to long-term excessive alcohol use

Sensory-perceptual alteration related to withdrawal from alcohol and liver dysfunction

Impaired skin integrity related to altered nutritional status and immobility

Anticipatory grieving (family) related to client's deteriorating status

Outcome identification	Nursing interventions	Rationale	Evaluation
Nursing diagnosis: Impaired gas exchange related to reduced hemoglobin and reduced lung function from aspiration			
1. Client will demonstrate adequate gas exchange as evidenced by alert and responsive mental status within 1 week.	1a. Give medications as ordered: • Lactulose 30 cc QID in NG tube • Omeprazole (Prilosec) 20 mg QD • Sucralfate (Carafate) 1 gm QID • Ceftazidime (Fazicef) 2 gm IV q 12 hours • Clindamycin (Cleocin) 600 mg IV q 8 hours • Albumin 12.5 gm IV q 6 hours • Ampicillin (Unasyn) 1.5 mg IV q 8 hours • Lorazepam (Ativan) 2 mg IV q 2-4 hours • Morphine sulfate 4-8 mg IV 2-4 hours • Dopamine, low dose	1a. For therapy • To treat encephalopathy • Antisecretory • Antiulcer agent • Antibiotic • Antibiotic • To decrease interstitial edema and bring fluid into vascular compartment • Antibiotic • For restlessness • For pain • To promote renal perfusion	1. Three weeks after admission, Raymond suffered an esophageal bleed that was described as "brisk." He was treated with octreotide acetate (Somatostatin) infusion at 100 μg/hr (suppresses gastrin). Raymond eventually developed renal insufficiency requiring ultrafiltration (a more gentle dialysis that uses the client's systolic pressure to perfuse the kidney instead of a pump). Ultimately, Raymond developed sepsis, metabolic acidosis, and multisystem failure. He succumbed to his disease 1 month and 21 days after admission. Client's mental status deteriorated during hospitalization. Goal not met.

Continued.

Care Plan 7-3

Hepatic Failure/Alcoholism—cont'd

Outcome identification	Nursing interventions	Rationale	Evaluation
Nursing diagnosis: Impaired gas exchange related to reduced hemoglobin and reduced lung function from aspiration—cont'd			
	1b. Monitor for signs of worsening lung status (↑R, ↑ anxiety/confusion, ↑rales, rhonchi, wheezes, ↓SaO$_2$, diaphoresis, hypertension).	1b. Early identification of worsening lung status provides opportunity for earlier remedial treatment.	
	1c. Provide pulmonary toilet (suction every 2 hours, chest PT every 4 hours if tolerated, turn every 2 hours).	1c. To keep the airway clear of blockage by secretions and avoid possible aspiration.	
	1d. Keep client comfortable to decrease anxiety and subsequent O$_2$ uptake increases.	1d. Anxiety increases O$_2$ usage.	
	1e. Monitor daily weights, serial CVP or PAP, PCWP to assess fluid status and treat with diuretics as needed.	1e. Weight increase may indicate congestive heart failure. Also monitors possible fluid overload or underload.	
Nursing diagnosis: Altered nutritional status related to long-term excessive alcohol use and impaired swallowing			
1. Client will maintain current weight throughout hospitalization.	1a. Monitor nutritional intake and supplements through TPN (hepatorenal formula) • Vitamin K in TPN • Fat emulsions 20% in TPN	1a. To provide adequate nutrition when client cannot eat. Vitamin K is given for his elevated Protime. Fat emulsions provide added calories and slow peristalsis.	1. Client lost weight throughout his hospitalization. Goal not met.

Outcome identification	Nursing interventions	Rationale	Evaluation
Nursing diagnosis: Sensory-perceptual alteration related to withdrawal from alcohol and liver dysfunction			
1. Client will maintain contact with reality throughout his hospital stay.	1a. Establish rapport and confidence by use of competent bedside care and warm, positive regard. Call the client by name.	1a. Persons respond positively when they feel respected and cared for.	1. Client's mental status deteriorated over the course of his hospitalization, he slipped into a coma 8 days after hospitalization and did not regain consciousness. Goal not met.
	1b. Monitor the client's vital signs, level of tremor and agitation.	1b. Level of tremors is an indicator of severity of withdrawal.	
	1c. Assess and record level of consciousness, mental status, orientation, presence of hallucinations or delusions, and coherence of speech patterns.	1c. Monitor course of mental status and withdrawal status. Deterioration in orientation is a sign of impending delirium tremens.	
	1d. Reorient the client daily.	1d. Helps prevent ICU psychosis, reduce anxiety.	
	1e. Reduce stimuli in the environment.	1e. Helps calm overactive CNS.	
Nursing diagnosis: Impaired skin integrity related to altered nutritional status and immobility			
1. Client will demonstrate skin integrity free of pressure ulcers throughout hospitalization.	1a. Turn client every 2 hours.	1a. Turning allows circulation to pressure points and prevents ischemia.	1. Client's skin did maintain integrity throughout his hospitalization. Goal met.
	1b. Pad bony prominences.	1b. Padding prevents pressure on bony areas and prevents chafing.	
	1c. Keep skin clean and dry.	1c. Wet skin causes increased breakdown.	

Continued.

Care Plan 7-3

Hepatic Failure/Alcoholism—cont'd

Outcome identification	Nursing interventions	Rationale	Evaluation
Nursing diagnosis: Anticipatory grieving (family) related to client's deteriorating status			
1. Family members will verbalize feelings about client's prognosis within 1 week.	1a. Determine the family members' perception of the prognosis.	1a. An accurate assessment of the family's perception assists the nurse in determining their needs.	1. Client's sister, Ellen, did discuss her feelings with the nurse. Goal met for her. Other family members did not deal with the situation well, and they did not want to discuss any of Raymond's care with the nurse. Goal not met for remaining family members.
	1b. Determine response of family members to prognosis.	1b. Observing the family members gives clues to how to give assistance.	
	1c. Provide open environment for expression of feelings.	1c. The first step of grieving is the expression of feelings.	
	1d. Permit expressions of anger and fear.	1d. Anger is a part of the grieving process and needs to be expressed.	
	1e. Be honest when answering questions, provide information.	1e. Honest response to the family fosters trust in the nurse.	
	1f. Provide hope within parameters of the specific situation. Do not provide false reassurance.	1f. If it is possible, hope provides strength to cope with difficult situations. False hope will only make coping more difficult, however.	
	1g. Include the family in problem solving.	1g. Problem solving will assist the family to mobilize energy from anxiety.	
	1h. Assist them to seek support from the chaplain or a minister with their permission.	1h. Many persons will find comfort and hope in talking to a clergyman.	

the stomach. The pancreas has both endocrine and exocrine tissues. Endocrine activities of the pancreas include release of glucagon and insulin. Exocrine activities include secretion of digestive enzymes, bicarbonate, and electrolytes. Pancreatic enzymes include amylase (used to digest carbohydrates), lipase (used to digest fats), and proteases (used to change proteins into amino acids) (Smith, 1991). The pancreas drains secretions from smaller ducts into the duodenum at the exit of the common bile duct.

Pancreatitis.   This condition is the self-destruction of the pancreas by its own enzymes, and it is associated with alcoholism. About 30% of clients with acute pancreatitis abuse alcohol and already have chronic pancreatitis when the acute disease begins (Dimagno, 1992). Pancreatitis proceeds from interstitial pancreatic edema to proteolysis, hemorrhage, parenchymal damage, and fat necrosis. As a result of pancreatic damage, increased levels of trypsin circulate in the blood and cause life-threatening complications such as hypotension, shock, acute respiratory distress syndrome, coagulation abnormalities, and hypocalcemia (Dimagno, 1992).

Clinical manifestations of pancreatitis include persistent midepigastric and left upper quadrant pain that may radiate to the back. Pain is aggravated by eating, drinking alcohol, and vomiting; it is decreased by fasting and leaning forward or assuming a fetal position. Other signs include nausea, vomiting, jaundice, fever, dyspnea, and tachypnea. Diagnostic tests are serum amylase, usually elevated in the first 24 to 48 hours; serum lipase, elevated after 48 hours and up to 7 days; amylase and myoglobin in the urine; elevations in serum bilirubin, lactate dehydrogenase (LDH), and alkaline phosphatase (indicators of impaired hepatic function); decreased serum calcium because calcium is deposited in pancreatic necroses; and abnormalities in prothrombin time (PT), partial thromboplastin time (PTT), and platelet count if coagulopathies develop (Smith, 1991). Ultrasound is used to detect gallstones, a distended common bile duct, pancreatic masses, or pseudocysts (collections of pancreatic juices that become encapsulated and pose risks for infection, hemorrhage, or obstructions). Abdominal X-rays and computed axial tomography scans reveal pancreatic distention, and chest X-rays identify atelectasis, pleural effusions, infiltrates, acute respiratory distress syndrome, and pneumonia (Smith, 1991).

Therapeutic interventions include drugs used to reduce pancreatic secretions, fluid replacement, pain management, and general measures to support respiratory and cardiovascular status. Surgical debridement and resection may be required for clients with vessel erosion, bleeding, or abscess formation (Smith, 1991). Clinical manifestations of acute withdrawal often accompany this disease and must be managed at the same time. Pancreatitis is a serious complication of alcohol abuse that can result in death.

Cardiovascular system

Alcohol affects the cardiovascular system in several ways. Alcohol is considered the most frequent identifiable cause of heart muscle disease, or cardiomyopathy, that is believed to occur in most chronic alcoholics (Rubin & Doria, 1990). *Alcoholic cardio-*

myopathy results in the abnormal distention, with blood, of one or more heart chambers. Alcoholic cardiomyopathy includes loss of contractility of myocardial cells, resulting in inefficient pumping action, and decreased cardiac output. The left ventricle becomes enlarged because of the excess blood after contraction. Hypertrophy of the muscle contributes to a further decrease in function, and signs and symptoms of congestive heart failure result. Because this process is indistinguishable from cardiomyopathies that are caused by other factors, the diagnosis is based on a history of alcohol consumption and the absence of other known causes such as infection, thiamine deficiency, or exposure to cardiac toxins (Rubin & Doria, 1990).

Clinical manifestations of alcoholic cardiomyopathy include dyspnea, orthopnea, fatigue, paroxysmal nocturnal dyspnea, weakness, and occasionally chest pain and cough. Diagnostic imaging of the heart reveals decreased cardiac output and distended left ventricle. Irregular heart beat and abnormal lung sounds are common. As the disease progresses, vital organs may be deprived of oxygen. Liver enlargement and ascites can occur. In the early stages, abstinence from alcohol may reverse the disease process. When congestive failure warrants hospitalization, the prognosis is poor. Complications include emboli and dysrhythmias (Rubin & Doria, 1990).

Medical treatment is the same as for other dilated cardiomyopathies. Diuretics, dietary sodium restriction, adequate diet, digitalis, and vasodilator may be prescribed. Abstinence from alcohol is essential. Nursing care includes promoting oxygenation with a semi-Fowler's position and providing oxygen as needed, monitoring fluid and electrolyte balance, giving prescribed medications, providing balanced rest and activity, assisting with nutritional intake, providing skin care to reduce risk of skin breakdown over edematous areas, and teaching the client and family about the disorder and the need for abstinence.

Moderate to excessive alcohol intake and binge drinking predispose individuals to *strokes* and sudden death. There is a strong association between alcohol consumption and stroke in people under 50. Although hypertension is a major risk factor in stroke, the clinical findings are often independent of hypertensive status (Altura & Altura, 1990). A major risk factor for stroke is eliminated or greatly reduced by the modification of drinking behaviors.

The link between alcohol abuse and *hypertension* is supported by epidemiologic, clinical, and laboratory evidence. Alcohol elevates blood pressure regardless of age, body weight, or cigarette smoking. The exact relationship between the quantity of alcohol consumed and the degree of hypertension is yet to be determined. Alcohol-associated hypertension may contribute to other cardiovascular complications in alcoholics. Friedman (1990) recommends treating this phenomenon as secondary hypertension that will respond to the treatment of alcoholism.

Alcohol ingestion is associated with a variety of *cardiac dysrhythmias*, particularly during intoxication and withdrawal. Atrial fibrillation, supraventricular tachycardia, isolated premature ventricular contractions, and nodal rhythms can occur (Woolf, 1991b). Atrial fibrillation in binge drinkers is called "holiday heart syndrome" because it often occurs during holiday seasons when alcohol intake increases (Woolf, 1991b; Lange et al, 1992). Alcohol abuse should be considered in hospitalized clients with *cardiomyopathy, hypertension,* and *stroke.* The risk of life-threatening *dysrhyth-*

mias accompanies excessive alcohol ingestion and withdrawal. Close monitoring of cardiovascular status is an important nursing intervention.

Musculoskeletal system

Acute and chronic *myopathies* occur as a result of alcohol consumption. Alcohol causes muscle inflammation and wasting. In chronic alcoholics, muscle wasting is noticed in the shoulders and hips (Schuckit, 1989). Jacobs (1992) reported that alcohol-induced *bone necrosis* results from fat embolism secondary to hyperlipidemia. In a study of alcohol-induced osteonecrosis, 45% of the clients experienced bilateral hip necrosis. Other sites of involvement included the humeral head, the knees, and the talus. He urges early diagnosis, using magnetic resonance imaging (MRI), in alcoholic clients who present with hip, shoulder, and knee pain. Treatment of hyperlipidemia through diet and medication may prevent the need for surgical intervention.

Alcohol and cancer

After tobacco, alcohol is the second most important substance that contributes to the development of cancer (Myers, 1991). Alcohol also works synergistically with tobacco to increase the risk of tobacco-related neoplasms (Blattner, 1992). Individuals who drink heavily develop cancers of the oral cavity, pyriform sinus, and esophagus. When excessive smoking and drinking are combined, the risk for all forms of *head and neck cancer* increases. Other problems that contribute to carcinogenesis, such as malnutrition, liver disease, and tooth decay, are associated with chronic alcoholism (Myers, 1991). Alcohol consumption is also associated with an increased risk of *liver cancer.* The tissue damage associated with cirrhosis may contribute to carcinogenesis (Blattner, 1992).

A careful history related to amount and duration of alcohol and tobacco use is important in the initial evaluation of clients presenting with these neoplasms (Snow, 1992). The major clinical sites of cancers of the head and neck are the mouth, larynx, and esophagus. Cancer of the *mouth* is usually asymptomatic with an initial inflammatory response that disappears. Leukoplakia (white patches) and erythroplasia (red patches) may precede cancer of the *larynx;* early symptoms include hoarseness, a lump in the throat, pain in the Adam's apple radiating to the ear, dyspnea, dysphagia, cough, and enlarged cervical nodes. *Esophageal* cancer produces progressive dysphagia, regurgitation, aspiration leading to pneumonia, malodorous breath, and a foul taste in the mouth (Phipps et al, 1995).

Surgery, radiation, chemotherapy, or a combination is used for malignancies associated with alcohol abuse. Particular attention should be given to improving nutritional status and assisting with cessation of alcohol and tobacco use. As with other problems associated with excessive intake of alcohol, nurses must consider the possibility of alcohol withdrawal syndrome in clients hospitalized for head and neck cancers. Other nursing care varies with the location and size of the tumor, as well as the nature of the treatment. General considerations include promoting optimal nutrition, monitoring respiratory status, promoting communication, assisting the client to cope with altered body image, promoting oral hygiene, promoting comfort (see section on pain management), and assisting the client to cope with the fear and anxiety associated with a diagnosis of malignancy.

Sequelae of other substances of abuse

Sequelae of other substances of abuse may be due to the substance itself, the route of administration, or the associated lifestyle. The major complications of drugs of abuse are summarized by organ system in Table 7-5.

Clients with substance abuse can sustain major health problems related to the technique used to administer drugs or to associated lifestyle factors. Infections and direct injury result in the majority of these health consequences. Drug abusers have increased risk for infection for the following reasons: (1) they are often carriers of staphylococcus aureus, (2) dirty needles and syringes are used to inject unsterile drugs, (3) dental hygiene is often poor, (4) decreased bacterial clearance of the tracheobronchial system during intoxication, (5) cell-mediated immunity may be impaired by HIV infection and by IV drug abuse itself, and (6) promiscuity and prostitution are often part of the lifestyle (Scheidegger and Zimmerli, 1989).

Nasal septum damage occurs from chronic snorting of cocaine through the nasal mucosa. Constriction of blood vessels in the mucosa ultimately results in destruction and perforation of the nasal septum. Chronic infections with the potential risk of sinus infections follow. Reconstructive surgery may be indicated.

Cellulitis, or infection of the skin and soft tissue, results from direct tissue damage or chemical irritation by the substance. Symptoms include local heat, redness, pain, swelling, and occasionally fever, chills, malaise, and headache. Staphylococcus aureus is the most common pathogen associated with cellulitis. Treatment with vancomycin hydrochloride (Vancocin) is recommended (Levine, 1991a). Moist compresses provide symptomatic relief.

Infective endocarditis is microbial invasion of the endocardium, usually the valvular endocardium, but potentially the interventricular septum or mural endocardium as well. Twenty-five percent of all cases are associated with IV drug abuse. Staphylococcus aureus is the predominant organism involved. Viridans streptococci, pseudomonas, and gram-negative bacilli may also cause this process.

The clinical features of endocarditis are caused by valvular defects, embolic or immune injury to other organs (splenic infarcts, arterial emboli), and disordered physiology (heart failure, renal failure). Clinical manifestations may be present in every organ system. Symptoms include myalgias, arthralgias, headache, nausea, vomiting, and diarrhea. Laboratory findings include positive blood cultures, anemia, leukocytosis, neutropenia, thrombocytopenia, elevated erythrocyte sedimentation rate, and abnormal blood chemistries (Cobbs & Douglas, 1992; Levine, 1991b).

Medical therapy consists of IV antimicrobials. Surgical intervention to replace valves may be lifesaving (Cobbs & Douglas, 1992). Nursing responsibilities include monitoring clinical manifestations of the disease and complications, administering antimicrobials, teaching clients measures to avoid recurrence, and providing for comfort and hygiene needs.

The following case example illustrates how complex it can be to care for a client with infective endocarditis and psychoactive substance abuse (Care Plan 7-4).

Acquired immune deficiency syndrome.   AIDS results from infection with *hu-*

Table 7-5

Summary: major complications of drugs of abuse

Organ system	Substance	Complications
Cardiac	Amphetamines Cocaine	Dysrhythmias, ischemia, infarction, sudden death related to increased oxygen demand and decreased oxygen supply (vasoconstriction); cardiomyopathy related to toxic effect of substance on muscle; endocarditis, myocarditis, cor pulmonale related to deposition of pathogens on heart valves (more common on right side of heart).
	Hallucinogens Solvents/aerosols	Dysrhythmias related to sensitization of heart to catecholamines.
	Marijuana	Ischemic pain caused by increased heart rate, decreased strength of contractions, and decreased delivery of oxygen to heart.
	Nicotine	Ischemia and infarction caused by decreased supply of oxygen to heart.
Vascular	CNS stimulants	Hypertension, rupture of aorta or heart secondary to hypertension.
		Parenteral drug abuse may result in air emboli, thrombophlebitis, and arteritis caused by air or impurities.
Pulmonary	Opiates Sedatives/hypnotics	Respiratory depression.
		Pulmonary edema in overdose related to permeability mechanisms (diffusion) rather than vascular pressure changes.
	Marijuana	Bronchitis caused by local irritation (reversible).
		Asthma-like syndrome with chronic use; decreased vital capacity.
		Head and neck tumors in young adults.
	Nicotine	Pneumothorax secondary to bullous disease; emphysema.
		Bronchitic changes, susceptibility to infection.
		Malignant tumors (associated with concomitant alcohol abuse).
		Parenteral drug abuse may result in foreign-body reactions, pneumothorax, infections.
Gastrointestinal	Opiates	Chronic constipation (abdominal cramping and diarrhea in withdrawal).
	Stimulants Nicotine	Anorexia.
	Hallucinogens	Anorexia, transient GI upsets.
	Solvents	Chemical hepatitis.
	Aerosols	Parenteral drug abuse associated with other viral hepatitis.
Neurologic	CNS stimulants	Seizures, cerebral infarction, intracranial hemorrhage, ischemia, stroke.
		Parenteral drug abuse leads to introduction of pathogens and CNS infections.
	Solvents Aerosols	Peripheral neuropathies.

From Lange, W.R., White, N., & Robinson, N. (1992). Medical Complications of Substance Abuse. *Post-graduate Medicine. 92*(3), 205-214.

Care Plan 7-4

Infective Endocarditis/IV Drug Abuse

Paul, a 44-year-old African-American male with a long history of IV drug abuse and recurrent infective endocarditis, was admitted to the hospital for reevaluation of his cardiac status.

ASSESSMENT
Relevant Information

Health history: Paul has a history of IV cocaine and heroin abuse. He is a heavy smoker who also abuses alcohol. Paul is a former truck driver who is disabled because of a motor vehicle accident 8 years ago that resulted in cardiac contusion. He also has arthritis. Approximately a year after the accident he developed infective endocarditis with tricuspid valve vegetation, regurgitation, and complete heart block. He had antimicrobial therapy, tricuspid valve replacement, and a permanent pacemaker placement. Three years later he required a second tricuspid valve replacement, as well as a mitral valve because of persistent endocarditis (he was noncompliant with anticoagulant regimen and continued to inject IV drugs). In the subsequent 4 years he has required surgery a third time for tricuspid valve replacement and for replacement of infected pacemaker wires. He has had wound-healing problems and worsening heart failure caused by recurrent vegetation on his tricuspid valve.

Psychosocial history: Paul is a divorced father of three. He has a history of suicide attempts and psychiatric treatment for depression and homicidal tendencies. He also has psychiatric diagnoses of borderline personality disorder and depression.

Medications: Buspirone hydrochloride (Buspar) 10 mg PO BID (anxiolytic); perphenazine (Trilafon) 2 mg PO BID (antipsychotic); doxepin hydrochloride (Sinequan) 50 mg PO HS (tricyclic antidepressant); hydroxyzine hydrochloride (Atarax) 50 mg PO HS (anxiolytic); morphine sulfate 4 to 6 mg IV q 2 to 4 hours for pain; antibiotic therapy; diuretics; inotropic agents.

NURSING DIAGNOSES

Altered cardiac output: decreased related to recurrent right and left ventricular failure
High risk for spread of infection related to sternal infection, IV drug abuse, debilitated
    state, chronic illness, poor nutrition, and poor hygiene
Impaired social interactions related to manipulative, hostile behaviors

Outcome identification	Nursing interventions	Rationale	Evaluation
Nursing diagnosis: Altered cardiac output: decreased related to recurrent right and left ventricular failure			
1. Client will exhibit no signs or symptoms of decreased cardiac output by 1 week.	1a. Assess cardiac status frequently.	1a. Frequent monitoring will discover changes in the early stages.	1. Paul had liver and spleen enlargement, caused by right ventricular failure. Cardiac output was decreased throughout hospitalization. Goal not met.
	1b. Administer medications as ordered.	1b. Provides support for compromised cardiac status.	
	1c. Encourage respiratory exercises.	1c. Prevention for pulmonary complications.	
Nursing diagnosis: High risk for spread of infection related to sternal infection, IV drug abuse, debilitated state, chronic illness, poor nutrition, and poor hygiene			
1. Client will not develop any additional infection while in the hospital.	1a. Administer antibiotics as needed.	1a. Treatment for infection.	1. Client's sternal infection resolved very slowly while in the hospital, and he did not develop any subsequent infection. Goal met.
	1b. Monitor wound frequently.	1b. Frequent monitoring will discover changes in the early stages.	
	1c. Provide sterile dressing changes.	1c. Sterile conditions necessary for controlling spread of infection.	
	1d. Maintain meticulous handwashing.	1d. Reduces exposure to contaminants.	
	1e. Instruct client and visitors on importance of cleanliness.	1e. Teaches client and family how to reduce exposure to contaminants.	

Continued.

Care Plan 7-4

Infective Endocarditis/IV Drug Abuse—cont'd

Outcome identification	Nursing interventions	Rationale	Evaluation
Nursing diagnosis: Impaired social interactions related to manipulative, hostile behaviors			
1. Client will cooperate with treatment while in the hospital.	1a. Facilitate psychiatric consultation.	1a. Psychiatric nurse can assist the med-surg nurse in planning care for the client with a psychiatric diagnosis.	1. Paul exhibited drug-seeking behaviors with frequent medication requests. He was given morphine via PCA, and he self-administered maximum dosages. He had many somatic complaints, each requiring diagnostic work-up to rule out complications of infective endocarditis (pulmonary embolus, gastrointestinal problems). He had recurrent constipation because of increased narcotic usage. Goal not met. Paul ultimately was discharged home with home health care planned. His prognosis is considered poor.
	1b. Administer medications as ordered.	1b. Psychiatric medications may be ordered.	
	1c. Maintain limits related to manipulative, hostile behavior.	1c. Manipulative clients will respond to consistent, firm limits administered in a kind, caring manner.	
	1d. Encourage family support if available.	1d. The client's acting-out behaviors likely hide a need for caring and support.	
	1e. Exhibit calm, nonjudgmental attitude.	1e. A calm, nonjudgmental manner will most likely elicit a positive response from the client.	

man immunodeficiency virus (HIV). The disease progresses through three stages: (1) an acute primary phase with flu-like symptoms, (2) an asymptomatic stage characterized by immune suppression (fever, night sweats, weight loss, diarrhea, neuropathy, fatigue, rashes, lymphadenopathy, cognitive impairment, oral lesions), and finally (3) AIDS with severe opportunistic infections, tumors, and neurological manifestations. Eighty to ninety percent of persons diagnosed with the complete syndrome die within 3 years (Grimes, 1991). The virus is present in blood and serum-derived body fluids. Contaminated needles and syringes and sexual encounters pose risks to the drug abuser. Diagnosis may be more difficult in clients with substance abuse because symptomatic phases are similar to withdrawal, "bad dope," or debilitated states caused by malnutrition or other neglect (Sobol, 1991). Antibodies do not appear in the blood for up to 6 months after infection. Nursing care for HIV/AIDS clients involves promoting good nutrition, preventing infection, administering medications, promoting self-care, and providing counseling. Prevention through education about modes of transmission is particularly important for this group of clients.

Tuberculosis.   The incidence of tuberculosis has increased in general, as well as secondary to immune suppression because of HIV/AIDS. This infection is more aggressive in HIV positive individuals. Diagnostic tests include a tuberculin skin test, sputum smear and culture, and chest X ray. Medical management includes antituberculosis drug therapy consisting of isoniazid (INH) 300 mg/day, rifampin 600 mg/day for 6 months, and pyrazinamide (PZA) 15 to 30 mg/kg/day up to a 3-gram maximum during the first 2 months of treatment. Nursing care includes teaching clients the importance of taking medications as prescribed and preventing the spread of airborne tubercle bacilli.

Viral hepatitis.   Viral hepatitis is the predominant cause of liver disease in non-alcoholic IV drug addicts (Mutchnick, Lee, & Peleman, 1991). Viral agents that can cause acute or chronic liver disease include hepatitis A, hepatitis B, non-A, non-B, and delta hepatitis. Transmission of hepatitis A occurs person-to-person through fecal contamination or from contaminated food or water. Hepatitis B, non-A, non-B, and delta hepatitis are spread through infected blood and parenteral drug abuse with contaminated needles and syringes.

Clinical manifestations occur in three phases and include fever, chills, nausea, vomiting, anorexia, headache, arthralgia, right upper quadrant tenderness, weakness, general malaise, weight loss, and enlarged lymph nodes (preicteric phase); jaundice, dark urine, clay-colored stools, anorexia, nausea, vomiting, weakness, malaise, and liver tenderness (icteric phase); and disappearance of signs and symptoms (posticteric phase). The preicteric phase lasts 4 to 6 weeks, and the posticteric phase may last as long as 4 months.

Medical management is supportive with fluids, electrolyte replacement, antihistamines for pruritus, and antiemetics. Nursing care consists of general supportive measures to promote rest and fluid balance; prevent injury, spread of disease, and skin breakdown; and provide information about self-care and adequate nutrition (Cassmeyer, 1995).

Sexually transmitted diseases.   STDs, diseases transmitted from person-to-person by sexual intercourse or intimate contact with genitalia, mouth, or rectum, have increased in incidence. Substance abusers may be at particular risk because of promiscuous behavior during intoxication or prostitution to support drug habits. STDs include syphilis, gonorrhea, chancroid, lymphogranuloma venereum, genital herpes infection, chlamydia, nonspecific urethritis, granuloma inguinale, trichomoniasis, candidiasis, pediculosis pubic, scabies, genital or venereal warts, hepatitis B infections, molluscum contagiosum, and bacterial vaginosis. Clinical manifestations include vaginitis, cervicitis, lower abdominal pain, urethritis, epididymitis, pharyngitis, proctitis, and lesions of skin or mucous membranes. Medical management is related to the causative organism. Nursing responsibilities include promoting self-care, teaching about transmission of disease and safe sex practices, providing emotional support, and promoting improved body image.

PERIOPERATIVE CARE FOR CLIENTS WITH SUBSTANCE ABUSE

The hazards and stress of surgery are intensified for clients who abuse psychoactive substances. The general health status is compromised by the chemicals or by attendant lifestyle factors. Common substances of abuse affect organ systems critical to general anesthesia. For example, smoking tobacco makes the airway more irritable to the introduction of endotracheal tubes or suction catheters. The thick secretions, chronic bronchitis, and pulmonary emphysema associated with smoking are added risks to respiratory status.

The effects of alcohol are more subtle and include increased tolerance to anesthetic agents, nutritional deficiencies, and in severe cases cirrhosis, esophageal varices, and coagulopathies, all of which can greatly compromise the surgical client (Larson, 1992). Tonnesen and colleagues (1992) found increased postoperative morbidity in a prospective study of symptom-free alcohol abusers. In a study of clients with colorectal surgery, there was a 67% rate of postoperative complications among alcoholics, as opposed to a 20% rate among controls. Average hospital stay was higher for the alcoholics than for their nonalcoholic counterparts. The authors speculate that the underlying mechanisms were subclinical cardiac insufficiency, immunosuppression, and decreased hemostatic function.

Cross-tolerance to and withdrawal from substances of abuse alter response to anesthetic agents and pose risks to safety and comfort during the perioperative period. The perioperative period is not an appropriate time to withdraw clients from addictive substances (Anderson, 1990). The emphasis is on achieving safe anesthesia, relieving postoperative pain, and preventing complications without precipitating withdrawal.

In the *preoperative* phase, it is essential to elicit a careful and complete history of substance use and abuse. Quantity and timing of chemical administration is particularly important when preparing clients for anesthesia. Thorough preoperative assessment to determine any health problems is key to guarding against complications. Clients who abuse alcohol and other drugs are at risk for trauma or diminished awareness of their health status. Obtaining an accurate history in an emergency situation, when denial may be a factor, can be a challenge. Friends and family may be consulted to provide information.

During the *intraoperative* phase, clients with substance abuse are monitored for signs of withdrawal (see Table 7-3). Anesthetic agents are chosen with regard to patterns of abuse, when known or suspected.

In the *postoperative* phase, pain is alleviated with appropriate analgesia. Baseline maintenance doses and flexible dose schedules of narcotics for clients addicted to those substances are used. Postoperative alcoholics often require benzodiazepines such as chlordiazepoxide (Librium) to control restlessness. Monitoring and controlling withdrawal occur simultaneously with routine postoperative care of these clients. Providing a safe environment is particularly important. Because of the heightened risk for postoperative complications, meticulous attention to respiratory and cardiovascular status is required.

Once the initial stress and discomfort of surgery have subsided, the nurse should discuss the relationship of addiction to pain and altered health status, as well as encourage the client to seek treatment. Teaching alternative pain management strategies such as deep breathing, guided imagery, and relaxation with audiotapes can be useful. Written materials on addiction, treatment options, and referral for treatment should be provided before discharge when appropriate. The client may be particularly receptive to treatment because of recent events (Anderson, 1990). (See Chapter 6 for more on the nurse's role in referring clients to treatment.)

PAIN MANAGEMENT

Individuals who abuse alcohol and other psychoactive substances have a higher incidence of traumatic injuries and other health problems than the general population (Agency for Health Care Policy and Research [AHCPR], 1992). Because pain is frequently a reason to seek health care and substance abuse is a common problem, coexistence of the two entities is likely (McCaffery and Vourakis, 1992). When surgery, trauma, or painful medical illnesses occur in substance abusers, pain management becomes a special challenge (Payne, 1989). A team approach, combining experts in pain management and addictions, is valuable in meeting that challenge. Ideally, such a team includes a physician experienced both in pain management and chemical dependency, an addictions nurse specialist, and a designated nurse on each hospital unit responsible for monitoring and coordinating care (McCaffery & Vourakis, 1992). Realistically, not every hospital has such expertise, so it becomes important that all nurses understand the basics of the dual problems.

A word of caution is needed regarding inadequate pain management. The prevalence of drug use and abuse coupled with legislation have led to public confusion regarding legitimate use of substances. These factors influence the attitudes of physicians and clients, and they have often led to inadequate pain management (Hill, 1989). Fear of addiction, among caregivers and clients, often results in undermedication (McCaffery & Vourakis, 1992). However, clients with painful conditions such as cancer, trauma, or surgery rarely develop psychological dependence during opioid administration (Gonzales & Coyle, 1992). When clients are inadequately medicated for pain, there is risk of pseudoaddiction. This phenomenon is characterized by escalation of analgesic demands, behavioral changes by the client to convince others of the severity of pain, and mistrust between the client and the caregivers (AHCPR, 1992). Hence, there is a need to distinguish "drug seeking" from "pain avoidance" behaviors when substance abuse is involved.

Another factor that may influence administration of medications is the attitude of caregivers toward substance abusers. Often, the desire to treat clients with substance abuse conflicts with a fear of contributing to abuse or of being duped into supporting addictive behaviors. McCaffery and Vourakis (1992) suggest examining personal values and institutional policies to assure that health care workers' feelings and opinions will not negatively impact care. Caregivers have a right to their personal opinions, as well as a professional responsibility to accept and respect the client's report of pain. The nurse must not permit negative attitudes to alter care of the client with substance abuse who is in pain.

The two main goals for pain management in the hospitalized client with substance abuse are to relieve pain and prevent or minimize withdrawal. Nursing responsibilities related to pain relief include early and accurate assessment of factors contributing to pain. In the postoperative or trauma client, infection, ischemia, or a new surgical diagnosis may be the primary cause for discomfort. Antibiotics, fasciotomy, or a reoperation may be needed and may greatly reduce the requirements and negotiations for opioids (AHCPR, 1992). Instruments such as pain rating scales to quantify pain and flow sheets to assist with titration of analgesics and identifying intervals between doses are useful in providing objective care. Furthermore, the nurse needs an accurate understanding of equianalgesic doses and the principles underlying addiction, tolerance, and dependence (see Table 7-3).

McCaffery and Vourakis (1992) suggest the following guidelines for care: avoid excessive negotiation but work with the client to determine analgesic, dose, and frequency; consider a client-controlled IV analgesia to give the client control and reduce anxiety; set limits and be consistent about expected behaviors and responsibilities of client and staff regarding medication; consider morphine for analgesia but avoid meperidine (Demerol) (tendency to accumulate in body), and pentazocine (Talwin), butorphanol (Stadol), buprenorphine (Buprenex), dezocin (Dalgan), and nalbuphine (Nubain) (antagonist activity of these drugs may precipitate severe withdrawal); and provide nonopioid and nonpharmacologic therapies for pain relief. They caution against giving psychoactive drugs with no analgesic effect, using pain relief as a bargaining chip, giving placebos, and using medications to precipitate withdrawal (McCaffery & Vourakis, 1992). Such practices destroy the client's confidence in the caregiver and may increase manipulative behaviors associated with drug seeking. Long-term treatment options are considered after the immediate need for pain management subsides and the client is ready for referral.

Clients who admit substance abuse

Managing pain is somewhat easier in clients with substance abuse who admit to past or current history of abuse. These clients may be predisposed to a reemergence of substance abusing behaviors with the stress of surgery or other painful illnesses. Their treatment does not differ from the nonaddict (AHCPR, 1992). The clients' and their families' fears about readdiction should be recognized and addressed openly (Gonzales & Coyle, 1992). Explain any psychoactive substances and respect the client's right to decide whether or not to comply. When opioids are unacceptable to the client, the nurse should consider alternatives such as nerve blocks or nonopioid analgesics. The nurse could suggest that the client contact the recovery program for support and give reassurance that physical dependence can be handled if it reoccurs (McCaffery & Vourakis, 1992).

Often it is difficult to determine the appropriate dose for the opiate addict even when the client provides a thorough history. Street drugs are subject to extreme variability. The nurse should expect the client to require larger amounts of medication and give it in sufficient amounts. Doses are titrated upward until pain relief is achieved without excessive sedation. Methadone is a good choice for treatment of acute pain in substance abusers. There is evidence that this drug also works well for clients with substance abuse who have chronic pain (Kennedy & Crowley, 1990).

When the pain-afflicted client is methadone-dependent as part of a recovery program, larger and more frequent doses of opioids are needed to achieve analgesia. If the client is NPO, methadone may be given IM in one half to one third of the total daily dose every 8 to 12 hours. Methadone may be supplemented with short-acting narcotics given parenterally. When pain subsides, supplemental narcotics are removed and the usual methadone maintenance dose is resumed (Tucker, 1990).

Clients who do not admit substance abuse

Clients who are actively abusing psychoactive substances may not admit to their use upon admission to the hospital. They may attempt to hide substance abuse for fear of punishment, unfair treatment, or legal reprisal. At the same time, these clients may be anxious about loss of control over self-medicating practices and the potential for withdrawal (McCaffery & Vourakis, 1992). The nurse must be alert to the obvious and subtle signs of addiction and its concomitant lifestyle. Specific indicators of possible abuse in the pain-afflicted individual include requests for higher and more frequent doses of injectable pain medication after the obvious cause for pain has subsided (e.g., several days after surgery), refusal to try oral medications, emotional lability, and abusive behavior. Tucker (1990) recommends tapering meperidine (Demerol), giving methadone in equivalent doses to prevent withdrawal discomfort, confronting the client to discuss pain management, and implementing a consistent plan in the presence of suspected abuse.

Nonopioid and nonpharmacological strategies

As with the nonaddicted client, nonopioid and nonpharmacologic pain management strategies are important to decrease or eliminate opioid requirements. Nonopioid analgesics such as ibuprofen (Advil, Motrin, Nuprin) are particularly effective for postoperative clients and those with orthopedic problems. Other nonopioid preparations include acetaminophen (Datril, Tylenol) and aspirin. Nonpharmacological approaches such as relaxation techniques (guided imagery, music), massage, applications of heat and cold, and transcutaneous electrical nerve stimulation (TENS) may be useful alternatives in pain management.

The following case illustrates a particularly challenging example of pain management in an addicted hospitalized client (Care Plan 7-5).

EMERGENCY CARE

The association between abuse of psychoactive substances and health crises requiring emergency care is well known. Alcohol intoxication is inextricably linked to suicides, homicides, motor vehicle accidents, drownings, burns, and falls (Skolnick, 1990; Gurney et al, 1992). Reports indicate that alcohol plays a significant causal role in at least 60% of vehicle-associated trauma (Skolnick, 1990). Trauma is also linked to abuse of other psychoactive substances, but the incidence may not be as well

Text continued on p. 184.

Care Plan 7-5

Chronic Pain/Narcotic and Benzodiazepine Addiction/
Interstitial Pulmonary Disease

Lucy, a 52-year-old Caucasian female, had been admitted to the hospital with complaints of nausea, vomiting, and shortness of breath. Lucy was diagnosed 3 years earlier with chronic interstitial pulmonary disease. She also had a history of cervical radiculopathy with chronic pain syndrome, migraine headaches, peptic ulcer disease, irritable bowel syndrome, IV narcotic abuse, and benzodiazepine abuse. Family history revealed that her father had died of abdominal carcinoma and her mother committed suicide.

ASSESSMENT

Hospital course: Lucy was cultured and found to be infected with multiple organisms: E. coli, group D enterococcus, serratia mercescens, staph aureus, candida albicans, and mycoplasma. Her lung biopsy was unremarkable, and she was HIV negative. Her IgG level was elevated.

Anti-infective therapy included: Vancomycin hydrochloride (Vancocin); fluconazole (Diflucan); clotrimazole (Mycelex) troches; ceftazidine (Fortaz); erythromycin (Erythrocin); trimethoprim sulfamethoxazole (Bactrim); and ciprofloxacin hydrochloride (Cipro).

NURSING DIAGNOSES

Impaired gas exchange related to lung failure
Alteration in comfort related to addiction, high tolerance, and increased anxiety
Ineffective individual coping related to drug addiction
Potential for infection related to IV drug use and lowered state of resistance to disease
Alteration in nutrition related to inadequate intake, poor choice of nutrients
Potential impaired skin integrity related to immobilization during hospitalization
Anticipatory grieving for client and family related to poor prognosis and limited options

Outcome identification	Nursing interventions	Rationale	Evaluation
Nursing diagnosis: Impaired gas exchange related to lung failure			
1. Client will maintain adequate gas exchange as evidenced by arterial blood gases within normal range and free from symptoms of respiratory distress in 2 weeks.	1a. See Care Plan 7-3 for nursing interventions for this nursing diagnosis. Medications: • Midazolam 5 mg q hr. • Fentanyl drip at 150 μg q hr. • Morphine sulfate (PCA and continuous mode) at 4 mg q hr.	1a. For therapy: • Anxiety management • Pain management • Glucocorticoid	1. Lucy developed acute respiratory distress syndrome (ARDS) with marked respiratory failure requiring intubation and maximum oxygenation. At one time her oxygenation was so poor that she required pancuronium bromide 4 mg per hour (nondepolarizing skeletal relaxant). She was worked up for a possible

Outcome identification	Nursing interventions	Rationale	Evaluation
Nursing diagnosis: Impaired gas exchange related to lung failure—cont'd			
	• Methylpred-nisolone sodium succinate 60 mg IV q 6 hrs.	• Anti-inflammatory	lung transplantation, but was not considered a candidate because of: active sepsis, increased doses of steroids, and history of IV narcotic abuse. A transesophageal echocardiogram was ordered to rule out endocarditis, but Lucy refused this procedure. She eventually required a tracheostomy to facilitate ventilation. Three months after hospitalization, Lucy died. Goal not met.
	• Sucralfate 1 gm PO q 6 hrs.	• Antiulcer agent	
	• Heparin sodium 5000 U subq q 12 hrs.	• Anticoagulant	
Nursing diagnosis: Alteration in comfort related to addiction, high tolerance, and increased anxiety			
1. Client will require no more than one medication for pain per 24 hours by 1 month.	1a. Administer analgesics and antianxiety medications as required.	1a. To assist with pain management.	1. Her initial medications of midazolam and fentanyl were not adequate for her to control pain so she was placed on morphine sulfate. Throughout her hospital stay Lucy required high levels of morphine sulfate (45 mg in 17 hours on PCA which increased at one point to 107 mg in 24 hours). She also received high doses of Soma Compound
	1b. Allow client to participate in medication decisions as appropriate (PCA pump).	1b. Client can supply pain medication as needed. Relieves pain before it becomes severe.	
	1c. Monitor effects of medications closely (pain rating scale, vital signs).	1c. Evaluates relief of pain from objective and subjective observations.	
	1d. Provide alternative pain control strategies (imagery).	1d. Teaches client to implement non-narcotic relief of pain.	

Continued.

Chronic Pain/Narcotic and Benzodiazepine Addiction/
Interstitial Pulmonary Disease—cont'd

Outcome identification	Nursing interventions	Rationale	Evaluation
Nursing diagnosis: Alteration in comfort related to addiction, high tolerance, and increased anxiety—cont'd			(carisoprodol, a skeletal muscle relaxant, and codeine) and benzodiazepines. Goal not met.
Nursing diagnosis: Ineffective individual coping related to drug addiction			
1. Client will cooperate with the treatment staff and assist in her own care by 2 weeks.	1a. Refer to psychiatric consultation.	1a. Psychiatrist can best prescribe psychiatric medications. Psychiatric nurse can assist with behavioral management.	1. A psychiatrist was called to evaluate Lucy's anxiety. The psychiatrist prescribed clonazepam, a benzodiazepine, 1 mg TID and 1.5 mg HS. Her basal rate of morphine was decreased slowly and visual imagery was suggested for pain control. Ultimately Lucy refused clonazepam and was returned to continuous morphine drip. The treatment team described Lucy as manipulative and uncooperative with her treatment regimen. Goal not met.
	1b. Set limits on manipulative behavior.	1b. Assists the client externally to control her behavior. (See Chapter 6 for steps.)	
	1c. Confront gently to motivate client to cooperate with treatment plan.	1c. Allows the client to face how her behavior affects others. (See Chapter 6.)	
	1d. Support efforts at alternative pain management.	1d. It is difficult for the client addicted to narcotics to use alternative methods, and she needs the nurse's support.	
	1e. Mobilize family support for client.	1e. The client needs support of family and friends to deal with severe illness, without her addiction.	
	1f. Provide support to client.	1f. The client needs the support of the nurse to deal with illness, etc.	

Outcome identification	Nursing interventions	Rationale	Evaluation
Nursing diagnosis: Potential for infection related to IV drug use and lowered state of resistance to disease			
1. The client will remain free from additional infections while in the hospital.	1a. Give medications as prescribed. 1b. Use sterile techniques. 1c. Frequent hand-washing.	1a. Combat infections. 1b. To prevent spread of infections. 1c. Same as above.	1. Client had unremitting sepsis. Goal not met.
Nursing diagnosis: Alteration in nutrition related to inadequate intake, poor choice of nutrients			
1. The client will regain her admission weight by discharge.	1a. Provide adequate nutrition either orally or parenterally.	1a. To supply needed nutrients.	1. Client's condition continued to deteriorate while in the hospital. Goal not met.
Nursing diagnosis: Potential impaired skin integrity related to immobilization during hospitalization			
1. Client maintains intact skin while in the hospital.	1a. Turn every 2 hours. 1b. Keep client clean and dry.	1a. To maintain adequate circulation to all areas of skin. 1b. To prevent infection.	1. Client's skin remained intact until 2 weeks before she died when she developed decubitus ulcers. Goal not met.
Nursing diagnosis: Anticipatory grieving for client and family related to poor prognosis and limited options			
1. Client verbalizes her feelings about her prognosis.	1a. Explain each procedure and rationale for use. 1b. Develop therapeutic relationship. 1c. Discuss prognosis with client. 1d. Reflect back feelings perceived or expressed. 1e. Encourage discussion of feelings.	1a. Helps client become aware of the reality of her situation. 1b. Helps client develop support from nurse. 1c. Helps the client become aware of her situation. 1d. Use of empathetic listening and responding skills helps the client feel supported. 1e. Allows the client to vent sad feelings.	1. Lucy refused to discuss her condition and her feelings with the nurse. She continued to deny the seriousness of her condition to the end. Despite the hopelessness of her situation, she insisted on being a full code. Goal not met.

documented (Brookoff et al, 1993). Trauma may be the most common indicator of alcohol and other drug abuse.

Substance abuse emergencies other than trauma include overdose and suicide. Overdose is a relatively common phenomenon, and there is an increased risk of suicidal behavior among substance abusers (Hasin et al, 1988). Hence the nurse in an emergency department must consider the possibility of alcohol and other drug abuse when clients present with traumatic injuries, as well as overdose and suicidal behavior.

General guidelines

There are some general guidelines that define treatment in substance abuse emergencies. The first priority is treating life-threatening problems such as airway obstruction, respiratory depression, cardiovascular collapse, and convulsions. Establishing a patent airway, providing ventilatory support (artificial respiration, respirator), maintaining adequate circulatory status (chest compressions, defibrillator, IV line), and controlling seizures (safety measures, IV diazepam) should be the first level of care. The second priority is gathering the most complete history of recent events as possible. This information may be elicited from a relative or friend, although most of these clients arrive unaccompanied. Routine blood chemistries, blood counts, urinalysis, and toxicological screens of blood and urine provide further clues to the clients' circumstances. Evaluation of HIV status, ECG, and chest X-ray are important also.

Safety precautions must be maintained during emergency care. Clients may exhibit varying levels of consciousness, convulsions, hallucinations, and combative behavior. The nurse should provide reassurance and support. A consistent, self-assured, calm demeanor and frequent eye contact help to reassure the client.

Client care procedures that address trauma and other medical problems are instituted as soon as feasible. Plans for transfer to another unit or for future treatment should be made when the client is stable.

Drug overdose

Drug overdose is an acute life-threatening emergency. Treatment follows the plan outlined in the general guidelines above. Specific interventions for drug classifications appear in Table 7-2. Respiratory depression and altered levels of consciousness are common in overdose. It is important to maintain a patent airway and assess vital signs every 15 minutes. After management of basic life support and establishment of IV access, the following medications are usually given: naloxone to immediately reverse coma induced by opiate overdose and 100 mg of thiamine because alcohol inhibits thiamine absorption. Inadequate thiamine in the presence of plentiful glucose may result in a complex mixture of neurological problems and memory deficits called *Wernicke-Korsakoff syndrome*. Maintaining hydration and monitoring fluid intake and output are important. An IV line should be established with the rate dependent on the client's needs. Drug overdose may be accompanied by stupor or agitation (or both with PCP or anticholinergics). Table 7-6 lists other clinical manifestations that assist in determining the substances responsible for the client's toxic state.

Table 7-6

Drug classifications and distinguishing clinical manifestations in stupor and agitation

Drug classification	Clinical manifestations
Stupor	
CNS depressants	Odor of alcohol, absence of other clinical manifestations presented below
Opiates/synthetic narcotics	Pinpoint pupils, diaphoresis
PCP	Hypersalivation, fixed stare, flushed skin
Solvents/aerosols	Dilated pupils, absence of dry mouth
Anticholinergics	Dilated pupils, fixed stare, flushed dry skin, dry mouth
Aspirin	Diaphoresis, tinnitus
Agitation	
Amphetamines	Dilated pupils, acute diaphoresis, fever, grinding of jaw
Cocaine	Absence of above clinical manifestations
PCP	Hypersalivation, fixed stare, flushed skin
Cannabis	Whites of eyes reddened
Anticholinergics	Dilated pupils, fixed stare, flushed dry skin, dry mouth
Hallucinogens	Dilated pupils, flushed skin, possible diaphoresis

A nursing care plan for two priority nursing diagnoses in drug overdose is presented (Care Plan 7-6).

Suicide attempts

Suicide may be attempted with a variety of means from intentional overdose to gunshot or knife wounds. Clients who attempt suicide require emergency care for life-threatening circumstances, as described, as well as evaluation for concomitant drug abuse. Psychosocial history is also extremely important in planning care. Often clients who have attempted suicide will deny the fact and attribute their injuries to an accident.

Other emergency care encounters

Alcohol intoxication is frequently encountered in an emergency setting. The nurse must recognize this condition and provide prompt, informed care. See Table 7-1 for clinical manifestations of intoxication and associated blood alcohol levels.

Substance abuse should always be considered in clients presenting for emergency care when there is *trauma* or with unexplained *CNS depression*. The possibility of *polydrug use* cannot be ignored. Again, prompt recognition and intervention are needed to assure client safety. Refer to Table 7-3 for summary of clinical manifestations and interventions in intoxication.

Drug-seeking behavior in the emergency room is not uncommon. Clients with substance abuse may feign injuries to obtain psychoactive substances. Because pain, a predominant symptom, is based on self-report, each situation must be carefully evaluated. These clients deserve support, reassurance, and understanding. A

Care Plan 7-6

Client Overdosed on Unknown Chemicals

John, about age 20, was brought to the emergency room by the police, who found him partially conscious on the sidewalk at a shopping center. There was no one around him when he was found.

ASSESSMENT

By the time John arrived at the emergency room, he was unconscious but could respond to extreme pain. He had no obvious cuts or bruises. Emergency procedures were begun.

NURSING DIAGNOSES

Ineffective airway clearance related to drug-induced respiratory depression
Potential for injury related to altered level of consciousness

Outcome identification	Nursing interventions	Rationale	Evaluation
Nursing diagnosis: Ineffective airway clearance related to drug-induced respiratory depression			
1. Client will maintain a patent airway throughout.	1a. Straighten or tilt head back.	1a. Prevents tongue from obstructing airway.	1. John maintained a patent airway during his hospitalization. Goal met.
	1b. Suction secretions if needed.	1b. Client is unable to clear secretions that block airway.	
	1c. Prepare for endotracheal tube insertion.	1c. Mechanical assistance may be required.	
2. Client will maintain adequate gas exchange as evidenced by arterial blood gases within normal limits within 1 hour.	2a. Continuously assess airway, respirations, capillary refill, vital signs, and mental status.	2a. Indicators of adequate gas exchange.	2. John's pO_2 was 65% at admission, but was 99% within 1 hour. Goal met.
	2b. Administer oxygen if ordered (used judiciously as it may decrease spontaneous respirations).	2b. To assist with ventilation.	
	2c. Keep client quiet, comfortable.	2c. Reduces oxygen needs.	

Outcome identification	Nursing interventions	Rationale	Evaluation
Nursing diagnosis: Ineffective airway clearance related to drug-induced respiratory depression—cont'd			
3. Client will maintain adequate tissue perfusion as evidenced by color return in extremities of 1 minute or less throughout.	3a. Establish IV access for fluids and emergency medications.	3a. Fluids and emergency medications (naloxone, physostigmine) may be ordered to restore circulation and reverse effects of drug.	3. John's tissue perfusion was maintained within normal limits throughout treatment. Goal met.
Nursing diagnosis: Potential for injury related to altered level of consciousness			
1. Client will sustain no injury while in the hospital.	1a. Assess for physical injuries on admission.	1a. Client may have sustained injury before admission.	1. As John began to regain consciousness, he became agitated but became calm after orientation by the nurse. Goal met.
	1b. Continuously assess level of consciousness.	1b. To assist in modifying interventions as changes are noted.	
	1c. Maintain NPO status.	1c. To prevent aspiration when consciousness is decreased.	
	1d. Promote safety (padded siderails, constant observation, check for dentures and contact lenses).	1d. Client may be restless, combative, and unable to maintain self.	
	1e. Maintain calm atmosphere and decreased sensory stimuli.	1e. Excessive stimuli may escalate anxiety or violence when present.	
	1f. Provide reassurance.	1f. Reassurance of the presence of the nurse helps maintain calmness in the client.	

calm, nonjudgmental attitude is important when approaching drug-seeking behavior. When confronted about alcohol or other drug abuse, clients may become hostile or manipulative. Referral to treatment is appropriate.

Discharge

Even though the association between substance abuse and emergency room admissions is well recognized, the opportunity for intervention is often missed. Lowenstein, Weissberg, and Terry (1990) found that few intoxicated clients treated for emergencies were referred for treatment. These authors suspect that underestimation of the problem, the hectic pace of an emergency setting, or the hostile nature of alcoholic clients may prevent intervention. Informed professional practice includes recognition and referral. Options for emergency room clients vary from brief intervention and appropriate written materials to referral to treatment professionals. When clients are transferred to other units, a careful documentation of actual or suspected patterns of abuse and interventions should accompany them. When clients are discharged home from the emergency room, they should have return appointments and referrals that address substance abuse and any other health problems. Often the life-threatening problem that brought a client with substance abuse to the emergency room serves as motivation for seeking help (see Chapter 6). Recognizing that denial is a major feature of substance abuse, the nurse should confront the client with objective evidence of the problem and offer support in obtaining treatment. Enlisting the cooperation of family and friends when possible will facilitate referral. Every emergency department or trauma center should have a comprehensive plan to evaluate and refer these clients with substance abuse.

SUMMARY

Because abuse of psychoactive substances poses a major health risk, nurses in hospital settings must be prepared to recognize the problem and intervene appropriately. To be effective, the nurse must be aware of the clinical manifestations and complications of drugs of abuse, as well as treatment options. A team approach that includes specialists in addictions is ideal for management of clients with substance abuse, but the abuse problem must first be recognized. Clients may be admitted to the hospital with the diagnosis of substance abuse or dependency, but they are more likely to have other medical conditions and undiagnosed substance abuse. Many medical conditions are results of the substance abuse. Clients may be seen on general medical-surgical units, ICUs, surgery units, or the emergency department.

REFERENCES

Acee, A.M. & Smith, D.C. (1987). Crack. *American Journal of Nursing, 98*(5), 614-617.

Agency for Health Care Policy and Research, Public Health Service. (1992). *Acute pain management: Operative or medical procedures and trauma. Clinical Practice Guideline* (AHCPR Publication No. 92-0032.) Rockville, MD: U.S. Department of Health and Human Services.

Altura, B.M. & Altura, B.T. (1990). Alcohol, stroke, and the cerebral circulation. *Alcohol World, 14*(4), 322-331.

Andersen, A.R. (1990). The postoperative client in withdrawal on a general medical-surgical unit. In L. Jack (Ed.) *Nursing care planning with the addicted client*, Vol. II, Skokie, IL: National Nurses Society on Addictions.

Benzer, D.G. (1990). Quantification of the alcohol withdrawal syndrome in 487 alcoholic patients. *Journal of Substance Abuse Treatment, 7*, 117-123.

Blattner, W.A. (1992). Etiology and epidemiology of malignant disease. In W.N. Kelley (Ed.) *Textbook of internal medicine* (2nd ed.). Philadelphia, PA: J.B. Lippincott Co.

Boro, J.K. (1989). Nicotine dependence and alcoholism epidemiology and treatment. *Journal of Psychoactive Drugs, 21*(3), 323-329.

Brody, S.L., Slovis, C.M., & Wrenn, K.D. (1990). Cocaine-related medical problems: Consecutive series of 233 patients. *The American Journal of Medicine, 88*, 325-331.

Brookoff, D., Campbell, E.A., & Shaw, L.M. (1993). The underreporting of cocaine-related trauma: Drug abuse warning network reports vs. hospital toxicology tests. *American Journal of Public Health, 83*(3), 369-371.

Cassmeyer, V.L. (1995). Management of persons with liver problems. In W.J. Phipps, B.C. Long, N.F. Woods, & V.L. Cassmeyer (Eds.) *Medical-surgical nursing: Concepts and clinical practice* (5th ed.). St. Louis, MO: Mosby.

Castaneda, R. & Cushman, P. (1989). Alcohol withdrawal: A review of clinical management. *Journal of Clinical Psychiatry, 50*(8), 278-284.

Cobbs, C.G. & Douglas, J.L. (1992). Approach to endocarditis, intravascular infections, pericarditis, and myocarditis. In W.N. Kelley (Ed.) *Textbook of internal medicine* (2nd ed.). Philadelphia, PA: J.B. Lippincott Co.

Crabb, D.W. & Lumeng, L. (1992). Alcoholic liver disease. In W.N. Kelley (Ed.) *Textbook of internal medicine* (2nd ed.). Philadelphia, PA: J.B. Lippincott Co.

Dans, P.E. (1987). Alcoholism: Defeatism in medical centers (letter). *Hospital Practice, 22*(11), 16.

Dimagno, E.P. (1992). Pancreatitis. In W.N. Kelley (Ed.) *Textbook of internal medicine* (2nd ed.). Philadelphia, PA: J.B. Lippincott.

Foy, A., March, S., & Drinkwater, V. (1988). Use of an objective clinical scale in the assessment and management of alcohol withdrawal in a large general hospital. *Alcoholism: Clinical and Experimental Research, 12*(3), 360-364.

Friedman, H.S. (1990). Alcohol and hypertension. *Alcohol World, 14*(4), 313-319.

Gawin, F.H. (1991). Cocaine addiction: Psychology and neurophysiology. *Science, 251*, 1580-1585.

Gonzales, G.R. & Coyle, N. (1992). Treatment of cancer pain in a former opioid abuser: Fears of the patient and staff and their influence on care. *Journal of Pain and Symptom Management, 7*(4), 246-249.

Greig, J.C. (1995). Intraoperative nursing. In W.J. Phipps, B.C. Long, N.F. Woods, & V.L. Cassmeyer (Eds.) *Medical-surgical nursing: Concepts and clinical practice* (5th ed.). St. Louis, MO: Mosby.

Grimes, D.E. (1995). *Infectious diseases.* St. Louis, MO: Mosby.

Gurney, J.G., Rivara, F.P., Mueller, B.A., Newell, D.W., Copass, M.K., & Jurkovich, G.J. (1992). The effects of alcohol intoxication on the initial treatment and hospital course of patients with acute brain injury. *The Journal of Trauma, 33*(5), 709-713.

Hasin, D., Grant, B., & Endicott, J. (1988). Treated and untreated suicide attempts in substance abuse patients. *The Journal of Nervous and Mental Disease, 176*(5), 289-294.

Hill, C.S. (1989). Pain management in a drug-oriented society. *Cancer, 63*, 2383-2386.

Holbrook, J.M. (1991). Hallucinogens. In E.G. Bennett & D. Woolf (Eds.) *Substance abuse: Pharmacologic, developmental and clinical perspectives* (2nd ed.). Albany, NY: Delmar Publishers, Inc.

Jacobs, B. (1992). Alcoholism-induced bone necrosis. *New York State Journal of Medicine, 92*(8), 334-338.

Kennedy, J.A. & Crowley, T.J. (1990). Chronic pain and substance abuse: A pilot study of opioid maintenance. *Journal of Substance Abuse Treatment, 7*, 233-238.

Lange, W.R., White, N., & Robinson, N. (1992). Medical complications of substance abuse. *Post-graduate Medicine, 92*(3), 205-214.

Larson, C.P. (1992). Evaluation of the patient and preoperative preparation. In P.G. Barash, B.F. Cullen, & R.K. Stoelting (Eds.) *Clinical anesthesia.* Philadelphia, PA: J.B. Lippincott Co.

Lee, E.W. & D'Alonzo, G.E. (1993). Cigarette smoking, nicotine addiction, and its pharmacologic treatment. *Annuals of Internal Medicine, 153*, 34-48.

Levine, D.P. (1991a). Skin and soft tissue infections in intravenous drug abusers. In D.P. Levine & J.D. Sobel (Eds.) *Infections in intravenous drug abusers*. New York, NY: Oxford University Press.

Levine, D.P. (1991b). Infectious endocarditis in intravenous drug abusers. In D.P. Levine & J.D. Sobel (Eds.) *Infections in intravenous drug abusers*. New York, NY: Oxford University Press.

Li, T.K. (1992). Approach to the patient with alcoholism. In W.N. Kelley (Ed.) *Textbook of internal medicine* (2nd ed.). Philadelphia, PA: J.B. Lippincott Co.

Lowenstein, S.R., Weissberg, M.P., & Terry, D. (1990). Alcohol intoxication, injuries, and dangerous behaviors—and the revolving emergency department door. *The Journal of Trauma, 30*(10), 1252-1258.

McCaffery, M. & Vourakis, C. (1992). Assessment and relief of pain in chemically dependent patients. *Orthopaedic Nursing, 11*(2), 13-27.

Mutchnick, M.G., Horchang, H.L., & Peleman, R.G. (1991). Liver disease associated with intravenous drug abuse. In D.P. Levine & J.D. Sobel. *Infections in intravenous drug abusers*. New York, NY: Oxford University Press.

Myers, E.M. (Ed.) (1991). *Head and neck oncology: Diagnosis, treatment, and rehabilitation*. Boston: Little, Brown & Co.

Payne, R.M. (1989). Pain in the drug abuser. In K.M. Foley & R.M. Payne (Eds.) *Current therapy of pain*. Philadelphia, PA: B.C. Decker, Inc.

Phipps, W.J., Long, B.C., Woods, N.F., & Cassmeyer, V.F. (Eds.) (1995). *Medical-surgical nursing: Concepts and clinical practice* (5th ed.). St. Louis, MO: Mosby.

Ray, O. & Ksir, C. (1993). *Drugs, society, and human behavior* (6th ed.). St. Louis, MO: Mosby–Year Book.

Robin, H. & Michelson, J. (1988). *Drug abuse and recognition*. Chicago, IL: Year Book Medical Publishers, Inc.

Rubin, E. & Doria, J. (1990). Alcoholic cardiomyopathy. *Alcohol World, 14*(4), 277-284.

Scheidegger, C. & Zimmerli, W. (1989). Infectious complications in drug addicts: Seven-year review of 269 hospitalized narcotics abusers in Switzerland. *Reviews of Infectious Diseases, 2*(3), 486-493.

Schenk, E. (1995). Addictive behaviors. In W.J. Phipps, B.C. Long, N.F. Woods, & V.L. Cassmeyer (Eds.) *Medical-surgical nursing: Concepts and clinical practice* (5th ed.). St. Louis, MO: Mosby.

Schuckit, M.A. (1989). *Drug and alcohol abuse: A clinical guide to diagnosis and treatment* (3rd ed.). New York, NY: Plenum Medical Book Company.

Shaw, J.M., Kolesar, G., Sellers, E.M., Kaplan, H.L., & Sandor, P. (1981). Development of optimal treatment tactics for alcohol withdrawal. 1. Assessment and effectiveness of supportive care. *Journal of Clinical Psychopharmacology, 1*, 382-389.

Skolnick, A. (1990). Illicit drugs take another toll—death or injury from vehicle–associated trauma. *Journal of the American Medical Association, 263*(23), 3122-3125.

Slade, J. (1989). The tobacco epidemic: Lessons from history. *Journal of Psychoactive Drugs, 21*(3), 281-291.

Smith, A. (1991). When the pancreas self-destructs. *American Journal of Nursing, 91*(8), 38-52.

Snow, G.B. (1992). Evaluation and staging. In G.B. Snow & J.R. Clark (Eds.) *Multimodality therapy for head and neck cancer*. New York, NY: Thieme Medical Publishers.

Sobel, J.D. (1991). Acquired immunodeficiency syndrome in intravenous drug abusers. In D.P. Levine & J.D. Sobel (Eds.) *Infections in intravenous drug abusers*. New York, NY: Oxford University Press.

Tonnesen, H., Petersen, K.R., Hojgaad, L., Stokholm, K.H., Nielsen, H.J., Knigge, U., & Kehlet, K. (1992). Postoperative morbidity among symptom-free alcohol misusers. *The Lancet, 340*, 334-337.

Tucker, C. (1990). Acute pain and substance abuse in surgical patients. *Journal of Neuroscience Nursing, 22*(6), 339-350.

Turrell, E.S., Schmetzer, A.D., Wright, J.J., & Scherl, E.K. (1988). Drug and alcohol withdrawal: Methods for patient management. *Indiana Medicine, 81*(5), 401-407.

Tweed, S.H. (1989). Identifying the alcoholic client. *Nursing Clinics of North America, 24*(1), 13-32.

Westermeyer, J. (1992). Substance use disorders: Predictions for the 1990's. *American Journal of Drug and Alcohol Abuse, 18*(1), 1-11.

Woolf, D.S. (1991a). Detoxification. In E.G. Bennett & D. Woolf (Eds.) *Substance abuse: Pharmacologic, developmental, and clinical perspectives* (2nd ed.). Albany, NY: Delmar Publishers.

Woolf, D.S. (1991b). CNS depressants: Alcohol. In E.G. Bennett & D. Woolf (Eds.) *Substance abuse: Pharmacologic, developmental, and clinical perspectives* (2nd ed.). Albany, NY: Delmar Publishers.

8 | Substance Abuse in Perinatal Care

There is no safe use of drugs or alcohol in the pregnant woman. Because social use of alcohol is prevalent and legal and illegal drug use is common among young adults, it is not surprising that use of these substances by pregnant women nears the prevalence of that of society as a whole. This chapter describes the effects of drug and alcohol use on the mother, the developing fetus, and the neonate, as well as the nursing care necessary for them.

Perinatal addiction results in grave consequences for the individual, family, and society. Planning and implementing a program to identify pregnant substance users and abusers and then treat them and their offspring is costly and cumbersome. The direct costs of administering such a program, however, are only a fraction of the total costs associated with ignoring the problem. Costs for crisis-related care, or care of the infant after exposure to substances of abuse, include hospitalization in neonatal intensive care units at an average daily charge of $1,500 (National Commission to Prevent Infant Mortality, 1990). Other costs include foster care, future medical care, counseling, special education, sheltered living, and lost earning potential.

Women who use or abuse substances and have repeated pregnancies wreak havoc in their own lives and those of their future children. The woman's general state of health deteriorates, she may incur further medical problems of her own, and she is at a higher risk for childbearing. If this vicious cycle can be stopped, the personal and societal suffering can cease.

Addiction crosses socioeconomic, geographic, and cultural lines. No one is immune from the problem. Chasnoff, Landress, and Barrett (1990) compared pregnant women obtaining prenatal care from private physicians with women who obtained prenatal care from a clinic. The groups had similar rates of urine toxicology positive for drugs (including alcohol). In a study of 30,000 women, 1 in 9 tested positive for drugs at delivery (National Council on Alcoholism and Drug Dependence [NCADD], 1993). Illicit drug use is not confined to urban, minority women according to Slutsker and others (1993), who found a 5% incidence of drug use (alcohol was not included) in a sample of all women giving birth in one state during one month.

Often, several substances (alcohol and other drugs) are used simultaneously; thus it is difficult to ascertain if the effects on the infant are caused by an isolated substance or the interaction of many substances. Lifestyle issues such as general nutrition, overall health, and risk-taking behaviors (e.g., engaging in unprotected intercourse with multiple partners) also influence the health of the woman and her fetus. These factors intertwine with the substance's direct effects, making it difficult to ascertain what maternal variable is responsible for which infant outcome.

In addition, many substances of abuse cause menstrual irregularities that obscure the early signs of pregnancy. Some substances interfere with pregnancy tests (Zuspan & Zuspan, 1991). This potential inability to recognize the state of pregnancy is concerning because some of the drugs of abuse are teratogens. A *teratogen* is a substance that interferes with embryologic development and produces defects in one or more organ systems.

Nurses who care for pregnant women with substance abuse should undergo a period of self-examination with respect to their feelings regarding addiction in childbearing women. Nonjudgmental, therapeutic relationships with these clients are impossible until the nurse's own feelings have been identified, contemplated, and resolved.

ALCOHOL

Alcohol consumption is pervasive in our society. Pregnant women's drinking patterns are of particular concern because alcohol is a teratogen. Knowledge about which beverages contain alcohol and an awareness of the harmful effects of its use can influence women to stop drinking. Numerous fetal problems can occur because of alcohol use (see Table 8-1). Many women do not realize that beer and wine coolers, especially those in 2-liter containers resembling soft drinks, contain alcohol. Because beer is inexpensive, it is commonly consumed by young women of childbearing age. Bingol and associates (1987) found Fetal Alcohol Syndrome (FAS) in children of drinkers whose beverage of choice was beer. Absolute alcohol is equally detrimental, whether it is derived from beer, wine, or liquor.

The consequences of maternal alcohol consumption depend upon factors such

---

Table 8-1

Risks associated with maternal alcohol ingestion

Drinks (no.)	Risks

2 or more drinks daily includes:
  2 mixed drinks, 1 oz. liquor each
  2 glasses of wine, 5 oz. each
  2 beers, 12 oz. each
	Intrauterine growth retardation
	Immature motor activity
	Increased rate of anomalies
	Decreased muscle tone
	Poor sucking pressure
	Increased rate of stillbirths
	Decreased placental weight

5 or more drinks on occasion	Increased risk of structural brain abnormalities
6 or more drinks daily	Fetal Alcohol Syndrome

From Bobak, I.M. & Jensen, M.D. (1995). *Essentials of maternity nursing: The nurse and the childbearing family.* (5th ed.). St. Louis: Mosby.

as genetic predisposition of the fetus, maternal health, women's metabolic rates, the amount, and timing of alcohol consumption with regard to stage of pregnancy.

Health status of the mother is influenced by age, nutritional status, exposure to infectious agents, and socioeconomic status (Schnoll, 1986). Chronic alcohol consumption causes the woman's general state of health to deteriorate. Also there is an increased incidence of FAS or fetal alcohol effects (FAE) when alcoholic mothers are older and have had several pregnancies. If a woman has one child with FAS or FAE and continues to drink, she has an increased likelihood of having another affected child (Streissguth, 1991).

Women achieve higher blood alcohol levels than men because they have less gastric alcohol dehydrogenase, the enzyme required for metabolism of alcohol. In addition, women have less body water; therefore they have a higher serum alcohol level. Pregnancy also affects maternal metabolism of alcohol (Brien, 1983).

No safe lower limit of alcohol consumption has been established. Some researchers believe that as little as one drink a day could result in FAS or FAE. For anomalies to occur, a "threshold level" must be present in the maternal system (Schnoll, 1986). Ernhart and others (1987) found a teratogenic maternal ethanol dose to be more than six drinks per day (i.e., more than 3 oz. of absolute alcohol), whereas Wright (1986) found the teratogenic dose of ethanol to be 80 grams of alcohol or about 8 large glasses of wine per day both before and during pregnancy. Conversely, despite excessive alcohol use, some women give birth to unaffected infants (Sokol, Miller, & Reed, 1980). In fraternal twin studies, Chasnoff (1986b) found different expressions of alcohol teratogenicity.

Timing of maternal alcohol consumption also determines the type of fetal effects. Ernhart and associates (1987) found a "critical period for alcohol teratogenicity to be around the time of conception." A *critical period* is a stage of fetal development when developing tissue is highly vulnerable to a teratogen. Typically, this occurs when cells are rapidly dividing and differentiating. Peak levels of ethanol play a more significant role in teratogenesis than chronic low levels (Chasnoff, 1986a), although chronic alcoholics have a higher rate of infants with FAS than women who drink socially.

Alcohol consumption before implantation may result in miscarriage. Exposure to ethanol early in the first trimester may disrupt organogenesis, causing the classic mid-facial anomalies associated with FAS. During the first half of this time, the woman may not know she is pregnant.

Alcohol exposure during the second trimester may cause spontaneous abortion. Kline and others (1980) found that as little as 2 ounces of absolute alcohol per week increased the likelihood of spontaneous abortion. Harlap and Shiono (1980) also compared the impact of drinking versus smoking on spontaneous abortion and found that maternal alcohol consumption much more greatly affects the rate of miscarriage. Alcohol consumption during the last trimester may cause fetal growth retardation and may interfere with the migration of neurons in the fetal central nervous system (CNS) (Miller & Robertson, 1993).

Placental transfer of alcohol

Alcohol's active ingredient, ethanol, and its metabolite, acetaldehyde, are of low molecular weight and are fat soluble; therefore they readily cross the placenta.

Maternal ethanol diffuses to the fetus, and the highest levels are deposited in the fetal liver, pancreas, kidney, lung, thymus, heart, and brain. The fetal circulatory pathway shunts most of the blood past the liver via the ductus venosus, thus limiting fetal detoxification. This action is compounded by an immature and inefficient fetal liver. The fetal circulatory pathway also enhances blood flow to the heart and brain, thereby increasing fetal exposure to ethanol and acetaldehyde. Once the alcohol has reached a state of equilibrium between the mother-infant system, the maternal system's concentration will drop, allowing the fetal ethanol to diffuse back to the mother. This metabolic lag causes the fetus to be bathed in ethanol-rich amniotic fluid. When an infant is delivered to a highly intoxicated woman, the amniotic fluid smells strongly of alcohol. The infant born with high ethanol levels may appear intoxicated until the immature liver can complete metabolism (Flandermeyer, 1993).

Lactation

Ethanol readily crosses into breast milk. The infant undergoes rapid brain growth during early infancy. This rapid growth includes cell division and replication of neurons in the CNS (Weiner & Larsson, 1987). Exposure of these neurons to ethanol may adversely affect the cells postnatally when alcohol is ingested via breast milk. Therefore women who breast-feed should not drink. If the woman cannot abstain from alcohol, then she should use infant formula.

In the past, lactating women were often advised to have a glass of wine or beer to relax, promoting the let-down reflex. It was thought to stimulate a richer, more abundant milk supply. Contrary to this advice, alcohol is of no benefit to enriching human milk, and such a suggestion may provide a heavy drinker with a rationalization to continue drinking.

FETAL ALCOHOL SYNDROME AND FETAL ALCOHOL EFFECTS

Fetal Alcohol Syndrome (FAS) was first described independently by Lemoine and associates (1968) and Jones and Smith (1973). Jones and Smith (1973) observed the clinical characteristics of 11 infants born to chronic alcoholic women, and distinct patterns of anomalies emerged. For the first time, alcohol was implicated as a teratogen that produced a specific pattern of anomalies. The term *Fetal Alcohol Syndrome* was coined. Unknown to Jones and Smith until later, Lemoine and others had studied 127 children of alcoholic parents and found similar anomalies. Since these landmark studies, over 2000 scientific reports have confirmed alcohol as an intrauterine teratogen that causes lifelong, irreversible disabilities (Table 8-2). FAS is now recognized as the leading cause of mental retardation and the only preventable form. *Fetal Alcohol Effects* (FAE) refers to children with less severe FAS anomalies.

Incidence

The incidence of FAS is estimated to be between 1.9 per 1000 to 3.7 per 10,000 births (Abel & Sokol, 1987; MMWR, 1993). The incidence of FAE is approximately twice that of FAS, depending on the criteria used to make the diagnosis (Streissguth,

Table 8-2

Manifestations of the principal features of Fetal Alcohol Syndrome

CNS dysfunction	Growth deficiency	Facial characteristics	Abnormalities in other systems
Intellectual	**Prenatal**	**Eyes**	**Cardiac**
Mild to moderate mental retardation	Less than 3% for length and weight	Short palpebral fissures (small eye openings)	Murmurs (atrial septal defects, ventricular septal defects, great-vessel anomalies, and tetralogy of Fallot)
Neurologic	**Postnatal**	Strabismus, ptosis, myopia	
Microcephaly (small head size)	Less than 3% for length and weight	**Nose**	**Skeletal**
Poor coordination	Failure to thrive	Short and upturned	Limited joint movements (especially fingers and elbows and hip dislocations)
Decreased muscle tone	Disproportionate-diminished adipose tissue	Hypoplastic philtrum (flat or absent groove above upper lip)	
Behavioral		**Mouth**	Aberrant palmar creases
Irritability in infancy		Thinned upper vermilion (upper lip)	**Renogenital**
Hyperactivity in childhood		Retrognathia in infancy (receding jaw)	Kidney defects
			Labial hypoplasia
			Cutaneous
			Hemangiomas

From Bobak, I.M. & Jensen, M.D. (1995). *Essentials of maternity nursing: The nurse and the childbearing family.* (5th ed.). St. Louis: Mosby.

1990). In spite of the difference in estimates, all indications are that FAS and FAE are far more common than generally expected.

Diagnosis

The diagnosis of FAS or FAE is not always easily made. A maternal history and physical examination of the offspring are necessary to correlate the physical findings with maternal alcohol consumption. Box 8-1 provides a checklist for determining FAS. FAS is diagnosed by some of the following features: (1) dysmorphic characteristics, (2) prenatal and postnatal growth deficiency, and (3) CNS dysfunction.

Some manifestations are subtle enough to escape detection until infancy or late childhood. Failure to thrive (FTT) or academic failure are often the impetus of a medical investigation in which a maternal history may reveal drinking during pregnancy.

Alcohol-induced aberrations fall on a continuum from mild to severe; some children manifest many characteristics, while others exhibit few. FAS is the severe

Box 8-1
Fetal Alcohol Syndrome Checklist

	Points assigned
A. History of maternal alcohol consumption during pregnancy	
1. None or minimal	0
2. Moderate (at least weekly or major binges)	30
3. Heavy	50
B. Radiologic findings (when available)	
4. Hypoplasia of diatal phalanges	4
5. Bone age one to two standard deviations below mean	1
6. Bone age more than two standard deviations below mean	3
C. Growth and development	
7. Prenatal growth deficiency	
a. Head circumference less than tenth percentile	10
b. Length less than tenth percentile	6
c. Weight less than tenth percentile	4
8. Postnatal slow growth	
a. Head circumference less than second percentile	10
b. Height less than fifth percentile	4
c. Weight less than fifth percentile	6
9. Delayed motor milestones (D.Q. or I.Q. less than 70)	10
10. Poor fine motor coordination (tremulousness)	2
11. Hyperactivity or irritability	6
12. Feeding problems (infancy)	2
D. Clinical observations	
General	
13. Generalized hirsutism (before 6 months)	2
14. Hypoplastic midface	4
Ear	
15. Prominent helical root	3
16. Protruding auricle	3
Eye	
17. Small palpebral fissures	5
18. Strabismus	2
19. Ptosis	4
Nose	
20. Short nose, manifested by	
a. Epicanthic folds	1
b. Low nasal bridge	1
c. Anteverted nostrils	2
Mouth	
21. Long philtrum	3
22. Smooth philtrum	4
23. Narrow, smooth vermilion border	4

From Clarren, S.K. & Aldrich, R.A. (1993). *A concise manual for fetal alcohol screening: fetal alcohol syndrome checklist*. (Grant No. U59-CCU0069120). Seattle, WA: USIHHS and U.S. Public Service and Washington State Department of Health.

Box 8-1
Fetal Alcohol Syndrome Checklist—cont'd

	Points assigned
D. Clinical observations—cont'd	
Mouth—cont'd	
24. Cleft palate (U-shaped)	3
25. Relative prognathism (after infancy)	2
Neck	
26. Short (may appear broad)	3
Chest	
27. Pectus excavatum	2
Arms and hands	
28. Inability to fully supinate forearm	3
29. Short fifth metacarpal (clinically or by X-ray)	3
30. Clinodactyly of fifth fingers	2
31. Camptodactyly (or contractures) of fingers	3
32. Sharply angulated distal palmar crease	3
Heart	
33. Heart murmur	2
34. Known cardiac malformation	4
Back	
35. Meningomyelocele	3

---

end of the continuum; FAE refers to children on the mild end of the continuum who manifest only a few characteristics of FAS.

Dysmorphic characteristics

Dysmorphic characteristics of FAS include a characteristic facies comprised of short palpebral fissures, flat midface, hypoplastic or long philtrum, thin upper lip, epicanthal folds, low nasal bridge, minor external ear anomalies, short nose, and micrognathia. Other facial abnormalities include ptosis, myopia, strabismus, a narrow receding forehead, and a short upturned nose. Other dysmorphic characteristics include abnormal palmar creases and cardiac and skeletal anomalies.

There is a dose-response relationship associated with the FAS facies. Russell and others (1991) found that the number of FAS facial features was twice as high in children born to very heavy drinkers compared with lighter drinkers. Ernhart and others (1987) report that craniofacial anomalies are often associated with prepregnancy and first trimester alcohol consumption. Streissguth (1990) states that the higher the fetal exposure to alcohol, the more severe the effects on the child.

However, the characteristic facies of FAS change over time. Streissguth and associates (1991) studied 61 patients aged 12 to 40 years with FAS or FAE and found that the characteristic facies become less distinctive in adolescence and adulthood. The areas of continued facial growth occurred in: (1) the height of the nasal bridge and the length of the nose from root to tip, (2) the midface region, (3) the soft tissue of the philtrum and upper lip, and (4) the chin.

Growth deficiency

Children diagnosed with FAS are smaller at birth and fail to demonstrate catch-up growth. Jones and Smith (1973) observed that all of the children suffered deficient prenatal growth, and 10 of the 11 subjects exhibited postnatal growth deficiency.

Consistent reports document reduced infant birth weight among alcohol-exposed infants; dose-response is correlated with birth weight. As maternal alcohol consumption increased, infant birth weight decreased (Ernhart et al, 1987; Russell et al, 1991). Little and associates (1980) noted infants born to abstaining alcoholics still had decreases in birth weight, but to a lesser degree.

Prenatal alcohol consumption affects subsequent growth patterns as well. Children with FAS are often diagnosed later in infancy when they present with failure to thrive (FTT) in spite of adequate caloric intake. Streissguth, Clarren, and Jones (1985) followed 11 children who were the basis of defining FAS. Boys remained extremely thin. Girls were short but gained weight during the transition into puberty. The Streissguth (1991) study of 61 adolescents and adults with FAS or FAE found that the weight deficiency was less striking. Height was most affected, but 16% were within the normal range. The researchers concluded that as children with FAS grew into adolescence and adulthood, short stature became a more distinguishing characteristic of FAS. The typical emaciated appearance of children with FAS often matured into a normal height-weight proportion and even pudginess in females.

Central nervous system dysfunction

The most profound effect of FAS is CNS dysfunction. There is a correlation between the extent of overt external manifestations of FAS and cognitive impairment. When a child displays severe physical dysmorphosis associated with FAS, significant mental retardation is often present as well, but the converse is not true. Children who have a normal appearance can be cognitively affected due to alcohol's influence on fetal brain structure and function (Clarren, Bowden & Astley, 1985).

Microcephaly.   Microcephaly is usually present in children with FAS and is indicative of smaller brain size. In the 11 patients with FAS originally described by Jones and Smith (1973), 10 of the 11 were microcephalic. Other studies of children born to women who drank during pregnancy found a large proportion to be microcephalic (Autti-Ramo, Gaily & Granstrom, 1992; Russell et al, 1991). Studies also indicated that head size is inversely affected by the amount of alcohol consumed during pregnancy (Day et al, 1991; Russell et al, 1991) and the duration of fetal exposure (Autti-Ramo et al, 1992; Day et al, 1991).

Microcephaly persists into adulthood. Day and others (1991) found that the head circumference of children exposed prenatally remained smaller than non-exposed children at 3 years of age. These findings were significant after controlling for current nutrition, environment, and alcohol exposure during lactation. The researchers concluded that head circumference does not catch up. Streissguth and associates (1991) came to the same conclusion in their study of 61 adolescents and adults with FAS or FAE. Head circumference for this study population was found to be two standard deviations below the norm, and it appeared that microcephaly was one of the principal deficiencies as these children with FAS grew older.

Cognitive impairment.   A quantifiable result of FAS is cognitive impairment, which can be categorized as: (1) minimally brain damaged, (2) mildly to moderately retarded, and (3) severely to profoundly retarded. Harwood and Napolitano (1985) compared these classifications to incidence. They found that of the children diagnosed with FAS, 52% are minimally brain damaged, 45% are mildly to moderately retarded, and 2.5% are severely to profoundly retarded. The level of cognitive impairment may be readily apparent or subtly expressed learning disabilities.

Streissguth and associates (1991) found the IQ range among adolescents and adults with FAS or FAE to be from 20 (severely retarded) to 105 (normal), but 58% of the subjects had an IQ score of 70 or below, within the classification of developmentally disabled. In a follow-up study of eight of the eleven patients identified by Jones and Smith in 1973, half were found to be mentally retarded. The other four, who had not been recognized as developmentally disabled, began having problems in the fourth grade (Streissguth, Clarren & Jones, 1985). Cognitive delays may not be evident until children are older and challenged with more complex cognitive tasks.

Behavioral manifestations.   Alcohol-exposed infants often display predictable behaviors after birth, including irritability, tremors, poor feeding, and hypersensitivity to external stimuli. Other behaviors include jitteriness, weak suck, hyperexcitability, opisthotonos, hypotonia, and fitful sleeping. Streissguth, Barr and Sampson (1990) studied 482 school-aged children who were moderately exposed to alcohol prenatally and reported on their attention deficits at one day of age. The more alcohol consumed by the mother, the more poorly the infant habituated to its environment and the longer the time required to initially attach to the nipple.

Feeding problems in infants with FAS are compounded by the infant's inability to focus, which necessitates reducing environmental stimuli during feeding. This distractibility and need to reduce stimuli during mealtime can persist as the child grows. These feeding problems are thought to be a result of a disruption in the neurophysiology of feeding (i.e., poor suck or swallow coordination, weak suck reflex) and are among the first signs of CNS impairment (Randels & Streissguth, 1992). These feeding difficulties can lead to failure to thrive (FTT). FTT was the initial finding in the children first diagnosed with FAS in 1973. Since that time, however, there has been a paucity of literature concerning FTT in children with FAS (Randels & Streissguth, 1992).

As children with FAS or FAE enter the preschool years, often they are alert, talkative, friendly, hyperactive, and overly sensitive to stimuli. They may have temper tantrums and difficulty making transitions. Learning disabilities emerge secondary to hyperactivity and attention deficit disorder (ADD). In spite of the prevailing ADD the children are friendly and outgoing. This gregariousness may mask deficient learning abilities, but cognitive deficits and learning disabilities become evident in the primary grades.

During middle childhood, children with FAS or FAE exhibit hyperactivity, distractibility, impulsivity, and memory deficits. They may be affectionate but lack social skills and have difficulty predicting the consequences of their behavior. These children are generally hypotonic and have increased minor motor movements that interfere with learning.

Adolescence and adulthood are also difficult periods for persons with FAS or FAE. They continue to exhibit traits such as attention deficits, poor judgment, and impulsivity that create barriers to independent living and employment. In adolescents and adults with FAS or FAE, Streissguth and associates (1991) found that lying and defiance were characteristic, and adaptive functioning was rare despite the appearance of being alert and verbal. This population also has been described as "innocent, immature, and easily victimized," which puts them at risk for "serious life adjustment problems, including depression, alcohol abuse, and pregnancy" (Olson, Burgess, & Streissguth, 1992).

Recognition and referral

Failure to diagnose FAS or FAE results in lack of treatment. A recent report from a large teaching hospital indicated a 100% failure rate to diagnose FAS in infants whose mothers had informed their doctors that they abused alcohol during pregnancy (Little et al, 1990). Physicians are reluctant to diagnose FAS because they feel the damage has already been done. However, this limits opportunities for early intervention (Streissguth, 1991).

Professional education, public awareness, and services designed for FAS and FAE clients are needed for effective intervention (Streissguth, 1991). Intervention needs to begin early and continue throughout the client's life. Early intervention may not overcome the disabilities associated with FAS and FAE, but it can reduce stress on the family and improve later outcomes.

FAS and FAE are preventable, and prevention can be enhanced by the provision of professional and public education concerning the effects of alcohol and alcohol treatment programs for pregnant women. However, for the child born with FAS or FAE, early intervention is essential and must include realistic expectations, redirection of behaviors, and long-term goals (Olson, Burgess & Streissguth, 1992).

HEROIN

Heroin is not considered a teratogen, but it still has detrimental effects on fertility, the mother, and the fetus. Obstetrical complications include pregnancy-induced hypertension (PIH), abruptio placentae, premature delivery, and postpartum hemorrhage. The lifestyle of heroin users also increases the risks of medical complications and infections.

Because heroin is of low molecular weight and is lipid soluble, it freely diffuses across the placenta from an area of higher concentration on the maternal side to an area of lower concentration on the fetal side. Heroin directly affects the fetus by reducing uteroplacental exchange and delivery of essential nutrients by vasoconstricting placental vessels and by reducing the number of organ cells. Thus heroin-addicted infants are at risk of being small for gestational age (SGA), low birth weight (LBW), and stillborn.

Interruption in the supply of heroin causes withdrawal in the fetus passively addicted to heroin. The fetus becomes irritable, agitated, and moves about in utero. This increased energy expenditure is met with increased oxygen demands. Concomitant withdrawal in the mother produces a reduction in uteroplacental exchange secondary to uterine cramping. The combination results in fetal hypoxia, which in turn induces deep breathing movements and fetal straining. During straining, meconium may be passed and subsequently aspirated.

Because of the danger of spontaneous abortion, detoxification of the mother is not recommended earlier than 14 weeks or later than 32 weeks gestation because of fetal distress. Generally the pregnant addict is placed on methadone maintenance and given prenatal care, nutritional assistance, and counseling. Once the child is delivered, detoxification may be attempted. Following delivery, the neonate often experiences withdrawal (see the Drug Addicted Neonate) within 48 hours of birth. Though congenital anomalies are not associated with heroin use, developmental delays and behavioral difficulties have been described (Wilson et al, 1979). Heroin-exposed infants are also at increased risk of sudden infant death syndrome (SIDS).

METHADONE

Pregnant women addicted to heroin can benefit by being maintained on methadone. Because methadone is prescribed by exact dose, a more constant drug level is maintained. An additional benefit is that women in methadone programs are provided with prenatal care and support services such as counseling and assistance for food and shelter.

The lowest possible dose that will not induce craving or withdrawal is sought so the woman will not seek other illicit drugs. The average methadone dose for pregnant women is 5 to 40 mg a day. Because infants addicted to methadone experience a more severe withdrawal that begins later and lasts longer than heroin, an attempt is made to gradually decrease the methadone dose throughout the pregnancy. It has been found that the degree of withdrawal appears to be dose-related. A dose of less than 20 mg a day produces milder, less frequent withdrawal symptoms (Bashore et al, 1981).

COCAINE

Cocaine is the best researched illicit drug in pregnancy. Like heroin users, the cocaine user often lives a lifestyle that places her at increased risk for sexually transmitted diseases. Poor nutrition is a common problem that results from the appetite suppression associated with cocaine use. A number of obstetrical complications are associated with cocaine. Spontaneous abortion (Chasnoff, Burns, Schnoll & Burns 1985) and premature labor (Oro & Dixon, 1987; MacGregor et al, 1987) are induced by uterine smooth muscle irritability. Placental abruption is related to the abrupt hypertensive crisis from intense vasoconstriction and is associated with a high incidence of neonatal mortality (Chasnoff, Burns & Burns, 1987; Townsend, Laing & Jeffery, 1988). Without an awareness of the dangers, some women who are *not* abusers will take cocaine near term in hopes of inducing labor.

Maternal cocaine abuse also has been associated with preterm labor and delivery of infants with LBW, SGA, abnormal fetal heartbeat patterns, and meconium staining (MacGregor et al, 1987; Chasnoff, Burns & Burns, 1987). LBW and SGA are a consequence of vasoconstriction, which reduces uteroplacental exchange of oxygen and essential nutrients necessary for growth. Intrauterine fetal hypoxic episodes may coincide with maternal cocaine ingestion. The total effects from these hypoxic episodes have yet to be documented.

Cocaine also passes through the placenta, causing vasoconstriction, hypertension, and tachycardia in the fetus. These result in both toxic and teratogenic effects, depending on timing during pregnancy. The most common anomalies described are prune belly syndrome, ileal atresia, and urogenital anomalies (Udell, 1989; Bingol et al, 1987). Toxic effects include cerebral infarcts and necrotizing enterocolitis (NEC). Cocaine has also been found to contribute to optic nerve malformation or atrophy, delayed visual maturation, and eyelid edema (Good et al, 1992). Maternal hyperpyrexia may indirectly cause anomalies by disrupting cellular proliferation.

The metabolism of cocaine also impacts the effects on the fetus. Cocaine is metabolized by the esterase enzymes produced in the liver and present in plasma. The rate of individual metabolism varies, according to the level of cholinesterase activity (Bingol et al, 1987). Pregnant women and their fetuses are slower to metabolize cocaine as a consequence of a lower level of plasma cholinesterase activity (Pritchard, 1955). This has practical implications when screening newly delivered mothers and their infants for cocaine metabolites. If a woman has ingested cocaine 2 to 3 days before delivery, the adult's urine will contain metabolites for 24 hours after delivery and the neonate's urine will test positive for 4 to 7 days after delivery (Chasnoff, Burns & Burns, 1987). However, the more immature the fetal liver, the longer cocaine's metabolites may linger in the fetal system (Udell, 1989).

After delivery, the cocaine-exposed infant does not experience withdrawal as described in the heroin- or methadone-addicted infant. Instead the neurobehavioral abnormalities that occur are the result of toxic effects on the central nervous system. The irritability, hypertonicity, and hyperresponsiveness to stimuli, as well as gaze aversion, decreased orientation to face or voice, and poor state control may last 8 to 10 weeks.

After delivery, attachment to the newborn may be difficult because of the infant's behavior, as well as the mother's impairment. A pattern of disturbed parent-infant interactions is common. This behavior increases the potential for child abuse and neglect. The situation may be further compromised because drug-exposed infants may be hospitalized in a neonatal intensive care unit. This separation of the infant and mother deprives them of the first few days or weeks together. If a woman does not attach to her infant, she might abandon the baby, resulting in a phenomenon known as a "boarder baby" in which the baby remains in the hospital awaiting foster placement. With an estimated 100,000 to 158,400 crack cocaine babies born each year in America (Pelham & DeJong, 1992), the potential for problems is immense.

Like alcohol, a number of long-term sequelae are associated with cocaine. Attention deficit disorders, affect and concentration anomalies, and abnormal play patterns have been described (Hurt, 1989). The risk of SIDS is 15 times that for the general population (Chasnoff, 1987).

Breastfeeding is contraindicated in women who use cocaine. Cocaine enters breast milk and directly affects the infant (Chasnoff, Lewis & Squires, 1987). Other recommendations are to abstain from exposing the infant to anyone who smokes cocaine to avoid passive inhalation of crack cocaine (Bateman & Heagarty, 1989). Children who are crawling may find and eat pieces of crack off the floors of their home (Udell, 1989).

MARIJUANA

Marijuana (including hashish) continues to be the most widely used illicit drug in the United States (National Institute on Drug Abuse [NIDA], 1990). Lifetime rates of marijuana use steadily increase with successive ages, beginning at age 12 and peaking among those aged 26 to 29 (NIDA, 1990). Marijuana use has been reported by 13% to 22% of pregnant women (Hingson et al, 1982; Greenland et al, 1982; Fried, 1982). Marijuana use has significant effects on the reproductive system. Anovulation and short luteal phases are common with frequent use (Asch & Smith, 1983). Preterm labor (Fried, Watkinson, & Willan, 1984; Hatch & Bracken, 1986) and the risks of precipitate or prolonged labor are high (Greenland et al, 1982).

Animal and human studies show that delta-9-tetrahydrocannabinol (THC), a component of marijuana, crosses the placenta (Blackard & Tennes, 1984). Maternal blood concentration may be 2.5 to 6 times higher than that found in fetal blood, and the length of exposure increases the fetal-maternal concentration ratio. Delta-9-tetrahydrocannabinol crosses the placenta more readily during early than late pregnancy (Indanpaan-Heikkila, Fritchie, & Englert, 1969). Because marijuana is fat soluble (Kreuz & Axelrod, 1973) and has a large enterohepatic recirculation (Klausner & Dingell, 1971), the amount ingested during one use may take as many as 30 days to excrete, with a tissue half-life of 7 days (Nahar, 1976). Therefore the fetus could be subjected to prolonged exposure secondary to even one-time marijuana use by the mother. Additionally the fetus is exposed to carbon monoxide levels five times that of a tobacco smoker (Wu et al, 1988).

The fetal effects of marijuana use are inconclusive. Elevations in maternal heart rate and blood pressure caused by marijuana use lead to uterine vasoconstriction (Wu et al, 1988); this may account for the increased incidence of meconium passage described by Greenland and others (1981). Several studies have described effects on birth weight or length (Hingson et al, 1982; Hatch & Bracken, 1986; Zuckerman et al, 1989). Linn and associates (1983) suggested an increase in congenital anomalies, and Hingson and others (1982) described features compatible with FAS. Further studies have failed to confirm these findings.

Limited data on mothers who use regularly, however, suggest an increase in tremors and startles, as well as altered visual responsiveness in the infant during the initial newborn period. These problems appear to resolve by 1 month of age, and occasional marijuana use by the mother does not appear to have the same adverse effects as regular use (Gal & Sharpless, 1984).

In a study by Hayes, Dreher, and Nugent (1988) infants of marijuana smokers had better state organization and were more alert and socially interactive at 1 month of age. These effects were attributed to the relaxed, social environment.

Our knowledge regarding marijuana use remains limited. Further research in this area is greatly needed. Part of the difficulty rests in the frequent use of tobacco and alcohol by marijuana users. Many also use illicit drugs. Marijuana use should be discouraged during lactation, as well as during pregnancy. Marijuana readily crosses into breast milk. If breastfeeding is attempted, difficulties may ensue because marijuana also decreases prolactin levels (Asch & Smith, 1983).

TOBACCO

Health concerns (cancer, stroke, myocardial infarction) associated with smoking are well documented (US Department of Health and Human Services [USDHHS], 1989). One in every six deaths in the nation is linked to smoking (USDHHS, 1989). In addition to these general health risks, women smokers also experience related earlier menopause, osteoporosis, reduced fertility, and increased risk of stroke when taking oral contraceptives (USDHHS, 1989). Tobacco is a highly addictive substance that often draws little attention as perinatal substance abuse. When cigarette tobacco is inhaled, more than 2000 chemicals are ingested (USDHHS, 1980). Approximately a third of all women enter pregnancy as smokers (Nowicki et al, 1984).

Substances in tobacco products that are of primary importance to pregnant women are nicotine, nitrosamine, carbon monoxide, cadmium, and cyanide; all readily cross the placenta and reach the fetus.

Nicotine

Nicotine reduces placental blood flow because of its vasoconstrictive qualities. Vasoconstriction is thought to be responsible for the propensity toward placental abruptio among heavy smokers. This vasoconstriction also reduces fetal-placental exchange.

Nitrosamine

Nitrosamines are known carcinogens. Multiple studies document increased cancer rates among smokers, and more current studies show elevated cancer rates among nonsmoking women married to smoking men. It is unknown if the fetus exposed to nitrosamine in utero will be more likely to develop cancer later in life (Enkin, 1984).

Carbon monoxide

Carbon monoxide is diffused across the placenta from high concentration to low concentration. Carbon monoxide competes with oxygen for binding sites on hemoglobin, thus inducing cellular hypoxia. Infant response to this chronic low level of oxygen results in several responses. First, more red blood cells are produced, often to the point of polycythemia, which increases blood viscosity, further reducing blood flow and hampering tissue oxygenation, hyperbilirubinemia, and venous thrombi during extrauterine life. Second, lung maturity is hastened by stimulating the fetal stress response, which increases secretion of glucocorticoids and facilitates surfactant production. Surfactant in turn stabilizes the alveolar membrane, which reduces the incidence of respiratory distress syndrome (Flandermeyer, 1993). Finally, changes in the placenta result in a larger, thinner placenta to increase maternal-fetal nutrient exchange.

Cadmium

Smokers have detectable cadmium levels after smoking. Kuhner et al (1982) found that the placenta traps cadmium during later gestation, although the efficacy of the placental barrier is unknown during early gestation. Because there is no known biological function of cadmium, the effects of elevated cadmium levels in the human fetus are unknown.

Cyanide

Cyanide crosses the placenta and inhibits cellular respiration. Cyanide is suspected to "contribute to retarded infant growth and increased perinatal mortality" (U.S. Department of Health and Human Services, 1980).

Consequences of tobacco use during pregnancy

Smokers have an increased incidence of spontaneous abortion, unexplained vaginal bleeding, abruptio placentae, and placenta previa. Pregnant women who smoke experience premature aging of the placenta, which encroaches on fetal-maternal nutrient exchange. The body attempts to compensate by enlarging and thinning the placenta. Placental infarctions and premature aging lead to a reduction in the infant's nutritional status.

The increased ratio of placenta weight to fetal weight is especially significant considering that the average birth weight of infants born to smokers is less than those of nonsmokers. This is a compensatory mechanism to facilitate fetal oxygenation. A large placental ratio also is seen in studies of infants born in high altitudes associated with fetal hypoxia.

Early pregnancy is an ideal time to support smoking cessation. Morning sickness with nausea causes smoking to be less enjoyable. If the woman is temporarily abstaining from tobacco use due to nausea, then her concern for the health of her developing fetus may sustain her motivation to quit smoking.

Fetal effects

Fetal tobacco syndrome.   *Fetal tobacco syndrome* is the term used to identify infants affected by maternal smoking (Nieberg et al, 1985). The following criteria are used to identify these infants:

1. The mother smoked five or more cigarettes a day throughout pregnancy,
2. The mother had no evidence of hypertension during pregnancy, specifically no preeclampsia and documentation of normal blood pressure at least once after the first trimester,
3. The newborn has symmetric growth retardation at term (up to or greater than 37 weeks), defined as birth weight less than 2500 grams and a ponderal index ([weight in grams] [length in milliliters]) greater than 2.32, and
4. There is no other obvious cause of intrauterine growth retardation (e.g., congenital infection or anomaly) (Bobak & Jensen, 1993).

Birth weight.   Tobacco is the single most frequent substance responsible for low infant weight. Tobacco affects infant weight directly by its vasoconstrictive properties and indirectly by suppressing the mother's appetite. The average birth weight of babies of smokers is consistently less than babies of equal gestation of non-smokers, and the average weight differential between infants of smokers and non-smokers is 200 grams (USDHHS, 1980). Furthermore, the infant's weight is reduced in accordance with the amount of cigarettes smoked. The infants also had smaller crown-to-heel lengths and smaller head, chest, and shoulder circumferences. Smoking during pregnancy is responsible for 14% of all LBW infants. Small infants are more prone to developing complicating factors such as asphyxia and atelectasis.

Morbidity and mortality. Infants who are intrauterine growth retarded (IUGR) or SGA account for a disproportionately large percentage of infant morbidity and mortality. *Placenta previa* and *abruptio placenta* contribute to the increased rate of stillborn infants among smokers (USDHHS, 1980). It is difficult to precisely track the underlying cause of infant morbidity and mortality, because infants are grouped by medical diagnoses such as prematurity, respiratory distress syndrome, or IUGR. Also, tobacco is commonly used in combination with other drugs such as alcohol.

Fetal heart rate. Fetal well being is commonly assessed by fetal heart rate (FHR) variability. FHR variability refers to the ability of the fetal heart to increase or decrease in rate 5 to 10 beats-per-minute in response to fetal activity. When Forss and associates (1983) examined FHR variability after the mother had smoked a standard filter cigarette, they found an acute decrease in FHR variability. Goodman, Visser, and Dawes (1984) measured the effects of smoking two low-tar filter cigarettes on fetal movement and FHR variability. They found that the fetus spent less time moving during the first 16 minutes of smoking.

Factors associated with smoking and infancy

Risk for increased infant morbidity and mortality continues into infancy and childhood. There is an increased incidence of sudden infant death syndrome (SIDS) among infants of mothers who smoked during pregnancy.

The infants of smoking women have more frequent episodes of *upper respiratory infections* and *otitis media* than their nonsmoking counterparts (Rantakallio, 1983). There is some controversy regarding whether this is caused by the actual fetal exposure to smoking during pregnancy or from passive smoking after birth. *Passive smoking* is exposure to the smoke emitted from a burning cigarette, known as sidestream smoke. Sidestream smoke has more toxins and carcinogens than mainstream smoke (McKool, 1987).

To document the effects of passive smoking on infants, Greenberg and others (1984) examined the saliva and urine of infants of smokers for cotinine, a byproduct of nicotine. The presence of nicotine in the saliva and urine reflect recent exposure, whereas cotinine is indicative of chronic exposure to tobacco. Both nicotine and cotinine were found in the excreta of infants exposed to passive smoking.

Lactation

In addition to exposure to nicotine and cotinine through passive smoking, cotinine present in the smoking mother's bloodstream diffuses into the breast milk and can be found in the milk and in the infant's urine. Schulte-Hobein and others (1992) found that breast-fed infants of mothers who smoke have the highest levels of cotinine, and partially breast-fed infants of smoking mothers have correspondingly lower levels of cotinine. Ten percent of nonsmoking women lived with partners who smoked and as a result had detectable amounts of cotinine in the breast milk. Women who smoke do not breast-feed as long as nonsmokers. This is thought to be related to nicotine-induced reduction of prolactin. Schulte-Hobein and associates (1992) found this to be true in their study of breast-feeding mothers; almost half of the smokers weaned within 4 weeks postpartum.

OTHER DRUGS

A woman's pregnancy can be compromised by other drugs, including narcotic analgesics, amphetamines, methamphetamines, phencyclidine (PCP), over-the-counter drugs, and prescribed medications, including narcotics. Heroin addicts may use alternative narcotics during pregnancy, believing there are less fetal and neonatal effects. All of these agents are capable of fetal addiction and can result in neonatal withdrawal. The major side effects are neonatal respiratory and cardiac depression. Urinary retention, constipation, vomiting, and drowsiness are other signs of narcotic effects. Pentazocine (Talwin) in particular may result in fetal addiction and neonatal withdrawal within the first 24 hours of life (Berkowitz, Coustan & Mochizuki, 1986).

The effects of *amphetamines* appear to be dose-related and include pregnancy-induced hypertension (PIH), prematurity, LBW, and postpartum hemorrhage. Newborns may be lethargic, jittery, or drowsy and may experience respiratory distress. Poor emotional and physical health, as well as delays in gross and fine motor development, may occur (Bobak & Jensen, 1993). Little is known about *methamphetamine* use during pregnancy. The neonatal course is often benign, but frontal lobe dysfunction has been suggested later in life (Dixon, 1989).

Phencyclidine (PCP) is a hallucinogen that causes delirium, confusion, and hallucinations. Its effects are unpredictable, putting both the mother and her fetus in danger. CNS disorders may occur in the newborn, resulting in neurobehavioral and motor problems.

Over-the-counter and prescribed medications may be used unwittingly. Today, rigorous testing of drugs should prevent the use of drugs dangerous to a fetus such as the sad consequences of thalidomide use a few decades ago. If a woman does not inform her physician that she might be pregnant or attempting to become pregnant, medications that could endanger her fetus may be prescribed inadvertently. Also, a woman may think that over-the-counter medications may be used safely during pregnancy.

NURSING CARE OF THE MOTHER

Prenatal care

Early prenatal care increases the likelihood of identifying women with substance abuse and getting them help to decrease the use of drugs. Yet many addicted women do not seek early prenatal care because of fear of identification, or they may not know they are pregnant. Amenorrhea is common with substance abuse; the woman may not associate her lack of menses with pregnancy. Nausea, another common symptom of pregnancy, is associated with withdrawal symptoms. Another symptom, fatigue, is an everyday occurrence caused by poor nutrition and a lifestyle centered around the next drink or dose of drugs. Often the woman with substance abuse does not recognize the pregnancy until she feels fetal movement around the 20th week of pregnancy. Even then fetal movements may mimic intestinal cramping common in withdrawal.

Another benefit is validation of the pregnancy so the beginning of maternal role attainment can occur. Maternal attachment is a process occurring over time with the development of enduring affectionate bonding and commitment to a child. During pregnancy the woman accepts the fetus into her self-system and an orderly sequence of emotional attachment occurs (Mercer et al, 1988). Maternal perceptions of the fetus change as pregnancy progresses, and these perceptions are reflected in the mother's developing awareness of the fetus as a person.

Identification of substance abuse

Nurses should systematically interview all pregnant women for signs of substance abuse. Should the client be using, she may deny use to the nurse and possibly to herself. A relationship of trust and an environment that promotes privacy is necessary. The nurse must use nonjudgmental phrasing and include sensitive questions in the same tone of voice and matter-of-fact manner used to elicit responses to more mundane questions. All use of drugs or alcohol needs to be assessed, including caffeine, tobacco, over-the-counter medications, prescription drugs, alcohol, and street drugs. Open-ended questions can be asked in a matter-of-fact, professional manner. Client responses need to be clarified with respect to frequency and quantity of consumption. Ambiguous responses such as "social drinking" or "recreational use" need further clarification. One of the best methods for identifying drug and alcohol use is to ask about use in the 6 months before becoming pregnant. Additional questions concern parental use, partner use, or past problems with drugs or alcohol. Asking "How many drinks does it take to make you feel high?" determines tolerance. An answer of three or more indicates heavy alcohol use. Corroboration of answers may be obtained by interviewing significant others. The T-ACE questionnaire, a modified version of the CAGE (Sokol, Martier & Agner, 1989), and the 4 P's questionnaire both can be used (Ewing, 1991). Boxes 8-2 and 8-3 illustrate these two questionnaires.

Once substance abuse has been identified, the nurse can begin educating the client about the consequences of continuing to use substances. Scare tactics and threats are counterproductive because they heighten maternal anxiety and may exacerbate substance use. Therefore the clinician should avoid dwelling on what damage may have already been sustained and instead focus on the potential good that could occur from detoxification or substituting heroin with methadone.

The lifestyle of women who abuse drugs contributes to their medical problems. Women who drink heavily often smoke and may be poorly nourished (Wright, 1986). Many ignore and neglect health care problems until they become severe. They may be admitted to the hospital because of medical problems related to their

---

Box 8-2
T-ACE Questionnaire

T-ACE questions

1. How many drinks does it **t**ake to make you feel high?   _____
2. Have people **a**nnoyed you by criticizing your drinking?   Yes   No
3. Have you felt you ought to **c**ut down on your drinking?   Yes   No
4. Have you ever had an **e**ye-opener first thing in the
   morning to steady your nerves?   Yes   No

Note: Persons who have two or more positive responses to these four questions are considered at risk for problematic alcohol use.

From Sokol, R.J., Martier, S.S., & Ager, J.W. (1989). The T-ACE questions: Practical prenatal detection of risk-drinking. *American Journal of Obstetrics Gynecology, 160*(7), 865.

use of drugs. The abuse of drugs may go unrecognized or if recognized untreated (see Care Plan 8-1).

Where drug abuse is known or strongly suspected additional information is helpful. Assess for illnesses and physical symptoms that are associated with drug use such as hepatitis, vaginal infections, anemia, nasal inflammation from cocaine use, track marks from drug injection, or stained fingers from cigarette smoking. Other assessments that indicate possible drug abuse are difficulties with previous pregnancies, including placental abnormalities, LBW babies, or a known FAS or FAE child.

Labor and delivery

With abbreviated hospital stays the admission protocol for all pregnant women should include a routine assessment for alcohol and other drug abuse similar to the prenatal assessment.

Box 8-3
Ewing's 4 *P*'s Screening Tool

Ewing's 4 *P*'s screening questionnaire

1. **P**arent with a drug or alcohol problem   ☐ Yes   ☐ No
2. **P**artner with a drug or alcohol problem   ☐ Yes   ☐ No
3. **P**ast problem with drugs or alcohol   ☐ Yes   ☐ No
4. **P**regnancy use of drugs, alcohol, or cigarettes   ☐ Yes   ☐ No

Note: These questions are weighted toward family ramifications of prenatal substance use. "Problem" is defined as continued use despite adverse consequences. *One or more positive answers* indicates a positive screening interview. A more in-depth diagnostic interview is recommended for patients who screen positive.

From Ewing, H. (1991). Management of the pregnant alcoholic/addict. Presented at American Society on Addiction Medicine, Medical Scientific Conference, Boston, April 20, 1991.

Care Plan 8-1

Early Pregnancy, Uncertain Drug or Alcohol Use

Tina, age 22 and 8 weeks pregnant, has come to the prenatal clinic for the first time. She has lived with her boyfriend, Roger, for 2 years and works as a secretary for a large advertising firm in a large city. The pregnancy, her first, was unplanned, but Tina expressed both apprehension and acceptance. Roger also accepted the pregnancy and thought he should now marry her. Tina wanted the marriage and was also cautiously enthusiastic about the baby as she expressed her lack of knowledge about having babies or taking care of them. She had been an only child of older parents. She acknowledged that she smoked a pack of cigarettes a day, drank "a drink or two" of alcohol several times a week, and smoked marijuana on social occasions or weekends. The times varied from several times a week to once a week.

ASSESSMENT

Gravida 1, para 0. Unmarried, living with boyfriend. Possibly they will marry. The baby is wanted. Smokes one pack of cigarettes a day, alcohol use about 6 to 10 drinks per week. Marijuana 4 to 8 times per month. Roger uses about the same amount of both alcohol and marijuana that Tina does. She states that it takes two drinks for her to feel "high." Tina's health status is within normal limits. She has had limited contact with babies and professes ignorance about them and demonstrates little knowledge about effects of substances upon pregnancy.

NURSING DIAGNOSES

Knowledge deficit: prenatal care and drugs related to expressed lack of knowledge and use of drugs and alcohol

Outcome identification	Nursing interventions	Rationale	Evaluation
Nursing diagnosis: Knowledge deficit: prenatal care and drugs related to expressed lack of knowledge and use of drugs and alcohol			
1. Client will state that drugs and alcohol enter the baby's bloodstream and interfere with fetal development within 1 week.	1a. Begin teaching client about healthy behaviors during pregnancy by talking about diet, exercise, rest, and a generally healthy lifestyle.	1a. The health of the baby is reinforced by the health and lifestyle of the mother. Teaching about drugs and alcohol in this framework places the focus on the health of both mother and baby.	1. Tina was astonished at the knowledge that drugs or alcohol entered the baby's bloodstream and interfered with the baby's development. She stated, "I didn't know that. I thought they were protected." Goal met.
	1b. Explain how nutrients and toxins pass from the mother's blood to the fetal blood.	1b. Understanding something of the process assists the mother to make more informed decisions.	

Outcome identification	Nursing interventions	Rationale	Evaluation

Nursing diagnosis: Knowledge deficit: prenatal care and drugs related to expressed lack of knowledge and use of drugs and alcohol—cont'd

Outcome identification	Nursing interventions	Rationale	Evaluation
	1c. Explain how chemicals may interfere with the growth and development of the fetus.	1c. Same as above.	
2. Client will agree to follow through with prenatal care throughout her pregnancy within 1 week.	2a. Discuss the importance of prenatal care with the client and explain the frequency of visits.	2a. Same as above.	2. Tina agreed to follow through with prenatal care and made an appointment for her second checkup. Goal met.
	2b. Praise client for her willingness to provide the best available care for her baby.	2b. Increases client confidence and willingness to do the best for her baby.	
	2c. Give the client literature about prenatal and infant care.	2c. Reinforces prenatal care information and begins preparations for the arrival of the infant.	
3. Client will agree to abstain from all drugs and alcohol throughout her pregnancy within 1 week.	3a. Ask the client if she is willing to make some changes in her lifestyle to ensure a healthier baby.	3a. Respects the mother's ability to make her own decisions.	3. Tina said she would gladly give up her marijuana use and that she could do that easily. She said she thought she could discontinue alcohol use. She said she knew that she couldn't quit smoking. She did agree to try to cut down on quantity. Goal partially met. Revision: Monitor tobacco use at each subsequent visit and try to assist her to quit.
	3b. Ask her if she is able to abstain from marijuana to help assure a healthy baby.	3b. Asking about each substance separately allows her to assess her own ability to abstain more clearly.	
	3c. Ask her if she is able to abstain from alcohol to help assure a healthy baby.	3c. Same as above.	

Continued.

Care Plan 8-1

Early Pregnancy, Uncertain Drug or Alcohol Use—cont'd

Outcome identification	Nursing interventions	Rationale	Evaluation
Nursing diagnosis: Knowledge deficit: prenatal care and drugs related to expressed lack of knowledge and use of drugs and alcohol—cont'd			
	3d. If she feels unable to abstain from use during the pregnancy, try to obtain her consent to cut down at each visit.	3d. Cutting down is not an appropriate goal, but it assists the nurse in determining if the client can control use.	
	3e. For each step she takes, support her strengths and commend her for working for a healthy baby.	3e. Helps her increase confidence in her own competence to provide for her baby.	
4. Client will remain drug and alcohol free throughout the remainder of her pregnancy.	4a. At each prenatal visit, assess the client's ability to maintain a substance-free lifestyle.	4a. Reinforces the importance of substance-free pregnancy. Assess for possible addiction.	4. Tina stated she quit marijuana and alcohol use throughout the pregnancy. She reduced her tobacco use from a pack a day to 1/2 pack a day but did not quit. Goal partially met.
	4b. Observe for possible objective clues that client is drinking or using.	4b. Clients may not be honest about use.	
	4c. In the event that it appears that the client cannot control use, refer for treatment.	4c. Nearly all mothers want their babies to be healthy. If the mother cannot control use, substance abuse treatment is indicated.	

Observation is another data-gathering technique that can be used in the hospital. The woman's first pregnancy-related contact with the health care profession may be during active labor. If a woman uses drugs before arriving at the hospital, behavioral manifestations will be related to the substance of abuse and according to the last dose of the drug (e.g., alcohol on the breath). (See Chapter 1 for symptoms of abuse.) Acute withdrawal symptoms should be treated in consultation with a chemical dependency specialist and neonatologist to avoid drug effects on the fetus and neonate. (See Chapters 7 and 11 for treatment of withdrawal symptoms.)

Sexually transmitted diseases (e.g., syphilis or gonorrhea), blood-borne illnesses such as hepatitis, and an overall picture of self-neglect (e.g., malnutrition or poor hygiene) should raise suspicions of drug use. Transient lifestyles and lack of consistent partners also are consistent with drug abuse. Other indicators of potential substance abuse include poor compliance with prenatal visits, prenatal care beginning after 20 weeks gestation, unexplained preterm labor, placental abruptio, intrauterine growth retardation, intrauterine fetal demise, history of family violence, other children in foster care, and a psychiatric history (Kaiser Foundation Hospital, 1989; Children's Hospital Medical Center of Northern California, 1990). If any of these factors are present, urine toxicology can be ordered for the mother or the neonate. (See Chapter 16 for more about drug testing.) Some institutions use meconium tests. Results are similar to urine toxicology studies but are reliable for all drugs up to 3 days after delivery (Ostrea et al, 1989). If narcotics have been given during or after labor, however, positive results for narcotics may be due to these medications. In some states the mother's consent is necessary before toxicology tests can be ordered.

Health care providers must be aware that mothers may self-medicate while in the hospital. Many women have IV infusions while they are in labor and may use this IV access for self-medication.

While in labor, close observation for complications is necessary. Abruptio placentae, abnormal labor patterns, and fetal distress are common. Some women may not be cognizant of the impending birth, others may repeatedly ask for pain medication. Appropriate analgesics and anesthetics should be provided. Following delivery the woman should be closely monitored for postpartum hemorrhage.

Postnatal care

Postnatal care for women who have substance abuse problems includes the elements of care for anyone who has given birth, in addition to some special considerations. Women who abused drugs during their pregnancy may not return for their postpartum visit, so it is important that birth control methods be discussed before discharge from the hospital. Breast-feeding is contraindicated in mothers who continue to use drugs after delivery.

After giving birth, the woman may leave the hospital against medical advice. She may fear exposure of her addiction and associated legal implications or worry over an insufficient supply of alcohol or drugs. Early discharge is a threat to the newborn's well being because the infant's onset of withdrawal may be somewhat delayed, hampering diagnosis and treatment.

Women with substance abuse problems often are unprepared for parenting and may have unrealistic expectations of their infant. They may look to the infant to meet their needs rather than caring for the infant. If the woman also returns to drug abuse after delivery, poor or abusive parenting may result. Drug-seeking behavior interferes with the individual's ability to function in society, including the ability to parent. Women who receive ongoing support during prenatal and postpartum periods are more aware of infant cues and needs and are better able to cope with parenting (Olds & Henderson, 1989).

The home environment of the mother with substance abuse may be chaotic and disorganized. The mother may have had poor parenting role models. She may avoid health care services for her infant for fear of losing custody of her child (Coles & Platzman, 1992). Other reasons for not getting health care include lack of transportation, lack of adequate child care, cultural barriers, the insensitivity of health care providers, and lack of money.

SUBSTANCE ABUSE TREATMENT FOR PREGNANT WOMEN

A pregnant woman who has a heart condition is treated by both an obstetrician and a cardiologist. Similarly a pregnant woman who has an addiction must have her care managed by both a specialist in obstetrics and a specialist in drug addiction.

Substance abuse treatment starts with an assessment of substance use and a diagnosis of abuse or dependency (see Chapter 3). Once a woman is diagnosed, she should be referred to an appropriate treatment program. It is critical that an expert in withdrawal manage that aspect of the woman's care. The benefits of remaining drug-free—decreased medical and obstetrical complications and decreased mortality and morbidity for the infant—must be stressed. Also mothers with substance abuse should be assured that they will be given medication or anesthesia as needed for labor and delivery.

Availability of treatment

Currently, few treatment facilities for substance dependent pregnant women exist in the United States. Many treatment programs were initially designed for men and continue to exclude pregnant women for fear of the legal ramifications of medical complications. In 1989 two thirds of the hospitals in 15 U.S. cities had no provisions for treatment of drug-exposed pregnant women (Miller, 1989). The lack of available treatment results in long waiting lists for admission. The substance dependent woman who is unable to obtain immediate treatment when psychologically ready runs the risk of continuing her drug use. In addition to the lack of treatment facilities, even fewer facilities provide space for children. If there is no provision for child care, the mother is other faced with the choice of treatment versus caring for her children. Unless treatment accessibility is addressed, there will continue to be an increase in the number of drug-exposed infants born in the United States.

Public policy

Public policy addresses pregnancy and substance abuse in women in several ways. The American Civil Liberties Union reports that about 50 women have been prosecuted and many spent time in jail for delivering a controlled substance to a minor via the umbilical cord (Kandall & Chavkin, 1992). Women also have been charged with child abuse or neglect after positive neonatal toxicology screens. Subsequent evaluation of parental fitness often results in loss of custody because of the mother's substance abuse. However, there are few available foster homes. Therefore some children are never removed or are returned after a short period of time. Obviously, few women will report their substance use during pregnancy when such threats loom. Offering treatment of course is the logical solution, but this option is limited by treatment availability.

THE DRUG ADDICTED NEONATE

Neonatal abstinence syndrome

The drug-exposed neonate's response to withdrawal from narcotics (neonatal abstinence syndrome) is directly related to the maternal pattern of abuse. The type, pattern, mix of substances, length of use, and timing of last substance use before delivery all determine what signs of withdrawal if any will be observable in the neonate. Onset of withdrawal can occur from birth to the sixth day of life (Reddy, Harper & Stern, 1971). With early discharges (in some cases 24 hours or less after the birth), withdrawal may begin after hospitalization. Infants exposed to narcotics in utero may or may not be sick or even small enough to be in a special care or newborn intensive care unit. Even in a special care nursery, they may not stay long enough for signs of withdrawal to begin; symptoms of withdrawal may be misdiagnosed as signs of immaturity, especially of the neurologic system.

Finnegan (1988) developed a scoring scale called the Neonatal Abstinence Syndrome Score (NASS) to identify infants at greatest risk for withdrawal from opiates (Figure 8-1). The American Academy of Pediatrics (1983) recommends using the NASS to identify infants at risk of withdrawal. Beginning at 2 hours of age, the infant is scored every 2 hours for the first 48 hours (Torrence & Horns, 1989).

In infants of mothers with substance abuse the vagal response, which is charged with maintaining homeostasis, is unpredictable. The infant may either be hypoactive or hyperactive, depending on the degree of effect the maternal drug use has had on the neonate. If the vagal tone is low the infant is more likely to experience apnea and concomitant bradycardia. When apnea and bradycardia are experienced with concomitant hypoxia and respiratory and metabolic acidosis, results can be fatal. If the vagal tone is high the infant will appear irritable, have more signs of gastrointestinal disturbances, and in general be more sensitive to external stimuli. The infant will experience signs of sleep-wake pattern disturbance, hyper- or hypo-irritability, shrill and persistent cry, inability to self-regulate or be easily soothed, poor suck-swallow coordination, weak suck, disturbed feeding patterns, temperature instability (usually elevated), frequent yawning and sneezing, attentional deficits, and almost incessant arousal (Brazelton, 1991; Flandermeyer, 1993). About 1.5% of heroin-exposed infants will experience seizures (Kandall, 1991).

CNS symptoms such as jitteriness, hypersensitive tendon reflexes, depressed normal neurological reflexes (e.g., Moro), or seizures are those that usually bring the infant to the attention of the health professional (Kandall, 1991). Phenobarbital can be used with or without paregoric to control seizures.

Gastrointestinal symptoms may accompany withdrawal from heroin or cocaine and appear after the onset of CNS problems. Vomiting and diarrhea make fluid, electrolyte, and nutritional management a priority for these infants. If these symptoms are accompanied by a crying, seemingly hungry infant, attempts are usually made to feed more than is tolerable, which leads to more vomiting and diarrhea.

Other signs of abstinence similar to adult withdrawal are nasal congestion, rhi-

Neonatal Abstinence Scoring System

Central Nervous System Disturbances				
Signs & Symptoms	Score	A.M.	P.M.	Comments
Excessive High Pitched (or other) Cry	2			Daily Weight
Continuous High Pitched (or other) Cry	3			
Sleeps <1 Hr After Feeding	3			
Sleeps <2 Hrs After Feeding	2			
Sleeps <3 Hrs After Feeding	1			
Hyperactive Moro Reflex	2			
Markedly Hyperactive Moro Reflex	1			
Mild Tremors Disturbed	1			
Moderate-Severe Tremors Disturbed	2			
Mild Tremors Undisturbed	3			
Moderate-Severe Tremors Undisturbed	4			
Increased Muscle Tone	2			
Excoriation (Specific Area)	1			
Myoclonic jerks	3			
Generalized Convulsions	3			

Metabolic/Vasomotor/Respiratory Disturbances				
				Daily Weight
Sweating	1			
Fever <101 (99-100.8° F or 37.2-38.2° C)	1			
Fever >101 (38.4° C and higher)	2			

Frequent Yawning (>3-4x/Interval)	1									
Mottling	1									
Nasal Stuffiness	1									
Sneezing (>3-4x/Interval)	1									
Nasal Flaring	2									
Respiratory Rate >60/min	1									
Respiratory Rate >60/min w/Retractions	2									

Gastrointestinal Disturbances

									Daily Weight
Excessive Sucking	1								
Poor Feeding	2								
Regurgitation	2								
Projectile Vomiting	3								
Loose Stools	2								
Watery Stools	3								

TOTAL SCORE:

INITIALS OF SCORER:

Fig. 8-1. Neonatal Abstinence Scoring System. (From Finegan L.P. (1986). Neonatal abstinence syndrome: Assessment and pharmacotherapy. In Rubalelli F.F. & Gronatel B. (Eds.) *Neonatal therapy: An update.* New York: Excerpta Medica.)

norrhea, and increased respiratory effort and rate. All of these symptoms increase the metabolic rate and usage of fluids, calories, and oxygen.

Respiratory depression

For the narcotic-exposed infant the danger of respiratory depression and further hypoxic episodes is great. Severe mental retardation, intraventricular hemorrhage, and CNS dysfunction are all potential outcomes. In the past this side effect was treated with a narcotic antagonist such as naloxone (Narcan). Although this medication is useful when there has been a narcotic exposure through analgesia during the intrapartal period, when given to an infant passively addicted to narcotics, narcotic withdrawal can be precipitated and results can be fatal (Berkowitz et al, 1986).

NURSING CARE OF THE INFANT

Withdrawal

Pharmacologic intervention is initiated if seizure activity is noted or the infant has a NASS greater than 12 on two occasions or greater than or equal to 8 on three occasions. For narcotic withdrawal, paregoric or tincture of opium is the drug of choice. For polydrug use or nonnarcotic drug withdrawal, phenobarbital is used (Torrence & Horns, 1989). Tincture of opium or paregoric can be added if the infant does not improve or persistent diarrhea is present.

Fluid balance

The ability to maintain a fluid and electrolyte balance is difficult for a drug-exposed infant, especially a preterm infant. The infant undergoing withdrawal has an increased metabolic rate and an increase in insensible water loss. Gastric mobility is increased and may result in decreased water or nutrient absorption. Fluids and electrolytes are lost through the GI tract, affecting this delicate balance. Loss of sodium, potassium, and chloride ions through vomiting and diarrhea further compromise the delicate electrolyte balance.

For the preterm infant, initial fluid requirements may be met with IV fluids, at first dextrose 10% and after the first 24 hours with electrolytes added. Fluids may be given at the level of 80 to 140 ml per kg per day. Intake and output records must be completed at least every 8 hours to determine fluid requirements.

If the infant is stable enough to be offered enteral feedings, these may be either gavage or nipple feedings, depending on the gestational age and respiratory status of the infant. With enteral feedings, more calories are used in the digestive process.

The infants often have suck-swallow incoordination and must be fed carefully to avoid aspiration. The infant may appear hungry and highly agitated. The tendency is to offer more formula or breast milk. Overfeeding will only lead to abdominal cramping, increased gastric motility, and increased fluid losses. Small trophic feedings (i.e., easily absorbed, growth-producing), every 2 to 3 hours either by nasogastric gavage or nipple, often are better tolerated than increased feedings or longer feeding intervals. Nonnutritive sucking should be offered to either the NPO or gavaged infant. This sucking is associated with increases in weight and reduced oxygen consumption (Lefrak-Okikawa & Meier, 1993). Pharmacologic intervention with paregoric or phenobarbital also may decrease gastric motility and accompanying fluid loss.

Because these infants are usually LBW (under 2,500 grams), they gain weight slowly. A 20-gram weight gain per day is the goal. It is essential for daily weights to be checked on the same scale and under the same circumstances in order to accurately measure weight fluctuations. Daily head circumferences should be done initially. When the infant is stable, these can be reduced to weekly.

Infection control

The drug-exposed infant may have been infected in utero with sexually transmitted diseases or secondary maternal infections acquired from the mother's compromised nutritional and immune status. Maternal infection, rather than drug use, may precipitate premature labor and delivery (Coyne & Landers, 1990). Due to a depressed immune system, premature infants are at increased risk of secondary infections. The infant also may be HIV positive or HIV exposed.

The danger of human immunodeficiency virus (HIV) is a very real possibility when risky behaviors such as IV drug use or multiple sexual partners have been exhibited. Neonates born to women who have engaged in such behaviors may or may not be HIV positive themselves at birth (Campinha-Bacote & Bragg, 1993). Eventually, 30% to 50% of infants born to HIV positive mothers actually develop the disease (Nanda, 1990).

The body's initial response to HIV exposure is to produce antibodies. These antibodies, either maternal or neonatal, form the basis of diagnostic testing.

The ELISA test is highly sensitive and specific for the antibody (99% if the double ELISA is used), but it cannot predict who will develop AIDS or the actual disease caused by the HIV. Passively acquired maternal antibodies interfere with the efficacy of this test in the neonate. Maternally derived antibodies may last 15 to 18 months (Bastin et al, 1992). As many as 20% of infants who eventually become HIV positive test negative via the ELISA test until after the first viral symptoms appear (Pitt, 1991).

The Western Blot is a better discriminator when separating maternal from infant infection (Pitt, 1991). The Western Blot will detect specific HIV antigenetic changes from one testing period to another. These changes usually represent the neonate's own changes in immune status.

The first suspicion of HIV may appear around 9 to 10 months of age. Symptoms will be vague and may include hepatosplenomegaly, lymphadenopathy, FTT, neurodevelopmental problems, persistent oral candidiasis or thrush, monilial or diaper infections, and extensive seborrheic dermatitis. If the HIV is severe, symptoms will include chronic parotitis, lymphocytic interstitial pneumonia, and a history of recurrent bacterial infections including pneumocystis carinii. There are noted dysmorphic facial features attributed to HIV, yet they are not often recognized until these other physical symptoms appear (Coyne & Landers, 1990).

Physical characteristics are similar to FAS—boxy appearance of the forehead, wide-spaced eyes, flattened nasal bridge, and flattened facies. If these signs or other symptoms are present, the infant should be tested. Even if the infant is asymptomatic but at risk for HIV, diagnostic tests should be run immediately.

Careful use of antimicrobials helps decrease the chances of secondary infections. The longer antimicrobials are given, however, the more likely that protective gastrointestinal flora will be disturbed and neutrophils depressed, leading to more chances for infection. Also, antimicrobial therapy decreases fluid and nutrient absorption because the flora loss further compromises nutritional status, fluid and electrolyte balance, and growth of the infant.

Close assessment for subtle signs of infection are necessary. These include temperature instability, mottling, cool extremities, paleness, sudden or periodic color changes, changes in feeding patterns, and possibly an increase in the signs of withdrawal.

Infantile flailing of extremities or vigorous rubbing of the skin against the bedclothes can lead to skin breakdown, which becomes a portal of entry for pathogens. Soft sheepskin may decrease the irritation. Positioning in a side-lying position also may help. Use of Tegaderm or a protective second skin that allows air circulation adds protection against further breakdown. Any obvious abrasions should be treated with topical ointments such as hydrocortisone creams or antimicrobial agents.

Respiratory care

Respiratory care or ventilatory support depends on gestational age, lung maturation, and symptoms of respiratory compromise. The goal is to maintain an arterial pH of 7.35 to 7.45, PaO_2 of 80 to 100, $PaCO_2$ of 35 to 45, and a base excess of plus or minus 2. The infant may require ventilatory support, head-hood oxygen, nasal cannula, or nothing at all. As the infant starts the withdrawal process, support of the respiratory system may change. The infant with suspected substance exposure in utero should be placed on a cardiopulmonary monitor. At discharge the caretaker should be taught cardiopulmonary resuscitation because of the increased possibility of SIDS.

Developmental assessment

The first step is to assess the infant, the environment, and the infant's response to environmental stimuli. Screening should focus on identification of developmental delays. There are a variety of standardized instruments that can be used for developmental screening (e.g., Bayley Scales of Infant Development [Bayley, 1969], Fagan Infatest [Fagan, Shephard & Knevel, 1991]). The purpose of the diagnostic assessment is to determine what if any developmental problems exist, especially in speech, hearing, or language development. The goal is to identify and intervene early for developmental problems to decrease long-term sequelae.

Oehler and associates (1993) have developed a scoring scale to determine those infants at highest risk for developmental delays (Figure 8-2). This score is based on seven neurobiological factors that are most often adversely affected when oxygenation has been diminished either in utero or postnatally. The seven factors are: ventilation, acidosis, seizures, intraventricular hemorrhage, periventricular leukomalacia, infection, and hypoglycemia. Each of these items is scored on a scale of 1 to 4. A score greater than or equal to 5 or 6 is considered high risk. The scoring can be done

Neurobiological Risk Score (NBRS)

	Points			
	0	1	2	4
Ventilation	No mechanical ventilation	<7 days	8-28 days	>28 days
pH	Never <7.15	<7.15 for < 1 hr (<7.15 < 2 x); or <7.15 all respiratory any duration	<7.15 metabolic for > 1 hour (<7.15 > 2 x); or <7.00 metabolic any duration	Cardiopulmonary arrest
Seizures	None	Controlled in one drug and normal interictal EEG	Not controlled on one drug or abnormal interictal EEG	Status epilepticus > 12 hours
Intraventricular hemorrhage	None	Germinal matrix only	Blood in one or both ventricles	Intraparenchymal blood or development of overt hydrocephalus
Periventricular leukomalacia	None	Questionable changes that resolve	Moderate or definite changes that resolve	Cyst formation or cerebral atrophy with large ventricles
Infection	None or antibiotics for possibility of infection with negative cultures	Highly suspicious or documented infection without changes in blood pressure	Septic shock (documented sepsis plys hypotension)	Meningitis
Hypoglycemia	No glucose readings <30 mg/dl	Glucose <30 mg/dl asymptomatic and <6 hrs duration	Glucose <30 mg/dl asymptomatic and >6 hrs; or symptomatic any duration	Glucose <30 mg/dl >24 hrs and symptomatic

Infant's name _____   Age in days _____   Total score: _____   (>5 at discharge is high risk)

Fig. 8-2. Neurobiological Risk Score (NBRS). (From Oehler-Goldsteen J.M., Catlett R.F., Boshkoff M., & Brozy J.E. (1993). How to target infants at highest risk for developmental delay. *Mat Child Nsg,* 18(1), 22.)

at the time of discharge, 2 weeks after birth, or later. A high-risk score has been correlated with later developmental problems. Use of such a risk score may lead to early intervention to support positive growth and development.

Developmental care

The goal of developmentally supportive care is to provide an atmosphere that avoids stressful reactions in infants. Actions of infants are really reactions or interactions caused by environmental (internal and external to the infant) stimuli. Care should not be reactionary but anticipatory. The outcome is to promote behavioral organization.

Disorganization in the physiologic state often leads to a number of cardiopulmonary changes, such as tachycardia, tachypnea, bradycardia, or apnea. Skin may go from pink to pale to mottled, depending on how the infant responds to a stimulus. Other signs of physiologic stress are gaze aversion, hiccupping, vomiting, gagging, spitting up, or changes in bowel patterns, including increased straining (VandenBerg & Hanson, 1993). Even in the busiest units, attempts can be made to support the infant's physiological state. For the drug-exposed infant the ideal room is quiet, isolated, and dimly lit with the infant observable and within range of a caregiver at all times.

Many drug- or alcohol-exposed neonates are born prematurely. Their neurologic development is immature and may even have been damaged by substance exposure in utero. These infants find it difficult to stay in synch with their environment. Interventions for these infants, whether in the nursery or at home, should be cue-based, supportive, and modulated to diminish environmental stresses. Als (1982) developed a syntactic model based on the premise that an infant's behavioral organization is related to its interaction with the environment. Five functional subsystems (physiologic, motor, state, attention, and self-regulatory) interact to result in behavioral organization.

Muscle tone may change from hypertonia or normal tone to hypotonia when sensory overload is experienced. Positioning the infant in the side-lying or the supine position, depending on the gestational age, prevents adduction of the hip, upper extremity retraction, flailing of the extremities, and back arching. Proper positioning promotes positive support of posture, enhances muscle development, and provides motoric control. Containment by swaddling, creating a nest in the bed, or moving the extremities to midline provides the infant with a sense of boundaries and security. The infant will gradually move from hypotonia to normal tone, but this process may take up to 2 years.

Premature and term neonates experience six sleep-wake states. These are *deep or quiet sleep, active sleep, drowsy, quiet alert, fussy,* and *robust crying* (VandenBerg & Hanson, 1993). This adaptation to the environment is referred to as state regulation or control. As previously described, the infant born to a mother with substance abuse has great difficulty in moving smoothly from one state to another. Wide state swings are typical. The adaptation or modulation of external stimuli is erratic and unpredictable.

The ideal state for the promotion of positive maternal-infant interaction is the quiet alert state; the infant is able to eat and ready to observe and interact with the world. If the mother is not mindful of the infant's stress signals such as decreased tone, color changes, gaze aversion, sneezing, hyperactivity, or hiccups, then the infant may progress to an agitated, irritable, vomiting baby (Sweeney, 1989). In addition to reducing environmental stimuli, positioning the infant toward the inside of the room in a dimly lit, quiet area also helps decrease stress. Techniques to calm a crying infant include turning the infant away from the caregiver's face and vertically rocking the baby (Miami Valley Hospital, 1992). Holding the infant's back against the caregiver's chest and stomach also will calm the infant by providing security and boundaries without overstimulation (Miami Valley Hospital, 1992).

Normally, attention span increases with gestational and postnatal age. The infant of a substance abusing mother, however, experiences shortened attention spans and more difficulty adapting to the surrounding environment. The caregiver can provide order in the infant's world by clustering activities. Attempts to cluster too many activities in a short span of time, however, can be as detrimental as interruptions several times per day. Again the infant must be observed for signs of stress and care-giving activities scheduled on these responses. Reactions to overstimulation for the substance-exposed infant may be habituation, shutting out of stimuli, or hyper-irritability and uncontrollable crying (Als, 1982; VandenBerg & Hanson, 1993).

Attempts at environmental self-regulation are less predictable in substance-exposed infants. These infants are dependent on caregivers to regulate or support their regulatory movements. Nonnutritive sucking devices, swaddling or containment within the bed, and allowing the infant to grasp a finger or a stuffed animal during a gavage or bottle-feeding are all supportive techniques (see Care Plan 8-2).

Parental support and education

Parents of drug-exposed infants, especially the mother, will need help to smooth the transition to home. The parents should be given an opportunity to express their fears and frustrations. Anticipatory guidance regarding withdrawal signs, infant care consoling activities, nutrition, feeding, and medication should be provided. The more emphasis placed on teaching the mother to notice and respond to the infant's cues, the better the chance that she will be able to care for her infant. Involving the parents in the care at the hospital also serves as a time for assessment of parent-infant interaction. Appropriate parenting behaviors should be identified and facilitated.

Consistent caregivers or case managers help provide the support needed by these families. Hospital-provided home follow-up, doula (laywoman who provides support to laboring women and early postpartum care), social service, and community health nurse referrals can facilitate the transition home and provide additional support.

PREVENTION

Community education

Community education is one method of alerting individuals to the problems related to use of legal and illegal drugs, to problems in individual and family

Text continued on p. 228.

Care Plan 8-2

Neonate Born with Crack Cocaine in Its System

Neonate Michael Jones was born 72 hours ago at 34 weeks and weighing 1420 grams. He is the third child born to a 24-year-old mother addicted to cocaine. She has had one child removed from the home and one die of SIDS at 4 months of age.

ASSESSMENT

Michael cries a great deal of the time and lies with his arms in the "W" position and his back arched. The amniotic fluid was meconium stained and he was placed on the respirator for 24 hours. His vital signs have stabilized, no longer necessitating the respirator. He has hypertonia, gaze aversion, a very poor suck, and is inconsolable. There is staining at each diaper change.

NURSING DIAGNOSES

Sensory-perceptual alterations related to withdrawal as manifested by increased sensitivity to stimuli
Ineffective airway clearance related to possible inhalation of meconium
Sleep pattern disturbance related to withdrawal effect
Altered nutrition: less than body requirements related to inability to ingest food
High risk of injury related to mother's history of cocaine use and inadequate care of previous infants

Outcome identification	Nursing interventions	Rationale	Evaluation
Nursing diagnosis: Sensory-perceptual alterations related to withdrawal as manifested by increased sensitivity to stimuli			
1. Infant will relax when stimuli are reduced after 1 week.	1a. Reduce noise in environment.	1a. Keep sound stimulation at a minimum.	1. Baby Michael was extremely irritable and inconsolable during his 3-month hospital stay. It was 1 month before he could relax when stimuli were reduced. Goal partially met.
	1b. Turn down lights.	1b. Keep light stimulation at a minimum.	
	1c. Swaddle infant in a cotton blanket in flexed position with arms close to body.	1c. Reduces hyperextension, and reproduces comfort of womb.	
	1d. Hold swaddled infant close.	1d. Same as above.	
	1e. Rock infant slowly and rhythmically, either horizontally or with head supported vertically, whichever soothes.	1e. SLOW rhythmic movement may recreate comfort of rocking motion of womb.	

Outcome identification	Nursing interventions	Rationale	Evaluation

Nursing diagnosis: Sensory-perceptual alterations related to withdrawal as manifested by increased sensitivity to stimuli—cont'd

	1f. Respond to stress cues by stopping activity with infant.	1f. This will give infant a respite from stimulation.	
	1g. Begin eye contact in small increments. Place infant outside of face to face contact when eye contact causes excessive stress.	1g. Eye contact may produce excessive stimulation, but learning to respond to care givers will enhance chances of receiving adequate care from mother.	
	1h. Provide firm, calm touch to the mid-chest, back, or sole of the infant's feet.	1h. A firm, calm touch to these areas reduces the likelihood of startle reactions.	
	1i. Provide background noise— try humming, soft music, or white noise such as fan or hair dryer. If all else fails, place infant in quiet, darkened room with no outside stimulation.	1i. Soft music or sustained background sound may soothe some babies.	

Nursing diagnosis: Ineffective airway clearance related to possible inhalation of meconium

| 1. Infant will maintain an open airway on an ongoing basis. | 1a. Have resuscitative equipment available. | 1a. May be needed if respiratory distress develops. | 1. The infant required careful monitoring of his respiratory status, especially during the first month. He did maintain an open airway. Goal met. |
| | 1b. Aspirate mouth and nose as indicated. | 1b. Keeping mouth and nose clear will assist in preventing aspiration. | |

Continued.

Care Plan 8-2

Neonate Born with Crack Cocaine in Its System—cont'd

Outcome identification	Nursing interventions	Rationale	Evaluation
Nursing diagnosis: Ineffective airway clearance related to possible inhalation of meconium—cont'd			
	1c. Assess breath sounds frequently.	1c. Monitoring status of airway.	
	1d. Report tachypnea or signs of respiratory distress.	1d. Signs of respiratory distress may signal need for physician intervention.	
	1e. Feed slowly in small amounts.	1e. Reduces possibility of aspiration of formula.	
	1f. Keep head elevated during feedings.	1f. Same as above.	
Nursing diagnosis: Sleep pattern disturbance related to withdrawal effect			
1. Infant will be able to remain asleep for 3 to 4 hours after 2 weeks.	1a. Organize care to provide long rest periods.	1a. Avoids interruptions in sleep.	1. Michael could only sleep fitfully for 20 to 30 minutes at a time for the first 3 weeks. By 6 weeks he could sleep 3 to 4 hours at a time. Goal met after extended time.
	1b. Provide warm bath.	1b. A warm bath is relaxing and conducive to sleep.	
	1c. Give child pacifier.	1c. A pacifier provides the child comfort.	
	1d. Reduce environmental stimuli.	1d. Reducing environmental stimuli enables the child to fall asleep and reduces the possibility of sleep interruption.	
	1e. Swaddle infant with blanket, cuddle, or hold close. When positioning infant on side, place with back against side of crib to provide support and prevent hyperextension.	1e. Provides a sense of comfort and safety. In addition, bringing the infant's arms close to center and near its mouth allows normal sucking.	

Outcome identification	Nursing interventions	Rationale	Evaluation
Nursing diagnosis: Altered nutrition: less than body requirements related to inability to ingest food			
1. Infant will regain birth weight within 2 weeks.	1a. Feed small frequent amounts.	1a. Helps prevent excessive stimulation or fatigue.	1. It took 4 weeks for baby Michael to regain his birth weight. Goal met after extended time.
	1b. Allow infant to rest frequently during feeding.	1b. Same as above.	
	1c. Have infant upright for feeding. After feeding, place infant in side-lying position.	1c. Helps prevent aspiration.	
Nursing diagnosis: High risk of injury related to mother's history of cocaine use and inadequate care of previous infants			
1. Child will remain free from injury on an ongoing basis.	1a. Examine infant in front of the mother, pointing out normal behaviors and those caused by cocaine.	1a. Helps mother learn that aversion of gaze, hyperextension, and irritability are results of cocaine and not rejection of mother.	1. Before Michael was discharged from the hospital, it was decided that his mother could not remain drug-free, so Michael was placed in a foster home. He remained safe. Goal met.
	1b. Teach and role model care needed to decrease cocaine-induced behaviors and increase healthy behaviors.	1b. Assists mother to learn appropriate care for infant.	
	1c. Refer to social services.	1c. Provides possibility of mother receiving drug treatment and also monitoring and protection of infant once it is discharged.	

functioning, and to physiological problems when drug use occurs in pregnancy. Community education can assist women and their families to become aware of resources available to assist them in overcoming substance abuse problems. Unfortunately, many communities either have no resources available to assist families with substance abuse problems or the resources available are not sufficient to meet the community needs.

Many of the physiological problems affecting drug-exposed children such as FAS can be prevented if drug use is halted. NAACOG (1987) recommends discussing substance abuse in childbirth classes. Unfortunately, many of these women may receive little prenatal care or education, particularly if they are of lower socio-economic status. The Indian Health Service launched a campaign to increase the awareness regarding effects of alcohol use in pregnancy (May & Hymbaugh, 1989). Similar efforts need to be made to educate the general public. The March of Dimes has a variety of materials regarding substance abuse in pregnancy for both professionals and the public.

Warning labels

Government warning labels regarding the effect of alcohol consumption now appear on alcoholic beverages and often are printed in business establishments that serve alcohol. The warning states, "According to the surgeon general, women should not drink alcoholic beverages during pregnancy because of the risk of birth defects." The more this message is spread to child-bearing women and their partners, the greater likelihood the warning will be heeded.

SUMMARY

Maternal usage of both legal and illegal substances affects not only the health of the mother, but her ability to conceive and the health of the fetus and neonate. For the nurse, this group of mothers and children presents a challenge and requires accurate assessment to anticipate potential problems. The complexity of caring for this population is increased due to the pattern of maternal polysubstance usage, thus each mother and child dyad may present with slightly different clinical manifestations. Each drug-exposed infant also presents a challenge to nursing care. The nurse plays a key role in identifying substance abuse and educating and assisting women to become substance-free. In the event that the mother cannot become substance-free, the nurse can refer her to and collaborate with others to assist and protect the child.

REFERENCES

Abel, E.L. & Sokol, R.J. (1987). Incidence of fetal alcohol syndrome and economic impact of FAS-related anomalies. *Drug and Alcohol Dependence, 19,* 51-70.

Als, H. (1982). Towards a research instrument for the assessment of preterm infants' behavior and manual for the assessment of preterm infants' behavior (APIB). In H.D. Fitzgerald, B.M. Lester, & M.W. Yogman (Eds.) *Theory and research in behavioral pediatrics.* New York: Plenum Press.

American Academy of Pediatrics Committee on Drugs. (1983). Neonatal drug withdrawal, *Pediatrics,* 72(6), 895-902.

Asch, R.H. & Smith, C. (1983). Effects of marijuana on reproduction. *Contemporary OB-GYN, 28,* 217-225.

Autti-Ramo, I., Gaily, E., & Granstrom, M.L. (1992). Dysmorphic features in offspring of alcoholic mothers. *Archives of Disabled Children, 67*(6), 712-716.

Bashore, R.A., Ketchum, J.S., Staisch, K.J., Barrett, C.T., & Zimmermann, E.G. (1981). Heroin addiction and pregnancy—interdepartmental clinical conference. UCLA School of Medicine. *Western Journal of Medicine, 134,* 506.

Bastin, N., Tamayo, O.W., Tinkle, M.B., Amaya, M.A., Trejo, L.R., & Herrera, C. (1992). HIV disease and pregnancy: Part 3: Postpartum care of the HIV-positive woman and her newborn. *JOGNN, 21*(2), 105-111.

Bateman, D.A. & Heagarty, M.C. (1989). Passive free base cocaine ("crack") inhalation by infants and toddlers. *American Journal of Diseases of Children, 143,* 25-27.

Bayley, N. (1969). *Bayley's scales of infant development.* New York: Psychological Corp.

Berkowitz, R.L., Coustan, D.R., & Mochizuki, T.K. (1986). *Handbook for prescribing medications during pregnancy.* (2nd ed.). Boston: Little, Brown & Company.

Bingol, N., Fuchs, M., Diaz, V., Stone, R., & Gromisch, D. (1987). Teratogenicity of cocaine in humans. *Journal of Pediatrics, 110*(1), 93-96.

Blackard, C. & Tennes, K. (1984). Human placental transfer of cannabinoids. *The New England Journal of Medicine, 311,* 797.

Bobak, I.M. & Jensen, M.D. (1995). *Maternity and gynecological care.* (5th ed.) St. Louis: Mosby.

Brazelton, T.B. (1991). What we can learn from the status of the newborn. In M.M. Kilbey & K. Asghar (Eds.) *Methodological issues in controlled studies on effects of prenatal exposure to drug abuse.* Research Monograph 114, Rockville, MD: NIDA.

Campinha-Bacote, J. & Bragg, E.J. (1993). Chemical assessment in maternity care. *MCN, 18*(1), 24-28.

Centers for Disease Control. (1993). Fetal alcohol syndrome—United States, 1979-1992. *Morbidity and Mortality Weekly Report, 42*(17), 339-341.

Chasnoff, I. (1986a). Alcohol use in pregnancy. In I. Chasnoff (Ed.). *Drug use in pregnancy: Mother and child.* Norwell, MA: M.T.P. Press.

Chasnoff, I. (1986b). Fetal alcohol syndrome in twin pregnancy. *Acta Genet Med Gamellol, 34,* 229-232.

Chasnoff, I.J. (1987). Cocaine use in pregnancy: Perinatal morbidity and mortality. *Neurotoxicology and Teratology, 9,* 291-293.

Chasnoff, I., Burns, K., & Burns, W. (1987). Cocaine use in pregnancy: Perinatal morbidity and mortality. *Neurotoxicology and Teratology, 9*(4), 291-293.

Chasnoff, I., Burns, W., Schnoll, S., & Burns, K. (1985). Cocaine use in pregnancy. *The New England Journal of Medicine, 313*(11), 666-669.

Chasnoff, I., Landress, H., & Barrett, M. (1990). The prevalence of illicit drug or alcohol use during pregnancy and discrepancies in mandatory reporting in Pinellas County, Florida. *New England Journal of Medicine, 322*(17), 1202-6.

Chasnoff, I., Lewis, D., & Squires, L. (1987). Cocaine intoxication in a breast-fed infant. *Pediatrics, 80*(6), 836-838.

Children's Hospital Medical Center of Northern California. (1990). *Toxicology screening protocol.* CA: The Center.

Clarren, S., Bowden, D., & Astley, S. (1985). The brain in the fetal alcohol syndrome: Observation in human and nonhuman primates. *Alcohol Health and Research World, 9*(3), 20-25.

Clarren, S.K. & Aldrich, R.A. (1993). *A concise manual for fetal alcohol screening: Fetal alcohol syndrome checklist.* (Grant No. U59-CCU0069120). Seattle, WA: USIHHS, PHS, and Washington State Department of Health.

Coles, C.D. & Platzmon, K.A. (1992). Fetal alcohol effects in preschool children. Research, prevention, and intervention. In OSAP monograph, *Identifying the needs of drug afflicted children: Public policy issues.* Rockville, MD: Office of Substance Abuse Prevention.

Coyne, B.A. & Landers, D.V. (1990). The immunology of HIV disease and pregnancy and possible interactions. *Obstetrics and Gynecology Clinics of North America, 17*(3), 523-544.

Day, N.L., Robles, N., Richardson, G., Geva, D., Taylor, P., Scher, M., Stoffer, D., Cornelius, M., & Goldschmidt, L. (1991). The effects of prenatal alcohol use on the growth of children at three years of age. *Alcoholism: Clinical and Experimental Research, 15*(1), 67-71.

Dixon, S. (1989). Effects of transplacental exposure to cocaine and methamphetamine on the neonate. *Western Journal of Medicine, 150,* 436-442.

Enkin, M. (1984). Smoking and pregnancy: A new look. *Birth, 11*(94), 225-229.

Ernhart, C., Sokol, R., Martier, S., Moron, P., Nadler, D., Ager, J., & Wolf, A. (1987). Alcohol teratogenicity in the human: A detailed assessment of specificity, critical period, and threshold. *American Journal of Obstetrics and Gynecology, 156*(1), 33-39.

Ewing, H. (1991). Management of the pregnant alcoholic/addict. Presented at American Society on Addiction Medicine. Medical Scientific Conference, Boston, April 20, 1991.

Fagan, J.F., Shepherd, P.A., & Knevel, C.R. (1991). Predictive validity of the Fagan Test of Infant Intelligence. Cleveland, OH: Case Western Reserve University.

Finnegan, L. (1988). The dilemma of cocaine exposure in the perinatal period. *National Institute of Drug Abuse Research: Monograph Series, 81*, 379.

Flandermeyer, A., (1993). The drug exposed neonate. In C. Kenner, A. Brueggemeyer & L.P. Gunderson (Eds.) *Comprehensive neonatal nursing care: A physiologic perspective.* Philadelphia: W.B. Saunders.

Forss, M., Lehtovirta, P., Rauramo, I., & Kariniemi, V. (1983). Midtrimester fetal heart rate variability and maternal hemodynamics in association with smoking. *American Journal of Obstetrics and Gynecology, 146*(6), 693-695.

Fried, P.A. (1982). Marijuana use by pregnant women and effects on offspring: An update. *Neurobehav Toxicol Teratol, 4,* 415-424.

Fried, P.A., Watkinson, B., & Willan, A. (1984). Marijuana use during pregnancy and decreased length of gestation. *American Journal Obstet Gynecol, 150*(1), 23-27.

Gal, P. & Sharpless, M.K. (1984). Fetal drug exposure—Behavioral teratogenesis. *Drug Intelligence and Clinical Pharmacology, 18,* 186-201.

Good, W., Ferriero, D., Golabi, M., & Kobori, J. (1992). Abnormalities of the visual system in infants exposed to cocaine. *Ophthalmology, 99*(3), 341-346.

Goodman, J., Visser, F., & Dawes, G. (1984). Effects of maternal cigarette smoking on fetal trunk movements, fetal breathing movements and the fetal heart rate. *British Journal of Obstetrics and Gynaecology, 91,* 657-661.

Greenberg, R., Haley, N., Etzel, R., & Loda, F. (1984). Measuring the exposure of infants to tobacco smoke. *The New England Journal of Medicine, 310*(17), 1075-1078.

Greenland, S., Staisch, K.J., Brown, N., & Gross, S.J. (1982). Effects of marijuana use during pregnancy. *American Journal Obstet Gynecol, 143,* 408-413.

Harlap, S. & Shiono, P. (1980). Alcohol, smoking, and incidence of spontaneous abortions in the first and second trimester. *Lancet, 2,* 173-176.

Harwood, H. & Napolitano, D. (1985). Economic implications of the fetal alcohol syndrome. *Alcohol Health and Research World, 9*(4), 38-43.

Hatch, E.E. & Bracken, M.B. (1986). Effect of marijuana use in pregnancy on fetal growth. *American Journal of Epidemiology, 42,* 566-567.

Hayes, J.S., Dreher, M.C., & Nugent, J.K. (1988). Newborn outcomes with maternal marijuana use in Jamaican women. *Pediatric Nursing, 14,* 107-110.

Hingson, R., Alpert, J.J., Day, N., Dooling, E., Kayne, H., Morelock, S., Oppenheimer, E., & Zuckerman, B. (1982). Effects of maternal drinking and marijuana use on fetal growth and development. *Pediatrics, 70,* 539-545.

Hurt, H. (1989). Medical controversies in evaluation and management of cocaine exposed infants. In Ross Laboratories (Ed.), *Special currents: Cocaine babies.* Columbus, OH: Ross Laboratories.

Idanpaan-Heikkila, J., Fritchie, G.E., Englert, L.F., Ho, B.T., & McIsaac, W.M. (1969). Placental transfer of tritiated 1-delta-9-tetrahydrocannabinol. *The New England Journal of Medicine, 281,* 330.

Jones, K. & Smith, D. (1973). Recognition of the fetal alcohol syndrome in early infancy. *Lancet,* 999-1001.

Kaiser Foundation Hospital. (1989). *Perinatal substance abuse protocol.* San Francisco, CA: The Hospital.

Kandall, S.R. (1991). Drug Abuse. In A.Y. Sweet & E.G. Brown (Eds.) *Fetal and neonatal effects of maternal disease.* St. Louis: Mosby.

Kandall, S.R. & Chavkin, W. (1992). Illicit drugs in America. History impact on women and children and treatment strategies for women. *Hastings Law Journal, 43,* 605-643.

Klausner, H.A. & Dingell, J.V. (1971). The metabolism and excretion of delta-9-tetrahydrocannabinol in the rat. *Life Sci,* Part I, 10:49-59.

Kline, J., Stein, Z., Shrout, P., Susser, M., & Warburton, D. (1980). Drinking during pregnancy and sponta-neous abortion. *Lancet, 2,* 176-180.

Kreuz, D.S. & Axelrod, J. (1973). Delta-9-tetrahydrocannabinol: Localization in body fat. *Science, 179,* 391-393.

Kuhner, P., Kuhner, B., Bottoms, S., & Erhard, P. (1982). Cadmium levels in maternal blood, fetal cord blood, and placental tissues of pregnant women who smoke. *American Journal of Obstetrics and Gynecology, 142*(8), 1021-1025.

Lefrak-Okikawa, L. & Meier, P. (1993). Nutrition: Physiologic basis of metabolism and management of enteral and parenteral nutrition. In C. Kenner, A. Brueggemeyer, & L.P. Gunderson (Eds.) *Compre-hensive Neonatal Nursing Care: A Physiologic Perspective.* Philadelphia: W.B. Saunders.

Lemoine, P., Harrousseau, H., Borteyru, J., & Menuet, J.C. (1968). Les enfants de parents alcooliques: Anomalies observées: A propos de 127 cas. *Ouest Med, 25,* 477-482.

Linn, S., Schoenbaum, S.C., Monson, R.R., Rosner, R., Stubblefield, P.C., & Ryan, K.J. (1983). The associa-tion of marijuana use with outcome of pregnancy. *American Journal of Public Health, 73,* 1161-1164.

Little, B.B., Snell, L.M., Rosenfeld, C.R., Gilstrap, L.C., & Grant, N.F. (1990). Failure to recognize fetal alcohol syndrome in newborn infants. *American Journal of Diseases of Children, 144,* 1142-1146.

Little, R., Streissguth, A., Barr, H., & Herman, C. (1980). Decreased birth weight in infants of alcoholic women who abstained during pregnancy. *Journal of Pediatrics, 96*(6), 974-977.

MacGregor, S., Keith, L., Chasnoff, I., Rosner, M., Chisum, G., Shaw, P., & Minogue, J. (1987). Cocaine use during pregnancy: Adverse perinatal outcome. *American Journal of Obstetrics and Gynecology, 157*(3), 686-690.

May, P.A. & Hymbaugh, K.J. (1989). A macro level fetal alcohol syndrome prevention program for Native Americans and Alaska natives: Description and evaluation. *Journal of Studies on Alcohol, 50,* 508-518.

McKool, K. (1987). Facilitating smoking cessation. *Journal of Cardiovascular Nursing, 1*(4), 28-41.

Mercer, R.T., Ferketich, S.L., De Joseph, J., May, K.A., & Saleed, D. (1988). Effect of stress on family, functioning during pregnancy. *Nursing Research, 37*(5), 268-275.

Miami Valley Hospital. (1992). *How to care for your affected baby.* Dayton, OH: The Hospital.

Miller, G. (1989). Addicted infants and their mothers. *Zero to Three, National Center for Clinical Infant Programs,* (June), *10,* 20-23.

Miller, M.W. & Robertson, S. (1993). Prenatal exposure to ethanol alters the postnatal development and transformation of radial glia to astrocytes in the cortex. *Journal of Comparative Neurology, 337,* 253-266.

Nahar, G.G. (1976). Marijuana: Chemistry, biochemistry, and cellular effects. New York: Springer-Verlag.

Nanda, D. (1990). Human immunodeficiency virus infection in pregnancy. *Obstetrics and Gynecology Clinics of North America, 17*(3), 617-626.

National Commission to Prevent Infant Mortality. (1990). *Troubling Trends: The Health of American's Next Generation.* Washington, D.C. NIAAA. (1990). Alcohol Alert. Screening for Alcohol. No. 8, PH 285, 1-4. Rockville, MD: National Institute on Alcohol Abuse and Addiction.

National Council on Alcoholism and Drug Dependence. (1993). One in nine pregnant women test posi-tive for drugs in California study. *The alcoholism report, 21*(9), 8-9.

National Institute on Drug Abuse. (1990). *National household survey on drug abuse: Main findings 1988.* U.S. Department of Health and Human Services. (DHHS Publication No. Adm90-1682). Rockville, MD: The Institute.

Nieburg, P., Marks, J.S., McLaren, N.M., & Remington, P.L. (1985). The fetal tobacco syndrome (commen-tary). *JAMA, 253,* 2998.

Nowicki, P., Gintzig, L., Hebel, R., Latham, R., Miller, V., & Sexton, M. (1984). Effective smoking interven-tion during pregnancy. *Birth, 11*(4), 217-224.

Nurses' Association of the American College of Obstetricians and Gynecologists. (1987). *Competencies and program guidelines for nurse providers of childbirth education.* Washington, D.C.: The Association.

Oehler, J.M., Goldstein, R.F., Catlett, A., Boshkoff, M., & Brazy, J.E. (1993). How to target infants at highest risk for developmental delay. *MCN, 18*(1), 20-23.

Olds, D.L. & Henderson, C.R. (1989). The prevention of maltreatment. In D. Cicchiti & V. Carden (Eds.), *Child maltreatment.* New York: Cambridge University Press.

Olson, H.C., Burgess, D.M., & Streissguth, A.P. (1992). Fetal alcohol syndrome (FAS) and fetal alcohol effects (FAE): A lifespan view, with implications for early intervention. *Zero to Three/National Center for Clinical Infant Programs, 13*(1), 24-29.

Oro, A. & Dixon, S. (1987). Perinatal cocaine and methamphetamine exposure: Maternal and neonatal correlates. *Journal of Pediatrics, 111*(4), 571-578.

Ostrea, E.M., Brady, M.J., Parks, P.M., Asensio, D.C., & Naluz, A. (1989). Drug screening of meconium in infants of drug-dependent mothers: An alternative to urine testing. *Journal of Pediatrics, 115,* 474-477.

Pelham, T. & DeJong, A. (1992). Nationwide practices for screening and reporting prenatal cocaine abuse: A survey of teaching programs. *Child Abuse and Neglect, 16,* 763-770.

Pitt, J. (1991). Perinatal human immunodeficiency virus infection. *Clinics in Perinatology, 18*(2), 227-239.

Pritchard, J. (1955). Plasma cholinesterase activity in normal pregnancy and in eclamptogenic toxemia. *South Am J Obstet Gynecol, 70,* 1083.

Randels, S.P. & Streissguth, A.P. (1992). Fetal alcohol syndrome and nutrition issues. *Nutrition Focus for Children with Special Health Care Needs, 7*(3), 1-6.

Rantakallio, P. (1983). A follow-up study up to the age of 14 of children whose mothers smoked during pregnancy. *Acta Paediatrica Scandinavica, 72,* 747-753.

Raskin, V. (1992). Maternal bereavement in the perinatal substance abuser. *Journal of Substance Abuse Treatment, 9,* 149-152.

Reddy, A., Harper, R., & Stern, G. (1971). Observations on heroin and methadone withdrawal in the newborn. *Pediatrics, 48,* 353-358.

Russell, M., Czarnecki, D.M., Cowan, R., McPhearson, E., & Mudar, P.J. (1991). Measures of maternal alcohol use as predictors of development in early childhood. *Alcoholism: Clinical and Experimental Research, 14*(5), 662-669.

Schnoll, S. (1986). Pharmacologic basis of perinatal addiction. In I. Chasnoff (Ed.). *Drug use in pregnancy: Mother and child.* Norwell, MA: M.T.P. Press.

Schulte-Hobein, B., Schwartz-Bickenbach, D., Abt, S., Plum, C., & Nau, H. (1992). Cigarette smoke exposure and development of infants throughout the first year of life: Influence of passive smoking and nursing on cotinine levels in breastmilk and infant's urine. *Acta Paediatr, 81,* 550-557.

Slutsker, L., Smith, R., Higginson, G., & Fleming, D. (1993). Recognizing illicit drug use by pregnant women: Reports from Oregon birth attendants. *American Journal of Public Health, 83*(1), 61-64.

Sokol, R.J., Martier, S.S., & Ager, J.W. (1989). The T-ACE questions: Prochial prenatal detection of risk-drinking. *American Journal of Obstetrics & Gynecology, 160*(7), 863-868.

Sokol, R.J., Miller, S.I., & Reed, G. (1980). Alcohol abuse during pregnancy: An epidemiological study. *Alcoholism: Clinical and Experimental Research, 4,* 135-145.

Streissguth, A.P. (1990). Fetal alcohol syndrome and the teratogenicity of alcohol: Policy implications. *Bulletin of the King County Medical Society, 69*(5), 32-36, 39, 42.

Streissguth, A.P. (1991). The Betty Ford lecture: What every community should know about drinking during pregnancy and the lifelong consequences. *Substance Abuse, 12*(3), 114-127.

Streissguth, A.P., Aase, J.M., Clarren, S.K., Randels, S.P., LaDue, R.A., & Smith, D.F. (1991). Fetal alcohol syndrome in adolescents and adults. *Journal of the American Medical Association, 265*(15), 1961-1967.

Streissguth, A.P., Barr, H.M., & Sampson, P.D. (1990). Moderate prenatal alcohol exposure: Effects on child IQ and learning problems at age 7½ years. *Alcoholism: Clinical and Experimental Research, 14*(5), 662-669.

Streissguth, A., Clarren, S., & Jones, K. (1985). A natural history of the fetal alcohol syndrome: A 10-year follow up of 11 patients. *Alcohol Health and Research World, 9*(A), 13-19.

Sweeney, L. (1989). Cocaine babies: The latest management dilemma. *NCAST National News, 5*(3), 1-2.

Torrence, C.R. & Horns, K.M. (1989). Appraisal and caregiving for the drug addicted infant. *Neonatal Network, 8*(3), 49-59.

Townsend, R., Laing, F., & Jeffrey, B., Jr. (1988). Placental abruption associated with cocaine abuse. *AJR, 150*(6), 1339-1340.

Udell, B. (1989). Crack cocaine. In Ross Laboratories (Ed.). *Special Currents: Cocaine Babies.* Columbus, OH: Ross Laboratories.

U.S. Department of Health and Human Services. (1989). *Reducing the health consequences of smoking: 25 years of progress.* A report of the Surgeon General (DHHS Publication No. CDC 90-8416). Washington D.C.: The Department.

U.S. Department of Health and Human Services. (1980). *The health consequences of smoking for women.* Public Health Service, Office on Smoking and Health. Washington, D.C.: The Department.

VandenBerg, K.A. & Hanson, M.J. (1993). *Homecoming for babies after the neonatal intensive care nursery: A guide for professionals in supporting families and their infants' early development.* Austin, TX: Pro-Ed.

Weiner, L. & Larsson, G. (1987). Clinical prevention of fetal alcohol effects—a reality: Evidence for the effectiveness of intervention. *Alcohol Health and Research World, 11*(4), 60-63.

Wilson, G., McCreary, R., Kean, J., & Baxter, C. (1979). The development of preschool children of heroin-addicted mothers: A controlled study. *Pediatrics, 63*(1), 135-141.

Wright, J. (1986). Fetal alcohol syndrome. *Nursing Times, 82*(13), 34-35.

Wu, T.C., Tashkin, D.P., Djahed, B., & Rose, J.E. (1988). Pulmonary hazards of smoking marijuana as compared with tobacco. *The New England Journal of Medicine, 318,* 347-351.

Zuckerman, B., Frank, D.A., Hingson, R., Amaro, H., Levenson, S.M., Kayne, H., Parker, S., Vinci, R., Aboagye, K., Fried, L.E., Cabral, H., Rimperi, R., & Bauchner, H. (1989). Effects of maternal marijuana and cocaine use on fetal growth. *The New England Journal of Medicine, 320,* 762-768.

Zuspan, F.P. & Zuspan, K.J. (1991). Drug addiction in pregnancy. In W. Rayburn & F. Zuspan. *Drug therapy in obstetrics and gynecology.* (3rd ed.). St. Louis: Mosby.

9

Substance Abuse in Families, Children, and Adolescents

Substance abuse affects the abusers, as well as others in their environment, especially family members. Thus substance abuse is considered a family disease, and when the primary substance of abuse is alcohol, use of the term *alcoholic family* is common. The number of individuals and families affected by alcohol and drug abuse or addiction is overwhelming. In a 1987 Gallup poll one in four families reported a problem with alcohol abuse in the home. Data from the National Institute of Mental Health's Epidemiologic Catchment Area Survey indicate that 13.7% of adults met current or lifetime criteria for alcohol abuse or dependence, and 5.9% met criteria for drug abuse or dependence (Raskin & Daley, 1991).

Health professionals are in prime positions to identify substance abuse and to help families face and deal with the problem, decrease enabling behaviors, and motivate the individual to seek treatment. This chapter focuses on family dynamics and the effects on family members, especially children, when one or more adults are substance abusers. Sections on substance abuse prevention and adolescent substance abuse are also included.

SUBSTANCE ABUSE AND THE FAMILY

When one member of a family becomes chemically dependent, the family organization must change for the family to survive. If the member with substance abuse is kept within the family constellation, the family must do two things. First, they must fulfill roles and responsibilities that were formerly carried out by the substance abusing member but currently are not. Second, they must cognitively explain the behavior of the substance abusing person. Generally, maintaining the dependent behavior is not compatible with family values and beliefs; therefore certain predictable patterns develop.

Dysfunctional family patterns

Isaacson (1991) describes the characteristics of a family system with substance abuse. A *functional* family system has a "hierarchical structure of leadership; roles that support individual and family goal achievement; rules for communication, problem solving, and intrafamily sub-group interaction; as well as interaction with the environment and support for separation and individuation of its members"

(Isaacson, 1991, p. 11). The family system in substance abuse has *dysfunctional* behaviors and interactions that inhibit differentiation and support continuation of substance abuse. There are five characteristics of addicted family systems (Isaacson, 1991).

1. The family resists change, and the interactions of its members support the stability of the dysfunctional system.
2. The individuals in the family behave and interact in ways that maintain a rigid, closed system, limiting interaction with the outside environment.
3. The family problems are repeated over generations.
4. The substance abuse covers up other family problems.
5. The family has rigid interactional patterns that do not change in response to changing circumstances.

As substance abuse progresses, subtle changes in the family system occur while the family "adjusts" to the insidious progression of the illness. Dysfunctional family patterns include changes in role behaviors within the family (Jacob et al, 1981), and ineffective problem solving (Steinglass et al, 1987); all family members behave in ways to regain homeostasis and control or resolve the crises created by substance abuse. For instance, if the mother is drinking and cannot prepare evening meals, the father may recruit a preteen daughter, who then may neglect her homework and have problems in school.

Kaufman (1985) summarizes some common factors related to both alcohol and drug abuse. He considers the use of alcohol or drugs a symptom of family dysfunction and identifies crises related to cohesiveness and fragmentation of the family system. Substance use is associated with fusion or overinvolvement between parents and children, and there is multigenerational addiction. The male parent is distant or uninvolved, while the female parent is overinvolved. The substance abuser is often the scapegoat of the family system, and family members use primitive defenses such as denial, projection, and rationalization to deal with conflict. There is a high incidence of loss in these families, either by death, separation, incest, or family violence. Others describe the alcoholic family as chaotic, inconsistent, and unpredictable, with unclear roles, arbitrariness, changing limits, frequent arguments, repetitious or illogical thinking, and perhaps violence and incest (Brown, 1988).

Difficulties with intimacy.   Coleman (1987) describes a relationship between substance abuse and intimacy dysfunction, the inability to develop close relationships with others. Intimacy dysfunction is related to difficulties with boundaries (Coleman & Colgan, 1986) that separate individuals from one another and clarify their identities. Boundaries are defined by rules that delimit appropriate behavior in relation to others. Healthy boundaries are flexible and open at times, yet rigid and closed at other times, depending on the circumstances. For instance, it is healthy to have high self-disclosure with a spouse but not with a casual acquaintance. It is healthy to maintain a half-block distance from a stranger on the street at night, but 12 inches or less is acceptable between intimates. Coleman describes three characteristics of boundaries in families with substance abuse. They are (1) too invasive of one another's boundaries, (2) too distant and rigid, or (3) so ambiguous that no family members know their standing with other family members. These boundary difficulties lead to intimacy dysfunction, and intimacy dysfunction leads to boundary difficulties. Indeed, adults reared in a family with substance abuse are more likely to become substance abusers or marry one (Brown, 1988). Black, Bucky, and Wilder-Padilla (1986) report higher divorce rates among children of alcoholics.

Role reversal. Most family behaviors revolve around the substance abuser. The abuser's behavior dictates how other family members interact inside and outside the family. As addicts become more involved with their substance use, they are less available to others. Consequently, individuals who previously played important roles in the addict's life are ignored. Spouses and children are emotionally abandoned as the substance becomes the primary relationship for the addicted individual. The addicted person's behavior becomes unfamiliar, unacceptable, and unpredictable, including angry outbursts, rages, and selfish, demanding behaviors. The family atmosphere becomes tense and fearful. The focus of the family is the addicted member. All of the nonaddicted parent's attention is often focused on controlling the addict, and this parent becomes less involved with the children. Parenting becomes inconsistent or sometimes nonexistent. Children may take care of parents or each other because parental attention is elsewhere. Thus children cross generational boundaries, functioning as parents in many situations (Kingery-McCabe & Campbell, 1991).

Clinebell (1968) reported four factors that produce damage in the lives of children of substance abusers. The first is *role reversal;* children may undertake parental duties either because the parents are unable or because adult responsibilities are forced on them. In incestuous families, daughter and mother switch roles. Second, an inconsistent and unpredictable relationship with the addicted parent is *emotionally depriving* to children. Third, the nonaddicted parent is struggling with major problems and personal unmet needs, and thus *cannot attend to the needs of the children.* The fourth factor is *social isolation* of the family. Because of embarrassment, the family discounts the importance of social relationships or adequate peer relationships for the children. Although these conditions do not occur in all families with substance abuse, they are damaging when they exist.

Denial system. Another component of the dysfunctional family system is denial. The denial system distorts reality to avoid identifying the family problem. Through the family denial system, ineffective problem solving, and role reversals, family members enable the substance abuser to continue using. Enabling is often unintentional, but until family members identify the substance abuse problem, it is inevitable.

Denial and family secrets pervade families with a parent who abuses substances. Because substance abuse is a secret inside and outside the family, children are made partners in the family denial (Woodside, 1986). Family members pretend everything is okay. Often, this is accomplished by invalidating the children's reality, which in turn may influence how they process information. That is, if a child is taught that pretending everything is okay and keeping family secrets is normal, consensual validation of a child's perceptions is not experienced and maladaptive psychological adjustment may result. Substance abusers use denial so consistently and subtly in their interactions that, in the absence of any intervention from outside the home, family members often question their own sanity.

In many instances, denial is based on the individual's genuine lack of recognition of and insight into the degree of substance use and the resulting problems (Weinberg, 1974). Denial permits the addicted person to continue using substances by screening the negative effects from awareness. The denial system interferes with the ability to realistically perceive the consequences of substance abuse for themselves and their families. The strength of the denial system is directly related to both the duration and extent of the harmful effects on the individual's life. Thus persons with mild substance abuse of recent origin are generally more able to recognize the relationship between their problems and their substance abuse. Confronting individuals in more advanced stages of addiction requires assertiveness and persistence. They must recognize the connection between their substance use and the problems it causes them and their families (Tweed, 1989).

Smith (1986) found that men and women differ in the process of facing the denial of substance abuse. Women described themselves as being aware of a problem long before others encouraged them to seek treatment. They described situations in which they had mentioned to others a potential problem with substance abuse and others had reassured them that no problem existed. Thus they continued to abuse and did not seek early treatment. In contrast, males were more likely to have substance abuse problems identified by others long before they identified the problems.

Role behaviors.   Family systems consistently seek homeostasis. Thus families alter how they function to accommodate the substance abuser's behavioral changes. As substance abuse progresses, the family is thrown off balance and must shift its functioning to survive. Satir (1967) identified role behaviors that family members play when they are under stress to preserve the family system at the expense of their own emotional and physical health. When these role behaviors fail and the stress continues, family members change roles in an attempt to cope.

Role behaviors specific to alcoholic families have been identified. (In this discussion the alcoholic family is generalized to families with substance abuse.) These roles disguise the illness, distracting family members from the real problems and their feelings. They serve as protection, allowing the family to function and individual members to achieve some security and stability for themselves. Meanwhile, the addiction progresses. Wegscheider (1981) identified the following role behaviors:

1. **Chief enabler**—Usually a spouse or parent plays the role of the chief enabler, who provides responsibility within the family system. As chief enablers protect substance abusers and compensate for loss of control, they enable the disease to continue but feel hurt, angry, guilty, and afraid.
2. **Family hero**—Usually the oldest child takes the role of the family hero, who provides self-worth for the family through hard work, achievement, and success in school. The family hero's job is to perform extremely well, proving that everything is normal at home. The hero has an overdeveloped sense of accomplishment, responsibility, and perfectionism. This individual's achievements are for others and the family; underneath the facade the hero feels inadequate.
3. **Scapegoat**—The role of the scapegoat is played by the child who acts out or

abuses alcohol or drugs, thus taking the focus off family problems. Although it appears that the child volunteers for this position, the scapegoat feels lonely and hurt.

4. **Lost child**—The lost child offers relief by not being a problem. These children withdraw and are quiet and independent, yet they feel lonely and inadequate.

5. **Mascot**—Often the youngest child is the mascot, who provides fun and humor to distract family members from the tensions of substance abuse. Although protected from what is really happening within the family, the mascot senses tension and feels insecure, frightened, and lonely.

Black (1981) defines role behaviors of children of alcoholics in the following two categories: (1) the misbehaving, obviously troubled child, and (2) the mature, stable, overachieving, behaving child who Black considers the majority. These "behaving" children develop survival roles to provide their own stability. As long as these children obtain some secondary gain from their role behaviors, they maintain a positive self-image. However, when a child's short-term goals become an adult's long-term goals, there is no foundation for self-worth. Later, this lack of self-worth may lead to alcohol abuse as a pain reliever.

Black (1981) divides "behaving" children into three types of role behaviors:

1. *Responsible* children are usually the oldest and they feel responsible for everyone. They provide structure for the family and become angry with themselves if they are not in control. They are adult-like, serious, rigid, and inflexible. They have little time for play or fun. Their self-reliance leads to loneliness, and they often marry alcoholics. Black's "responsible children" are similar to Wegscheider's "family hero."

2. *Adjusters* follow directions and must be flexible to adjust to the fighting, separation, and multiple life changes within the alcoholic family. They feel they have no power over their own lives. They work hard at taking care of others and deny any feelings of their own. They are adaptable and can adjust to many situations, but they are easily manipulated by others and often experience low self-esteem.

3. *Placaters* are emotionally sensitive children. They take care of others, neglecting their own feelings and needs. They smooth over conflicts and are rewarded for their help.

These role behavior categories are not mutually exclusive. Children may blend several of these behaviors and use different ones at different times or switch roles. A family hero who goes away to college, is influenced by a peer group to drink abusively, and does poorly in school can quickly become the scapegoat. If a scapegoat leaves home, the next youngest may fill that position. Once role behaviors become the norm, they continue even after the child leaves the family or the addict achieves sobriety.

Although these role behaviors are clinically appealing, investigators have been unable to validate them. Rhodes and Blackham (1987) used Black's categories to compare adolescents from alcoholic homes with those from nonalcoholic homes. They found that the acting-out role was the only role more prevalent in adolescents from alcoholic homes. Similarly, Manning, Balson, and Xenakis (1986) did not find a prevalence of type-A personalities (equated with the hero role) among school-age and adolescent children of alcoholics. Scavnicky-Mylant (1988) studied coping among young adult children of alcoholics and was unable to identify specific role behaviors. Devine and Braithwaite (1993) found that parental alcoholism contributed to children adopting the acting-out role and predicted the responsible child role.

CODEPENDENCY

The term *codependency* originally described the spouse of the chemically dependent person. While the person with substance abuse focused on the substance, the spouse focused on the substance abuser. The definition of codependency has broadened and proliferated, but currently there is no consistent definition. Generally the codependent develops an unhealthy pattern of relating to others, low self-esteem, a need to be needed, a strong urge to change and control others, and a willingness to suffer as a result of being closely involved with someone who has an alcohol or drug problem (Zerwekh & Michaels, 1989).

Codependents are usually dealing with unresolved family of origin issues that may include substance abuse. For example, Friel and Friel (1988) described codependency as a dysfunctional pattern of living, emerging from one's family of origin, that produces arrested identity development. Wegscheider-Cruse (1985) described codependence as a specific condition characterized by preoccupation and extreme emotional, social, and sometimes physical dependence on a person or object. Codependence has the following characteristics: (1) It is learned and acquired, (2) it involves alteration of normal personality development, (3) it is externally focused, (4) it is a disease of lost selfhood, (5) it includes personal boundary distortions, and (6) it is a feeling disorder manifested by emptiness, low self-esteem, shame, fear, anger, confusion, and numbness (Whitfield, 1987).

Cermak (1986) proposes that codependence is a pattern of personality traits that can create sufficient dysfunction to warrant the diagnosis of Mixed Personality Disorder. These traits are most likely to develop in individuals reared in families with substance abuse. According to Cermak, the diagnostic criteria for codependence include the following:

1. Continued investment of self-esteem in the ability to control both oneself and others despite serious, adverse consequences;
2. Assumption of responsibility for meeting others' needs to the exclusion of one's own needs;
3. Anxiety and boundary distortions concerning intimacy and separation;
4. Enmeshment in relationships with personality disordered, chemically dependent, and impulse disordered individuals; and
5. At least three of the following: excessive reliance on denial, constriction of emotions, depression, hypervigilance, compulsions, anxiety, substance abuse, recurrent physical, sexual, or emotional abuse, stress-related medical illness, or involvement in a primary relationship with an active alcoholic or other drug addicted person for at least 2 years without seeking outside support.

Even though there is no agreement on a definition of codependency, there has been widespread response from people who personally recognized the characteristics and the subsequent pain. Many find it explained their life experiences. There are many books, lectures, and workshops available, including self-help groups such as Co-dependents Anonymous and Adult Children of Alcoholics Anonymous (see Care Plan 9-1).

Text continued on p. 248.

Female Spouse of Husband with Substance Abuse

Agnes, age 38, appeared frequently in an outpatient mental health clinic. She had been having anxiety attacks, palpitations, and insomnia and had a medical diagnosis of irritable bowel syndrome. Her husband, John, age 45, has been drinking heavily for many years. They have three children, John, Jr, age 15, Arlene, age 12, and Derek, age 9. In spite of everything, she wanted to save her marriage.

ASSESSMENT

Agnes presents to the clinic in an attractive outfit. When complimented, she states that she is fat and ugly, as well as tired. She works all day, caring for the children, taking care of the house, and picking up after John, and she gets no gratitude. She complains that she and John never go out anymore. All he does is drink and yell. She states, "I am tired of being sick and tired."

NURSING DIAGNOSES

Knowledge deficit: alcoholism related to lack of exposure to concepts of alcoholism and codependence

Ineffective family coping: compromised related to changes made in response to husband and father's drinking patterns

Anxiety related to role overload as a result of husband's heavy drinking

Sleep pattern disturbance related to high anxiety levels

Social isolation related to husband's drinking and her role overload

Outcome identification	Nursing interventions	Rationale	Evaluation
Nursing diagnosis: Knowledge deficit: alcoholism related to lack of exposure to concepts of alcoholism and codependence			
1. Client will list signs and symptoms of the disease of alcoholism in 1 week.	1a. Teach client signs and symptoms of the disease of alcoholism.	1a. Knowledge of the disease of alcoholism will give the client better understanding of her husband's behavior.	1. Agnes was interested in hearing about her husband's problem. After a week, she listed the signs and symptoms of alcoholism demonstrated by John. Goal met.
	1b. Give client literature about the disease.	1b. Since this is new knowledge, it will need reinforcement, hence the literature.	
2. Client will describe three ways in which these changes affect the family after 2 weeks.	2a. Ask her how her husband's drinking affects her and her family.	2a. Learning about one's own behavior has a significant emotional impact. One must start from the client's perspective.	2. After two weeks, Agnes responded with the same complaints about her husband. She said, "I don't think this other stuff describes me,

Outcome identification	Nursing interventions	Rationale	Evaluation
Nursing diagnosis: Knowledge deficit: alcoholism related to lack of exposure to concepts of alcoholism and codependence—cont'd			
	2b. Point out commonalities between her experiences and those of other spouses of alcoholics.	2b. It is easier to receive information when one is not alone.	though." Goal not met. *Revision:* Continue to gently teach Agnes about codependence.
	2c. Describe how a spouse's alcoholism can become the central focus of the family; do not blame the family or wife.	2c. This information can be threatening and is received better if given in a matter-of-fact manner.	
	2d. Give her additional literature about family changes in substance abuse.	2d. Again, repetition and varied formats enhance learning.	
3. Client will list resources for family support after 4 weeks.	3a. Describe Al-Anon and give her literature and contact numbers.	3a. Introduction of Al-Anon will give her an additional source of information and support.	3. After 4 weeks Agnes was able to discuss Al-Anon, Al-Ateen, and Al-Atot. She decided to attend a few meetings herself before "involving my children." Goal met.
Nursing diagnosis: Ineffective family coping: compromised related to changes made in response to husband and father's drinking patterns			
1. Client and children will maintain safety through the next 6 months.	1a. Assess for abuse in the family.	1a. Sometimes somatic complaints are a symptom of abuse in the family.	1. Agnes was emphatic when she said that John did not physically abuse them. She insisted there was no sexual abuse but said he yelled at everyone a lot. She said that she would try to find ways to keep the children out of John's way when he was drinking
	1b. If abuse is found, take steps to assure safety for the client and the children.	1b. Family may require outside help to assure safety of members.	

Continued.

Care Plan 9-1

Female Spouse of Husband with Substance Abuse—cont'd

Outcome identification	Nursing interventions	Rationale	Evaluation
Nursing diagnosis: Ineffective family coping: compromised related to changes made in response to husband and father's drinking patterns—cont'd			
	1c. Help her find ways to protect the children against John's verbal attacks such as serving them dinner before John's arrival home.	1c. It has been found that children are protected when they have routines and holidays free from disruption by substance abuse.	heavily. Goal partially met.
2. Client will state that she did not cause nor can she cure John's alcoholism.	2a. Elicit from client ways in which she attempts to control John's drinking. Ask her if this was successful (it won't be).	2a. Agnes is likely to be operating under the erroneous assumption that if she does the right thing and tries hard enough, she can keep him from drinking.	2. After 3 weeks, she reports not trying to control his drinking. She still feels very guilty and responsible for his drinking, as well as guilty and irresponsible for failing to control the drinking. Goal only partially met.
	2b. Ask her if her life would be less stressful if she would quit attempting this control. Request that she try not to do so for a set period of time.	2b. These repeated attempts to control the drinking take a severe toll.	
	2c. Discuss how she feels when John drinks excessively. Reassure her that whatever feelings she experiences are okay.	2c. Allowing her to ventilate feelings will reduce stress and identify the guilt and anger she feels. These feelings are normal under the circumstances.	
	2d. Assure her that she neither causes the drinking nor can she control it. Help her "let go."	2d. She will need to hear this repeatedly. Once she can accept this fact, it will reduce her stress level a great deal.	

Outcome identification	Nursing interventions	Rationale	Evaluation
Nursing diagnosis: Ineffective family coping: compromised related to changes made in response to husband and father's drinking patterns—cont'd			
3. Client will list her needs and family members' needs and identify which of these she has power to meet by 3 weeks.	3a. Have her make a list of responsibilities she has been meeting in her family. Compliment her for being so responsible.	3a. She has been complaining of role overload. It is helpful for her to see just what she has been doing. Compliment shows respect for client's efforts.	3. With a great deal of difficulty, Agnes identified that she needed to have some time for herself. She required much help to make a list that included her own needs. When she did identify her needs, she placed them at the bottom. After 4 weeks, she could include her own needs with much help. Goal partially met.
	3b. Help her identify her own priority needs.	3b. Codependent clients have difficulty identifying their own needs. She will need assistance to do this.	
	3c. Help her prioritize responsibilities and needs, both hers and others'.	3c. She will also need assistance to give high enough priority to her own needs with that of others'.	
	3d. Help her assess her power to meet these responsibilities.	3d. These clients need assistance to let go of responsibilities for which they realistically have no control.	
	3e. Help her with guilt feelings for those she cannot meet.	3e. These steps will not be easy. It is likely she will feel very guilty about these changes. She needs to know that it is common to feel guilty, but it is healthy for her and others to meet some of their own needs.	

Continued.

Outcome identification	Nursing interventions	Rationale	Evaluation
Nursing diagnosis: Ineffective family coping: compromised related to changes made in response to husband and father's drinking patterns—cont'd			
4. Client will take steps to do two things for herself that she enjoys by 4 weeks.	4a. Help client identify her own interests, talents, and strengths.	4a. She likely has very low self-esteem. It is self-esteem–raising to begin to know positive aspects of the self.	4. Agnes stated she likes to sew, but would like to take a class to learn some advanced techniques. She enrolled in the class. Agnes has missed her sister who lives in a city 200 miles away. She has wanted to visit, but has been unable because of home circumstances. She found a friend who would keep the children for a long weekend so she could make the visit. Goal met.
	4b. Ask her to identify two things she would like to do.	4b. Doing something one enjoys raises mood and self-esteem.	
	4c. Encourage her to take these steps for herself.	4c. The nurse's encouragement will allow the client to have the courage to follow through with wished-for activities.	
5. Client will begin to establish clear boundaries between family members and herself by: a. Allowing appropriate privacy of space and property by 2 months.	5a1. Have the client draw a "family floor plan" of the home. Have her identify spaces that are private for each person.	5a1. A picture allows a clearer view of the family's use of privacy.	5a. Agnes was able to identify areas in which she had not been allowing privacy but reported few changes. Goal only partially met.
	5a2. Discuss the importance of privacy of thoughts, mail, and relationships with others.	5a2. Without discussion, the client may not be aware of invasions of privacy. Discussion will assist the nurse to assess whether this is happening.	
b. Communicating directly with the person for whom the message is intended by 2 months.	5b1. Teach the importance of sending the "mail to the right person."	5b. In dysfunctional families, it is common for members to communicate through someone other than the one for whom the message is intended.	5b. It is difficult to assess her performance at home, but she was able to discuss some medication changes directly with her doctor. Goal partially met.
	5b2. Role-model communicating directly and appropriately.		

Outcome identification	Nursing interventions	Rationale	Evaluation

Nursing diagnosis: Ineffective family coping: compromised related to changes made in response to husband and father's drinking patterns—cont'd

Outcome identification	Nursing interventions	Rationale	Evaluation
c. Refusing to be a go-between for other family members by 2 months.	5c1. When meeting with the family, do not allow one member to speak for another. 5c2. Teach tolerance for differences and differences of opinion. 5c3. Help client identify times when she becomes a go-between. 5c4. Assist her to practice responding to attempts to draw her into this and reinforce her successes.	5c. Boundaries are established between members when each speaks only for himself. Frequently, in these families there are attempts to control communication of unacceptable realities and family secrets.	5c. With difficulty, when family members met with the nurse, they were prevented from speaking for one another. There was much anxiety as a result. It will be difficult to follow through at home. Goal partially met. Revision: Continue to follow through with these interventions.

Nursing diagnosis: Anxiety related to role overload as a result of husband's heavy drinking

Outcome identification	Nursing interventions	Rationale	Evaluation
1. Client will report reduced anxiety by 4 weeks.	1a. Continue to assist client to assume only her own responsibilities. 1b. Point out how assuming responsibilities for her husband enables him to continue drinking. 1c. Explore techniques she can use when anxiety becomes overwhelming, e.g., relaxation techniques, getting away for a while, talking to someone, etc.	1a. Anxiety is precipitated by her role overload. 1b. Ceasing to enable relieves stress on family members and assists the addicted individual to face the consequences of the chemical abuse. 1c. Sometimes the stressful events cannot be alleviated; therefore she needs to learn new ways of coping with her stress.	1. Agnes reported a somewhat lowered level of anxiety by 4 weeks, but still considered it intolerable even though she had been attempting to work with the nurse to alleviate this tension. Goal partially met.

Continued.

Care Plan 9-1
Female Spouse of Husband with Substance Abuse—cont'd

Outcome identification	Nursing interventions	Rationale	Evaluation
Nursing diagnosis: Sleep pattern disturbance related to high anxiety levels			
1. Client will report feeling rested in the mornings after 4 weeks.	1a. Assess factors that may disturb sleep such as husband's drunkenness, children's sleep/wake schedule, bed comfort, room quietness, level of darkness, and temperature.	1a. Environmental conditions strongly influence quality of sleep.	1. Client reported feeling more rested after 4 weeks. She has been following good sleep hygiene practices and reducing role overload with good results. Goal met.
	1b. Teach sleep hygiene: a. Importance of arising at the same time. b. Controlling environmental conditions. c. Do not take daytime naps. d. Eat only lightly late in the evening such as warm milk or cereal. e. If sleep doesn't come after 20 minutes, get up and do something quiet. Return when sleepy, Again, arise if sleep doesn't come.	1b. Many times insomnia will respond to good sleep hygiene.	
	1c. Use relaxation techniques, especially in the evening.	1c. Relaxation facilitates sleep.	
	1d. Avoid sleep medications if at all possible.	1d. Most sleep medications alter the normal structure of sleep. In addition, many sleep	

Outcome identification	Nursing interventions	Rationale	Evaluation
Nursing diagnosis: Sleep pattern disturbance related to high anxiety levels—cont'd			
		medications will have a rebound effect after use and will cause insomnia, tolerance develops to many, and many are addictive.	
Nursing diagnosis: Social isolation related to husband's drinking and her role overload			
1. Client will attend Al-Anon family group by 6 weeks.	1a. Teach client about Al-Anon.	1a. Al-Anon provides social support to family members of substance abusers.	1. Client attended four Al-Anon meetings and reported enjoying them. Goal met.
2. Client will establish friendship with one person by 4 weeks.	2a. Encourage client to seek out someone whose company she enjoys.	2a. Everyone needs other persons. The social isolation of the substance abusing family adds to the stress and anxiety.	2. Client invited her neighbor over for coffee. She said they mostly talked about the children, the community, and external things. Goal partially met.
	2b. Help her work through her anxieties about spending time with someone outside of the family.	2b. She has been overresponsible and may feel guilty "shirking" her responsibilities long enough to spend time with someone else.	
	2c. Help her work through her anxieties about talking about family concerns with someone outside of the family.	2c. A common injunction of substance abusing families is "Don't talk, don't trust, don't feel." It may produce much excess anxiety to share concerns with someone outside of the family.	

Adult children of alcoholics

Typical adult children of parents with substance abuse have an excessive need for control, avoid feelings, mistrust others, feel overresponsible, and ignore their own needs (Cermak & Brown, 1982). These individuals are described as failing to identify their own strengths and assets, instead perceiving only their weaknesses; this leads to decreased self-esteem and compulsive needs to be perfect and to achieve (Robinson, 1989). Woititz (1985) states that adult children of alcoholics have problems with identity and intimacy. These descriptions strongly resemble the descriptions of codependents.

Cermak (1988) describes Post Traumatic Stress Disorder (PTSD) in Adult Children of Alcoholics. A diagnosis of PTSD is usually given to those who have experienced war or a natural disaster. Cermak maintains that the trauma for children of alcoholic families is just as severe, but it is the result of events that occur over a lengthy period of time. Examples include being left alone at a very young age; not being picked up from school, a friend's house, or other trip; failure to provide meals; lack of proper dress for weather conditions; and emotional, physical, or sexual abuse. Most children of alcoholic parents experience at least several of these stressors.

Adult children of alcoholics experienced more abandonment and loss than those who grew up in nonalcoholic homes (Brown, 1988; Cermak, 1988). In addition to grieving for deaths and abandonment, adult children of families with substance abuse may also have grief issues from growing up in a perpetually stressful environment. These issues may center around a lost childhood and lost relationships with a parent, both parents, or siblings.

The most frequent result of growing up in an alcoholic family is increased frequency of substance abuse in the second generation (Wampler et al, 1993). In addition, Bekir and others (1993) reported intergenerational transmission of role reversal. They studied 50 adults in a methadone program. Of the subjects, 42 had parents who were substance misusers and 32 of the parents were also adult children of alcoholics. The number of subjects with absent fathers was 40; 30 of them had been abandoned, and had taken on adult roles as children. As adults they abandoned their own children.

Family problems when the substance abuser recovers

Although family members are both relieved and optimistic when the substance abuser seeks treatment and stops using, they are also skeptical about the possibility of continued recovery. During early recovery, the family is in transition and is highly vulnerable. Sobriety for the addict without alterations in family functioning may end in relapse. The degree to which a family makes necessary adjustments in relationships and implements effective coping strategies influences the extent to which treatment effects are maintained. Strategies for recovery should focus on the entire family. Realigning family members according to parent and child hierarchies is necessary to foster role-appropriate behaviors. Issues regarding trust and responsibility should be addressed. Interventions should be directed toward improving family interactions, communication skills, problem-solving abilities, and identification and expression of feelings (Captain, 1989). Even though a parent receives treatment, the role behaviors of children or the problems do not magically disappear. Children need help adjusting to changes that occur in the family once a parent is no longer abusing substances (Moos & Billings, 1982).

Nursing care of families with substance abusing adults

Nurses interact with family members of a substance abusing individual in many different settings. Understanding the particular difficulties of and behaviors commonly exhibited by those family members helps the nurse understand the stressors encountered by those members, as well as plan nursing interventions to assist them (Box 9-1).

Box 9-1
Characteristics of Optimal Families

1. **Open-system orientation**
   Multiple causation of events
   Need for each other and other people
2. **Boundaries**
   Touching
   Interaction between family members
   Allocation of space in household
   Clear links to society
3. **Contextual clarity**
   Clear generational lines
   Strong parental coalition
   Communication
       Clear, direct, honest, specific
       Congruent
4. **Power**
   Flows from parental coalition
   Delegated to children, appropriate to age
   Clear role definition
5. **Encouragement of autonomy**
   Differentness accepted
6. **Affective issues**
   Warmth-caring
   Empathy
   Feelings attended to
   Amount of conflict
   Resolution of conflict
   Self-esteem of members high

7. **Negotiation and task performance**
   Input from all members
   Led by parents
   Little amount of conflict
8. **Transcendent values**
   Expect loss
   Recover from and prepare for loss
   Hopeful
   Altruistic
9. **Health measures**
   Healthy diet
   Freedom from drugs and chemicals
   Regular exercise and recreation
   Concern for the environment
   Abstinence from dangerous activities
   Family history of health

Modified from Hogarth, C.R. (1993). Families and family therapy. In B.S. Johnson, *Psychiatric–mental health nursing: Adaptation and growth* (3rd ed.). New York: JB Lippincott Co.

EFFECTS ON CHILDREN

An estimated 7 million children live with an alcoholic parent (Children of Alcoholics Foundation, 1985). In addition, 21 million adults were reared by a parent with substance abuse and are coping with the long-term effects (Gravitz & Bowden, 1986).

Consequences for children, adolescents, and adults

School, behavioral, emotional, and physical problems. Children of families with substance abuse have more school problems such as lower academic achievement, less skill in math and abstract reasoning, lower levels of reading recognition and comprehension, and less verbal proficiency (Marcus, 1986; Tarter, Alterman & Edwards, 1985). Similarly, these children display more restlessness, impulsiveness, emotional detachment, social aggression, emotional lability, and decreased attention span (Schulsinger et al, 1985). Parental substance abuse is also associated with conduct disorder, anxiety, and depression (Chassin, Rogosch & Berrera, 1991; Sher et al, 1991), as well as somatic problems such as migraines, asthma, and weight problems (Moos & Billings, 1982) for children and adolescents. Russell, Henderson, and Blume (1984) followed sons of alcoholics from preschool through adolescence and found that this group sustained 60% more injuries than their peers from non-alcoholic families, and daughters of alcoholics were 3 times as likely to be hospitalized.

Distress and pathology in the children may result from the family disorganization and dysfunction, as well as the substance abuse (Devine & Braithwaite, 1993; Hill, Nord & Blow, 1992). The extent of the children's difficulty depends on the ability of the family to function despite the substance abuse, the age of the child at the onset of the addiction, the personality of the child, and the availability of other adults to nurture and protect the child (Brown, 1988).

Resiliency protective factors. Although research describes children and adults from families with substance abuse as being at high risk for psychological problems, the vast majority of individuals from these environments do not develop negative psychological adjustment (Roosa et al, 1993). Werner (1986) identified some characteristics that differentiate "resilient" individuals, including average intelligence, adequate communication skills, achievement orientation, internal locus of control, responsible attitude, and absence of parental conflict during the first 2 years of life.

Wolin and associates (Bennett, Wolin & Reiss, 1988) have searched for evidence of protective factors that prevent the transmission of alcoholism. They reason that the family derives a sense of identity from ceremonies such as weddings and funerals, celebrations such as national and religious holidays, traditions such as celebration of birthdays and family vacations, and patterned routines such as mealtimes and weekend activities. If the family rituals persisted despite the alcohol abuse, they were protective for the children.

Family growing-up experiences. Hecht (1973) describes communication in families with substance abuse as often incongruent and unclear. Spouses try to protect the child with half-truths about the substance abuser; the children learn that parents cannot be trusted. Children learn to ignore verbal messages and observe parental behavior. Children may also imitate the parental communication style of fighting and hostile sarcasm, often acting out their impulses. Booz-Allen and Hamilton (1974, p. 73) concluded that, "If children do not resolve the problems created by parental alcoholism, they will carry them the rest of their lives." The two most frequent disturbances they found were emotional neglect of the children and family conflict (defined as aggression, fighting, arguments in the home, and spouse abuse). These families also experienced many other problems, including lack of fulfillment of parental responsibilities, instability, divorce, separation, and physical abuse. The children in this study felt that they did not have "normal" parents, expressed embarrassment, and did not bring their friends home because of the chaos. They also expressed a wide range of ambivalent feelings, including love, admiration, respect, fear, anger, hate, guilt, and loneliness. Children were at higher risk of developing problems when they (1) belonged to a lower socioeconomic group, (2) witnessed or experienced physical abuse, (3) were 6 years old or younger at the onset of parental substance abuse, (4) were an only or oldest child, and (5) lived in a nonsupportive family situation (Booz-Allen & Hamilton, 1974).

Cork (1969) interviewed 115 children from alcoholic families and found that the children were dealing with adult problems and had not expressed their feelings to others. The children's primary concern was not alcohol consumption but parental fighting and quarreling and a lack of interest in them by both parents. Two thirds of the children stated they would never drink. Ironically, research suggests that 50% to 60% of children of alcoholics become alcoholics (Lawson, Peterson & Lawson, 1983). Although this points to a genetic component, the conflictual family environment may be a strong contributor as well.

Childhood abusive experiences.   Although emotional, physical, and sexual abuse have been associated with substance abuse, child abuse studies report contradictory findings. Kempe and Helfer (1980) reported that alcoholism played a role in about one third of all child abuse cases; Gil (1970) reported that alcohol intoxication rather than alcoholism was more often a precipitating factor in child abuse. However, more children from alcoholic families than from nonalcoholic families responded affirmatively to the question, "Have either of your parents ever hit you so hard that you had bruises?" Alcoholics in treatment described themselves as aggressive and sometimes physically abusive toward their spouse and children (Wing, 1991). Victims of physical or sexual abuse during childhood experience long-lasting negative consequences into adulthood (Brown & Garrison, 1990; Gil, 1988; Pope & Brucker, 1991).

Both clinicians and researchers report that emotional abuse is common in families with substance abuse. Examples of emotional abuse include harsh discipline, unresponsiveness, emotional unavailability, rejection, threatened abandonment, and inconsistent expectations (Cook, 1988; Tweed, Ryff & Cranley, 1990). Children are particularly vulnerable to negative psychological symptoms when parental problems impinge on or involve the child in some way (Rutter and Quinton, 1984). Perceptions of rejection and low levels of nurturance, affection, acceptance, and concern from parents during childhood were associated with depression in adulthood (Lefkowitz & Tesiny, 1984).

Interpretations of family experiences. Children in families with substance abuse see themselves as being *responsible* or *to blame* for parental problems (Grisham & Estes, 1986). Children need to believe that their parents are good. When reality disproves this assumption, children alter their beliefs about themselves to preserve a belief in parental integrity. Thus children often conclude that they are to blame for family problems, and this affects their perceptions of future experiences. Easley and Epstein (1991) found that adult children of alcoholics who blamed themselves for their parent's alcoholism had higher levels of psychopathology than those who did not blame themselves.

Children in alcoholic families are confronted with the *unpredictability* of the substance abusing parent's behavior (Black, 1981; Wegscheider, 1981). Inconsistencies in discipline and frequent changes in family rules make it difficult for children to see cause and effect. The child may receive markedly different reactions from the parent for the same behavior. Under these circumstances, some children may come to believe that consequences are unrelated to actual behaviors. *Worry* is another factor for children in alcoholic families. They often feel a sense of impending doom; apprehension and fear become normal for children in unpredictable situations (Black, 1981). Thus worry may be another filter through which children in alcoholic families interpret their reality.

Perception of *social and emotional support* is another important dimension along which children of alcoholics may assign meaning to their early family experiences. Both clinicians (Black, 1981; Brown, 1988; Wegscheider, 1981) and researchers (Benson & Heller, 1987; Black, Bucky & Wilder-Padilla, 1986) describe children and parents in alcoholic families as isolated from external social support. Normal friendships are often impaired because children in alcoholic families may try to hide their parent's drinking, or they avoid bringing friends home for fear of embarrassing parental behavior. Lack of social and emotional support can lead to feelings of helplessness and depression, whereas adequate support that encourages and reinforces coping efforts promotes positive psychological adjustment (Werner, 1986).

Finally, research has shown that individuals who discover something positive in a negative situation show less distress than those who do not (Silver & Wortman, 1980). Children who interpret difficult and painful situations within their family as a *challenge* might have more positive psychological adjustment. Easley and Epstein (1991) found that adult children of alcoholics who used positive reappraisal rather than escape-avoidance as a coping strategy experienced more positive psychological adjustment. Thus how a child interprets and assigns meaning to experiences within the family may influence psychological adjustment.

Therapy for children in families with substance abuse. Children who live in a family with substance abuse may be identified as "the problem," or they may seem perfect. Both of these roles remove the focus from the family's central problems and the tension resulting from the substance abuse. The best way to help children from such families is to improve the functioning of the nuclear family. Improving family communication patterns, rebuilding marital and parental relationships, reestablishing trust and respect, and facilitating emotional contact will change the environment positively (Lawson, Peterson & Lawson, 1983). If the substance abuser continues to abuse, working with the nonaddicted spouse establishes one parent who can protect and care for the children. When children have a positive relationship with the nonaddicted parent, they are protected from the negative psychological consequences of having a substance abusing parent (Obuchowska, 1974). If non-using parents stop taking responsibility for substance abuser's behavior, they can begin to care for themselves and parent the children.

In addition to family therapy, group work with other children is beneficial. The group provides a place where role behavior is not necessary. Children also find that they are not alone and they can establish relationships with peers. Ackerman (1978, p. 109) states, "Helping children of alcoholics to work through their feelings and establish effective relationships with others will be very helpful in overcoming the impact of an alcoholic parent." When children develop self-confidence, they feel they can control themselves and influence the outcome of their own lives. Black (1981) recommends using group work with children from families with substance abuse to let them know that they are not alone, their parent's addiction is not their fault, the parent can get help, and they need to take care of themselves. She recommends having children draw pictures of their family life and their views on addiction to help them express the problem in their family. Treatment for addiction must include children if the intergenerational transmission of addiction is to be interrupted (Lawson, Peterson & Lawson, 1983).

Nursing care of the child from a family with substance abuse

When the nurse encounters the child of a substance abusing parent, the nurse may not have information about the parent's problem. The child may present behavior problems, health problems, or neglect. Assessment of the child is always comprehensive, addressing all spheres of the child's life and using major sources of information. This includes obtaining information from the child, parents, siblings, teachers, other health professionals, and other persons involved with the child. Information from (1) health perception or management, (2) nutrition, (3) elimination, (4) activity levels, (5) ability to perform ADL's, (6) sleep or rest patterns, (7) cognitive development and perception of current issues, (8) self-perception and self-concept, (9) role relationships within and without the family, (10) coping and stress tolerance, and (11) values and beliefs. This information is compared with normal guidelines for growth and development to determine areas of difficulty. Assessment also includes the usual assessment of the parent's substance abuse. An older child's perception of this can be assessed by the Children of Alcoholics Screen Test (CAST) (Jones, 1982). The wording in this test can be changed to include both drugs and alcohol. CAST consists of 30 frequent experiences of children of alcoholics. Positive responses to six or more items suggest that this child has an alcoholic parent.

When working with a child from a family with substance abuse, the nurse must be cautious about inadvertently reinforcing the child's distorted worldview. The nurse can develop enabling behaviors because of lack of knowledge. Examples of enabling behaviors include (1) becoming overinvolved, which would be joining the child's family system, (2) accepting the child's worldview, which is that the child can control those things, (3) reinforcing overly compliant behaviors, or (4) reinforcing the scapegoated child's perception that he or she is causing the problem in the family (see Care Plan 9-2).

SUBSTANCE ABUSE IN ADOLESCENTS

During the past several decades, there has been a growing concern in the United States about adolescent use of alcohol and other substances. Substance abuse among the young constitutes a major public health problem (Bennett, 1991). Alcohol-related accidents are the leading cause of death for those between 15 and 24 years of age. The National Council on Alcoholism estimates that as many as 3 million adolescents have serious alcohol problems. However, the majority of adolescent drug use involves experimentation that can be viewed as a developmental process that does not inevitably lead to addiction. Any use of an illicit drug or use of alcohol by under-aged adolescents is considered abuse (DuPont, 1989).

Substance use as a developmental phenomenon

In our society, experimentation with substances seems to be a normal part of growing up. More than 50% of high school freshmen have tried alcohol, and by their senior year, 93% have tried it (Raskin & Daley, 1991). Adolescents experiment with a wide range of behaviors and lifestyle patterns. This experimentation is part of the natural process of separating from parents, developing a personal identity, feeling a sense of independence and autonomy, and learning the necessary skills for becoming an adult. These developmental processes may influence adolescents to engage in risk-taking behaviors that include substance abuse. Adolescents tend to feel immortal and invulnerable, which increases the risk of substance abuse. Adolescent substance users show a remarkable absence of concern about the adverse consequences of their use. Instead, engaging in illicit behaviors provides a way to be part of a particular peer group and to rebel against parental authority; these factors seem more important to the adolescent than warnings from parents, teachers, and health professionals (Schinke, Botvin & Orlandi, 1991).

Patterns of adolescent substance use

Recent epidemiologic research indicates that the onset of alcohol and other drug use is between the ages of 12 and 20, and the peak-age for first use is around 15 (DuPont, 1989). However, in some inner-city environments, and especially among school dropouts, substance use may begin even earlier. The younger an individual when a drug is first used (outside family or religious rituals), the more likely substance abuse problems will occur.

Adolescents have various patterns of substance use. Experimental use is intermittent and presents few problems. Recreational users tend to use the gateway drugs—alcohol, cigarettes, and marijuana—for the purpose of relaxation or intoxication. The most problematic type of use is by compulsive users who engage in polydrug use and have intoxication as their goal. Particular dangers for compulsive abusers are overdose or addiction. If addiction occurs, the adolescent may become involved in criminal behavior, prostitution, or drug trafficking (Glassner & Loughlin, 1987).

Influencing factors

Clinical experience and empirical research indicate that drug abuse cannot be explained by any one factor. Drug abuse is more likely to occur and to be more severe as the number of risk factors to which the adolescent is exposed increases (Newcomb, Maddahian & Bentler, 1986). Risk factors include *biogenetic influences, intrapsychic factors,* and *environmental influences* such as family and peers.

Biogenetic influences.   Genetic studies support the significance of biological factors in substance abuse. Adoptees raised apart from their biological alcoholic parents have a higher risk of developing alcoholism than offspring of nonalcoholics even if the latter were adopted into homes of alcoholics (Cloninger, Bohman & Sigvardsson, 1981; Goodwin, 1984). These genetic studies are limited; they fail to explain the mechanisms by which genetic vulnerability precipitates alcoholism in some offspring of alcoholic parents but not others. Genetic researchers agree that the development of substance abuse may be caused by the interaction of predisposing genetic factors and environmental stressors.

Intrapsychic factors.   Low personal control, meaninglessness in life (Newcomb & Harlow, 1986), emotional distress, and life dissatisfaction, are associated with adolescent substance abuse (Newcomb, Maddahian & Bentler, 1986). Other intrapsychic factors that influence adolescent substance abuse include low self-esteem, apathy, pessimism, personal alienation, and depressed mood (Kandel, 1978). Unconventional attitudes and behavior, rebelliousness, and deviance have been identified as both antecedents and consequences of adolescent substance use (Johnston, O'Malley & Bachman, 1987).

Parental influences.   Parental influence is a multifaceted phenomenon (Bennett, 1991). Parental attitudes and behavior regarding substance use and abuse influence a child's substance abuse behavior. Other parental influences include agreement between parents on what constitutes proper use, degree of parental supervision, and quality of parent-child relationships. Poor parent-child relationships predict use of illicit drugs (Kandel, 1978), and heavy drinking by parents is associated with earlier substance abuse (Chassin, Rogosch & Berrera, 1991; Sher et al, 1991). Other family influences include social isolation, deprivation, cynicism, and antisocial behavior within the family system.

Peer group influences.   Research shows that substance use patterns and drug-related attitudes of peers are strong predictors of drug involvement (Kandel, 1978). Parental influence begins to decline during early adolescence, while there is a corresponding increase in the influence of peers. Most adolescents who report substance abuse also report that their friends are users (Johnston, O'Malley & Bachman, 1987). Adolescents who become substance abusers are often participating in a peer group that significantly influences their drug involvement (Bennett, 1991).

Text continued on p. 260.

Care Plan 9-2

Child with Stress-related Symptoms

Recently, 9-year-old Gina was making increasingly frequent visits to the school nurse's office. She complained of "stomach aches." No other changes were found. She said, "Everything's okay at home." Her classroom performance had dropped, and she frequently fought with other students. A family conference was requested.

ASSESSMENT

Gina's father, Jim, smelled of alcohol, and the speech of her mother, Sharon, was slurred. She apologized, explaining that she had been sick and the medicine was making her groggy.

NURSING DIAGNOSES

Potential for altered growth and development related to parent's use of intoxicating substances

Potential for altered protection related to impairment in functioning of both parents

Self-esteem disturbance related to dysfunctional home situation

Outcome identification	Nursing interventions	Rationale	Evaluation
Nursing diagnosis: Potential for altered growth and development related to parent's use of intoxicating substances			
1. Gina will establish a relationship with the school nurse as evidenced by coming to her with concerns in 2 weeks.	1a. Develop a relationship with the child.	1a. Often children of alcoholic homes do not trust others. They can learn that the nurse is someone they can trust.	1. Gina comes into the nurse's office nearly every day and talks to the nurse about concerns. Goal met.
	1b. Don't pass judgment on what the child reveals.	1b. Trust develops as a result of positive regard and acceptance by the nurse.	
2. Gina will demonstrate trust in the nurse by sharing two feelings with the nurse in 4 weeks.	2a. Encourage expression of feelings.	2a. Children of alcoholics (COAs) first learn to suppress expression of feelings, then to suppress feelings altogether.	2. Gina was able to identify two feelings after drawing pictures of her family and her other relationships. Goal met.
	2b. Use drawings, puppets, and role-playing to assist her to express feelings.	2b. Children are able to express feelings much more readily graphically than verbally.	

Outcome identification	Nursing interventions	Rationale	Evaluation
Nursing diagnosis: Potential for altered growth and development related to parent's use of intoxicating substances—cont'd			
3. Gina will no longer fight with other children at school by 4 weeks.	3a. Place Gina in a group to discuss behaviors and problem solving.	3a. Group gives the children an opportunity to discuss conflicts in a supervised setting. COA's often feel they are not normal. The group gives her an opportunity to feel more normal.	3. Gina's acting-out behavior ceased immediately upon establishment of a relationship with the nurse. Goal met.
	3b. Encourage verbal expression of feelings instead of acting on them.	3b. Teaching children to verbally express feelings may relieve the need to act them out.	
	3c. Teach problem-solving and conflict resolution.	3c. Children acquire these skills by learning.	
	3d. Role play conflict resolution with Gina.	3d. Allows the child to practice the skill.	
4. Gina will declare that her stomach no longer hurts by 4 weeks.	4a. Use third-person storytelling to discuss suspected alcoholism with Gina.	4a. COA's learn early not to reveal the family secret of alcoholism. They can listen safely to another person's story.	4. Gina's stomach aches slowly became less frequent over time. By 4 weeks, she was complaining less than once a week. Goal partially met.
	4b. Use posters and literature in the school to teach all the children about the disease of alcoholism.	4b. This allows Gina to learn about the disease in a nonthreatening manner.	
	4c. Administer the CAST assessment instrument.	4c. This can assist the nurse and the child to identify the parental AODA.	

Continued.

Care Plan 9-2

Child with Stress-related Symptoms—cont'd

Outcome identification	Nursing interventions	Rationale	Evaluation
Nursing diagnosis: Potential for altered growth and development related to parent's use of intoxicating substances—cont'd			
	4d. Help her identify parental alcoholism. Reinforce that she did not cause it, nor can she cure it.	4d. Use of the CAST and books such as Black's text for children can assist the nurse in helping the child to face parental AODA.	
	4e. Reinforce that parents love her even though they have a disease.	4e. Children need to realistically assess parental behaviors as a result of the disease and not the child's fault or lack of love from the parent.	
Nursing diagnosis: Potential for altered protection related to impairment in functioning of both parents			
1. Gina will verbalize when to get help if needed and a plan of action by 6 weeks.	1a. Teach Gina emergency numbers and how to contact an operator in times of emergency.	1a. Because of family isolation and denial, she may not recognize that she can call to receive help.	1. and 2. Gina remained safe. She quickly learned emergency numbers and demonstrated how to contact the operator. She verbalized both circumstances and contact persons appropriately for help. Goals met.
2. Gina will remain safe on a continuing basis.	2a. Help her identify times when she should call for help, e.g., fire, if a parent becomes violent, or if she needs a ride and the parent does not show up.	2a. The child's perception is often negated in an alcoholic family, and she needs help to identify when she needs help.	
	2b. Help her identify reliable persons in her environment to whom she may turn if she needs help.	2b. Because of the family's isolation, she needs assistance in determining who is safe and who is not.	

Outcome identification	Nursing interventions	Rationale	Evaluation
Nursing diagnosis: Self-esteem disturbance related to dysfunctional home situation			
1. Gina will raise her school performance by one grade by 9 weeks.	1a. Give Gina opportunities to assist the nurse.	1a. Being seen as a valuable assistant raises self-esteem.	1. Gina's grades returned to her previous level by the next 9-week report period. Goal met.
	1b. Praise her sincerely for a job well done.	1b. Praise for a job well done raises self-esteem.	
	1c. Praise her for the courage to discuss her concerns with the nurse or with the group.	1c. It takes courage for a COA to share concerns with others.	
Parental interventions			
	1. Assess for parental substance abuse.	1. The nurse can use knowledge of AODA to help this family identify the substance abuse.	
	2. Assess and use the parents for interventions with Gina as much as possible.	2. Help to place the parents in charge, relieve the child from parental responsibility.	
	3. Help them set appropriate rules and consequences for violations for Gina and affirm the need to be consistent.	3. Help them establish protection for the child.	
	4. Refer to AA, Al-Anon, or Al-Atot.	4. The best source for help for their AODA problems is through these self-help programs.	
	5. Refer for family therapy.	5. The family needs assessment for further therapy.	

Combined psychosocial factors. Jessor and Jessor (1977) described how intrapsychic, family, and peer influences interact to contribute to adolescent deviance and problem behaviors such as substance abuse. *Behavior* is the outcome of the interaction between *personality* (intrapsychic factors) and *perceived environment* (family and peer influences). In this theory the perceived environment is more important than the environment as defined by demographic variables. When the adolescent's perceived environment is characterized by weak parental control, incongruence between peer and parental expectations, and dominance of peer over parental influences *and* the adolescent's personality is characterized by tolerance of deviance, low religiosity, independence, and low academic interest, substance abuse is most likely to occur.

Identifying the adolescent substance abuser

Although there is no single accepted definition of adolescent substance abuse, it generally includes behaviors ranging from frequent intoxication to interpersonal and school-related complications related to substance abuse. Adolescents who abuse substances have more trouble with the law as a result of driving while intoxicated, possession of drugs, and drug-related auto accidents. Negative consequences related to substance abuse include trouble with teachers, difficulties with friends, driving while intoxicated, criticism from someone they date, and trouble with the police (Donovan & Jessor, 1978).

Identifying a teenager's problem with substance abuse involves a careful assessment. Teenagers rarely acknowledge concern about their alcohol or drug abuse. Most often they are referred to a health care professional by parents, teachers, school counselors, or the courts. Therefore to identify substance abuse in adolescents, it is necessary to observe behavioral changes. Estes and associates (1980) identified the following clues to substance abuse in adolescents: drop in school grades; truancy; disinterest in sports or hobbies that the adolescent previously enjoyed; changes in personal habits such as decreased interest in dress, shaving, or bathing; nervousness or depression; suicidal tendencies such as frequent expressions of hopelessness or failure; hidden liquor bottles; use during the day at school or elsewhere; withdrawal from family and friends; changes in social life; drinking alone; and the adolescent's own concern that his or her substance use is different from that of friends.

Snow (1989) stated that substance abuse during adolescence reflects in part a way of coping with chronic stress within the family system. Thus intervention must involve the entire family yet recognize the unique developmental issues of the adolescent (see Care Plan 9-3).

Current trends

Widespread use of illegal drugs among middle-class youth is declining. The use of marijuana and cocaine among high school seniors has decreased (Johnston, O'Malley & Bachman, 1989). Although no specific prevention strategy has been linked to this decrease in drug use among middle-class youth, possible explanations include increased interest in healthier lifestyles, return to more traditional values, and drug prevention programs (Rhodes & Jason, 1990).

Although this decline in substance abuse by middle-class youth is a promising trend, lower socioeconomic and minority youth in urban areas are experiencing an increase in substance abuse, dealing, and violence. Many urban youth experience a variety of disadvantages. For example, more than 80% of African-American youth live in families below the poverty level. Inner-city schools often lack resources, and the dropout rate among minority youth approaches 50%. Many of these young people must confront gang membership, crime, violence, pregnancy, drug use, and drug dealing (Rhodes & Jason, 1990). These behaviors may be quite functional when the alternative is continued poverty and impoverished neighborhoods. For example, although drug dealing is delinquent behavior, it offers status, money, and mobility. Of course, there are also negative consequences. Violence, homicide, and juvenile arrests have tripled in many of the nation's largest cities. Of major concern is that more urban young people are being inducted into drug abuse and addiction.

PREVENTION EFFORTS

Twenty years ago, the primary emphasis in prevention was on providing adolescents information about the dangers of substance use and abuse. It was assumed that youth lacked adequate information about alcohol and other drugs and that knowledge about drugs would lead to changes in behavior. However, the inadequacy of antidrug campaigns that involve information alone became evident (Benard, 1990).

In the mid-1970s prevention programs focused on values clarification and affective education. The assumption behind these programs was that young people used alcohol and other drugs because they had not thought through their values or learned how to express their feelings. When these approaches failed to deter drug use, there began a period of pessimism about preventing substance abuse among youth (DuPont, 1989).

Recent years have brought renewed optimism about prevention, largely sparked by new prevention programs that use life-skills training and peer-refusal techniques. Some successes from the previous information and affective programs have been included in these prevention programs. In addition, environmental approaches such as raising the legal drinking age to 21 have begun to reduce alcohol-related fatalities among youth. Although initially developed to prevent cigarette smoking, the life-skills programs have been adapted for the prevention of marijuana and alcohol use. At the same time these programs were developed, a new communitywide prevention approach was becoming increasingly acknowledged as an important and integral strategy to counter teenage drug abuse (Benard, 1990; DuPont, 1989).

Community-wide prevention is defined as the application of prevention strategies throughout the community in a sustained, highly integrated approach (Benard, 1990). It must target and involve diverse social systems such as families, schools, workplaces, media, government institutions, and community organizations. Inherent in this approach are three critical attributes that distinguish community-wide efforts from other prevention approaches. First, it is comprehensive in that it targets multiple systems and uses multiple strategies. The following five

Text continued on p. 266.

Care Plan 9-3

Adolescent Abusing Alcohol and Marijuana

Seventeen-year-old Ronald was court-ordered for treatment at the Mental Health Clinic after he was arrested for destroying property. He and a friend were found camping in a city park and had broken picnic tables to use for firewood. They had also broken into a house and extensively vandalized the property.

ASSESSMENT

Ronald's parents had divorced when he was 5 years old, and he had lived with his father, Richard, who had remarried Frieda. Three months ago, Richard and Frieda filed for divorce. Ronald, who had experimented with marijuana and drank in binges with friends at parties, then left home to live with his mother, Joan. At that time, he began smoking marijuana several times a day and increasing alcohol use. At the time he was arrested, his girlfriend, Mona, was 2 months pregnant.

NURSING DIAGNOSES

Altered role performance related to substance abuse
Ineffective individual coping related to substance abuse
Altered family processes related to father's divorce and changed living arrangements

Outcome identification	Nursing interventions	Rationale	Evaluation
Nursing diagnosis: Altered role performance related to substance abuse			
1. Ronald will verbalize the signs and symptoms of substance abuse by 1 week.	1a. Teach Ronald signs and symptoms of substance abuse.	1a. Knowledge assists him to understand his own behaviors.	1. Ronald was able to verbalize signs and symptoms of substance abuse. Goal met.
2. Ronald will agree to treatment for substance abuse within 1 week.	2a. Use intervention techniques if necessary to get Ronald to go for substance abuse evaluation.	2a. See Chapter 11.	2. With the assessment information from the nurse and the substance abuse evaluator, the court-ordered him into treatment. Goal met.
3. Ronald will agree to go to AA meetings on the treatment unit within 1 week.	3a. Encourage him to attend unit AA meetings. Explain benefits for him.	3a. AA provides social support in recovery.	3. Ronald was also court-ordered to attend AA meetings. Goal met.

Outcome identification	Nursing interventions	Rationale	Evaluation
Nursing diagnosis: Ineffective individual coping related to substance abuse			
1. Ronald will verbalize problematic situations to the nurse by 3 weeks.	1a. Establish therapeutic relationship with Ronald.	1a. Therapeutic relationship helps establish trust between client and nurse.	1. Ronald verbalized problem behaviors to the nurse without any difficulty. Goal met.
	1b. Elicit Ronald's cooperation by discussing his behavior along with the consequences of that behavior. Ask him if he would like to change that.	1b. Adolescents have difficulty connecting behavior to its consequences. They often change the behavior to avoid the consequences.	
	1c. Ask him to verbalize one situation in which he feels uncomfortable.	1c. He will be able to talk about the situation as one with discomfort before he can take the next step to discuss the feelings involved.	
2. Ronald will verbalize feelings associated with problematic situation to the nurse by 6 weeks.	2a. Ask him what he does in that situation.	2a. The next step in assisting him to identify feelings is to ask for his response as he has been acting-out feelings.	2. With difficulty, Ronald verbalized several feelings related to difficult situations. Goal met.
	2b. Help him select a feeling that he feels in that situation from a list.	2b. He may not be able to name his feelings. He can begin to develop this skill by identifying a feeling from a list.	
	2c. Repeat the above on other situations.	2c. Adding new situations helps him name additional feelings.	

Continued.

Outcome identification	Nursing interventions	Rationale	Evaluation
Nursing diagnosis: Ineffective individual coping related to substance abuse—cont'd			
3. Ronald will name alternative solutions to problematic situations by 6 weeks.	3a. Help Ronald to list alternative solutions to the first situation he produced.	3a. The first step in changing behavior is to identify alternatives to the behavior.	3. Ronald seemed to enjoy learning to problem-solve and quickly responded. Goal met.
	3b. Help him list the consequences to each alternative.	3b. Connecting the consequences to the behavior assists him in developing competent judgment.	
	3c. Help him select the most appropriate response to the situation.	3c. This thinking process also assists in developing competent judgment.	
4. Ronald will practice appropriate solutions to problematic situations by 6 weeks.	4a. Role play the situation with Ronald so that he can practice responding.	4a. Practice will add the new behaviors to his repertoire.	4. Ronald practiced the newly acquired behaviors and did well. Goal met.
Nursing diagnosis: Altered family processes related to father's divorce and changed living arrangements			
1. Ronald will choose an appropriate living arrangement from available options by discharge.	1a. Meet with Ronald's parents to determine which living arrangements are viable.	1a. An adolescent cannot decide this alone, and parents must be in on the choice.	1. Ronald indicated that he had a good relationship at times with his father, and they both wanted Ronald to live with him. The court agreed. Goal met.
	1b. Provide options with pros and cons to the court.	1b. In the case of court-ordered care, the court will ultimately make this decision.	
	1c. Meet with Ronald and his parents to mutually decide upon the most appropriate living arrangements. Make sure Ronald will agree to the living arrangements.	1c. If this decision will be made by the adolescent and his parents, the nurse can mediate the decision. In the case of an older adolescent, any decision will not work without the adolescent's agreement.	

Outcome identification	Nursing interventions	Rationale	Evaluation
Nursing diagnosis: Altered family processes related to father's divorce and changed living arrangements—cont'd			
2. Ronald will agree to abide by decisions on family rules by discharge.	2a. Meet with Ronald and parent or guardian to determine appropriate rules and responsibilities for Ronald.	2a. Many times, behavior problems arise because of unclear or inappropriate rules or responsibilities.	2. Ronald was very unhappy about the rules that were decided upon. He signed the agreement but said the only reason was because he would have to go to jail if he didn't. He felt he could make his own decisions. Goal partially met.
	2b. Determine consequences for failure to abide by rules or to complete responsibilities.	2b. Adolescents need clear rules and responsibilities and clear knowledge of what will happen if rules are not followed.	
	2c. Have rules and responsibilities in writing and have all parties sign the agreement.	2c. Compliance is more likely when all parties are clear about what has been agreed upon and have made a commitment.	
3. Ronald will identify at least one person as a role model and support person by discharge.	3a. Talk to Ronald about whom he feels comfortable talking with; use persons already in his life if possible, e.g., father, coach, youth leader, pastor, or neighbor.	3a. All adolescents need both a role model and a confidant. Someone with whom he already has a relationship would be ideal.	3. Ronald wanted to have his father as a support person and also identified his basketball coach as someone he admired a lot. It was agreed that Ronald and his father would receive therapy to facilitate the further development of their relationship. Goal met.
	3b. Be the support person for him until another can be found.	3b. There may not be anyone available for him at this time. The nurse can serve as a bridge.	
	3c. Help him develop guidelines for evaluating the reliability of support persons.	3c. An adolescent rarely has the ability to evaluate the trustworthiness of a support person without help.	

strategies have been identified as necessary for prevention efforts: (1) involving and training significant individuals and role models in the community, (2) providing information and educational materials, (3) developing life-skills that promote healthy personal functioning, (4) creating alternatives, and (5) influencing policy. Another attribute is that prevention is collaborative, involving representatives of all systems in the community (Benard, 1990).

The rationale for such a prevention approach is twofold. First, from more than a decade of prevention research the conclusion has been that the causes of drug abuse and other social problems are multiple, involving personality, environment, and behavioral variables, and that prevention efforts focused on a single system and a single strategy will probably fail (Benard, 1990).

SUMMARY

Parents with substance abuse have a profound effect on the family. The family must either alter its functioning and accommodate the substance abusing parent or exclude the parent from the family to survive. Children's stereotyped roles have been described by Wegscheider and Black, and criteria for a possible psychiatric diagnosis of codependency has been developed by Cermak. Children growing up in homes with substance abuse may have school, behavioral, emotional, or physical problems. However, many children from these homes show little difference in psychological functioning when compared with children from nonsubstance abusing homes. Resiliency factors include average intelligence, adequate communication skills, achievement orientation, internalized locus of control, responsible attitude, and absence of parental conflict during the first 2 years of life. Substance abuse in adolescents may be experimental, intermittent, or problem use. Drug abuse by adolescents is more likely to occur and to be more severe as the number of risk factors to which the adolescent is exposed increases.

REFERENCES

Ackerman, R.J. (1978). *Children of alcoholics: A guidebook for educators, therapists, and parents*. Holmes Beach, FL: Learning Publications.

American Psychiatric Association. (1987). *Diagnostic and statistical manual of mental disorders*, (3rd ed., Rev.). Washington, D.C.: The Association.

Bekir, P., McClellan, T., Childress, A.R., & Garite, P. (1993). Role reversals in families of substance misusers: A transgenerational phenomenon. *International Journal of Addictions, 28*(7), 613-630.

Benard, B. (1990). An overview of community-based prevention. In *Prevention Research Findings: 1988*. OSAP Prevention Monograph 3. Rockville, MD: Office for Substance Abuse Prevention.

Bennett, G. (1991). Substance abuse among the young. In G. Bennett & D.S. Woolf (Eds.) *Substance abuse: Pharmacologic, developmental, and clinical perspectives*. (pp 142-156). Albany, NY: Delmar.

Bennett, L., Wolin, S., & Reiss, D. (1988). Deliberate family process: A strategy for protecting children of alcoholics. *British Journal of Addiction, 83*, 821-829.

Benson, C.S. & Heller, K. (1987). Factors in the current adjustment of young adult daughters of alcoholic and problem drinking fathers. *Journal of Abnormal Psychology, 96*, 305-312.

Black, C. (1979, Fall). Children of alcoholics. *Alcohol Health and Research World, 4*, 23-27.

Black, C. (1981). *It will never happen to me!* Denver: MAC Printing.

Black, C., Bucky, S.F., & Wilder-Padilla, S. (1986). The interpersonal and emotional consequences of being an adult child of an alcoholic. *The International Journal of the Addictions, 21*, 213-231.

Booz-Allen & Hamilton, Inc. (1974). *An assessment of the needs of the resources for children of alcoholic parents*. Rockville, MD: NIAAA.

Brown, B.E. & Garrison, C.J. (1990). Patterns of symptomatology of adult women incest survivors. *Western Journal of Nursing Research, 12*(5), 587-600.

Brown, S. (1988). *Treating adult children of alcoholics: A developmental perspective.* New York: Wiley.

Captain, C. (1989). Family recovery from alcoholism: Mediating family factors. *Nursing Clinics of North America, 24,* 55-67.

Cermak, T. (1986). *Diagnosing and treating co-dependence.* Minneapolis, MN: Johnson Institute.

Cermak, T.L. & Brown, S. (1982). Interactional group therapy with the adult children of alcoholics. *International Journal of Group Psychotherapy, 32,* 375-388.

Chassin, L., Rogosch, F., & Berrera, M. (1991). Substance use and symptomatology among adolescent children of alcoholics. *Journal of Studies on Alcohol, 53,* 306-319.

Children of Alcoholics Foundation. (1985). *Report of the conference on research needs and opportunities for children of alcoholics.* New York: The Foundation.

Clinebell, N.J. (1968). Pastoral counseling of the alcoholic and his family. In R. Catanzaro (Ed.), *Alcoholism: The total treatment approach.* Springfield, IL: Charles C Thomas.

Cloninger, R., Bohman, M., & Sigvardsson, S. (1981). Inheritance of alcohol abuse: Cross-fostering analysis of adopted men, *Archives of General Psychiatry, 38,* 861-867.

Coleman, E. (1987). Marital and relationship problems among chemically dependent and codependent relationships. Special Issue: Chemical dependency and intimacy dysfunction. *Journal of Chemical Dependency Treatment, 1*(1), 39-59.

Coleman, E. & Colgan, P. (1986). Boundary inadequacy in drug dependent families. *Journal of Psychoactive Drugs, 18*(1), 21-30.

Cook, D.R. (1988, October). *Family of origin measures: Validating a new scale.* Paper presented at the annual conference of the American Association for Marital and Family Therapists, New Orleans, LA.

Cork, R.M. (1969). *The forgotten children: A study of children with alcoholic parents.* Toronto, Canada: Paperjacks.

Devine, C. & Braithwaite, V. (1993). The survival roles of children of alcoholics: Their measurement and validity. *Addiction 88*(1), 69-78.

Donovan, J.E. & Jessor, R. (1978). Adolescent problem drinking: Psychosocial correlates in a national sample study. *Journal of Studies on Alcohol, 39,* 1506-1524.

DuPont, R.L. (Ed.) (1989). *Stopping alcohol and other drug use before it starts: The future of prevention.* OSAP Prevention Monograph 1. (DHHS Publication No. ADM 89-1645). Rockville, MD: Office for Substance Abuse Prevention.

Easley, M.J. & Epstein, N. (1991). Coping with stress in a family with an alcoholic parent. *Family Relations, 40,* 218-224.

Estes, N.J., Smith-DiJulio, K., & Heinemann, M.E. (1980). *Nursing diagnosis of the alcoholic person.* St. Louis: C.V. Mosby.

Friel, J. & Friel, L. (1988). *Adult children: The secrets of dysfunctional families.* Deerfield Beach, FL: Health Communications.

Gil, D.G. (1970). *Violence against children.* Cambridge, MA: Harvard University.

Gil, E. (1988). *Treatment of adult survivors of childhood abuse.* Walnut Creek, CA: Launch Press.

Glassner, B. & Loughlin, J. (1987). *Drug in adolescent worlds: Burnouts to straights.* New York: St. Martin's Press.

Goodwin, D.W. (1984). Studies of familial alcoholism: A growth industry. In D.W. Goodwin, K.T. Van Dusen, & S.A. Mednick (Eds.) *Longitudinal research in alcoholism* (pp. 97-105). Boston: Kluwer-Nijhoff.

Gravitz, H. & Bowden, J. (1986). Therapeutic issues of adult children of alcoholics: A continuum of developmental stages. In R.J. Ackerman (Ed.) *Growing in the shadow: Children of alcoholics* (pp. 187-195). Pompano Beach, FL: Health Communications.

Grisham, K.J. & Estes, N.J. (1986). Dynamics of alcoholic families. In N.J. Estes & M.E. Heinemann (Eds.) *Alcoholism: Development, consequences, and interventions* (3rd ed., pp 303-314). St. Louis: Mosby.

Hecht, M. (1973). Children of alcoholics are children at risk. *American Journal of Nursing, 73,* 1764-1767.

Hill, S. & Hruska, D. (1992). Childhood psychopathology in families with multigenerational alcoholism. *Journal of the American Academy of Child and Adolescent Psychiatry, 31*(6), 1024-1030.

Hill, E., Nord, J., & Blow, F. (1992). Young adult children of alcoholic parents: Protective effects of positive family functioning. *British Journal of the Addictions, 87*(12), 1677-1690.

Hogarth, C.R. (1993). Families and family therapy. In B.S. Johnson, *Psychiatric–mental health nursing: Adaptation and growth* (3rd ed.). New York: JB Lippincott.

Isaacson, E.B. (1991). Chemical addiction: Individuals and family systems. *Journal of Chemical Dependency Treatment, 8*(1), 7-27.

Jacob, T., Ritchey, D., Cvitkovic, J.F., & Blane, H.T. (1981). Communication styles of alcoholic and non-alcoholic families when drinking and not drinking. *Quarterly Journal of Studies on Alcohol, 42,* 466-482.

Jessor, R. & Jessor, S.L. (1977). *Problem behavior and psychosocial development.* San Diego, CA: Academic Press.

Johnston, L.D., O'Malley, P.M., & Bachman, J.G. (1987). *National trends in drug use and related factors among American high school students and young adults, 1975-1986.* (DHHS Publication No. ADM 87-1535.) Rockville, MD: National Institute on Drug Abuse.

Johnston, L.D., O'Malley, P.M., & Bachman, J.G. (1989). *Drug use, drinking, and smoking: National survey results from high school, college, and young adult populations: 1975-1988,* (DHHS Publication No. ADM 89-1638). Rockville, MD: National Institute on Drug Abuse.

Jones, J.W. (1982). *Children of alcoholics screening test.* St. Paul, MN: Family Recovery Press.

Kandel, D.B. (1978). Convergences in prospective longitudinal surveys of drug use in normal populations. In D.B. Kandel (Ed.) *Longitudinal research on drug use: Empirical findings and methodological tissues* (pp 3-38). Washington, D.C.: Hemisphere.

Kaufman, E. (1985). Family systems and family therapy of substance abuse: An overview of two decades of research and clinical experience. *Journal of Studies on Alcohol, 42,* 466-482.

Kempe, C.H. & Helfer, R.E. (Eds.) (1980). *The battered child* (2nd ed.). Chicago: University of Chicago Press.

Kingery-McCabe, L.G. & Campbell, F.A. (1991). Effects of addiction on the addict. In D.C. Dailey & M.S. Raskin (Eds.) *Treating the chemically dependent and their families.* (pp 57-78). Newbury Park, CA: Sage.

Lawson, G., Peterson, J.S., & Lawson, A. (1983). *Alcoholism and the family: A guide to treatment and prevention.* Rockville, MD: Aspen.

Lefkowitz, M.M. & Tesiny, E.P. (1984). Rejection and depression: Prospective and contemporaneous analyses. *Developmental Psychology, 20,* 776-785.

Manning, D., Balson, P., & Xenakis, S. (1986). The prevalence of type A personality in the children of alcoholics. *Alcoholism: Clinical and Experimental Research, 10,* 184-189.

Marcus, A. (1986). Academic achievement in elementary school children of alcoholic mothers. *Journal of Clinical Psychology, 42,* 372-376.

Moos, R.H. & Billings, A.G. (1982). Children of alcoholics during the recovery process: Alcoholic and matched control families. *Addictive Behaviors, 7,* 155-163.

Newcomb, M.D. & Felix-Ortiz, M. (1992). Multiple protective and risk factors for drug use and abuse: Cross-sectional and prospective findings. *Journal of Personality and Social Psychology, 63,* 280-296.

Newcomb, M.D. & Harlow, L.L. (1986). Life events and substance use among adolescents: Mediating effects of perceived loss of control and meaninglessness in life. *Journal of Personality and Social Psychology, 51,* 564-577.

Newcomb, M.D., Maddahian, E., & Bentler, P.M. (1986). Risk factors for drug use among adolescents: Concurrent and longitudinal analyses. *American Journal of Public Health, 76,* 400-401.

Obuchowska, I. (1974). Emotional contact with the mother as a social compensatory factor in children of alcoholics. *International Mental Health Research Newsletter, 16,* 2, 4.

Pope, C. & Brucker, M.C. (1991). Adolescents as victims: An overview of the special impact of sexual abuse. In M.C. Brucker (Ed.) *Clinical issues in perinatal and women's health nursing.* (pp 263-269). Philadelphia: JB Lippincott.

Raskin, M.S. & Daley, D.C. (1991). Overview of addiction. In D.C. Daley & M.S. Raskin (Eds.) *Treating the chemically dependent and their families.* (pp 1-21). Newbury Park, CA: Sage.

Reich, W., Earls, F., & Powell, J. (1988). A comparison of the home and social environments of children of alcoholic and nonalcoholic parents. *British Journal of Addiction, 83,* 831-839.

Rhodes, J. & Blackham, G.J. (1987). Differences in character roles between adolescents from alcoholic and nonalcoholic homes. *American Journal of Drug and Alcohol Abuse, 13,* 145-155.

Rhodes, J.E. & Jason, L.A. (1990). A social stress model of substance abuse. *Journal of Consulting and Clinical Psychology, 38,* 395-401.

Robinson, B.E. (1989). *Working with children of alcoholics.* Lexington, MA: D.D. Heath.

Roosa, M.W., Tein, J.Y., Groppenbacher, N., Michaels, M., & Dumka, L. (1993). Mothers' parenting behavior and child mental health in families with a problem drinking parent. *Journal of Marriage and the Family, 55,* 107-118.

Russell, M., Henderson, C., & Blume, S. (1984). *Children of alcoholics: A review of the literature.* New York: Children of Alcoholics Foundation.

Rutter, M. & Quinton, D. (1984). Parental psychiatric disorder: Effects on children. *Psychological Medicine, 14,* 853-880.

Satir, V. (1967). *Conjoint family therapy.* Palo Alto, CA: Science and Behavior Books.

Scavnicky-Mylant, M.L. (1988). The process of coping and emotional development of young adult children of alcoholics: A nursing study. *Dissertation Abstracts International, 49.*

Scheitlin, K. (1990). Identifying and helping children of alcoholics. *Nurse Practitioner, 15*(2), 34-43, 46-47.

Schinke, S.P., Botvin, G.J., & Orlandi, M.A. (Eds.) (1991). *Substance abuse in children and adolescents: Evaluation and intervention.* Newbury Park, CA: Sage.

Schulsinger, F., Goodwin, D., Knop, J., Pollock, V., & Mikkelsen, U. (1985). Characteristics of young men at higher risk for alcoholism. In U. Rydberg (Ed.) *Alcohol and the developing brain.* (pp 193-205). New York: Raven Press.

Sher, K.J., Walitzer, K.S., Wood, P.K., & Brent, E.E. (1991). Characteristics of children of alcoholics: Punitive risk factors, substance use and abuse, and psychopathology. *Journal of Abnormal Psychology, 100,* 427-448.

Silver, R.L. & Wortman, C.B. (1980). Coping with undesirable life events. In J. Garber & M.E.P. Seligman (Eds.) *Human helplessness: Theory and application.* (pp 279-340). New York: Academic Press.

Smith, A.R. (1986). Alcoholism and gender: Patterns of diagnosis and response. *Journal of Drug Issues, 16,* 407-420.

Snow, D. (1989). The client who is an adolescent. *Nursing care planning with the addicted client,* Vol. 1, Skokie, IL: National Nurses Society on Addictions.

Steinglass, P., Bennett, L.A., Wolin, S.J., & Reiss, D. (1987). *The alcoholic family.* New York: Basic Books.

Tarter, R., Alterman, A., & Edwards, K. (1985). Vulnerability to alcoholism in men: A behavior-genetic perspective. *Journal of Studies on Alcohol, 46,* 329-356.

Tweed, S.H. (1989). Identifying the alcoholic client. *Nursing Clinics of North America, 24*(1), 13-31.

Tweed, S.H., Ryff, C.D., & Cranley, M.S. (1990, November). *Adult children of alcoholics: Their views of past family and parental relationships.* Presented at the annual meeting of the National Council on Family Relations. Seattle.

Wampler, R., Fischer, J., Thomas, M., & Lyness, K. (1993). Young adult offspring and their families of origin: Cohesion, adaptability, and addiction. *Journal of Substance Abuse, 5*(2), 195-201.

Wegscheider, S. (1981). *Another chance: Hope and health for alcoholic families.* Palo Alto, CA: Science & Behavioral Books.

Wegscheider-Cruse, S. (1985). *Choicemaking.* Pompano Beach, FL: Health Communications.

Weinberg, J.R. (1974). Interviewing techniques for diagnosing alcoholism. *American Family Physician, 9*(3), 107-115.

Werner, E.E. (1986). Resilient offspring of alcoholics: A longitudinal study from birth to age 18. *Journal of Studies on Alcohol, 47,* 34-40.

Whitfield, C.L. (1987). *Healing the child within.* Pompano Beach, FL: Health Communications.

Wing, D.M. (1991). Goal setting and recovery from alcoholism. *Archives of Psychiatric Nursing, 5*(3), 178-184.

Woititz, J.G. (1985). *Struggle for intimacy.* Pompano Beach, FL: Health Communications.

Woodside, M. (1986). Children of alcoholics: Helping a vulnerable group. *Public Health Reports, 103,* 643-647.

Zerwekh, J. & Michaels, B. (1989). Co-dependency: Assessment and recovery. *Nursing Clinics of North America, 24*(1), 109-120.

10 Nursing Care of Clients with Substance Abuse in Community Settings

The community health nurse plays a vital role in primary, secondary, and tertiary prevention of substance abuse in public health agencies, homes, schools, industry and various outpatient settings. Because of the long-term, caring relationships established with clients in community settings, nurses are especially important for finding and referring clients with alcohol and drug problems, as well as providing care to recovering individuals. This chapter describes caring for clients with substance abuse in urban and rural settings. The nurse's role in all levels of prevention in a variety of lifestages and populations is described. Also, substance abuse issues are discussed as they relate to home, school, and industrial settings.

The devastating effects of substance abuse have ramifications in all areas of the community health nurse's practice. In the community these effects include violence, abuse, bankruptcy, juvenile delinquency, and felonious crimes. It is estimated that up to 80% of the prison population is there because of substance abuse related crimes (Burns, Thompson, & Ciccone, 1991b). In schools, underage use of alcohol, use of illegal drugs, drug dealing, lack of performance, and loss of the student's potential for optimal achievement are concerns. Students under the influence of alcohol or drugs may disrupt the classroom, be truant or delinquent, or be involved with an unplanned pregnancy. Alcohol or drug abuse leads to increased absenteeism and tardiness, decreased productivity, and an increased incidence of work-related injuries.

Comprehensive knowledge of the community is essential for the community health nurse to be effective in assisting clients with substance abuse problems. Knowledge about such areas as shopping centers with heavy drug traffic, local bars in the neighborhood, or at-risk housing complexes are important. The community health nurse must be well-informed about community resources that help prevent substance abuse, as well as resources that provide assessment and treatment services. The nurse may serve as a community resource, sharing information with community groups, treatment centers, or self-help groups.

SPECIAL NEEDS IN URBAN POPULATIONS

Nursing care of individuals in the urban inner city poses special challenges to the community health nurse. Community problems already described (poverty, unemployment, homelessness, unplanned pregnancies, HIV infection, and violence) increase in urban areas.

Poverty

Poverty is related to substance abuse because of the extensive hopelessness of people without adequate income, housing, or employment. Alcohol or drugs are a way to escape the dreariness of daily life. Chronic use or abuse leads to more hopelessness as the possibility of employment decreases. Without adequate treatment services and necessary social supports in the community (e.g., adequate education, enough employment, satisfactory housing), solving the problems of poverty and substance abuse is unlikely.

Unemployment

Unemployment may occur as a result of sustained alcohol or drug abuse. The person who is addicted is usually unable to meet the demands of a job and as a result is fired or let go. In addition, the person who is actively using drugs or alcohol may not be interested in working. Drug dealing or prostitution, which sometimes accompanies substance abuse, may supply more money than the average job. Unemployment also may cause depression or low self-image. This then contributes to the development of substance abuse; people use alcohol or drugs to escape the reality of a life of poverty or frustration.

Homelessness

Another negative consequence of drug abuse and addiction is financial devastation that results in a loss of housing. Addicts are often unable to make mortgage or rent payments and consequently lose their homes or are evicted. Some are thrown out of housing by their families or by landlords as a result of drug use, prostitution, theft, or violence. Many of these addicts and their young children end up in homeless shelters. Their drug use usually continues and is supported by crime.

Unplanned pregnancies

Unplanned pregnancies are commonly associated with alcohol or drug abuse. Pregnancies may result from irresponsible sexual practices or prostitution. Conception may occur when a woman is under the influence of alcohol or drugs and has not taken precautions to prevent pregnancy. In other situations the woman may see pregnancy as a way to feel better about herself. Adolescents who are experimenting with alcohol, drugs, *and* sex are especially vulnerable. (See Chapter 8 for further discussion of substance abuse during pregnancy.)

HIV/AIDS

People who use drugs intravenously are at high risk for human immunodeficiency virus (HIV) infection, which has become an epidemic in the United States. By May of 1991, 132,510 cases of acquired immune deficiency syndrome (AIDS) had been reported in America and it was estimated that another 1 to 1.5 million people are infected but asymptomatic (Long, B., 1993). Populations at risk for HIV exposure include intravenous drug users who often share needles.

The problem of HIV and AIDS infection in drug-addicted women is steadily increasing. Currently, women comprise 12% of the AIDS population, approaching 20,000 women. Half of this group uses drugs intravenously. An increasing number of HIV positive clients are manifesting AIDS and AIDS-related complex. HIV infection affects black and Hispanic women unequally; women of color represent only 19% of all women nationwide, but they comprise 72% of all women with AIDS (Dumas, 1992).

Violence

Violence is increasingly prevalent, especially in cities, and it is associated with substance abuse in several ways. First, arguments between drug users, dealers, and suppliers often erupt into violence. Second, some people may resort to crime (and related violence) to pay for drugs. Third, people who abuse alcohol or drugs are more likely to handle disagreements with violence.

SPECIAL NEEDS IN RURAL POPULATIONS

The nurse working in a rural setting is in an excellent position to be involved in the primary, secondary, and tertiary prevention of alcoholism and substance abuse. The nurse's visibility in the community provides an opportunity for assessing needs specific to health-promotion activities. The nurse often is seen as the resource for the community on health issues. Often there is a level of trust between the nurse and the people of the community.

It is important for the nurse who is working with rural clients to be aware of the cultural biases of the area. The rural community is characterized by the history, values, beliefs, and cultural practices of its people. Biases can have a tremendous impact on a community's health status and are a critical factor in program development.

The health problems that plague rural communities of today are related to limited resources and inaccessible or inappropriate services. For example, the absence of a viable public transportation system is problematic when planning and scheduling outpatient services. The adolescent or adult whose license has been suspended for driving under the influence may have a very difficult time arranging transportation to an outpatient substance abuse program. Generally, trends in rural populations that have increased responsibilities of the community health nurse include the deemphasis on farming as the means of livelihood, rural poverty, and decentralization of government (Anderson & Yuhos, 1993).

A study of rural health nurses in Nebraska revealed sources of stress reported by clients. Stress was caused by changes in the rural way of life, aging farm families, children moving away, increased use of alcohol and drugs, elder, spouse, and child abuse, loneliness, and depression (Anderson & Yuhos, 1993).

All of these characteristics of rural areas pose special problems for the community health nurse working to implement prevention and treatment services for persons with substance abuse problems. Creativity is important, as well as involvement of community leaders in a cooperative effort. If the nurse is a member of the rural community, providing such care is easier.

AVAILABILITY OF TREATMENT SERVICES

Treatment services for the addicted person are most effective when they are offered in conjunction with other community services. Community-based services include hospitals, ambulatory care departments, shelters, home care agencies (such as visiting nurse organizations), neighborhood health centers, public health departments, and special programming (e.g., maternal-child health grant programs). It is important for the community health nurse to be familiar with all of the community resources for treatment.

The availability of treatment services varies in different communities. One source of help available in virtually every community is the self-help group. The most common groups are twelve step programs such as Alcoholics Anonymous, Narcotics Anonymous, and Al-Anon. Meetings are held in a variety of places (e.g., churches) at various times of the day so they are usually accessible to anyone. The twelve step approach teaches a process for dealing with alcohol and other drug problems on a daily basis. Major lifestyle changes can result from this approach. (See Chapter 4 for more about twelve step programs.)

Another possible source of help in the community is the church. Some churches have organized efforts to educate people about the risks of alcohol and drug use, as well as to offer assistance to those who are addicted. Pastors may be specially trained in counseling, or they may have persons on their staff who are able to work with abuse problems.

Detoxification is another service that is needed. Detoxification takes place in general hospitals and drug and alcohol treatment centers. In most cases treatment follows detoxification. (A detailed description of treatment may be found in Chapter 4.)

Individual or group counseling may be needed to assist the client and family in making necessary life changes. Counseling may not be readily available to some people because of lack of third-party coverage. Some community agencies offer counseling on a sliding-fee scale basis.

Another treatment option for clients with substance abuse problems is a halfway house or three-quarter house. These programs are available for persons who need a longer period of treatment to maintain recovery and a healthy lifestyle. The program length is usually 3 months to a year, and the focus is on remaining drug-free while learning skills for living in a supervised setting. Often, the resident returns to work while living in the house.

Financing treatment

Finances for inpatient alcohol and drug treatment have become much less available recently. This has resulted from a concerted effort on the part of third-party payers (e.g., the federal government through Medicare, HMOs, and insurance companies) to decrease the cost of treatment. In most cases outpatient treatment is required before inpatient treatment will be approved. Also, many payers only pay for detoxification. Other policies allow for a maximum number of treatments in a lifetime or only a certain number of admissions for detoxification per calendar year. As with other illnesses, hospitalization for drug or alcohol abuse often requires precertification. (Chapter 15 describes financing treatment in detail.)

PRIMARY PREVENTION

Primary prevention aims to prevent nonusers from initiating use and to prevent individuals who are experimenting with substance use from progressing to chronic and abusive use of substances. Community education is the most common method of primary prevention. Methods of education vary widely; they include the following: (1) warning labels on containers of alcohol or prescription drugs, (2) signs that warn about alcohol's effects on pregnancy located in establishments serving alcohol, (3) required notices on cigarette packages, (4) pamphlets placed in well-traveled areas such as health clinics, physicians' offices, hospital waiting rooms, and grocery stores, (5) public service messages on radio and television, and (6) community education presentations by health professionals. Frequent attention to the topic of prevention is necessary for long-term attitude and behavior changes.

Primary prevention related to substance abuse has had varying rates of success. The antismoking campaign, begun more than 20 years ago, has resulted in a reduction in smoking and has limited the public areas where people may smoke. The tobacco lobby, however, has vigorously opposed efforts to curtail smoking just as the alcohol industry has resisted attempts to reduce alcohol consumption. The illicit drug industry operates outside the law and therefore is tax exempt. International attempts to eliminate opium and cocaine trafficking have been unsuccessful.

Nursing role

The nurse's role in primary prevention includes education about alcohol and drugs, as well as promotion of healthy alternatives to recreational drug use and other ways to cope with stress. The community health nurse plays a vital role in educating individuals about their prescriptions. Nurses can explain the additive, synergistic, or antagonistic effects of drugs with each other and with alcohol.

Educating people about avoiding the initial introduction of alcohol or other drugs is ideal. Education about responsible, intermittent use of alcohol should be provided. For example, if a youth can be persuaded to "just say no" to drugs, a great deal of later anguish and agony may be avoided. Therefore preventive measures should be targeted for children between the ages of 10 and 13 and their parents. In addition to information about the specific negative effects of alcohol and drugs and the problems encountered with specific substances, efforts need to focus on values clarification, decision-making, and peer group pressure. (See Chapter 9 for more information on prevention in adolescents.)

The nurse has a pivotal role in home care, schools, industry, and other settings in the community to teach individuals healthy recreational activities and offer advice about coping with stress without using alcohol or drugs. Community, church, or school recreational activities (e.g., sports, camp, after-school programs) are especially useful for children and teens. Stress reduction classes may be offered by a local hospital or the community health nurse. Charity runs, for example, challenge community members to get in shape, while reducing stress and raising funds for needed programs. Because of the nurse's long-term relationship with community members and the community's respect for the nurse, the nurse's opinions and advice are taken seriously.

SECONDARY PREVENTION

Secondary prevention involves screening and treatment to minimize the health and social consequences of substance abuse. Some groups of individuals are of special concern because of their vulnerability for substance abuse. They require vigilant attention by the community health nurse. These groups are *adolescents, minorities, pregnant women* who use drugs, the *mentally ill,* and the *elderly.* The issues with each group are initiated here, and the reader is referred to other chapters for additional information.

Adolescents

Adolescents in all population groups (e.g., urban poor, suburban wealthy) are vulnerable to substance abuse because of the developmental need to explore and experiment that is characteristic of this age. Concern about the dangers inherent in alcohol and drug abuse by adolescents (e.g., traffic accidents, violence, unplanned pregnancies), however, requires intervention. Twenty years ago it was thought that providing information about the dangers of substance use to adolescents would discourage them from experimenting. Today, prevention efforts use multiple strategies, including building self-esteem, improving decision-making skills, clarifying values, training in life skills, and teaching peer refusal strategies. Furthermore, it is recognized that a community-wide effort is required, targeting homes, schools, businesses, churches, and community organizations. (Chapter 9 includes more information about adolescents.)

Minorities

Minority populations are at risk for substance abuse because of concomitant poverty, violence, and lack of opportunity that may be present in the community. Alcohol and drugs may be used to cope with a continually disruptive environment.

The four major racial and ethnic minority groups in the United States are African Americans, Hispanics, Asian Americans, and Native Americans. Diverse cultural patterns exist within each group and between the groups. An awareness of cultural differences is needed to develop prevention and intervention strategies to meet the special needs of any minority population. (Chapter 13 includes more information about minority populations.)

Part of the problem in identifying addicted persons is that a majority of health care professionals are middle class and white, and they tend to identify people as addicts when they are different or do not share the same values. For example, low-income women of color are more likely to be identified as addicts, while middle-class, white women may be underreported (Dumas, 1992).

Pregnant women

Pregnant women are at risk because their use affects themselves and also their unborn children. It is important to identify *pregnant women* who abuse drugs as early as possible. Without treatment, their babies risk being born addicted. Also, these women often deliver prematurely and have complications associated with childbirth. (See Chapter 8 for information about the pregnant woman and her baby.)

Mentally ill

The mentally ill are especially vulnerable to substance abuse for several reasons. They may use alcohol or drugs to mitigate the symptoms of their illness or their medications. Because of the manifestations of their illness they may not be able to learn about the problems with substance use, or they may not be able to recall and use previously learned information. Overall difficulty in functioning may leave the mentally ill person homeless as well. In addition, some individuals suffer from mental illness *and* substance abuse (see Chapter 12).

Elderly

The elderly are at risk because they may drink to fill voids brought on by ill health, loneliness, or feelings of low self-worth (Iber, 1990). The stress of retirement includes a loss of positive self-image and a loss of daily structure. "Ageism" in society also leads some elderly people to feel useless and powerless. The elderly may be isolated from others, including family (see Chapter 13).

The elderly who are alcoholic and started their use in their younger years often are chronically ill as a result of their years of use. Other alcoholics may start drinking later in life. Called *late-onset alcoholics* (Burns, Thompson & Ciccone, 1991a and b), these individuals generally drink alone, hiding their drinking from others. Members of these individuals' families may have difficulty admitting that their parent or grandparent has a problem with drugs or alcohol (Krach, 1990). The elderly also may abuse prescription drugs.

Alcohol-induced impairments in the elderly include decreased alertness, poor judgment, impaired memory, increased forgetfulness, and mental confusion. Depression, irritability, social isolation, insomnia, poor hygiene, falls, and lack of physical coordination also may be present. At times the symptoms of alcohol and drug use, such as poor nutrition and incontinence, may be confused with normal aging, which can prohibit the problem from being identified and hinder the individual from receiving needed help (see Care Plan 10-1). (See Chapter 13 for more about the elderly.)

Families

Families play a crucial role in substance abuse problems. The community health nurse's assessment of the family plays a vital role in identification. Families frequently deny the problem and minimize the degree to which the family member abuses drugs or alcohol. The family often becomes protective and attempts to hide the problem from those outside of the family. They make excuses for absences from or tardiness to work, school, or social activities and support rationalizations about the use of substances. Children often cope with alcoholism or substance abuse by fleeing, fighting, or being a perfect child. During times of violence, they may flee by escaping physically (such as hiding under the bed or retreating to a closet) or flee mentally by emotionally insulating themselves from their family (Levy & Rutter, 1992).

In families, substance abuse becomes a self-perpetuating cycle. The abuser often blames the family for troubles or for the substance abuse, instilling guilt and feelings of inadequacy in the family. The more the family attempts to control the abuser's use, the more the dependent person uses substances, and the more inadequate the family feels. Family members of substance abusers often experience feelings of hurt, guilt, shame, loneliness, inadequacy, and low self-esteem. A common psychiatric disorder that affects family members is depression. Physical symptoms also are common in family members, including palpitations, vague aches and pains, weakness, headaches, gastritis, and irritable bowel syndrome. More serious problems include hypertension, peptic ulcer disease, ulcerative colitis, and asthma (Stanhope & Lancaster, 1992).

It is not only physical and psychological problems that are more common in families of substance abusers. Physical violence, abuse (sexual, physical, and emotional), and incest also may be present in these families. Health care costs have been found to be significantly higher for families with a member receiving treatment for alcoholism than for families without a member with an alcohol problem. It is believed that the health care costs of untreated chemical dependency are double the health care costs of those who are not dependent on substances (Burns, Thompson & Ciccone, 1991a and b).

Families also are being affected because many children, including newborns and infants, are being abandoned by their parents. This seems to be more common with crack cocaine use. Crack addiction has led to the creation of the "boarder-baby" (babies boarded in maternity and pediatric units and other settings). This has also led to an increase in "kinship" foster care placement in which blood relatives are licensed and paid to be foster parents. In other cases grandparents, especially grandmothers, often of advanced age are being forced to care for their children's children. (More about families can be found in Chapter 9.)

TERTIARY PREVENTION

Tertiary prevention is aimed at preventing relapse of those individuals already treated for substance abuse problems. The community health nurse encounters recovering individuals in homes, industry, schools, and outpatient settings. Ongoing education and care of these clients requires the nurse to be fully informed about the recovery process, relapse prevention, and especially the use of medications to avoid compromising the recovery (see Chapter 5).

Care of recovering clients

Recovery for alcohol- and drug-dependent clients is not an overnight process. It requires tremendous effort for a person to change an established dependency on drugs or alcohol. Rehabilitation takes a long time. During this time, the nurse can play an important role in monitoring the client's physical condition, psychological health, and medications.

Monitor physical conditions.   The community health nurse monitors the physical condition of clients, helps them adapt to their condition, and facilitates medical care. Many persons who enter treatment for alcohol or drug illnesses may be in poor physical condition. Many years of abuse may have taken their toll. For some, other chronic diseases such as AIDS, tuberculosis, or cirrhosis may necessitate med-

Text continued on p. 284.

Care Plan 10-1

Elderly Man in Home, Alcoholism

Fred Smith, age 77, has lived alone since the death of his wife 3 years ago. He has three children; two live out of the city and a 45-year-old daughter, Beth, lives nearby. Fred prepares his own meals and does his own laundry. He reports that he likes a little drink occasionally and has done this all of his life. Before his wife's death, they traveled together and enjoyed fishing, visiting with friends and family, and playing cards with several friends. Since her death, he has stayed home alone most of the time. Fred was hospitalized 2 months ago for broken ribs and torn cartilage in his knee. He takes medication for blood pressure and for ulcers. Beth reported that she cleans his house monthly and looks in on him at least once a week. She is concerned about his increasing confusion, lack of personal hygiene, and a smoldering fire he started in his living room divan with a cigarette. Fortunately, a neighbor visited, smelled smoke, and called the fire department. The neighbor told the nurse that he smelled alcohol on Fred's breath, as he did most of the time. Beth also validated that her father "likes to have a drink in the evening," but didn't think his drinking was a problem. She is considering insisting that her father be placed in a nursing home because of his "increasing senility."

ASSESSMENT

Fred appeared thin, frail, and disheveled. His breath smelled of alcohol. Multiple bruises were apparent on his arms. Fred couldn't remember when or what he ate last night. He reported that he had been sleeping poorly for several days.

NURSING DIAGNOSES

High risk for injury related to alcohol ingestion
Knowledge deficit: Alcohol use in the elderly related to evidence that he used excessively
Impaired home maintenance management related to drinking alcohol and cognitive impairment

Outcome identification	Nursing interventions	Rationale	Evaluation
Nursing diagnosis: High risk for injury related to alcohol ingestion			
1. Client will remain safe on a continuing basis.	1a. Assess client's home for hazards.	1a. An elderly client may have impaired balance and sight, as well as impaired cognition requiring special safety precautions.	1. After discussing the situation with the client's daughter, it was decided to have a home health aide live with him until he could be safe alone or until other arrangements could be made. He remained safe. Goal met.
	1b. Assess the client's mental status carefully.	1b. The client's mental status may be impaired sufficiently that an in-home caretaker may be required.	

Outcome identification	Nursing interventions	Rationale	Evaluation

Nursing diagnosis: High risk for injury related to alcohol ingestion—cont'd

| | 1c. Take steps to assist the client to change living arrangements if safety cannot be reasonably assured. | 1c. Impairment may be severe enough that he requires other living arrangements. | |

Nursing diagnosis: Knowledge deficit: Alcohol use in the elderly related to evidence that he used excessively

1. Client will state that alcohol makes his stomach and blood pressure problems worse in 2 weeks.	1a. Carefully assess the client's alcohol use. Ask him when he drinks. Ask him if his drinking changed after his wife's death. Does he drink when he feels lonely? What does he use to help him fall asleep?	1a. The older client who has an alcohol problem usually does not recognize it. Asking specific questions about how and when it is used provides more useful information.	1. At the first home visit after assessment, client stated he was amazed that alcohol made his blood pressure and stomach problems worse. Goal met.
	1b. Discuss client's drinking with his daughter. Ask specifically if she has observed a change since her mother's death. Has she found a number of bottles around when she cleans his house?	1b. It is common for family members to not recognize a parent's drinking problems. It is more helpful to use specific questions.	
	1c. Relate to client that alcohol can cause his physical problems and will certainly exacerbate them.	1c. This is likely new information to the client and is usually well received by the older client.	

Continued.

Elderly Man in Home, Alcoholism—cont'd

Outcome identification	Nursing interventions	Rationale	Evaluation
Nursing diagnosis: Knowledge deficit: Alcohol use in the elderly related to evidence that he used excessively—cont'd			
2. Client will express hope that his memory and confusion will improve without alcohol use in 4 weeks.	2a. Ask client if he has observed difficulties with his memory in recent weeks.	2a. Obtains information about the client's perception of his mental status in a non-threatening way.	2. At the first home visit, Fred also stated that he was amazed that he could hope for improved memory at his age. He asked if he stopped using alcohol, could he expect to think better. Goal met.
	2b. If he acknowledges that he has observed difficulties with memory, relate this and other thinking difficulties to the use of alcohol; and explain that reducing the use of alcohol will likely improve his thinking.	2b. Again, new information to assist the client to understand his problem. This is shared in a non-threatening way and gives the client hope that he may regain at least some of his thinking abilities.	
3. Client will abstain from drinking for 1 week by the fourth week.	3a. Elicit agreement from the client to try to abstain from drinking for 1 week.	3a. This will test the client's ability to abstain from alcohol without treatment.	3. At the second week, client stated that he decided to drink a couple more times before attempting to abstain. After the next visit, he presented unshaven, depressed, and very shame-faced when he admitted that he had been drinking again. Goal not met.
	3b. Teach client's daughter that many of the client's physical and mental problems may be caused by his drinking, and that if he is able to abstain from drinking, he may make a remarkable recovery. Elicit her collaboration in assisting the client.	3b. This is new information for her and supplies much hope. Includes the daughter in care of her father.	
	3c. Explain to the daughter that the plan is to first allow the client to try to quit drinking on his own.	3c. Includes the family in the plan of care.	

Outcome identification	Nursing interventions	Rationale	Evaluation

Nursing diagnosis: Knowledge deficit: Alcohol use in the elderly related to evidence that he used excessively—cont'd

Outcome identification	Nursing interventions	Rationale	Evaluation
	3d. Explain to the client and daughter that his problems will be unlikely to abate unless he is able to completely abstain from drinking.	3d. Factual information that the client needs in order to make an informed decision about his care.	
	3e. If the client was not successful, inform him matter-of-factly that it is an indication of his need for outside help for his problem. If he refuses help, try an additional week of abstinence.	3e. Introduces the idea that treatment may be needed and lets him make the decision to seek treatment now. It is important to be nonjudgmental.	
4. Client will agree to enter an alcohol treatment unit by the fourth week.	4a. Tell client that two unsuccessful attempts at abstinence indicates the need for him to obtain treatment for his drinking. Relate again how his drinking is causing many of his problems and they likely will improve with treatment. Tell him that he likely will be able to go fishing again with treatment. Elicit assistance from daughter if needed.	4a. Usually in an older person, relating the consequences with drinking and presenting the reality of hope for improvement in his quality of life will produce a positive response. Including a benefit of treatment that he especially wants will improve compliance.	4. Client agreed to treatment without much objection upon the third visit by the nurse. He said it would really be great if he could go fishing again. Goal met.

Continued.

Care Plan 10-1

Elderly Man in Home, Alcoholism—cont'd

Outcome identification	Nursing interventions	Rationale	Evaluation
Nursing diagnosis: Impaired home maintenance management related to drinking alcohol and cognitive impairment			
1. Client will maintain adequate nutrition as demonstrated by weight maintenance by 2 months.	1a. Evaluate adequacy of meals by eliciting a detailed daily intake. 1b. If it is determined that he cannot provide his own meals, arrange for Meals on Wheels.	1a. Assessing daily intake will assist the nurse in determining adequate diet. 1b. Meals on Wheels provides one balanced meal a day.	1. This intervention was not attempted until after the client returned home from treatment. His meal preparation was barely adequate. He was enthused about the possibility of Meals on Wheels and did maintain his weight by 3 months. Goal partially met.
2. Client will take medication as prescribed and only take OTC medications with approval from the nurse by 2 months.	2a. Evaluate all medications taken by the client by having him show the nurse all of his medication containers including OTC. 2b. Contact the physician and pharmacist if there are medication-related problems. 2c. Assist the client to take medications in a safe manner, e.g., distribute a week's supply of medications in a compartmentalized pill container.	2a. The nurse can determine interacting medications, those prescribed by multiple physicians, and those OTC that would impair functioning. 2b. This should ensure appropriate prescriptions for the client. 2c. A compartmentalized pill container helps the client keep straight what medication to take when.	2. It was found that he had medications from two different physicians. This was discussed with his primary physician and his pharmacist, and his medications were adjusted appropriately. His daughter agreed to help him keep his medicines straight. Because he had just returned from treatment, there was inadequate time to assess goal. After 3 months the goal was met, however.

Outcome identification	Nursing interventions	Rationale	Evaluation
Nursing diagnosis: Impaired home maintenance management related to drinking alcohol and cognitive impairment—cont'd			
	2d. Teach the client's daughter to set up the week's supply of medication.	2d. Enlistment of family member's help reduces dependence upon the nurse, helps assure safety of medication use.	
3. Client will attend AA meetings regularly by 2 months.	3a. Encourage the client to attend AA meetings.	3a. AA is important for social support and continued recovery from alcoholism.	3. Client began attending an AA group upon discharge from treatment. The group had a large number of older persons and Fred stated that he enjoyed the group. Goal met.
	3b. Assist the client to find an AA group with which he feels comfortable.	3b. An AA group that is tolerant of older individuals and whose members are compatible with the client is best.	
4. Client will maintain an alcohol-free environment by engaging in hobbies and interests and finding a satisfying social group by 3 months.	4a. Discuss with client and daughter interests and hobbies that he would like to pursue and the means to do so.	4a. Engaging in meaningful activities will enhance his quality of life.	4. Within 3 months, Fred had gone fishing several times and had begun taking advanced woodworking classes at a nearby community college. He played cards with some men in the neighborhood and went out to eat with friends from his AA group. Goal met.
	4b. Ask the client who his friends are. Encourage him to seek out and find others whose company he enjoys.	4b. Satisfying relationships with other people enhance his quality of life.	

ical treatment. Nutritional status may be compromised, and a consultation with a dietitian may be required. The client may have had little physical exercise and may benefit from appropriate activities to improve strength and endurance.

Monitor psychosocial health.   The recovering individual may be dealing with a variety of psychological changes and problems. The individual may be angry about the changes required and the realization that sobriety is necessary. Many alcohol and drug dependent persons go through a grieving process for the loss of alcohol or drugs. For the recovering person the sense of loss and sadness can be quite intense. The nurse can facilitate grieving by encouraging the client to talk about feelings and express grief or anger. Letting the person know that these feelings are normal and expected is helpful (Long, K., 1993).

Depression also may occur as the client recognizes and accepts the illness. Although the decision to stay clean and sober will bring relief and assurance in the long run, the individual may have times when the desire for a drink or drug will be very strong. For some, giving up the substance may also mean giving up friends who use substances as well.

Some individuals who have concomitant psychiatric problems will continue to manifest symptoms after treatment. These persons may need a psychiatric evaluation and counseling or psychiatric care. (See Chapter 12 for more about comorbidity of substance abuse and mental illness.)

The community health nurse also may be able to help the client regain a sense of hope. People dependent on alcohol or drugs enter treatment with a great deal of hopelessness. They may have attempted treatment before without success. They also may feel that they will never be able to achieve sobriety. In addition, many alcoholics or drug abusers have used substances to block feelings of hopelessness, especially about the loss of family, friends, or perhaps a job. Often the best way to aid clients in regaining hope is by encouraging participation in support groups such as AA or NA; there they will get to know recovering people who have maintained sobriety, changed their lifestyle, and regained hope. Also, support groups offer a social network of new, nonusing people to help with loneliness.

Monitor medications.   The community health nurse may assist clients to monitor medications after treatment. This is important for several reasons. For persons dependent on substances, cross-addiction is common. For example, a person who has been treated for alcoholism and later is placed on pain medications for a physical illness is at risk of becoming dependent on the medication.

Also, it is important for the nurse to help educate the client about medications to avoid. Many over-the-counter medications contain alcohol (e.g., cough medicine and mouthwash). Medications available as elixirs also contain alcohol. Pain or sleep medications also may be inadvertently abused by a recovering person.

Clients also may be on prescribed medication as part of their treatment program (e.g., methadone). A drug antagonist that causes an extremely unpleasant reaction when used with alcohol, such as disulfiram (Antabuse), may be prescribed. It disrupts the metabolism of alcohol in the liver and produces a severe reaction that includes stomach and head pain, extreme nausea, and vomiting. For someone on

Antabuse, milder reactions can be triggered by a number of products that contain alcohol such as mouthwash or perfume. Another drug, naltrexone hydrochloride (Trexan) blocks the euphoric response to the use of opiates. (See Chapter 2 for more about drug substitutes and antagonists.)

It is important to monitor medications to ensure that the recovering alcohol or drug dependent person continues to take therapeutic medications necessary to regain and maintain health. Many in recovery fear using *needed* medications for short periods and need guidance and support.

NURSING CARE IN THE HOME SETTING

Individual and family assessment

In ongoing work with individuals and families in the home, the community health nurse can observe for signs and symptoms of drug or alcohol abuse. In assessing the individual and family the nurse should use a standardized tool for recording data (Chapters 3 and 6 provide examples). The assessment should include an inventory of all alcohol and drugs used, including amounts and frequency. Signs and symptoms of withdrawal (see Chapter 4) may be one of the first indications of a substance abuse problem. The nurse should remember that one of the common symptoms of substance dependence is denial of the problem; information provided by the individual may minimize actual use. Additional information can be gathered, with the client's permission, from family members, employers, friends, and health care personnel.

In addition to the individual assessment, the family should be assessed. A current nuclear family history should be obtained that includes the following (Stanhope & Lancaster, 1992):

1. Family's sociodemographic profile;
2. Family's environment—strengths and problems regarding home, neighborhood, and community;
3. Family structure, processes, functions—strengths and limitations, existing and potential problems, interaction styles;
4. Family's coping ability—conflict management, support systems, life changes, and life satisfaction profile; and
5. Family's health behaviors—health history, status of health, ability to carry out activities of daily living, health risk profile, health beliefs, ability to care for self, resources for health care, and use of community health nursing services.

Also, a three generation family health history should be completed, including information about substance abuse, the presence of significant physical illness, social behaviors such as difficulty with the law, and any history of physical violence or child abuse.

Clues in the home

Many clues to substance abuse may be observable during home visits. Empty liquor or pill bottles may suggest substance abuse. Drug paraphernalia may be found. Behavior and problems of family members may yield evidence of substance abuse in the home. Children may appear neglected or may be undernourished, anemic, or hungry. The appearance of the home may be unkempt and dirty. Furniture may be lacking, and there may be evidence of a lack of food or other necessities. The home also may show signs of pest infestation. It is important, however, to note that not all homes of persons with substance abuse will show these characteristics. The spouse of an alcoholic, for instance, may overcompensate for the problem and keep the house clean and tidy.

Financial complaints are common in homes where substance abuse occurs. Money is often spent on alcohol or drugs rather than on the necessities of life. An abusing person may spend an entire paycheck during a cocaine binge, for example. Financial complaints also may be magnified because of unemployment.

Abuse

Abuse is commonly found in homes in which one or more members abuse drugs or alcohol. Abuse may include physical, emotional, and sexual abuse. Abuse tends to occur most often when the substance abuser is under the influence of alcohol or drugs. At other times the abuser may treat family members well. If the abuse occurred during a blackout, recollection of the incident may be absent. If there is memory of abusing, the alcoholic or drug addict may feel remorse and shame. As a result the person may overcompensate, showering those they harm with gifts, positive words, or outings. This cycle is difficult for those who are abused because they never know what to expect. If parents, for example, pretend that abuse did not occur, children may begin to feel that they did something to deserve the abuse. The startling contrast between behaviors and the lack of predictability keep family members confused. Children especially have difficulty understanding how a parent can seem like a cruel, overbearing monster one day and come home all smiles and bearing gifts the next (Prentice Hall Personnel Manager, 1989).

Physical abuse. Physical abuse refers to episodes of extreme discipline or displaced anger and frustration, often resulting in serious physical damage to the internal organs, bones, central nervous system, or sense organs of the abused person. This form of abuse is most often seen in child abuse as beating, burning, kicking, branding, or shaking. Box 10-1 illustrates some factors that may indicate child abuse, and Box 10-2 shows behavioral indicators of abusive parents.

The abuse found in families of substance abusers includes children and spouses. Children are frequently victims of abuse because they are small and powerless. Spouse abuse often accompanies child abuse and is an increasing problem. Spouse abuse is defined as any physical attack by one partner against another, ranging from a slap to homicide. Women are more often the victim of the abuse, but men also are abused by their wives.

Battered women often have bruises, lacerations, and broken bones. Frequently the injuries are carefully inflicted on parts of the body that can easily be concealed with clothing such as the abdomen, upper thigh, and back. Women stay in abusive relationships because they hope the spouse will reform, have no place to go, have financial problems, fear reprisals, or fear being alone.

Box 10-1
Factors That May Indicate Presence of or Potential for Child Abuse

1. Unexplained injury such as
   a. Skin—burns, old or recent scarring, bruising, swelling, bite marks
   b. Fractures—recent or healed
   c. Subdural hematomas
   d. Trauma to genitals
   e. Whiplash (caused by shaking young children)
2. Dehydration and malnourishment without apparent cause
3. Being given inappropriate foods or drugs (alcohol, for example)
4. Evidence of general poor care—poor hygiene, dirty clothes, unkempt hair, dirty nails
5. Unusual fear of nurse or other adults
6. Being considered a bad child
7. Inappropriate dress for season or weather conditions
8. Evidence or report of sexual abuse
9. Injuries not mentioned in history
10. Tendency to take care of the parent

From Stanhope, M. & Lancaster, H. (1992). *Community health nursing.* (2nd ed.). St. Louis: Mosby.

Emotional abuse.   Emotional abuse includes extreme debasement of another person's feelings, so that the person being abused feels inadequate, inept, uncared for, and worthless. An example of this is constant criticism and ridicule directed toward a spouse or child. As a result the person may ultimately believe that he or she is a bad person. Victims of emotional abuse learn to hide their feelings to avoid additional scorn. These repressed feelings then can lead to symptoms of hyperactivity, withdrawal, overeating, psychosomatic problems, vague complaints, stuttering, truancy, general hostility, or aggression toward others or themselves (Stanhope & Lancaster, 1992).

Box 10-2
Behavioral Indicators of Potentially Abusive Parents

1. Family beset by stress and numerous crises
2. Isolation from family, neighbors, or friends
3. Evidence of poor impulse control or fear of losing control
4. Contradictory history
5. Appearance of detachment
6. Use of drugs or alcohol
7. Shopping for hospitals or health care providers—often move around
8. Unrealistic expectations of a child

From Stanhope, M. & Lancaster, H. (1992). *Community health nursing.* (2nd ed.). St. Louis: Mosby.

Sexual abuse.   Sexual abuse ranges from fondling to rape. A particularly destructive form of sexual abuse sometimes found in families where substance abuse occurs is incest. Although incest is a problem of great magnitude, it often remains a family secret. It has been estimated that one of every four girls is molested sexually during childhood or adolescence (Stanhope & Lancaster, 1992). In more than one-third of the cases, the perpetrator is related to the victim (Stanhope & Lancaster, 1992). Many women who turn to drug or alcohol use are victims of incest. Many cases of parental incest go unreported because the victim fears punishment, abandonment, or family rejection.

INTERVENTION AND REFERRAL

One of the prime considerations for the nurse working with the substance abuser is to break through the denial that often exists regarding the substance abuse. Once this occurs, attempts to treat the abuser can occur. Often this requires either a brief intervention or a more structured intervention. Addressing denial is also discussed in Chapters 4 and 6.

Brief intervention

At times a substance abuser may be convinced to seek treatment on the basis of a brief intervention. A brief intervention is when a health professional presents clear data on the effects of the substance on the client's health and recommends a reduction in or abstinence from the substance. The community health nurse is in an ideal position to do this. Some general guidelines are helpful in these situations. First, the focus should be on developing a warm, accepting relationship. Informal teaching about physiological effects of substance abuse should be done whenever possible. The nurse should consider substance abuse an important health issue and be conscious of his or her own level of awareness and attitudes concerning substance abuse. It is important to avoid aiding the denial of the substance abuser. Finally, the nurse should be aware that life in an alcoholic family is unstable and unpredictable and that, as a professional, the nurse must be stable and predictable.

Structured intervention

If brief intervention techniques are ineffective, further efforts may be necessary. Some believe that only when the alcohol or drug dependent person desires and seeks help (that is, "hits bottom") can treatment be effective. A structured intervention is done to assist the person to recognize the problem. Recovering people call this "raising the bottom." The advantage of a planned intervention is that presenting concerns as a collective unit minimizes additional defensiveness and does not allow the abuser to manipulate individuals. Specific steps are listed here.

1. **Elicit family support**—Interventions are planned group confrontations by people who care about an individual who is abusing alcohol or drugs. Most often these people are family members. Their support and help for the intervention needs to be gathered for the intervention to be as successful as possible.

   One of the most difficult tasks for the nurse helping to elicit family support is breaking through the denial of family members. Even when they see the extent of the problem, the thought of confronting the substance abuser may be intimidating. Family members may require a great deal of support before, after, and during the intervention. A referral to Al-Anon may help prepare family members for this process.

2. **Obtain physician support, if possible**—Involvement of the substance abuser's physician often has a positive effect on the outcome of the intervention. Physicians often bring objective and subjective data indicating the need for treatment.

3. **Determine needed resources**—In planning an intervention, it is necessary to determine the type of treatment that will be suggested. This treatment should be arranged before the intervention so the substance abuser can receive help immediately. Often the subject of an intervention is brought to the point of readiness to accept help. Treatment should be offered before the denial can resurface. Planning for treatment may mean that the person is transported directly from the intervention to treatment.

4. **Assemble intervention team**—Members of the intervention team may include family members, clergy, physicians, neighbors, employers, coworkers, and other friends. The intervention team should be chosen and assembled before the actual intervention, and if possible at least one practice session should take place. This allows the members of the team to get comfortable with each other and practice stating the information they have to contribute. It is usually helpful to have those involved in the intervention write down their concerns. This helps maintain organization in the midst of the intense feelings often generated during an intervention (Burns, Thompson & Ciccone, 1991b). Additionally, members of the team need to determine the possible consequences if the individual fails to accept help. For example, will the person lose a job or be unwelcome at home? Often the consequences need to be great enough to encourage the person to receive help. If, during the intervention, the individual declines treatment, the consequences are immediately enforced.

5. **Use an expert, if needed**—Unless the community health nurse has been trained in the process of intervention, expert help should be obtained. This is available through counseling services, treatment centers, and some clergy. Without expert guidance the intervention can easily deteriorate into an exchange of insults, and the end result can be destructive rather than helpful.

Intervention process

The following are general rules for the process of intervention (Johnson, 1987):

1. Meaningful persons present facts or data.
2. The data presented is specific and describes events that have occurred or conditions that exist.
3. The tone of the confrontation is nonjudgmental.
4. Chief evidence should be tied into alcohol or drug abuse.
5. Behavior is presented in detail and should be explicit.
6. The goal of the intervention is for the substance abuser to see and accept reality so the need for help can be accepted.
7. Choices for treatment should be offered and should be available if at all possible (Johnson, 1987).

Follow-up

Follow-up for the person in treatment is both short- and long-term. Once a person enters treatment, it is helpful for the nurse to keep in contact. This will depend on the individual, however, because the individual must initiate contact and sign a release. Otherwise, confidentiality laws prevent the treatment staff from revealing any information about an individual. The nurse may become involved again when the individual returns home.

NURSING CARE IN SCHOOL SETTINGS

Primary prevention in schools

The school nurse can play an integral role in the primary prevention of drug and alcohol abuse. A quality school health education program should provide factual information about the harmful effects of drugs, support and strengthen students' resistance to using drugs, and carry out collaborative drug abuse prevention efforts with parents and other community members. It is important that the program be supported by school policies, as well as procedures for referral of students to treatment when substance abuse is detected. The alcohol or drug education program should help young people develop positive attitudes about themselves.

Educating students.   Educating students about substance abuse is an essential component of a comprehensive strategy to reduce demand for and use of drugs in the United States. In the past decade there has been a concerted effort to prevent substance abuse problems by educating the nation's students. The federal government first mandated prevention programs with the Drug-Free Schools and Community Act of 1986. This legislation requires elementary, middle, and high schools to have programs emphasizing a drug-free school environment. It also requires schools to provide drug education programs. In 1990 an amendment to the 1986 act required that colleges and universities also develop alcohol and drug prevention programs and evaluate the effectiveness of the program on a biennial basis. It also mandates that the university provide education to its faculty including the following:

1. Information about drugs and alcohol,
2. Information about available treatment programs,
3. Information about sanctions for unlawful possession or distribution of alcohol or drugs, and
4. Information about sanctions for persons who violate the standards of conduct.

"Healthy People 2000" is a federal initiative developed by the U.S. Public Health Service to promote health and prevent major illnesses, injuries, and infectious diseases throughout the coming decade. Measurable targets to be achieved by the year 2000 were established with the input of health care professionals, other disciplines, and consumers. One of the objectives of "Healthy People 2000" is the education of children regarding substance abuse. This objective states (National Institute on Drug Abuse, 1990),

Provide to children in all school districts and private schools primary and secondary school educational programs on alcohol and other drugs, preferably as part of quality school health education. (Baseline: 63% provided some instruction, 39% provided counseling, and 23% referred students for clinical assessments in 1987.)

Traditional alcohol and drug abuse programs have been aimed at junior and senior high school students. Because data show that the average age of first use for the gateway drugs (alcohol, tobacco, and marijuana) often occurs during the later elementary years, education also must be directed to elementary-age students.

Project DARE (Drug Abuse Resistance Education) is a program used in many school districts aimed at equipping fifth, sixth, and seventh graders with the skills and motivation to resist peer pressure to use alcohol, drugs, and tobacco. This program began as a joint project of the Los Angeles Police Department and the Los Angeles Unified School District. DARE instructors are uniformed police officers assigned to the project. The DARE project includes lessons about building self-esteem and avoiding the use of drugs. It ends with the reading of DARE pledges the students have written. The use of uniformed police officers is a key element in the success of the program; because the officers are in positive, nonpunitive roles, students are more likely to develop positive attitudes toward them (DeJong, 1987).

Peer training.   Peer training has become an important part of substance abuse programs for older students. Junior and senior high school students are trained as peer counselors or peer tutors. The peer counselors meet with students on a one-to-one or small-group basis to listen, inform, refer, and help peers solve their problems. Volunteer community service also may be a part of the program. The nurse may be involved in sponsoring or providing training for this program.

Educating other professional staff.   The school nurse has a responsibility and opportunity to educate other professional staff, including teachers, guidance counselors, and administrators. Teachers who are in frontline positions may be the first to detect alcohol and drug use in students, and they must be especially knowledgeable about signs and symptoms of abuse. They must be prepared to make referrals to the nurse or guidance counselor. This education can take place informally but is more effective as inservice education. The school nurse also may arrange for written literature to be made available to the school staff.

Secondary prevention in schools

Recognizing substance abuse in students.   Often the school nurse is the first person to notice signs of substance abuse in adolescent elementary students.

Characteristics of students who abuse drugs have been identified. These characteristics are listed in Box 10-3.

Teenage abusers often lag behind their peers in accomplishing the adolescent tasks necessary to reach emotional maturity. The lack of judgment that results from substance abuse may lead to unwanted pregnancy or to sexually transmitted diseases. Relationships with peers, parents, and teachers are often disrupted by abrupt personality and behavior changes. Because the child may attempt to hide use from

---

Box 10-3
Characteristics of Children Who Abuse Substances

Impaired school performance
Increased absenteeism and tardiness
Declining interest in academic work
Failure to do or complete assignments
Severe mood swings
Change in extracurricular participation
Sunglasses worn when not appropriate
Unusual outbursts of temper
Needle-track scars or trail of ecchymosis along course of veins on arms and hands
Continually wearing clothing with long sleeves
Deteriorating grooming habits and physical appearance
Stealing or unusual borrowing of money from parents or others
Frequenting of odd places such as closets or storage rooms
Shunning of responsibility
Noticeable personality changes
One long fingernail, especially males (used to spoon up cocaine)
Inability to stop drinking until inebriated
Constant depression
Change in peer group to include people who receive disapproval of family
Numerous accidents or driving tickets
Difficulty with authorities, including police
Chronic fatigue

From Lewis, K. & Thomson, H. (1986). *Manual of school health.* Menlo Park, CA: Addison-Wesley Publishing Co. Inc.

teachers and parents, peers may have the first insight into the change. When a relationship of trust exists between the student and the school's teaching or administrative staff, these changes are most likely to be reported (Lewis & Thompson, 1986).

While all youth are at risk for use and abuse of drugs, some are considered to be at high risk. These include children who have dropped out of school, have become pregnant, have economic disadvantages, or have a chemically dependent parent. Other categories of at-risk children include those that have been victims of any kind of child abuse, have been in trouble with police, have attempted suicide, or have had a long history of pain (Burns, Thompson, & Ciccone, 1991a, 1991b).

Rationales given by young people for the use of drugs and alcohol include curiosity, peer group pressure, insecurity, escape from reality, boredom, a sense of rebelliousness, and the desire for "kicks." Many adolescents experiment with drugs or alcohol to see how it feels. Some will become recreational or situational users. A few will cross into addiction and compulsive use.

Emergency care. The school nurse may have to provide emergency care for the student who has ingested alcohol or drugs. Symptoms will vary, depending on the kind and amount of the drug taken. Serious symptoms include the following (Creswell, 1989):

1. Lethargy
2. Confusion
3. Stupor
4. Combativeness
5. Self-destruction
6. Seizures
7. Unconsciousness
8. Derangement

Depending on the severity of these symptoms, it may be necessary to summon emergency help. The nurse should attempt to find out what drug was taken, the route of administration, and the dosage. Vital signs should be monitored until the ambulance arrives. Any pills, syringes, or drug paraphernalia found on the student should be sent to the hospital with the student. If the student is awake, emotional support should be provided. The nurse should provide reassurance and talk in a calm voice. Stimuli should be reduced. The student should be oriented to time, place, and circumstances. If the student is combative, physical restraint should be used only as a last resort. However, when offering aid to a student with a PCP-induced psychosis, precautions should be taken to minimize danger to school personnel. This includes ensuring that faculty have an emergency exit when confined with the student, that all items that could be used as weapons are removed from the area where the student is being examined, and that calmness and minimal contact with the student are maintained.

Treatment for students.   An intervention with a student with drug abuse should involve other members of the school staff such as the teachers, school psychologist, and guidance counselor, as well as the parents. The student should be referred to a treatment program that specializes in the care of children or adolescents.

Recognizing parental substance abuse.   As many as 6.5 million children under the age of 18 live in households where parents abuse substances (Rivinus, 1991). Some symptoms have been found to occur with greater frequency in these children; these include stuttering, bed wetting, fears, and social isolation after the age of six. Complaints of abdominal pain occur often. Also, school difficulties include temper tantrums, difficulty with school work, and fighting with other children.

A student may share concerns about parental drinking or drug use if he or she has developed a relationship with a teacher, nurse, guidance counselor, or other school official. These admissions should be taken seriously. Also, school officials should be aware of the correlation of abuse or neglect and familial substance abuse. This abuse may include neglect of the child, who may appear unkempt, malnourished or compliant (Rivinus, 1991). See also Chapter 9.

Tertiary prevention in schools

When a student has been treated for substance abuse and returns to school, it is important to provide support and encouragement for progress. The student should be encouraged to explore personal abilities and to determine ways of coping at home and at school. Counseling should be supported and a respected adult should be established as a role model. Some schools offer support groups for students in recovery.

NURSING CARE IN OCCUPATIONAL SETTINGS

Most corporations are well aware of the costs they incur as the result of substance abuse. These costs include higher health care rates, absenteeism, turnover, loss of productivity, and accidents caused by an employee under the influence of drugs or alcohol (Rice, 1990). The United States Chamber of Commerce estimates that annual drug abuse costs to the business community range from $30 billion to $100 billion (National Institute on Alcohol Abuse and Alcoholism, 1990).

In response, many companies have instituted drug and alcohol programs. These range from punitive policies (e.g., drug-testing procedures designed to identify and terminate drug-using employees) to programs that encourage employees to seek treatment and return to work (e.g., employee assistance programs). See Chapter 16 on drug testing.

Primary prevention in the workplace

Occupational health nurses often function as an integral part of an occupational alcohol or drug program. Their involvement in primary prevention includes advising management personnel of the need for a definitive policy to handle employees with substance abuse, as well as educating employees, including frontline supervisors, about identification, intervention, referral, treatment, and reentry of employees with substance abuse.

Company policies. The occupational health nurse must be familiar with the company's policies regarding substance abuse or be involved in developing them. Many employers give chemically dependent employees a chance to seek treatment, and in some cases they create a diversion program that circumvents the normal disciplinary process. In other cases the employee is encouraged to receive treatment, but also is given appropriate disciplinary action. Generally speaking, it is more advantageous to offer an employee treatment than to implement disciplinary action.

It is important that the following guidelines are included in policies regarding substance abuse (Shawe & Rosenthal, 1993; Prentice Hall Personnel Manager, 1989):

1. Adopt a policy statement that explains the company philosophy, taking into account concerns for employees' safety and well-being.
2. Define standards of conduct for use, possession, transfer, or sale of illicit drugs or alcohol on company premises or on company time. Include the consequences of improper use of prescription medication or being under the influence and use of alcohol or drugs on company premises.
3. Define methods of detection and the circumstances under which drug tests will be administered, including decisions about testing conditions and procedures, supervisory observations, searches, and confidentiality.

4. Describe how the policy will be enforced.
5. Define alternatives to discipline such as rehabilitative leaves of absence or referral to an employee assistance program.
6. Make sure the program has appropriate safeguards (proper notice, consent, releases, test levels, and confirmation of positive results).
7. Train all managers, especially frontline supervisors, to deal properly with substance abuse problems.
8. Provide all employees with a copy of the policy, and be certain they are familiar with it.

Employee assistance programs.   Employee assistance programs (EAPs) are designed to address a wide range of family and personal problems that affect or can affect job performance. The program's objectives are usually to reduce absenteeism and restore productivity of the worker. A reduction in work-related accidents also is a goal. Problems that can be dealt with by an EAP include (Rosow & Zager, 1985):
1. Emotional, psychological, marital, family, or financial problems that affect job performance or have the potential to do so,
2. Problems caused or aggravated by stress on the job, and
3. Problems for which the normal treatment is counseling or a change in lifestyle.

One of the most common problems handled by EAPs is substance abuse. Referral for treatment is often recommended if the EAP counselor suspects substance abuse. The employee who seeks help voluntarily may avoid disclosure to the employer. If performance problems become serious enough and the substance abuse becomes known by the employer, the employee assistance program can support the employee and monitor recovery at the same time.

An employer may have an in-house EAP or a contract for external EAP services. The internal or in-house EAP has several advantages. The staff can understand corporate policy and how it is interpreted, deal with problems as soon as they occur, and more easily lend counseling expertise and educational services to other company programs and supervisors. An external EAP, on the other hand, offers a greater degree of confidentiality and may be more cost-effective for a small company (Prentice Hall Personnel Manager, 1989).

Wellness programs.   Wellness programs are one part of a program of primary prevention that is especially well-suited to the workplace. Occupational health nurses can play an important role in instituting and maintaining such programs and emphasizing healthy alternatives to alcohol and drug use. Prevention can reduce absenteeism, lessen long-term health care costs, decrease the number of disability claims, increase productivity, and improve morale. The increase in wellness programs is in response to a number of factors, including employee concerns over rising health insurance premiums, public awareness of the effects of lifestyle changes on health, and incentives offered by insurance companies.

Wellness programs may include education, health counseling, nutritional guidance, exercise and fitness activities, and stress reduction programs, to name a few of the many options available. Some of the earliest wellness programs dealt with substance abuse. Evaluation of the success of these programs is often difficult because of a time lag between program activities and a measurable change in health status. It is also difficult to separate the effects of multiple interventions on improvements.

Secondary prevention in the workplace

Early identification of the employee with a substance abuse problem is important for successful treatment and rapid return to the job. Identification, however, is not easily accomplished because the signs and symptoms may not be readily apparent on the job or the employee may attempt to disguise use, fearing disciplinary action.

Assessment.   There are certain clues to substance abuse that are commonly seen in the workplace. Some substances are easier to detect than others. Supervisors can smell alcohol on an employee's breath, see the person staggering, and hear slurred speech. Other drugs are more difficult to detect.

The alcoholic or drug-addicted employee will often be absent from work, especially on Mondays or Fridays, days that adjoin a weekend off. Absenteeism also is more likely to occur around payday. The employee also may be increasingly late offering no excuses or unusual excuses. There may be early departures from work or extended lunch hours. There may be a change in performance noted after lunch.

The employee also may show a deterioration in quality and quantity of work done. Dependability may decrease. Physical appearance may deteriorate; the person may look unkempt at times. A change in interpersonal relationships may be apparent; conflicts may occur with coworkers. Health problems may increase. Finally, there is usually an increase in accidents both on and off the job.

The occupational health nurse will most likely interact with employees when seeing them for health screening or when providing care for injuries or illnesses sustained on the job. Most of the time the use of drugs and alcohol will not be easily apparent. The nurse will more likely see physical complaints that result from substance use or withdrawal such as intestinal problems, headache, or shakiness. Combined with job performance problems, these symptoms may indicate a substance abuse problem. An evaluation of performance that indicates possible substance abuse is the basis of the intervention strategy.

Counseling or intervention.   Initial counseling may be provided by the occupational health nurse directly, or the employee may be referred to either an employee assistance program or an outside counseling agency. The nurse also may be asked to take part in an intervention or may actually have responsibility for planning an intervention. Guidance from professionals in substance abuse treatment is recommended before conducting an intervention, unless the nurse has preparation in this area.

An intervention in the workplace is structured very much like that described for family members except events at work are used as a basis to persuade the individual that an evaluation is needed. (See previous section on intervention in a home setting.) The goal of the intervention is to get the employee to agree to an assessment of a possible substance abuse problem. The occupational health nurse may work with management or union officials to prohibit an employee from working until such an assessment is done. Because of the importance of employment in most people's lives, the employer is a persuasive force for motivating employees to seek an evaluation of substance abuse and to receive treatment if needed.

After an intervention in which the individual agrees to a substance abuse assessment, plans should be made. If the employee is under the influence of alcohol or drugs, he or she must be removed from work but should not be allowed to drive. If the intervention is unsuccessful, the usual disciplinary actions are taken.

Referral.   One of the occupational health nurse's primary roles with persons with substance abuse is referral for treatment. If the assessment results in a recommendation for treatment, satisfactory completion of treatment usually is required before the employee can return to work.

Negotiating treatment services.   The occupational health nurse may be involved in negotiating treatment for individual employees. This should be done carefully, maintaining fairness to all employees. The nurse may serve as the case manager for the employee and be involved in determining what treatment is offered. Repeat treatments may come under special scrutiny; this is especially important because relapse is a common feature of addiction and recovery.

Tertiary prevention in the workplace

Supervising return to work.   Once an employee completes treatment, it is important to supervise the return to work. Employee agreements and random urine screens are often used and job performance is monitored.

Employee agreements.   Many employers will ask that an employee sign an agreement upon return to work. In this contract the employee agrees to remain substance-free and to continue in any recommended follow-up treatment. The employee also may be asked to agree to random urine screens. As part of most agreements the employee understands that the expectations for work performance are the same as for other employees.

The employer may agree to allow the employee to attend support groups or other meetings during work time or arrange work schedules to allow such attendance. Some employers have someone such as an EAP counselor who helps provide support to the employee. The union also may assign a person for this role.

Supportive versus monitoring role.   At times the occupational health nurse is torn between the desire to support the substance abuser and the need to monitor the use of substances. On one hand, the nurse is an official of the company and as such is required to help maintain a drug-free workplace, which might involve reporting drug use. On the other hand, the nurse is a provider of care and as such is an advocate of the employee or patient. The nurse needs to understand the reason for monitoring and the importance of assisting employees to get the help required. The nurse should realize that some dependent persons will not seek help voluntarily, and the nurse cannot "fix" people. A deep sense of the importance of treating substance abuse as a danger to the abuser and other employees helps the nurse develop a professional role (see Care Plan 10-2).

Care Plan 10-2

A Monitoring Program in a Work Setting for a Client Recovering from Alcoholism

Harry is a 34-year-old engineer who was referred for treatment of alcohol and marijuana abuse by his employer through the employee assistance program. He had been missing days of work frequently, projects were completed late, and the project just before treatment was not completed at all despite repeated time extensions. Formerly an employee noted for few errors and flawless detail, errors were found frequently in the past few months. After an intervention carried out by his supervisor, the nurse, and the EAP counselor, he agreed to enter treatment. He has completed treatment and just returned to work. He is married and has four children.

ASSESSMENT

Harry was excited and anxious to return to work. He expressed appreciation for referral to treatment. He reported that things at home were going better than they have in years. He hoped he could improve things at work also.

NURSING DIAGNOSIS

Potential for ineffective individual coping related to recent cessation of substance use and new acquisition of alternative coping skills

Outcome identification	Nursing interventions	Rationale	Evaluation
Nursing diagnosis: Potential for ineffective individual coping related to recent cessation of substance use and new acquisition of alternative coping skills			
1. Client will remain free from alcohol and drug use on a continuing basis.	1a. Develop therapeutic relationship with the client.	1a. Therapeutic relationship is necessary to develop trust.	1. Harry expressed appreciation for the nurse's interest in his concerns. He remained free from drugs and alcohol throughout the two-year period. Goal met.
	1b. Examine values and feelings about alcohol use.	1b. The nurse's feelings and values may interfere with the therapeutic process for the client.	
	1c. Listen to the client's progress and demonstrate concern and support.	1c. The nurse can function as a support person for the recovering client.	
	1d. Reinforce the advantages of ongoing sobriety to the client's health and job security.	1d. The nurse reinforces the need for ongoing measures to maintain sobriety. AODA is a chronic disease and prone to relapse.	

Outcome identification	Nursing interventions	Rationale	Evaluation
Nursing diagnosis: Potential for ineffective individual coping related to recent cessation of substance use and new acquisition of alternative coping skills—cont'd			
	1e. If the client doubts the need for ongoing measures to maintain sobriety, gently relate previous problems and lack of control with consequences.	1e. Same as above.	
	1f. Offer help if the client is having difficulty coping.	1f. Offers the nurse as a resource person.	
	1g. Encourage client to talk about his difficulties.	1g. Talking about difficulties affords the opportunity to find solutions and elicit support from others.	
	1h. Help client develop a plan of action to resolve difficulties.	1h. One key to maintaining sobriety is moderating stress levels.	
	1i. Teach healthy lifestyle—adequate sleep, nutrition, exercise, and social interaction.	1i. A healthy lifestyle helps decrease stressful feelings and increase a sense of well-being.	
	1j. Refer client for additional treatment or therapy if needed.	1j. Some of the client's difficulties may be beyond the scope of the nurse's practice.	

Costs

Insurance. The occupational health nurse needs to know provisions for alcohol and drug treatment by the health care insurers of the company. In most instances, insurers' provisions are spelled out and should be followed to facilitate maximum coverage and treatment. Some insurance companies require precertification for treatment, some need proof of a failed outpatient treatment, and many only cover outpatient treatment. The occupational health nurse can act as a liaison to make sure needed information is provided and the best choice is made. The nurse working in an occupational health setting must be aware of the insurance options workers have and help facilitate approval for treatment if appropriate.

Impact on workers' compensation. The occupational health nurse should be aware that intoxication is one of the several defenses available to employers facing potential liability for worker's compensation. Some states disallow benefits entirely when the injury resulted from drug or alcohol intoxication. The following questions commonly arise when intoxication is a question:

1. Whether intoxication was the sole cause of the injury or whether the cause was work-related,
2. Whether the injury occurred in the normal course of employment, and
3. Whether the injury occurred accidentally.

Documentation of all facts and observations concerning the injury is important. If company policies and procedures allow for drug and alcohol testing in this circumstance, it should be done.

Employees' rights

Preemployment drug and alcohol screening. In an effort to prevent future problems with substance abuse, more and more companies are requiring drug testing of job applicants. Preemployment screening may identify that a person has used the substance in the recent past. Even with preemployment testing, drug or alcohol dependency is difficult to detect.

Random drug testing. In some industries with the potential to harm the public, random drug testing of employees is allowed. These industries include employees of the Department of Defense, some federal contractors and grantees, and the Department of Transportation. Other employers vary in their approach to drug testing (see Chapter 16).

Confidentiality. Confidentiality is extremely important when dealing with employees with substance abuse. Results of drug testing should be released only on a need-to-know basis and with written consent of the employee tested. Confidentiality protects the company and prevents damage to an employee's reputation or work history. Also, federal confidentiality laws prohibit drug treatment providers from releasing information about a person's treatment without written releases.

Americans with Disabilities Act of 1990. The Americans with Disabilities Act of 1990 (ADA) is a comprehensive effort to eliminate discrimination against persons with disabilities (see Chapter 15 for more about ADA provisions). According to the ADA, a *qualified individual with a disability* is an individual with a disability who can perform the essential functions of the employment position that they hold or desire, with or without reasonable accommodations. The employer must provide reasonable accommodation, as long as it does not impose an "undue hardship" on the operations of the business. This *undue hardship* is an action requiring significant difficulty or expense. This is determined by considering several factors, including the financial cost and the resources of the organization.

The most notable exclusion from the definition of "qualified individual with a disability" is for current users of illegal drugs and alcohol. Once an employee has successfully participated in a "supervised drug rehabilitation program," has "otherwise been rehabilitated," or is participating in such a program and is no longer engaging in drug use, the person is qualified to be protected under ADA. This is also true for persons who have been "erroneously regarded" as using drugs. Also, ADA provides that an employer may hold drug users and alcoholics to the same standards of performance as other employees. The ADA further provides that an employer may

1. Ban the use of alcohol or the illegal use of drugs at the workplace,
2. Require that employees are not under the influence of alcohol or illegal drugs at the workplace, and
3. Require that employees abide by federal workplace requirements regarding alcohol and the illegal use of drugs.

Communication with others

It is important for the occupational health nurse to establish a working relationship with others in the organization, including supervisors, union representatives, and the human resources department. Effective treatment and reentry of employees are facilitated when such positive working relationships are developed.

Supervisors.   The occupational health nurse needs to maintain good communication with supervisors in the workplace. Supervisors are likely to be the first to recognize performance problems in an employee who may be abusing drugs and alcohol, and they will be monitoring the employee returning to work after treatment. Education of supervisors includes teaching them signs and symptoms of drug and alcohol abuse and how to confront an employee. The supervisor also should be educated about provisions made for employees returning to work after receiving help.

Unions.   Unions have a direct interest in health care management because union members are the recipients of health care benefits and because inflating health care costs displace other benefits, perhaps even wage increases. Union members are interested in quality of care, coverage, and accessibility of benefits, especially when health care is costly and employment security is doubtful. Nationally, union-management cooperation on cost containment in health care remains strong, although individual employers and local unions may clash on this issue. One area of disagreement is the inclusion of benefits for drug and alcohol treatment.

Human resources department. It is important for the company's human resources department to be involved in all cases of employee substance abuse. The department can be a real asset to the occupational nurse, ensuring that employees are treated as fairly as possible and that the company is also protected. Policies and procedures regarding substance abuse should be developed with the help of this department.

Treatment providers. In addition to maintaining a positive working relationship with internal constituents, communication between the occupational health nurse and treatment center personnel is important. The nurse should request that a release be signed by the client so information regarding treatment outcomes and recommendations is available to the employer. Open communication enables planning for the employee's return to work. The occupational health nurse may be involved in discharge planning at the treatment center.

NURSING CARE IN OUTPATIENT SETTINGS

The nurse working in outpatient settings plays an integral role in case finding and referral of those with substance abuse problems.

Prenatal and well-baby clinics

Prenatal and well-baby clinics provide opportunities for the nurse to identify substance abuse problems in parents and future parents. Pregnant women may be more receptive to the need for treatment because of the child they are carrying. Prenatal and well-baby clinics are also a logical place to offer educational programs about alcoholism and drug abuse. Appropriate literature can be shared with the people attending the clinic, also. (Several chapters in this book provide information about nursing in outpatient settings, including Chapter 8.)

Surgi-centers

Surgi-centers were first developed as an alternative to the traditional hospital surgical stay. Surgeries that do not require an overnight stay can be performed at a surgi-center. Patients with substance abuse problems may be detected during preoperative screening, while observing the actual operative procedure, or by monitoring the postanesthesia period. Patients who abuse alcohol and drugs may require additional anesthesia or pain medication. Surgi-centers should have policies and procedures for the referral of clients for treatment of detected drug and alcohol abuse. (See Chapter 7 for care of the surgical client.)

Urgent care centers

Urgent care centers have become the primary medical care providers in many areas. They are designed to treat patients with immediate health care problems (e.g., symptoms of influenza) that do not require the hospital emergency room. Many persons with injuries or with physical ailments caused by substance abuse may first present to these settings. Proper referral of the patient when substance abuse is suspected is important.

Primary care

Primary care settings are the best source for assessment and detection of substance abuse. The relationship with primary care physicians, nurse practitioners, and office nurses often leads the patient to admit to use. Also, knowledge of the patient over a period of time allows the staff to recognize signs and symptoms of substance abuse (e.g., suspicious illnesses, frequent accidents, recurring family problems) and to recommend early treatment for substance abuse. Screening of new clients and periodic rescreening for substance abuse are paramount to providing quality care.

SUMMARY

The nurse who works in a community may encounter substance abuse issues in any setting, with any population, and at all levels of prevention. The community health nurse may be involved with primary prevention in the schools, the workplace, the home, and the community at large. Nurses working in the community play a key role in identifying the client who is abusing drugs or alcohol in any of these settings, referring the client for support groups or treatment, or assisting in a planned intervention to move the client into treatment. Frequently, it is the nurse who identifies abuse or other sequelae of substance abuse and initiates protection or intervention for the child or older adult. In addition, the nurse's knowledge about the disease of substance abuse can assist the nurse in supporting those persons who are recovering.

REFERENCES

Anderson, J. & Yuhos, R. (1993). Health promotion in rural settings: A nursing challenge. *Nursing Clinics of North America, 28*(1), 145-155.

Burns, E., Thompson, A., & Ciccone, J. (1991a). *An addictions curriculum for nurses and other helping professionals. Level A: Basic knowledge and practice.* Columbus, OH: The Ohio State University College of Nursing.

Burns, E., Thompson, A., & Ciccone, J. (1991b). *An addictions curriculum for nurses and other helping professionals. Level B: Advanced knowledge and practice.* Columbus, OH: The Ohio State University College of Nursing.

Creswell, W. (1989). *School health practice.* St. Louis: Mosby.

DeJong, W. (1987). A short-term evaluation of Project DARE: Preliminary indications of effectiveness. *Journal of Drug Education, 17,* 279-294.

Dumas, L. (1992). Addicted women: Profiles from the inner city. *Nursing Clinics of North America, 27*(4), 901-915.

Iber, F. (1990). Alcoholism and associated malnutrition in the elderly. *Nutrition and Aging,* 157-173.

Johnson, V. (1987). *Intervention.* Minneapolis: Johnson Institute.

Krach, P. (1990). Discovering the secret: Nursing assessment of elderly alcoholics in the home. *Journal of Gerontological Nursing, 1611,* 32-38.

Levy, S. & Rutter, E. (1992). *Children of drug abusers,* New York: Lexington Books.

Lewis K. & Thomson, H. (1986). *Manual of school health.* Menlo Park, CA: Addison-Wesley Publishing Co Inc.

Long, B. (1993). *Medical-surgical nursing: A nursing process approach.* St. Louis: Mosby.

Long, K. (1993). The concept of health: Rural perspectives. *Nursing Clinics of North America, 28*(1), 123-131.

National Institute on Alcohol Abuse and Alcoholism. (1990). *Seventh special report to the U.S. Congress on alcohol and health: From the Secretary of Health and Human Services.* (DHHS Publication No. ADM 90-1656). Alexandria, VA: Edelmeal Experts, Inc.

National Institute on Drug Abuse. (1990). *National household survey on drug abuse: Main finding.* DHHS Publication No. (ADM 90-1681). Washington, D.C.: US Government Printing Office.

Prentice Hall Personnel Manager. (1989). *Policies and procedures.* Englewood Cliffs, NJ: Prentice Hall.

Rice, D. (1990). *The economic costs of alcohol and drug abuse.* San Francisco: Institute for Health and Aging.

Rivinus, T. (1991). *Children of chemically dependent parents.* New York: Brunner/Mazel Inc.

Rosow, J. & Zager, R. (1985). *Improving health-care management in the workplace: A work in American institute policy study.* New York: Pergamon Press Inc.

Shawe & Rosenthal Firm. (1993). *Employment law deskbook.* Baltimore, MD: Matthew Bender & Co, Inc.

Stanhope, M. & Lancaster, H. (1992). *Community health nursing.* (3rd ed). St. Louis: Mosby.

11 Nursing Care in Chemical Dependency Treatment Settings

This chapter focuses on nursing care in a substance abuse treatment setting; however, clients with substance abuse are seen in a variety of health care settings. This chapter covers the factors that affect nursing care in substance abuse treatment, the interdisciplinary aspects of substance abuse treatment, including the use of recovering personnel, and nursing care during detoxification and treatment.

FACTORS AFFECTING NURSING CARE IN SUBSTANCE ABUSE TREATMENT

The type of nursing care and the role of the nurse in substance abuse varies widely from treatment facility to treatment facility. This variety in nursing roles is a result of many factors including the following:

1. The philosophy of the treatment setting,
2. The number of nurses educated in substance abuse and their level of education,
3. The program's values related to education and certification,
4. Organizational structure regarding to whom nursing and other team members report, and
5. The level of nursing leadership on the substance abuse treatment team.

Philosophy

A wide variety of philosophical beliefs result in the treatment modalities used in specific treatment settings. The program's philosophy identifies beliefs about the etiology of substance abuse, its appropriate treatment, the location for treatment, client goals, and plans for long-term follow-up. These philosophies affect the structure of the setting, its functioning, and the role of the nurse. Some of the major opposing philosophies are described here.

Social versus medical model concerns whether the program is developed around a medical model or a social model of treatment. Medical model programs are usually located in hospitals and have traditional staffing patterns. Social model programs are common in the community and use nurses minimally. Other health care professionals are used to treat medical problems, often through an emergency room.

Detoxification versus rehabilitation versus habilitation concerns whether the program's focus is primarily treating withdrawal, returning the individual to prior functioning, or helping the client develop a higher level of functioning. For example, adolescent substance abusers, particularly those who began use at an early age, fail to develop age-appropriate social, academic, and vocational skills, and need habilitation to develop those skills.

Abstinence versus maintenance concerns long-term goals for clients. While abstinence from all substances is the most common treatment goal in the United States, some programs, such as methadone maintenance, have the treatment goal of maintaining the client on a substitute substance.

Step-down versus long-term care refers to the type of program and services offered. A *step-down program* has a continuum of treatment modalities and places clients according to the best match of client needs and program availability. The client might progress from detoxification to partial-day hospitalization to outpatient counseling. Other options may include a halfway house or assisted living. A *long-term care program* implements a traditional 28-day program for all clients.

Inpatient versus outpatient treatment involves whether the client is admitted for a hospital stay or treated on an outpatient basis during the day or evening while living at home. The intensity of the program varies, as well as staffing needs.

Disease versus illness model is a philosophical controversy that affects the type of program. The disease model defines substance abuse as a primary disease in and of itself (IOM, 1990). This model is closely tied to Alcoholics Anonymous (AA) and the inpatient mode of treatment. The illness model of substance abuse is more closely tied to a psychological model of substance abuse and may result in a social or outpatient model of treatment that includes individual or group psychotherapy.

Twelve step programs versus other treatment modalities refer to the treatment approach used. When a twelve step program is the primary modality, recovering counselors and AA volunteers are often responsible for much of the program. This results in an orientation that may be less broad-based than that of a program based on an interdisciplinary team approach.

These philosophic differences dramatically affect the number of nurses employed in the treatment facility. Social detoxification units may or may not hire nursing personnel, while social rehabilitation programs may hire only one nurse (1.0 full-time equivalent [FTE]) or one nurse per shift per day (4.2 FTEs). Hiring is often guided by accreditation standards, which are minimal regarding nurse staffing. Unless nurses can clearly demonstrate their versatility in this setting, nursing will continue to have limited involvement in social detoxification settings.

Medical detoxification units vary in the numbers of nurses per shift based on a number of factors, including (1) whether the program involves medical detoxification only or medical detoxification and a rehabilitation or treatment program; (2) whether the setting is a free-standing facility without intensive care capabilities, a unit within a medical center, or allocated beds on another primary unit; (3) whether budget limitations create a climate in which nurses are perceived as expensive and only the minimum required are hired (this is a short-sighted approach, however, because nurses are a much more versatile and cost-effective employee), and (4) the type of system used to determine the acuity of clients and the recommended staffing patterns related to that acuity, particularly regarding the type of nursing personnel and shift.

Education of nurses in a substance abuse practice

Another critical factor is the educational level of nurses employed in the treatment setting. Not only does the level of formal education impact the roles and costs of nursing personnel, but, more important, education increases the nurse's substance abuse knowledge and skills. A variety of initiatives have been developed to increase substance abuse knowledge in nursing schools and among practicing nurses. At the national level, these initiatives include model curriculum grants, faculty development grants, and an American Nurses Association (ANA) position paper.

Model curriculum grants in three schools of nursing were funded by the Office of Substance Abuse Prevention (now the Center for Substance Abuse Prevention [CSAP]) and administered by the National Institute of Alcohol Abuse and Alcoholism (NIAAA) and the National Institute for Drug Abuse (NIDA). These grants funded the development of three model substance abuse curricula that are now available to all nursing schools. The curricula are particularly convenient because they are complete, containing overhead masters, student handouts, and references (Naegle, 1991, 1992; Church, Fisk & Neafsey, 1992; Burns & Thompson, 1993).

Faculty development grants in 11 schools of nursing also were funded by CSAP and directed by NIAAA and NIDA. These grants allowed three to five faculty fellows in each grantee school to develop expertise in substance abuse. The fellows were required to represent different clinical areas; as a result of this requirement, breadth of substance abuse expertise was developed within each school (Gerace et al, 1992).

An ANA *position paper* calls for substance abuse education in every nursing curriculum and every setting where nurses are employed, including content specific to the ages of the clients served. Additionally the paper calls for more substance abuse-related items on state board examinations, mandatory substance abuse courses in states that require continuing education for relicensure, and an increased number of substance abuse specialty tracks in graduate nursing programs (ANA, 1991).

Education and certification.   Currently, variations in formal education for nurses employed in substance abuse treatment settings are further complicated by variations in the certification with which nurses validate their competency in substance abuse. Nurses may be certified in addictions nursing practice (Certified Addictions Registered Nurse, CARN), chemical dependency nursing (Certified Chemical Dependency Nurse, CCDN), substance abuse counseling at the state or national level (National Certified Addictions Counselor, NCAC I or II), or as Certified Employee Assistance Program Counselors (CEAP).

Educational requirements for nurses in substance abuse vary dramatically across treatment settings and geographic locations. Urban areas have greater access to certified and master's-prepared nurses. Organizational budgets may impact employment requirements and salary levels and therefore the ability to attract qualified nurses.

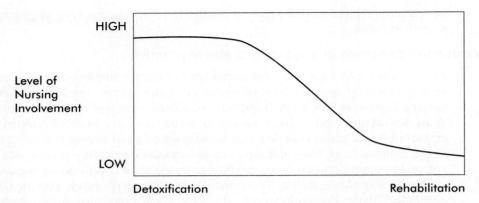

Fig. 11-1. Nursing involvement in traditional model of medical treatment.

Role of the nurse in the organization

Different models of treatment and organizational structure affect the level of nursing involvement. Figure 11-1 illustrates nursing involvement in a traditional model, and Figure 11-2 is an example of a social model that includes both detoxification and rehabilitation. In a traditional medical model program, nurses are highly involved in client care during the detoxification phase but scarcely involved in rehabilitation. Medical model programs are more common in traditional inpatient institutional settings and attract clients with more serious health problems. Detoxification of these clients requires greater nursing care.

In the social model, detoxification is often handled without medication. There may be moderate nursing involvement in detoxification because the clients are likely to be healthier and the setting is often in the community. Nursing may have little involvement in rehabilitation.

Each organizational structure has assets and liabilities. During major organizational restructuring, nurses must weigh the strengths of the organizational struc-

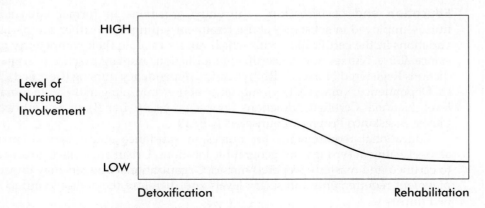

Fig. 11-2. Nursing involvement in social model of treatment.

ture in which they seek or continue employment, especially in regard to where nursing fits in the structure and thus its ability to carry out the nursing role effectively. Regardless of the formal structure, it is critical that nurses determine the scope of nursing practice and participate in defining the role of nursing in the treatment setting. When nurses actively participate in determining their roles on the interdisciplinary team, they are in better positions to control their practice, promote the development of nursing expertise in substance abuse, and demonstrate the value of their nursing knowledge.

Treatment programs with nurses in key administrative positions encourage and promote the fullest use of nursing abilities. In this case nurses are more likely to be actively involved in both detoxification and rehabilitation. Also, nurse administrators are better able to move nurses from a strictly detoxification model to integrated members of the interdisciplinary treatment team. Figure 11-3 illustrates a model of desired nursing involvement.

How can nurses entering the substance abuse field identify the best setting for practicing nursing? How do experienced nurses assess a treatment setting to see if their interests and the facility's interests match? The philosophies and characteristics discussed previously should be explored from the perspective of the organization and the nurse. The better the fit between the nurse and the facility's philosophy and values, the more likely it is that the nurse will blossom professionally in the setting.

INTERDISCIPLINARY ASPECTS OF SUBSTANCE ABUSE TREATMENT

Nursing involvement in interdisciplinary collaboration is a standard in the *Standards of Addictions Nursing Practice* (ANA & NNSA, 1988). Although the terms *interdisciplinary* and *multidisciplinary* are sometimes used interchangeably, McGivern (1991) makes a useful distinction based on team interactions. According to her schema, *multidisciplinary interaction* involves several disciplines that rarely interact, and the members represent only their respective disciplines. *Interdisciplinary interactions* involve mutual problem solving in which members learn from each other

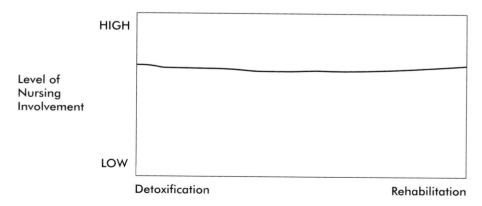

Fig. 11-3. Nursing involvement in desired model of treatment.

through team interaction. *Transdisciplinary interaction* refers to interactions that transcend disciplinary boundaries. The term *interdisciplinary* is used here because the goal of the team is mutual problem-solving.

A substance abuse treatment program assembles a unique team from various disciplines to provide care. Interdisciplinary team members contribute to the program from three perspectives: (1) the unique perspective of their professional discipline, (2) the unique skills and talents of the individual members, and (3) the members' unique personal experiences with substance abuse.

Each discipline has its own perspective, language, and approach that direct the practitioner's approach to substance abuse. The initial task of the treatment team is for members to share this information and enhance their understanding of each other's perspective. Embedded in the discipline-specific perspective is the individual's unique skills, interests, and talents, which are often developed within the framework of the discipline. It is important for the team to identify and use these individual talents.

The third component is the individual's unique experience with substance abuse. Some team members may be recovering from substance abuse and are affected by their personal use, treatment, and recovery experiences. Other team members may have personal experiences with substance abuse of significant others. These personal experiences are often the impetus for working in the field, and they may influence the effectiveness of the individual positively or negatively. These experiences need to be carefully processed by the individual before entering the substance abuse field. Personal counseling or therapy may be necessary to resolve personal experiences sufficiently before the team member can respond appropriately to clients.

This combination of training, individual skills, and unique experiences allows the team to identify and use the unique aggregate of talents within the team (Mariano, 1989b). *Role conflict* describes situations in which factors other than discipline determine which team member performs specific tasks (Mariano, 1989a). Potential role conflict also occurs in substance abuse treatment settings; who runs a specific group may depend on who can do it best, has the most interest, or has the time available, assuming that several team members are educationally prepared for the task. This can be either threatening or exhilarating to team members.

One reason for role diffusion in substance abuse treatment is that the knowledge base is not unique to any one discipline, although each discipline has its own perspective. For example, nursing process and the use of nursing diagnoses are unique nursing perspectives; however, they can be interpreted and used in a manner that has meaning for the total team. Historically, no discipline has clearly included substance abuse content in its basic program, thus many professionals have learned their skills on the job. Because of the blending of skills, health care professionals are not necessarily given leadership by virtue of their discipline, as is typical in traditional hospital settings (e.g., physicians in charge of total client care).

A component that may affect role diffusion is the development of the demonstrated competency standard by the Joint Commission on the Accreditation of Health Care Organizations (JCAHO). According to this standard, staff members must demonstrate competency in selected skills before using the skills in the workplace. Whether certification itself will demonstrate competence has not yet been determined. Many group treatment modalities fall under this standard. Health care organizations may limit use of these skills to those who demonstrate competency upon employment, develop internal or external training programs to develop the skills, or develop mechanisms to measure performance.

The first task of a treatment team is to identify its unique individual skills and talents, then determine optimal use of these talents in client care. The current health care climate, with its increasing emphasis on cost-effectiveness, adds cost as a factor in deciding who delivers care. Often salary differential between nurses and substance abuse counselors becomes an issue. Counselors' salaries are generally lower than nurses', although nurses have more health care knowledge and a broader perspective.

The disciplines involved in substance abuse treatment include *nursing* (generalists and specialists), *medicine, psychology, social work,* and *substance abuse counseling.* Their preparation and their most common roles are described as follows.

Nurse generalists.   Substance abuse nurses often are drawn to the specialty through personal experiences. Because students have inconsistent educational experiences with substance abuse, they are rarely exposed to it. When student clinical experiences in substance abuse become more common, earlier entry into the specialty should result.

Another reason for relatively few generalist nurses in substance abuse is that, historically, nursing education on substance abuse has been minimal. One study reported an average class time of 5 hours allocated to alcohol and drug content (Hoffman & Heinemann, 1987). Today, nursing educators are making attempts to increase substance abuse content and clinical experiences, and through continuing education, practicing nurses are also receiving content on substance abuse.

Nurse specialists.   Several routes lead to nursing specialization in substance abuse. Often, specialty knowledge has been obtained on the job and through continuing education. The advent of nursing certification in substance abuse has created a mechanism to recognize that skill and knowledge.

Three specialty nursing organizations currently represent nurses in substance abuse and offer certification. The National Nurses Society on Addictions (NNSA) has interpreted addictions broadly to include chemical and process addictions (gambling, sexual addiction, and food addictions). NNSA sponsors certification as a CARN through the Addictions Nursing Certification Board. Two other nursing organizations also sponsor certification (see Chapter 17).

Many substance abuse nurses are also credentialed as substance abuse counselors. Some nurses function in counselor rather than nursing roles or in combined roles. Some nurses maintain both credentials for maximum flexibility. Whether counselor certification will be replaced by nursing certification depends on the particular work role and the evolving significance of nursing certification. Salary and work factors will undoubtedly impact which route nurses take in credentialing.

A few nursing schools have graduate programs with substance abuse concentrations. This concentration may be independent or a subspecialty of psychiatric nursing. Research on substance abuse nursing also is developing through doctoral study by nurses specializing in substance abuse. As graduate programs produce faculty knowledgeable in substance abuse, education of all nurses, especially those practicing in substance abuse, should improve. (See Chapter 14 for more about education for substance abuse nursing.)

Other professional roles in substance abuse treatment

Medical practice. Addictions medicine is not the purview of any particular medical specialty, although psychiatrists often have the most exposure to substance abuse treatment and treatment settings in their clinical training. Actual practice roles are determined by physician interest, training, and the treatment setting. Often, a physician or physician group acts as medical director of a treatment program and provides medical care for clients. For reimbursement purposes, third-party payers usually require a medical director (IOM, 1990).

Specialty training and certification in addictions medicine is available through the American Society on Addictions Medicine (ASAM), formerly the American Medical Society on Alcoholism and Other Drug Dependencies (Galanter, 1989). A survey of ASAM-certified physicians indicates that the most frequent medical specialties represented are general and family practice, psychiatry, and internal medicine (Schnoll et al, 1993).

Psychology. The role of psychology in substance abuse treatment varies from conducting psychological testing to full participation in the treatment program as a therapist. Psychologists typically have a doctorate in either clinical or counseling psychology, and their substance abuse experience may be from internships or work in a treatment program. While most psychology curricula have some content on alcohol and drug abuse, the amount varies considerably. Psychologists with master's preparation may function as substance abuse counselors. State regulations control the education and practice of psychology, and these regulations vary from state to state.

Social work. Social work curricula do not routinely cover substance abuse. Although some social work programs specialize in substance abuse, others barely mention it (Corrigan & Anderson, 1985). Social workers in substance abuse usually have additional credentials in substance abuse counseling. Their role is often as a primary therapist or case manager.

Substance abuse counseling. Substance abuse counselors also are termed alcohol, drug, or addictions counselors. Credentials vary greatly. As an emerging group, consensus on academic content and credentialing is still developing. Accreditation can be through national counselor organizations or state organizations. Most states have a mechanism to accredit substance abuse counselors through a required course of study and supervised clinical experience. Because state credentials vary, a variety of certifications exist. National certification is available as a Nationally Certified Addictions Counselor (Level I or II) through examination.

The role of the substance abuse counselor involves many components of substance abuse treatment. Counselors can provide individual and group counseling, as well as other facets of treatment. In some settings, they act as case managers.

Using recovering personnel in treatment.   Many substance abuse personnel have prior personal experience with substance abuse. This experience may be personal, through family, or through significant others. A recent survey of nationally accredited substance abuse counselors found that 63% were in recovery (NCADD, 1993).

The use of recovering practitioners is somewhat unique to the substance abuse field. There are few other clinical areas in which treatment professionals have experienced the disease. In substance abuse the converse is true; recovering personnel are so common that nonrecovering personnel are unusual.

Often a specific period of sobriety, usually 2 to 3 years, is required by an employing treatment facility before the recovering professional is eligible to work with clients. The treatment setting also may apply this mandate to AA volunteers. Volunteers in treatment programs usually are involved in integrating twelve step groups into the treatment program. Treatment programs commonly integrate an ongoing twelve step group or offer an introduction to AA, Narcotics Anonymous (NA), or other appropriate twelve step group.

It is somewhat unclear what effect the Americans with Disabilities Act (ADA) may have on the use of recovering personnel. Because the act bars employment discrimination against those with disabilities, and recovery from substance abuse is a disability, it may affect the usual mandate regarding length of time in recovery before hiring. Overall, this issue remains to be resolved. (See Chapter 16 for further discussion of the ADA.)

There are advantages and disadvantages of using recovering personnel to care for substance abuse clients. One advantage is the powerful impact they have on clients as role models. They speak with experience and have worked out the same issues. Historically, recovering alcoholics have reached out to fellow substance abusers, often as part of their own twelve step programs, but also out of understanding and compassion.

There are potential disadvantages. It is important for recovering personnel to see clients' needs more broadly than their own experience. Otherwise, they may see their recovery as the only "right way." While their recovery provides valuable experience, clients have varying needs and experiences of their own. The need to broaden one's perspective can be met by observing and learning as a member of the treatment team and through additional education.

Also, recovering personnel need to continue their own program of recovery. The term "recovering," rather than "recovered," presents substance abuse as a chronic disease in which there is always risk of relapse. Helping professions are often at risk of neglecting their personal well-being, and in this case personal well-being is crucial to maintain recovery.

As a practical matter, treatment programs need policies concerning relapse of recovering personnel. Organizational responses should help the person return to recovery in a timely fashion. The effect of the relapse on clients should be responded to appropriately (Kinney, 1983).

NURSING CARE IN DETOXIFICATION

Substance abuse treatment is a multistage process. The first stage, *detoxification,* focuses on stabilizing the client physiologically and psychologically in a substance-free state. The second stage, *rehabilitation or treatment,* focuses on addressing the actual substance abuse problem through an organized treatment program. The third stage, *aftercare or continuing care,* focuses on assisting the client in remaining substance-free in their own environments and includes relapse prevention strategies (see Chapter 5).

Detoxification involves reestablishing homeostasis in the absence of the abused substance or substances. Long-term substance abuse causes physiologic and psychologic symptoms when the substance is withdrawn, particularly when withdrawal is abrupt. This is true physical dependence; that is, the body has adjusted to the substance so that withdrawal symptoms occur when the substance is removed. These withdrawal symptoms can vary greatly.

Assessment of withdrawal

In general the symptoms of withdrawal are the opposite of the drug effect. For example, clients with alcohol abuse accustomed to the depressant effects of alcohol may experience increased stimulation, particularly in the autonomic nervous system. Clients accustomed to the stimulant effect of cocaine experience depression and lack of energy. This reversal of symptoms is thought to be due to a rebound phenomenon related to reversal of the effect of the substance on neurotransmitters (Woolf, 1991a).

The presence and degree of withdrawal symptoms is poorly understood but thought to be related to (1) the *substance or substances used,* (2) the *patterns of use,* including amount and length of use, and (3) the *physiological and psychological status of the client.* Even with an accurate drug use history, prediction of withdrawal symptoms is very imprecise, thus close monitoring of the client during detoxification is essential.

Substances used.   Because the symptoms of withdrawal are determined by the substance used, it is important that the nurse and the treatment team have a detailed substance use history (see Chapter 3) and a current, working knowledge of usual withdrawal symptoms. The amount of the substance used, time of last use, and half-life of the substance predict when withdrawal symptoms are likely to occur. The most dangerous substances for detoxification are the central nervous system depressants—alcohol, benzodiazepines, and barbiturates. In each case the body develops a true physiological tolerance to the substance, and withdrawal can result in severe physiological reactions or even death.

Patterns of use.   The patterns of use also affect withdrawal symptoms. A substance that has been used daily over a prolonged period with increasing dosage is more likely to produce withdrawal symptoms, and the symptoms are more severe than withdrawal from a drug used less regularly. Because many drugs interact, both in effect and tolerance, combinations of substances deserve particular caution. Depending on the substances, it may be necessary to address withdrawal of each substance sequentially. Again, an accurate substance use history is imperative.

Client characteristics.   Characteristics of clients, particularly those that are health related, also affect withdrawal symptoms. Age, nutritional status, liver function, concurrent illness, and past history of withdrawal are important assessment areas to determine clients' potential for withdrawal symptoms. Clients with prior withdrawal symptoms are likely to repeat them; this is particularly true for clients who have experienced severe alcohol withdrawal syndrome with seizures or delirium tremens in the past. Each withdrawal episode produces neurological changes that "kindle" or sensitize the sympathetic nervous system to the next episode. With each occurrence of withdrawal, greater sympathetic activity results, with accompanying withdrawal symptoms (Linnoila, 1987). Animal research indicates that this increased sensitivity is independent of the amount of alcohol consumed or the client's current health status (Becker & Hale, 1993).

When clients have used substances to self-medicate for a psychiatric problem, that problem, often depression or schizophrenia, may reappear or intensify during detoxification. Skilled nursing assessment and time are needed to distinguish psychiatric symptoms from withdrawal. Similarly, medical problems that have been masked by substance use also may reappear. Frequently, it is not clear which symptoms are withdrawal-related and which represent medical or psychiatric problems until the client is stabilized.

Detailed alcohol, drug, and medical histories are vital. A drug history records the substances used, amount used, frequency, duration, and last use. On admission a body fluid screen may identify other substances. Because of the tendency for clients to minimize or deny use, the nurse must be alert to indicators that substances not yet identified or much larger quantities of substances identified are involved. Developing a clinical sense of the usual presentation and behavior of clients helps the nurse detect variations that merit further investigation. The nurse also must be alert for other emerging medical problems. An observant and holistic nursing approach is crucial. A baseline mental status examination should be done on admission, using an objective assessment tool such as the Mini-Mental Status (Folstein, Folstein & McHugh, 1975) or a withdrawal assessment scale (see next paragraph), so subsequent changes in mental status can be determined.

A scale to assess alcohol withdrawal symptoms, the Clinical Institute Withdrawal Assessment of Alcohol (CIWA), can quantify alcohol withdrawal symptoms and guide the use of withdrawal medications (Sullivan et al, 1989). The revised version of the scale (CIWA-Ar) (Box 11-1) monitors 10 symptoms of withdrawal on a 0- to 4- or 7-point scale. The assessment takes 2 minutes and can be repeated every 30 minutes. The maximum score is 67. Scores of less than 20 indicate mild withdrawal, 20 to 25 indicate moderate withdrawal, and greater than 25 indicates severe withdrawal with potentially pending delirium tremens (DTs). The importance of closely monitoring clients for alcohol withdrawal symptoms cannot be overemphasized; early treatment can prevent the more serious withdrawal syndromes such as DTs, which can be life-threatening.

Withdrawal patterns

Different categories of drugs elicit specific withdrawal symptoms and patterns. Table 11-1 displays the most common withdrawal symptoms of selected substances. Also see Chapter 7 for more on withdrawal.

Box 11-1

Addiction Research Foundation Clinical Institute Withdrawal Assessment for Alcohol (CIWA-Ar)

Patient: _____ Blood pressure _____/_____ Pulse or heart rate, taken for one minute _____

Date: _____
(yy   mm   dd)

Time: _____:_____
(24-hour clock, midnight = 00:00)

Nausea and vomiting—Ask, "Do you feel sick to your stomach? Have you vomited?" Observation.

0 = no nausea and no vomiting
1 = mild nausea with no vomiting
2
3
4 = intermittent nausea with dry heaves
5
6
7 = constant nausea, frequent dry heaves, and vomiting

Tremor—Arms extended and fingers spread apart. Observation.

0 = no tremor
1 = not visible, but can be felt fingertip to fingertip
2
3
4 = moderate, with patient's arms extended
5
6
7 = severe, even with arms not extended

Paroxysmal sweats—Observation.

0 = no sweat visible
1 = barely perceptible sweating, palms moist
2
3
4 = beads of sweat obvious on forehead
5
6
7 = drenching sweats

Anxiety—Ask, "Do you feel nervous?" Observation.

0 = no anxiety, at ease
1 = mildly anxious
2
3
4 = moderately anxious, or guarded, so anxiety is inferred
5
6
7 = equivalent to acute panic states as seen in severe delirium or acute schizophrenic reactions

Agitation—Observation.

0 = normal activity
1 = somewhat more than normal activity
2
3
4 = moderately fidgety and restless
5
6
7 = paces back and forth during most of the interview, or constantly thrashes about

Tactile disturbances—Ask, "Have you any itching, pins and needles sensations, any burning, any numbness, or do you feel bugs crawling on or under your skin?" Observation.

0 = none
1 = very mild itching, pins and needles, burning or numbness
2 = mild itching, pins and needles, burning or numbness
3 = moderate itching, pins and needles, burning or numbness
4 = moderately severe hallucinations
5 = severe hallucinations
6 = extremely severe hallucinations
7 = continuous hallucinations

Auditory disturbances—Ask, "Are you more aware of sounds around you? Are they harsh? Do they frighten you? Are you hearing anything that is disturbing to you? Are you hearing things you know are not there?" Observation.

0 = not present
1 = very mild harshness or ability to frighten
2 = mild harshness or ability to frighten
3 = moderate harshness or ability to frighten
4 = moderately severe hallucinations
5 = severe hallucinations
6 = extremely severe hallucinations
7 = continuous hallucinations

From Sullivan, J.T., Kykora, K., Schneiderman, J., Naranjo, C.A., & Sellers, E.M. (1989). Assessment of alcohol withdrawal: The revised clinical institute withdrawal assessment for alcohol scale. *British Journal of Addiction, 84,* 1353-1357.

Box 11-1

Addiction Research Foundation Clinical Institute Withdrawal Assessment for Alcohol (CIWA-Ar)—cont'd

Visual disturbances—Ask, "Does the light appear to be too bright? Is its color different? Does it hurt your eyes? Are you seeing anything that is disturbing to you? Are you seeing things you know are not there?" Observation.

0 = not present
1 = very mild sensitivity
2 = mild sensitivity
3 = moderate sensitivity
4 = moderately severe hallucinations
5 = severe hallucinations
6 = extremely severe hallucinations
7 = continuous hallucinations

Headache, fullness in head—Ask, "Does your head feel different? Does it feel like there is a band around your head?" Do not rate for dizziness or lightheadedness. Otherwise, rate severity.

0 = not present
1 = very mild
2 = mild
3 = moderate
4 = moderately severe
5 = severe
6 = very severe
7 = extremely severe

Orientation and clouding of sensorium—Ask, "What day is this? Where are you? Who am I?"

0 = oriented and can do serial additions
1 = cannot do serial additions or is uncertain about date
2 = disoriented for date by no more than 2 calendar days
3 = disoriented for date by more than 2 calendar days
4 = disoriented for place and/or person

Total CIWA-Ar Score _____
Rater's Initials _____
Maximum Possible Score = 67

Table 11-1

Substances and withdrawal symptoms

Substance	Withdrawal symptoms
CNS depressants	
Alcohol	Tremors, hallucinosis, seizure disorder, delirium tremens
Barbiturates	Postural hypotension, tachycardia, fever, insomnia, tremors, agitation, anxiety; rapid withdrawal causes apprehension, weakness, tremors, postural hypotension, anorexia, grand mal seizures
Benzodiazepines	Tremors, agitation, anxiety, grand mal seizures, abdominal cramps, vomiting, diaphoresis
Opiates	Watery eyes, dilated pupils, anxiety, abdominal cramps, piloerection, yawning, diaphoresis, rhinorrhea, achiness, anorexia, insomnia, fever, nausea, vomiting, diarrhea
CNS stimulants	
Amphetamines	Depression, fatigue, lethargy, irritability
Cocaine	Depression, fatigue, anxiety
Other substances	
Hallucinogens	None
Marijuana	None
Phencyclidine	None

Modified from Stuart, G.W. & Sundeen, S.J. (1995). *Principles and practice of psychiatric nursing.* (5th ed.). St. Louis: Mosby.

Central nervous system depressants.   This category of related substances includes alcohol, barbiturates, and benzodiazepines. Alcohol is the prototype for this category.

With alcohol dependence, withdrawal symptoms can occur within 6 to 12 hours after the last drink. A three-stage progression of symptoms can be identified (Fleming, 1991). Stage 1, or minor withdrawal, is characterized by restlessness, anxiety, agitation, and tremor. Tachycardia, elevated temperature, diaphoresis, and elevated blood pressure also may occur. Stage 2, or major withdrawal, includes the signs of stage 1 plus visual or auditory hallucinations without disorientation. The client often is aware of hallucinating and may exhibit agitation, increased tremors, and nausea and vomiting. This may occur 24 to 72 hours after the last drink. Stage 3, or delirium tremens (DTs), is characterized by confusion and disorientation. Diastolic blood pressure and temperature increase. Mortality at this stage ranges from 2% to 5%, thus this is a serious medical emergency. Delirium tremens can occur from 48 hours to 10 days after drinking ceases. Seizures can occur at any time but are most frequent during Stage 2.

This three-stage progression generally occurs in sequence, but there are exceptions, and stages may overlap. Prevention of Stage 3 best occurs through close observation and early pharmacologic intervention. The process is difficult to interrupt once begun. Table 11-2 shows the elements of all three stages and their progression.

Table 11-2

Stages of alcohol and sedative withdrawal

	General signs	Hallucination	Delirium
Stage 1	Mild	No	No
Stage 2	Moderate	Yes	No
Stage 3 (Delirium tremens)	Severe	Yes or No	Yes

From Fleming, M.F. (1991). Medical detoxification for sedatives, stimulants, and opiates. In M. Fleming (Ed.) *Substance abuse education for family physicians*. Kansas City, MO: Society of Teachers of Family Medicine.

Withdrawal from barbiturates and benzodiazepines follows a similar pattern to withdrawal from alcohol. With barbiturates in particular, seizures can occur independently of other symptoms. Onset of symptoms depends on the substance, its half-life, the amount of the substance to which the body has developed tolerance, and the duration of dependence. With short-acting benzodiazepines, withdrawal may occur suddenly and progress rapidly; longer acting benzodiazepines may produce withdrawal symptoms 5 to 10 days after last use. Pharmacologic treatment is usually necessary.

Opiate withdrawal is characterized by a progression of symptoms that can be classified by grades (Fleming, 1991). Withdrawal begins with drug craving and anxiety (Grade 0), then progresses to yawning and sweating (Grade 1), followed by gooseflesh, muscle twitching, and anorexia (Grade 2), and in the last stage, insomnia, increased pulse and blood pressure, abdominal cramps, nausea, and diarrhea occur (Grade 3). The degree of progression on this continuum in 24 hours is an indicator of the severity of withdrawal. Clients who do not progress past Grade 0 within 24 hours have limited dependence and can be withdrawn with supportive care. Those who develop Grade 1 or 2 symptoms will need treatment, and those with Grade 3 symptoms should be observed for more severe withdrawal symptoms. The various substances in this category vary in the severity and type of withdrawal symptoms, according to drug potency, physical tolerance, and duration of action. Propoxyphene, codeine, and pentazocine have the lowest incidence of withdrawal.

Stimulants.   The most frequently abused stimulants are cocaine and amphetamines. They are particularly problematic when used intravenously (amphetamines) or smoked (crack cocaine; ice or methamphetamine). Acute intoxication can produce psychological symptoms typical of paranoia or psychosis that are related to prolonged, intense use. This psychosis usually clears within a week. Cocaine withdrawal may involve intense craving or depression with severe anhedonia. Both symptoms may continue for some time. Regular monitoring of suicidal ideation and drug-seeking behavior is crucial. Clients who use stimulants often alternate them with CNS depressants such as alcohol or barbiturates, thus polydrug use should always be assessed.

Delayed withdrawal syndrome.   During early sobriety, it is critical that the nurse monitor clients for a secondary or delayed withdrawal syndrome. Clients who require large doses of medications while detoxifying may experience a secondary withdrawal syndrome that is less dramatic but also requires intervention. Additionally, clients dependent on longer-acting substances such as diazepam may appear stable, but then experience a severe withdrawal syndrome as long as 2 weeks after the last use.

Management of detoxification

The length of time needed for detoxification varies according to the substance, characteristics of use, and client characteristics. For some clients, withdrawal may last only a few hours; for others, it could last several days to a week or longer. Longer-acting substances such as long-acting benzodiazepines produce a longer withdrawal phase. The time allocated in treatment programs for detoxification is usually 1 to 3 days, although often this must be revised for particular clients.

Formats for detoxification.   Two formats for detoxification have emerged—medical and social detoxification. The formats differ in the degree of medical supervision, the site of detoxification, and the use of medications. Criteria are currently being developed for assigning clients to specific programs. Sometimes the distinction is described as outpatient versus inpatient because many outpatient programs are based on a social detoxification format. Social detoxification programs are usually housed in a community setting that may or may not include a treatment program. Sometimes detoxification may be supervised at home by a family member through daily contact with a professional. When stabilized, clients are referred to a treatment program. In social settings a protocol for assessment of withdrawal symptoms needs to be in place and rigorously followed because the program is less health-care oriented and could potentially overlook early withdrawal symptoms. State regulations determine the minimum nursing and medical personnel required. A client with good health and moderate substance abuse would be an excellent candidate for social detoxification. Some studies estimate that 90% of clients with alcohol abuse or dependence can be safely detoxified socially (Hayashida, Alterman, & McLellan, 1989), and social detoxification clearly decreases the cost of treatment. A back-up medical system such as an emergency room or a treatment program is necessary when severe withdrawal symptoms occur (see Care Plan 11-1).

Medical detoxification is indicated for clients with more acute or longer addictions; addictions to multiple substances; unsuccessful prior attempts at recovery; those who pose a danger to self or others; severe medical, psychiatric, or other problems; or poor social support (Barker & Whitfield, 1991). Medical detoxification usually occurs in hospital settings and more often uses a medication protocol. Dependent health care professionals often require medical detoxification because the purity of the substances used, their high tolerance, and polysubstance use complicate withdrawal. An alcohol-dependent client with a history of severe alcohol withdrawal syndrome or a client with barbiturate or benzodiazepine abuse also is a candidate for medical detoxification.

Pharmacologic treatment.   Pharmacologic treatment of withdrawal can involve several protocols. The most common protocol uses a cross-tolerant substance in decreasing doses to lessen the effect of withdrawal symptoms and to prevent se-

Text continued on p. 328.

Nursing Care of the Client with Alcohol Dependence in a Social Detoxification Setting

Bob, age 52, was brought to the community alcohol and drug treatment center by his brother, John. Bob's speech was slurred, and he staggered slightly as he walked. They both stated that Bob had agreed to treatment, that he was "sick and tired of things as they were." Bob lost his job as a new car salesman a month ago, after he wrecked his demonstrator vehicle. He has a long history of DWIs. This is the third job that he has lost in the past 5 years. In addition, 5 years ago, his wife of 25 years left him, saying that she couldn't take it anymore.

ASSESSMENT

John described Bob's drinking as episodic, saying that at one time he had abstained for 6 months. The current drinking episode began 3 days ago when his rent came due and he didn't have enough money to pay. At that time, he arrived at John's door, disheveled and crying because he wasn't going to have a place to live. He shut himself in the bedroom and spent the time watching TV and drinking, consuming two fifths of whiskey.

NURSING DIAGNOSES

Sensory-perceptual alteration related to withdrawal from alcohol
Ineffective individual coping related to use of alcohol for coping, to the detriment of other aspects of his life
Spiritual distress related to change in value system contrary to that established in childhood

Outcome identification	Nursing interventions	Rationale	Evaluation
Nursing diagnosis: Sensory-perceptual alteration related to withdrawal from alcohol			
1. Client will be withdrawn safely from heavy alcohol use by the end of the second week as evidenced by stable vital signs and minimal tremor.	1a. Assess the client's physical status.	1a. Physical status is an indicator of progress of withdrawal.	1. Bob's vital signs were stable at the end of 1 week and his tremor was only slight. Goal met.
	1b. Establish rapport and confidence by use of competent bedside care and warm, positive regard.	1b. Reduces anxiety and enhances both biological and emotional stability.	
	1c. Treat the client with dignity and respect.	1c. All clients, regardless of behavior or condition, are worthy of dignity and respect.	
	1d. Monitor the client's vital signs and degree of tremor.	1d. Vital signs and tremor are indicators of the progress of withdrawal.	

From Jack, L. (1990). *Nursing care planning with the addicted client,* Vol II, (pp 50, 54, 203). Skokie, IL: National Nurses Society on Addictions.

Outcome identification	Nursing interventions	Rationale	Evaluation
Nursing diagnosis: Sensory-perceptual alteration related to withdrawal from alcohol—cont'd			
	1e. Assess the client's mental status according to the level of impairment. Record his orientation to person, place, and time; the presence of hallucinations or delusions; and the coherence of his speech pattern.	1e. Hallucinations may be a reason to transfer this client to a medical detoxification. Difficulties with orientation indicate impending delirium tremens and an emergency situation.	
	1f. Reorient the client daily.	1f. Slight confusion will clear up with reorientation.	
	1g. Supervise activities of daily living.	1g. Client's self-esteem will be raised if groomed and clean.	
	1h. Educate the client as to the process of withdrawal and the purpose of medication.	1h. Knowledge of the meaning of symptoms the client is experiencing will reduce anxiety.	
	1i. Reduce stimuli in the environment.	1i. His CNS is already hyperexcited; small stimuli may evoke large responses.	
	1j. Call the client by name.	1j. Increases self-respect.	
	1k. Reinforce behaviors that are reality-oriented.	1k. This begins the process of treatment. Typically the chronic substance abuser blames others in his environment for his own problems.	

Continued.

Care Plan 11-1

Nursing Care of the Client with Alcohol Dependence in a Social Detoxification Setting—cont'd

Outcome identification	Nursing interventions	Rationale	Evaluation
Nursing diagnosis: Sensory-perceptual alteration related to withdrawal from alcohol—cont'd			
	1l. Institute measures to help the client sleep, such as relaxation techniques.	1l. Most persons withdrawing from CNS depressants will have difficulty sleeping.	
	1m. Do not confront about substance abuse at this time.	1m. Client is physically ill during withdrawal, and confrontation at this time leaves the client feeling unsupported and anxious, both counterproductive.	
Nursing diagnosis: Ineffective individual coping related to use of alcohol for coping, to the detriment of other aspects of his life			
1. Client will identify how alcoholism has affected his behavior and relationships within 3 weeks.	1a. Establish a therapeutic one-to-one relationship.	1a. This establishes trust so that the nurse can assist the client.	1. After 3 weeks, Bob tearfully related how his excessive alcohol use had impacted his marriage, his other relationships, his legal status, and his jobs. Goal met.
	1b. Demonstrate acceptance of the client's worth as a human being.	1b. Acceptance from others assists the client to accept self as worthy of making the effort to change.	
	1c. Spend time with the client to convey interest and acceptance.	1c. This establishes trust and self-worth, both necessary in order to work in the treatment program.	
	1d. Teach the client about the effects of alcohol on the body.	1d. This knowledge assists the client to make the connection between the alcohol use and consequences.	

Outcome identification	Nursing interventions	Rationale	Evaluation
Nursing diagnosis: Ineffective individual coping related to use of alcohol for coping, to the detriment of other aspects of his life—cont'd			
	1e. Reinforce the client's socialization efforts.	1e. Establishing a bond with other clients undergoing treatment provides social support while facing the painful realities of his drinking behavior.	
	1f. Encourage the client to discuss the consequences of drinking behaviors.	1f. Begins to assist the client to face the realities of his problem drinking.	
	1g. Encourage the client to verbalize his feelings honestly.	1g. To identify painful feelings is the first step to dealing with stress. The chronic substance abuser medicates feelings.	
2. Client will participate in structured treatment program activities by the end of 2 weeks.	2a. Help the client recognize and focus on his strengths and positive accomplishments.	2a. Provides basis for beginning to find new ways to cope by addressing his current coping resources.	2. By 2 weeks, Bob was participating in activities in the treatment program. Goal met.
	2b. Explore alternative ways of reaching out to other people without the use of alcohol.	2b. Many clients continue to use alcohol because of the belief that alcohol enhances sociability.	
	2c. Help the client identify stress-producing situations.	2c. Stress-producing situations are often triggers for alcohol use and abuse.	

Continued.

Care Plan 11-1

Nursing Care of the Client with Alcohol Dependence in a Social Detoxification Setting—cont'd

Outcome identification	Nursing interventions	Rationale	Evaluation
Nursing diagnosis: Ineffective individual coping related to use of alcohol for coping, to the detriment of other aspects of his life—cont'd			
	2d. Teach the client methods for coping with stress, such as problem solving, relaxation techniques, and cognitive restructuring.	2d. Not only does the client need to identify his own resources for coping, but he will need to learn additional methods of coping.	
	2e. Provide positive feedback for the client's independent decision making and effective use of problem-solving skills.	2e. Positive feedback for successes reinforces use of these skills.	
	2f. Promote the client's participation in a twelve-step program on the unit.	2f. Beginning work in a twelve-step program enhances the probability that he will follow through with this upon discharge.	
	2g. Help the client obtain a sponsor in the community before discharge.	2g. Acquiring a sponsor before discharge will provide support for relapse prevention immediately at a stressful time.	
Nursing diagnosis: Spiritual distress related to change in value system contrary to that established in childhood			
1. The client will identify the value system with which he currently lives and his feelings connected with it within 3 weeks.	1a. Help the client examine the personal spiritual or belief dimension in his own life.	1a. The nurse, already viewed as a support person, is in a position to assist the client to discuss his distress.	1. Bob discussed his religious upbringing and expressed much guilt about how he had left these teachings. He wasn't sure

Outcome identification	Nursing interventions	Rationale	Evaluation
	Nursing diagnosis: Spiritual distress related to change in value system contrary to that established in childhood—cont'd		
	1b. Encourage the client to attend spiritual activities set up by the program.	1b. Most programs have spiritual treatment, and alcoholism is viewed as a disease of the spirit.	about whether he wanted to follow these beliefs at the present time, but expressed contradictory beliefs and confusion currently. After 3 weeks, goal not met.
	1c. Encourage the client to write about his spiritual distress in a journal.	1c. Writing down his concerns in a private manner will allow the client to examine his spiritual confusions and concerns.	*Revision:* Continue to assist him to clarify his values.
	1d. Help the client complete steps 1 through 3 in the AA twelve-step program.	1d. Working these steps aids the client in addressing his spiritual distress (e.g., experiencing own powerlessness to control own life, becoming willing to turn to a higher power for help, and actually doing this).	
	1e. Explore with the client his past religious practices and how they might or might not fit into his present lifestyle or belief system.	1e. Frequently the substance abusing client will hold a confusing collection of conflicting views from childhood, which upon examination he will reexamine and return, revise, or reject.	

rious withdrawal symptoms. Substances used for withdrawal have a longer duration of action than the abused substance, so they can be administered less frequently, producing a lessened substance effect. With alcohol abuse or dependence, the substance usually is administered on a symptom-based protocol, but sometimes it may be routinely prescribed. Close monitoring is essential. The drugs used for alcohol detoxification vary among treatment settings based on the training of the medical director and the philosophy of the treatment program. No clear drug of choice has been identified, although most protocols use a long-acting benzodiazepine in decreasing doses over 3 to 5 days. For clients with liver disease, a short-acting benzodiazepine not metabolized by the liver may be more appropriate. Table 11-3 shows common medication regimens.

Detoxification from barbiturates and benzodiazepines uses phenobarbital, diazepam, or Tegretol gradually withdrawn over a period of up to 10 days, depending on the client's tolerance. Determining the appropriate substitution dose initially may be done through a drug challenge and a thorough drug-use history. In a drug challenge, also called a tolerance test, a predetermined amount of diazepam or pentobarbital is given to a client who is *not* experiencing withdrawal. The client is examined in 1 hour for signs of sedation. If none are noted, a repeat dose is given in 2 hours, and the procedure is repeated until a drug effect is noted. This challenge estimates the client's tolerance and daily substance use and helps the treatment team determine what dose is appropriate to begin withdrawal (Woolf, 1991a). This is particularly useful for a client who gives an unreliable substance abuse history or has polysubstance use.

Table 11-3
Drugs used in alcohol withdrawal

Drug	Routes of administration*	Common dosage range†
Chlordiazepoxide (Librium)	PO	25-100 mg q4-6h
	IM‡	50-100 mg q4-6h
Diazepam (Valium)	PO	5-20 mg q4-6h
	IV	2.5 mg/min
	IM‡	5-10 mg q4-6h
Phenobarbital	PO	30-120 mg q4-6h
	IM	60-120 mg q4-6h
Paraldehyde§	PO	5-15 ml q4-6h
Clorazepate (Tranxene)	PO	30 mg initially, then 30-60 mg in divided doses/d
Lorazepam (Ativan)	PO	1-5 mg q6h
	IM	2 mg q6h

From Woolf, D.S. (1991a). Detoxification. In E. Bennett & D. Woolf (Eds.) *Substance abuse.* (2nd ed.). Albany, NY: Delmar.
*PO—oral; IM—intramuscular; IV—intravenous.
†Dosage for first day. Dosages may be lower in the elderly or clients with liver disease.
‡IM absorption is erratic and not preferred.
§For reference only. Its use is not recommended.

Stimulant dependence may require antipsychotics to treat resulting psychiatric symptoms such as amphetamine psychosis. Use of psychotropic medications may continue until the symptoms disappear. The depression associated with cocaine withdrawal frequently requires tricyclic antidepressants. A variety of medications have been used to treat craving; bromocriptine is common. However, no medications are clearly superior to treat craving (Fleming & Barry, 1992).

Opiate withdrawal often involves methadone. Methadone may be used for detoxification only or for maintenance. Methadone is a long-acting opiate and can be used to taper the opiate dose gradually with a minimum of withdrawal symptoms. This detoxification may take 10 to 21 days, depending on the amount and type of opiate used. Methadone also is used in maintenance programs in which the client is tapered to a dose that alleviates drug craving then maintained indefinitely on that dose. This use is controversial because it represents continued dependence. Clonidine has also been used for opiate withdrawal, but it ameliorates only selected symptoms.

Nursing management.   Nursing diagnoses that guide nursing interventions are determined from the assessment and the nurse's knowledge of the withdrawal patterns of the identified substance(s). Common nursing diagnoses include sensory-perceptual alteration, alteration in comfort, and potential for injury (NNSA, 1990). The first two clearly relate to the withdrawal symptoms, and the last emphasizes the potential for harm that exists during withdrawal.

Continued assessment for withdrawal symptoms and changes in symptom level is mandatory. Changes in vital signs or orientation level may indicate increased severity of withdrawal or other physiological problems. Interaction with the client during detoxification should focus on the immediate goal of safe withdrawal, as well as physiological and psychological stabilization. The nursing approach should be factual, supportive, and reality-enforcing. Client education about withdrawal is important to allay anxiety; however, the content needs to be consistent with the client's level of orientation and comprehension. During detoxification, memory may be impaired and information needs repetition. It is important to emphasize that detoxification is a short-term phenomenon. Hydration and nutrition need to be monitored carefully by the nurse and are important client teaching elements. Nutritional and vitamin supplements are often part of alcohol withdrawal protocols.

One component of nursing care is to closely monitor the client's physiological status and to provide appropriate medication without unduly alarming the client, encouraging somatization, or reinforcing drug-seeking behaviors. This requires a balanced and objective approach by the nurse. Often, this is best accomplished by collecting data indirectly during an interaction with the client. Client teaching about withdrawal and the purpose of withdrawal medications is important. Overdependence of the client on the medication can replace one substance with another, which defeats the purpose of treatment.

Environmental manipulation is another focus of nursing interventions. For clients experiencing withdrawal symptoms that impair reality testing, a quiet environment with appropriate lighting is helpful. Frequent and orienting interactions help maintain client orientation. Because frequent monitoring of vital signs is important, these interactions and vital signs can be integrated. Clients experiencing anxiety may need to walk or engage in light activity as tolerated.

It is important for nurses to be familiar with the treatment protocol, implement it consistently, and note client variances from the usual response. In programs that do not use medications for withdrawal, the nurse must be particularly alert for symptoms that may indicate withdrawal or physiological problems.

As the detoxification period ends and the client becomes more stable and mentally alert, the nurse can encourage the client to focus on the treatment recommended for the client. The nurse can introduce information, encourage interaction with other clients in treatment, and answer questions as they arise.

While detoxification is time-limited, data indicate that return to physical and psychological homeostasis is extremely variable and some ongoing long-term physiological and psychological symptomatology is common (Box 11-2) (DeSoto, O'Donnell & DeSoto, 1989).

NURSING CARE IN SUBSTANCE ABUSE TREATMENT

Nursing roles in the treatment phase of substance abuse vary according to institution, locale, and the organizational factors discussed earlier. Nurses provide care in every domain of life—physical, psychosocial, spiritual, and cognitive—for clients and their families. These dimensions were identified in a survey of nurses working in substance abuse (ANA & NNSA, 1988), and they collectively represent nursing the whole person (see Care Plan 11-2).

Dimensions of care

Physical dimension. Once the client has been safely detoxified, the nurse has a major role in the ongoing assessment of the client's physical needs. This may include monitoring vital signs as indicated. Urine drug screens may continue throughout treatment; other diagnostic procedures may also be used. The nurse's astute assessment skills continuously monitor known health problems and identify problems secondary to substance abuse. See Box 11-2 for examples of potential health problems related to substance abuse.

Two physical problems associated with early recovery are (1) *withdrawal seizures*, which may occur when a client detoxifies too quickly, has a known seizure disorder, or has decreased magnesium levels and (2) *blood sugar stabilization*. A major concern during detoxification, particularly with alcohol and other depressants, is the potential for seizures. The purpose of a withdrawal medication protocol is to prevent seizures and other symptoms. A good health history and prior withdrawal experiences provide clues to this potential. Withdrawal seizures are usually grand mal and single episodes. Phenobarbital or diazepam are the medications of choice.

A variety of factors impact the recovering client's blood sugar in early recovery. These include but are not limited to the high caloric content of alcohol, sporadic eating habits while using, and nausea during detoxification. Known diabetics and clients with hypoglycemia require frequent monitoring and a stable intake of appropriate foods during this time. Small-framed females detoxifying from benzodiazepines may have an especially difficult time with hypoglycemia.

Text continued on p. 340.

Box 11-2
Effects of Alcohol Abuse

Chronic alcohol abuse can lead to many physical and psychological complications, including the following:

Cardiovascular complications
- Alcoholic cardiomyopathy
- Increased systolic and pulse pressure
- Tissue damage, weakened heart muscle, and heart failure

Gastrointestinal complications
- Abdominal distention, pain, belching, and hematemesis
- Acute and chronic pancreatitis
- Alcoholic hepatitis, leading to cirrhosis
- Cancer of the esophagus, liver, or pancreas
- Esophageal varices, hemorrhoids, and ascites
- Gastritis, colitis, and enteritis
- Gastric or duodenal ulcers
- Swollen, enlarged fatty liver

Genitourinary complications
- Swelling of prostate gland, leading to prostatitis and interference with voiding or sexual function
- Prostate cancer

Hematologic complications
- Abnormal red blood cells, white blood cells, and platelets
- Anemia and increased risk of infection
- Bleeding tendencies, increased bruising, and decreased clotting time

Neurologic complications
- Wernicke-Korsakoff syndrome, Marchiafava-Bignami disease, cerebellar degeneration, and peripheral neuropathy

Respiratory complications
- Cancer of the oropharynx
- Impaired diffusion, chronic obstructive pulmonary disease, infection, and tuberculosis
- Respiratory depression, causing decreased respiratory rate and cough reflex and increased susceptibility to infection and trauma

Miscellaneous complications
- Acute and chronic myopathies
- Alcoholic amblyopia
- Beriberi
- Electrolyte abnormalities
- Osteoporosis
- Scars, burns, and repeated injuries

From Krupnick, S.L.W. & Wade, A.J. (Eds.) (1993). *Psychiatric care planning.* Springhouse, PA: Springhouse Corp.

Care Plan 11-2

Client with Bulimia, Cocaine Abuse

June, age 30, who is married and has one 6-year-old child, was brought to a substance abuse treatment center by her husband, Craig, who said, "Her behavior is out of control."

ASSESSMENT

After assessment, she was diagnosed with cocaine abuse. According to her husband, her housekeeping was immaculate even when she held a full-time job, which she did until 3 months ago. She had received an award for Outstanding Employee 1 year ago. Her behavior changed when she began going out with a girlfriend. She began staying out all night and neglecting her husband, her home, and her child. In addition, she had lost 25 pounds during the 3 months. She presented as slightly disheveled and cachectic. Her parotid glands are swollen, and she has tooth erosion on her molars. She revealed that she vomited after meals to maintain her weight but considers herself "too fat." Craig disclosed that June's father was an alcoholic, and she had been sexually abused as a child. Detailed initial assessment of June's eating habits revealed she sometimes ate large quantities of food and was obsessed with her weight, but had maintained normal weight until she began using cocaine. She was found inducing vomiting after a meal while on the unit and obtained the additional diagnosis of bulimia nervosa.

NURSING DIAGNOSES

Body image disturbance related to the belief that she is "too fat"
Ineffective individual coping related to the cocaine use
Personal identity disturbance related to childhood dysfunctional family and history of sexual abuse

Outcome identification	Nursing interventions	Rationale	Evaluation
Nursing diagnosis: Body image disturbance related to the belief that she is "too fat"			
1. Client will eat meals with other clients while on the unit and will not engage in self-induced vomiting during her stay on the treatment unit.	1a. Maintaining safe environment for client.	1a. Often these clients feel like victims. For them to risk self-disclosure, they must feel safe.	1. During the first week on the unit, June was found in the bathroom inducing vomiting. Thereafter, she was placed under observation for 2 hours after mealtime. No more incidences occurred. Goal met at discharge.
	1b. Insist the client only eat at mealtime, in the dining room, with other clients.	1b. The client with bulimia may have a pattern of eating when others are not present, then binging, followed by feeling guilty, then inducing vomiting.	
	1c. Monitor her after meals.	1c. This is to prevent vomiting.	

Outcome identification	Nursing interventions	Rationale	Evaluation
Nursing diagnosis: Body image disturbance related to the belief that she is "too fat"—cont'd			
	1d. Assist her to achieve balance in sleep, eating, work, and play.	1d. These clients often indulge in activities excessively and compulsively.	
	1e. Monitor elimination.	1e. With both self-induced vomiting and withdrawal from cocaine abuse, constipation may be a problem.	
	1f. Encourage her to seek long-term treatment for her eating disorder.	1f. This disorder most frequently arises as a result of dysfunction in the family of origin and long-term psychotherapy is needed for treatment.	
2. Client will gain 5 pounds within 3 weeks of admission to the unit.	2a. Encourage nutritious food eaten in moderate quantities at mealtime with others.	2a. Client is cachectic and is in need of nutrition. Social interaction enhances digestion and helps reduce anxiety about eating.	2. June had gained 1 pound at the end of 3 weeks. Goal not met. Continue as planned.
	2b. Assist her to discuss feelings that arise when she eats.	2b. This begins the self-examination process, as one of the sources of the binging-purging cycle is the feelings about her body image and about eating.	

Continued.

Care Plan 11-2

Client with Bulimia, Cocaine Abuse—cont'd

Outcome identification	Nursing interventions	Rationale	Evaluation
Nursing diagnosis: Body image disturbance related to the belief that she is "too fat"—cont'd			
	2c. Enlist the assistance of a dietitian to plan an appropriate diet to use long-term to maintain her weight at a healthy level.	2c. Because of her anxiety about weight gain, she has an unrealistic fear of eating. It will be essential for her to find a realistic and appropriate diet for weight control and health.	
Nursing diagnosis: Ineffective individual coping related to the cocaine use			
1. Client will acknowledge that she cannot control her cocaine use by 3 weeks.	1a. Teach the client the disease concept of chemical dependency.	1a. This assists the client in accepting the idea that she needs treatment.	1. Client did state that she thought cocaine was ruining her life and that she could not control its use. Goal met.
	1b. Ask her to write a chemical use history beginning at age 12.	1b. Histories and autobiographies are useful in assisting clients to make connections with life events and use of chemicals. This can be threatening to someone abused as a child; therefore it should be limited to chemical use after 12.	
	1c. Go easy on the concept of powerlessness.	1c. For someone sexually abused as a child, the concept of powerlessness terrifies them.	
	1d. Assist her to identify situations and problems that indicate cocaine use was problematic.	1d. Helps to connect her use with problems. Avoid generalization of life being unmanageable.	

Outcome identification	Nursing interventions	Rationale	Evaluation
Nursing diagnosis: Ineffective individual coping related to the cocaine use—cont'd			
	1e. Use dialogue, videos, and literature to explain to her how cocaine affects the brain.	1e. Cocaine is highly addictive, and clients have difficulty maintaining abstinence. She needs all of the information that she can obtain.	
	1f. Insist that the client maintain abstinence after discharge.	1f. Because of cocaine's highly addictive quality, abstinence is essential.	
2. Client will participate in the treatment program by 1 week.	2a. Use high levels of structure for this client.	2a. These clients have difficulty making decisions for themselves, so they function better with higher levels of structure.	2. June began attending treatment classes and groups on the third day after admission to the facility. Goal met.
	2b. Plan for how to respond if and when the client acts out or attempts self-harm.	2b. Often these clients will act out feelings if stressed.	
	2c. Use self-awareness for own family of origin issues.	2c. Often clients struggling with family of origin issues will trigger these conflicts in the nurse.	
	2d. Use matter-of-fact, here-and-now approach.	2d. Acceptance without emotional demands works best with this client. Here-and-now is important because old issues from family of origin may trigger overwhelming feelings.	

Continued.

Care Plan 11-2

Client with Bulimia, Cocaine Abuse—cont'd

Outcome identification	Nursing interventions	Rationale	Evaluation
Nursing diagnosis: Ineffective individual coping related to the cocaine use—cont'd			
	2e. Assign client to a women's-only treatment group part of the time.	2e. She will be able to address women's issues with other women. Problem-specific interventions are possible in a nonthreatening atmosphere.	
3. Client will attend AA or NA meetings on unit during treatment.	3a. Do not push this client to work steps.	3a. Pushing will cause her to act out.	3. June attended AA meetings on the unit, but stated that she did not like them and at discharge, she reluctantly stated she would go for a while. Goal met.
	3b. Ask how using was "insane."	3b. Less threatening. Defines the using as the problem, in no way does it attack her.	
	3c. Ask her to name three positive things that have occurred since not using.	3c. Gives her concrete examples of benefits.	
	3d. Allow her the freedom to say (when feeling threatened), "I feel unsafe or overwhelmed and want to stop for now."	3d. Overwhelmed feelings may prevent this client from completing treatment.	
	3e. Require her to supply equal amount of positive attributes as negative ones during working on step 4.	3e. Step 4 requires an "inventory" of self, and this client has such low self-esteem that she probably would focus only on the negative—again triggering overwhelming feelings.	

Outcome identification	Nursing interventions	Rationale	Evaluation
Nursing diagnosis: Ineffective individual coping related to the cocaine use—cont'd			
	3f. Predict that she may not like some meetings.	3f. Predicting a possible unpleasant experience at some time will help her to expect and protect herself from overwhelming feelings.	
	3g. Encourage her to find a group with which she can feel comfortable after discharge.	3g. Gives her hope that there will be a group with which she can feel compatible.	
	3h. Discourage her from attending Adult Children of Alcoholics groups at this time.	3h. These groups may revive painful feelings for her, and she needs to undergo therapy before she can manage them.	
	3i. Recommend that she find a same-sex sponsor.	3i. She has a hard time trusting males as a result of her sexual abuse.	
Nursing diagnosis: Personal identity disturbance related to childhood dysfunctional family and history of sexual abuse			
1. Client will state that she is a survivor by discharge.	1a. Help her to feel safe by using firm limits and explaining this as helping to protect her.	1a. Client is prone to act out and then distrust the nurse because she wasn't protected.	1. At the last group meeting before discharge, June stated that she did not feel like a survivor. She had agreed to obtain psychotherapy. Goal not met. _Revision:_ Goal is probably too advanced to be met by discharge for most clients.
	1b. Use anti-harm contracts.	1b. Contracts assist the client to assume responsibility for her behavior.	
	1c. Start discussions about her behavior at the intellectual level.	1c. Feelings may be overwhelming causing her to drop out of treatment.	

Continued.

Care Plan 11-2

Client with Bulimia, Cocaine Abuse—cont'd

Outcome identification	Nursing interventions	Rationale	Evaluation
Nursing diagnosis: Personal identity disturbance related to childhood dysfunctional family and history of sexual abuse—cont'd			
	1d. Avoid expressive, feeling-oriented approaches.	1d. Same as above.	
	1e. Teach about dysfunctional families, using videos, literature, and didactic.	1e. Helps her to intellectually understand dynamics of dysfunctional families.	
	1f. Help her learn about use of secrets and family thought-control in abusive families.	1f. Helps her see that she is not alone.	
	1g. Give her permission to control how much emotion she experiences by closing the book, leaving the class, or switching the topic when it gets too painful.	1g. Gives the client some intentional control over experiencing painful feelings.	
	1h. Gently and explicitly question client's thinking errors, specifically focusing on the role of victim that this client often takes.	1h. Helps her see that she has taken the role of victim. Also gives her the hope that she can change that and assume the role of survivor.	
2. Client will relate three steps to take when she does not feel safe by 2 weeks.	2a. Help her identify support persons and use them for support.	2a. She has difficulty trusting anyone, so also has difficulty assessing who is safe and who is not.	2. June could relate the three steps she could take to feel safe, but doubted that she would be able to follow

Outcome identification	Nursing interventions	Rationale	Evaluation
Nursing diagnosis: Personal identity disturbance related to childhood dysfunctional family and history of sexual abuse—cont'd			
	2b. Help her identify situations or events that trigger self-destructive behavior and plan and practice alternative behaviors.	2b. Helps the client learn safe behavior to replace self-destructive behavior.	through and do them. Goal met. *Revision:* Have her practice taking these steps with safe persons on the unit.
3. Client will list three strengths which she has by 2 weeks.	3a. Be a role model of appropriate behavior.	3a. Client usually has difficulty determining what is appropriate.	3. June stated that she was a good worker, a good housekeeper, and she loved her husband. Goal met.
	3b. Emphasize accomplishment.	3b. Seeing her accomplishments raises her self-esteem.	
	3c. Teach time management to structure day or week.	3c. Raises self-esteem, lowers risk of self-destructive behavior.	
	3d. Help her identify recreational outlets.	3d. Frequently, children from dysfunctional families feel guilty if they are having fun.	
	3e. Teach positive self-talk and affirmations.	3e. Affirmations such as "I am glad I am here" raise self-esteem.	
	3f. Teach assertiveness training.	3f. Helps them use words rather than actions to express anger. It is empowering as it allows her to meet some of her own needs.	

The challenge is to accurately manage the client's withdrawal symptoms, as well as the low blood sugar. General protocols for physiological symptoms include first checking vital signs then testing blood sugar. If blood sugar is low, first feed the client then medicate per protocol. Blood sugar management warrants ongoing nursing observation and monitoring. If vital signs are elevated (BP more than 20 mm above baseline and pulse greater than 100), follow the protocol for detoxification medications. Physician orders or unit protocols will set the levels of specific dietary and pharmacologic interventions.

The client's physical condition and mental status are monitored; frequency of monitoring depends on the stability of the client's status. Common conditions that require frequent monitoring include abnormal laboratory findings, hypertension, elevated temperature, and other alterations in physical assessment findings.

Health teaching with each nursing intervention is an "umbrella" concept throughout substance abuse treatment; that is, it is routinely included with all nursing interventions. Specific content for health teaching is discussed in the section on cognitive dimensions of care.

Psychosocial dimension. Nursing is key in managing the treatment milieu. In a health care environment, nurses are role models for clients in treatment. Healthy social interaction is encouraged in community meetings where dysfunctional behaviors are identified and more appropriate behaviors suggested.

Family-style dining fosters healthier nutritional intake, as well as offering another social setting for role modeling and practicing functional behaviors. Evening relaxation or study time fosters healthy interaction with self. Again, nursing staff may facilitate the initial introduction of these concepts to clients early in treatment.

Emotionally, clients share their feeling status daily. This enhances self-identification of feelings, provides feedback when incongruence between feelings and behavior is identified, and supports developing and enlarging a vocabulary to describe feelings.

Treatment may be very emotional for clients due to several factors. The recency of detoxification and physiological stabilization creates a physiological and psychological instability in the client. The client in treatment has accepted the need for treatment and given up denial of the illness at some level. Being substance-free requires coping with daily life without the numbing effects of substances, thus clients may be particularly aware of their emotions. Also, identifying and facing the consequences of substance abuse elicits emotional responses.

The treatment phase is an optimal time to help clients become aware of their emotions and develop coping skills. In programs that use a twelve step model, the steps can be used to organize client care because the twelve steps are a logical sequence in accepting and understanding substance abuse. Also, clients progress through the steps at individual rates.

Nursing care in treatment involves individual and group counseling and the clinical skill to select the best modality for specific client issues. While a preponderance of treatment occurs in groups, each client has a personal set of issues and responses. Thus the nurse and other treatment personnel must be sensitive to which client issues can be met in groups and which need individual counseling. In most settings, clients are assigned to a particular team member, either in addition to or including the nursing staff, who is responsible for identifying whether group or individual therapy is most appropriate. Nursing personnel, particularly those on evening and night shifts, may identify issues not apparent during the day. They need to address those issues and bring them to the awareness of the other members of the treatment team.

Some client issues may involve the client as a member of a special population such as women or minorities. Depending on the client mix, this may call for groups that target particular issues of these populations. Because a history of physical or sexual abuse often occurs in women with substance abuse, the treatment program should include a protocol for addressing abuse. The treatment program must be flexible enough to meet specific client needs.

Family counseling is another dimension of nursing care. As the client changes, family changes are necessary for the client to reenter the family milieu. These needs can be met through individual nursing interventions with the family, group orientations for families, and individual or group sessions for the client and the family. It is very important that the family is involved in the client's treatment program and planning.

As the client progresses the treatment focus becomes preparing the client to continue recovery upon discharge and prevent relapse (see Chapter 5). Vocational assessment and intervention may occur at this stage if needed, and appropriate use of leisure time can be explored.

Spiritual dimension.   Although spirituality is approached with reluctance in this culture, it is an important component of treatment and recovery for the client with substance abuse. Clients should examine their own religious framework to meet this spiritual need. However, spirituality and religion are related but separate concepts, and the clients may choose other frameworks.

Time is spent exploring the client's concept of spirituality. A key area of focus is developing a clearer understanding of spiritual self versus religion per se. Many clients enter treatment angry with their concept of a higher being and negative about the rudiments of formal religion. Daily relaxation, meditation, and quiet time provide self-exploration along this dimension.

The importance of spirituality in recovery is that clients identify a higher power than themselves. Because substance abuse is an individually oriented illness, recovery requires clients to expand their vision beyond themselves. It also is a response to the hopelessness often experienced by recovering clients regarding their ability to maintain recovery and return to their previous lifestyle.

Nursing care in this dimension often involves opening the topic for discussion and ascertaining the client's understanding of spirituality. The nurse needs to accept the client's thoughts and perceptions. Often, reading materials are encouraged to assist the client in developing the concept and finding a direction. Interacting with the nurse or other clients on this topic may open up new ideas. Visits from clergy and clergy-run groups on spirituality may be helpful. It is important that involved clergy understand substance abuse and the role of spirituality in recovery.

Cognitive dimension. Often neurological functioning, particularly cognition, is impaired, which has implications for participation in treatment. Nursing and program variations that accommodate cognitive impairment include informing clients of potential memory problems, repeating important information, encouraging clients to record information and ask for clarification, visual displays or handouts of significant information, and short information sessions (20 minutes) with summaries (Friedrich & Kus, 1991).

Health education is a critical component of all substance abuse treatment to address knowledge deficits. Many clients, with the exception of clients who have been in treatment previously, enter the treatment setting with little or erroneous information regarding substance abuse. It is wise to assess clients' knowledge base rather than assume a knowledge deficit regarding substance abuse. Ongoing program and performance assessment keeps the educational components of treatment relevant. Specific educational content addressed in the treatment setting includes the following:

Knowledge of alcohol and other mood-altering substances
Knowledge of real and potential health problems
Current medications and future use of medications
Stress management
Assertiveness skills
The relationship between HIV/AIDS and substance abuse
Psychosocial adaptation in recovery
Emotional symptoms that require additional therapy
Relapse risks in relation to all of the above

Nursing also plays a key role in educating other members of the substance abuse team about nursing-specific components of treatment and related health issues of substance abuse. A current focus is HIV-AIDS and drug-resistant tuberculosis.

Role modeling for clients

To clients, each treatment team member is a role model of acceptable behavior in recovery. Appropriate role modeling and understanding of that role require ongoing clinical supervision to continually assess and provide feedback that promotes program stability and staff development. This may occur in individual or group interactions, through case presentations, or in program meetings.

Nonaddictive lifestyles are the best role modeling staff can provide. This includes food and nicotine abuse. The nursing staff should be perceived as respected, approachable health care professionals who are members of the treatment team.

SUMMARY

A variety of factors are involved in identifying the nature of the nursing role in substance abuse. Many of these factors relate to the nature of the particular substance abuse treatment setting and its organization. A nurse entering the field or seeking employment in substance abuse should carefully review the characteristics of the setting being considered.

There are a number of disciplines involved in substance abuse care, and often the treatment team experiences role diffusion when roles are defined based on experience and individual characteristics rather than discipline. Treatment personnel may include recovering members, which is somewhat unique to the substance abuse field.

Throughout the stages of the client's treatment, nurses are involved in coordinating the care of the client. Nursing care during detoxification requires knowledge of potential withdrawal patterns. Nursing care during treatment requires that the nurse assess and address the physical, psychosocial, spiritual, and cognitive domains of care.

REFERENCES

American Nurses Association & National Nurses Society on Addictions. (1988). *Standards of addictions nursing practice with selected diagnoses and criteria.* Kansas City, MO: The Association.

American Nurses Association Task Force on Substance Abuse and Addictions. (1991). *Statement on substance abuse and addictions.* Kansas City, MO: The Association.

Barker, L.R. & Whitfield, C.L. (1991). Alcoholism. In L.R. Barker, J.R. Burton, & P.D. Zieve (Eds.) *Principles of Ambulatory Medicine.* (3rd ed, pp 204-231). Baltimore: Williams & Wilkins.

Becker, H.C. & Hale, R.L. (1993). Repeated episodes of ethanol withdrawal potentiate the severity of subsequent withdrawal seizures: An animal model of alcohol withdrawal "kindling." *Alcoholism: Clinical and Experimental Research, 17,* 94.

Burns, E. & Thompson, A. (1993). *An addictions curriculum for nurses and other helping professionals.* New York: Springer.

Church, O.M., Fisk, N.B., & Neafsey, P.J. (1992). *Project NEADA: Curriculum for nursing education in alcohol and drug abuse.* Storrs, CT: University of Connecticut.

Corrigan, E.M. & Anderson, S.C. (1985). Graduate social work education in alcoholism. In E. Freeman (Ed.) *Social work practice with clients who have alcohol problems.* (pp 335-350). Springfield, IL: Thomas.

DeSoto, C.B., O'Donnell, W.E., & DeSoto, J.L. (1989). Long-term recovery in alcoholics. *Alcoholism: Clinical and Experimental Research, 13,* 693-697.

Fleming, M.F. (1991). Medical detoxification for sedatives, stimulants, and opiates. In M. Fleming (Ed.) *Substance abuse education for family physicians.* Kansas City, MO: Society of Teachers of Family Medicine.

Fleming, M.F. & Barry, K.L. (1992). *Addictive disorders.* St. Louis: Mosby.

Folstein, M.F., Folstein, S.E., & McHugh, P.R. (1975). Mini-mental state: A practical method for grading the cognitive states of patients for the clinician. *Journal of Psychological Research, 12,* 189.

Friedrich, R.M. & Kus, R.J. (1991). Cognitive impairments in early sobriety: Nursing interventions. *Archives of Psychiatric Nursing, 5*(2), 105-112.

Galanter, M. (1989). Alcohol and drug abuse as a subspecialty. *Alcohol Health and Research World, 13,* 42-47.

Gerace, L., Sullivan, E.J., Murphy, S., & Cotter, F. (1992). Faculty development and curriculum change in alcohol and other drug abuse. *Nurse Educator, 17*(1), 24-27.

Hayashida, M., Alterman, A.I., & McLellan, A.T. (1989). Comparative effectiveness and costs of inpatient and outpatient detoxification of patients with mild-to-moderate alcohol withdrawal syndrome. *New England Journal of Medicine, 320,* 358.

Hoffman, A. & Heinemann, M.E. (1987). Substance abuse education in schools of nursing. *Journal of Nursing Education, 26,* 282-287.

Institute of Medicine. (1990). *Broadening the base of treatment for alcohol problems.* Washington, D.C.: National Academy Press.

Jack, L. (1990). *Nursing care planning with the addicted client, Vol. II.* Skokie, IL: National Nurses Society on Addictions.

Kinney, J. (1983). Relapse among alcoholics who are alcoholism counselors. *Journal of Studies on Alcohol, 44*(4), 744-748.

Krupnik, S.L.W. & Wade, A.J. (Eds.) (1993). *Psychiatric care planning.* Springhouse, PA: Springhouse Corp.

Linnoila, M. (1987). Alcohol withdrawal and noradrenergic function. *Annuals of Internal Medicine, 107,* 875.

McGivern, D.O. (1991). The role of the nurse on the interdisciplinary treatment team. In M.A. Naegle (Ed.) *Substance abuse education in nursing,* Vol. III, New York: National League for Nursing.

Mariano, C. (1989a). The case for interdisciplinary collaboration. *Nursing Outlook, 37,* 285.

Mariano, C. (1989b). Interdisciplinary collaboration in the treatment of addictions. *Addictions Nursing Network, 1*(4), 7.

Naegle, M. (1991). *Substance abuse education in nursing, Vols. I, II, III,* New York: National League for Nursing.

Naegle, M. (1992). *Substance abuse education in nursing, Vols. I, II, III,* New York: National League for Nursing.

National Council on Alcoholism and Drug Dependence publishes salary study. (1993). *The Alcoholism Report, 21*(5), 8.

National Nurses Society on Addictions. (1990). *The core curriculum of addictions nursing.* Skokie, IL: Midwest Education Association.

Schnoll, S., Durburg, J., Griffin, J., Gitlow, S., Hunter, R.B., Sack, J., Stimmel, B., deWit, H., & Jara, G.B. (1993). Physician certification in addiction medicine 1986-1990: A four-year experience. *Journal of Addictive Diseases, 12,* 123.

Stuart, G.W. & Sundeen, S.J. (1995). Principles and practice of psychiatric nursing. (5th ed.). St. Louis: Mosby.

Sullivan, J.T., Kykora, K., Schneiderman, J., Naranjo, C.A., & Sellers, E.M. (1989). Assessment of alcohol withdrawal: The revised clinical institute withdrawal assessment for alcohol scale. *British Journal of Addiction, 84,* 1353-1357.

Woolf, D.S. (1991a). Detoxification. In E.G. Bennett & D. Woolf (Eds.) *Substance abuse* (2nd ed., pp 214-227). Albany, NY: Delmar.

Woolf, D.S. (1991b). CNS depressants: Alcohol. In E.G. Bennett & D. Woolf (Eds.) *Substance abuse* (2nd ed., pp 13-29). Albany, NY: Delmar.

12 Dual Diagnosis: A Challenge for Mental Health and Substance Abuse Caregivers

This chapter describes the phenomenon of "dual diagnosis," or clients diagnosed with both substance abuse and a psychiatric disorder. The characteristics of such clients, approaches to treatment, and the nurse's role in the care of these clients are discussed.

DEFINITION OF DUAL DIAGNOSIS

Dual diagnosis is defined as the concurrent existence of both substance abuse or dependency and one or more psychiatric disorders (NIDA, 1991). Improvement in one disorder is not necessarily associated with improvement in the other. According to DSM IV, a mental disorder is a "clinically significant behavioral or psychological syndrome or pattern that occurs in an individual and that is associated with present distress (a painful symptom) or disability (impairment in one or more important areas of functioning)" (APA, 1994, p. xxi). Substance abuse is the maladaptive pattern of use (i.e., causing or exacerbating a physical, psychological, social, or occupational problem) not meeting the criteria for dependence. Substance *abuse* and *dependence* differ diagnostically but both involve continual use of alcohol or other substances that cause physical, mental, social, occupational, or family problems. Individuals who meet DSM-IV criteria for substance abuse or dependency *and* a mental disorder are considered to have dual pathology.

Problems in individuals with both psychiatric disorders and substance abuse occur on a continuum of severity and complexity. A young schizophrenic man who lives in a residence and smokes marijuana rather than taking his medication is one example. Those who work with him may not view this occasional drug use as a problem, even though it seems that his intense paranoia worsens and he is often readmitted after a weekend of heavy smoking. Another example is the middle-aged woman with a bipolar illness who, during a manic episode, skips her medication, drinks heavily in bars, and becomes sexually promiscuous. Her private psychiatrist and a clinical nurse-specialist therapist realize her drinking is a problem but their only alternative is to have her readmitted to an inpatient psychiatric unit. A severely personality-disordered man who mutilates himself after a night of drinking alcohol and snorting cocaine also has dual problems. Every time he's admitted to an inpatient unit he is detoxified and told to stop his substance abuse, but no referral is made for substance abuse counseling. Still another example is that of an alcoholic woman who continues to feel depressed and discouraged, sleeps poorly, and has already had one relapse two months into sobriety. Her alcoholism counselor tells her to attend more AA meetings and to "keep it simple," and she will feel better. She is beginning to entertain ideas of suicide. All of these individuals can be "dually diagnosed" but each has highly individualized problems. Their treatment will differ in length and complexity; their risk for relapse and complications, as well as prognosis for recovery, differ dramatically.

Until recently, both mental health and substance abuse treatment providers have avoided this kind of client. However, in the past few decades, as a result of deinstitutionalization, more chronic mentally ill clients have been released into the community. Often lacking adequate care and supervision, many drank and/or took drugs and many became homeless. Even though individuals who are chronically mentally ill and abusing substances are more obvious today, they are not the only, or even majority of, clients with a dual diagnosis.

What do we know about these clients with a dual diagnosis? According to the National Institute of Mental Health Epidemiologic Catchment Area Study, clients with either a psychiatric or substance abuse disorder are at increased risk for the other problem (Reiger et al, 1990). Among those with a mental disorder, 29% also had an alcohol or drug abuse disorder. Similarly, 37% with an alcohol disorder also had a mental disorder. The highest occurrence of comorbidity was among those with a drug (other than alcohol) disorder. More than half (53%) with a drug disorder also had a mental disorder.

It has been estimated that about one third to one half of psychiatric clients seen for admission, crisis intervention, or in emergency rooms following suicide attempts are there as a direct result of alcohol and/or drug consumption (Galanter, Casteneda, & Ferman, 1988). These estimates probably are low because of both client and clinician denial and minimalization. One study found that 75% of hospitalized schizophrenics who also were abusers of alcohol were not diagnosed for the alcohol abuse (Drake & Wallach, 1989).

Clinical reports and research support the view that psychiatric clients are especially vulnerable to psychoactive substances and that the course of a psychiatric disorder is adversely affected by substance abuse. Major mental illness is a disease of the brain and its neurotransmitters; medications are used to improve functioning. When alcohol or other mind-altering drugs are added, managing an already difficult illness is significantly compromised. Schizophrenics who use alcohol or drugs have more delusions, hallucinations, depressions, suicidal behavior, hostility, aggression, housing difficulties, and homelessness (Wilen, O'Keefe, & O'Connell, 1993).

Many problematic relationships between psychoactive substance abuse and its deleterious effect on mental health or illness have been reported (GAP, 1991). The report substantiates that the prognosis is much less favorable when substance abuse occurs in conjunction with mental illness.

In addition, the disorders exacerbate each other. Confused and delusional clients are more confused and delusional and the suicidal are more suicidal. Impulse control and judgment are severely impaired; depression and agitation are increased. Substance abuse clients who experience psychiatric symptoms may self-medicate with psychoactive substances in an attempt to relieve their symptoms. (See Evans & Sullivan, 1990, for more information about dual disorders.)

PRIMARY AND SECONDARY DIAGNOSES

A major issue in treating the client with a dual diagnosis is that of determining primary and secondary diagnoses. The traditional mental health view is that substance abuse is a symptom of an underlying psychiatric disorder (e.g., "When his depression improves, he won't drink"). Given that view, the main target for intervention is the psychiatric problem. The traditional substance abuse view is that substance use is the primary problem and that achieving sobriety and recovery will result in the other symptoms dissipating (e.g., "His depression will lift when he stops drinking").

Knowing which came first—the substance abuse or the psychiatric illness—is important in the early stages of treating anxiety disorders, depressions, bipolar illness, and first-break schizophrenia. Wallen and Werner (1989) suggest that there are five categories of interconnection between substance abuse and mental illness disorders. These are:

Category 1   Mental illness comes first and increases the risk for environmental influences that result in substance abuse.
Category 2   Substance abuse comes first and results in secondary mental illness, especially organic-affective syndromes, organic-delusional disorder, and antisocial behaviors.
Category 3   Substance abuse and mental illness occur simultaneously with no apparent relationship to each other.
Category 4   Substance abuse precipitates the occurrence of a primary mental illness.
Category 5   Mental illness precipitates substance use in an effort to self-medicate to relieve symptoms.

How much impact substance abuse had on the development of a depression, for example, will determine when and if antidepressant medications are started. Miller and Gold (1991) encourage clinicians to delay starting psychiatric medications as long as possible after alcohol and drugs have been discontinued so the individual's sensorium and thinking can stabilize. There is danger, however, of a return to drinking because of untreated depression or severe anxiety. Once the individual has stabilized, if psychiatric symptoms abate a trial period during which the client is free of alcohol, drugs, and medication can determine the need for additional treatment of psychiatric problems. Clients should be monitored closely during this time.

TREATMENT OF THE CLIENT WITH DUAL DIAGNOSIS

Dual diagnosis is difficult for both the client and the clinician. The clinician must be skilled and knowledgeable in treating both substance abuse *and* psychiatric illness. Traditionally, mental health professionals have been reluctant to treat clients with substance abuse. Some addictions professionals have complained that mental health providers ignored or underdiagnosed substance abuse, inappropriately prescribed minor tranquilizers, or hospitalized alcoholics in mental institutions rather than in alcohol treatment facilities. Furthermore, mental health facilities may refuse to treat clients with substance abuse histories, and substance abuse programs may reject those with psychiatric histories.

A clash occurs generally about the selection of a client's primary goal; in mental health it is often stabilization first, followed by increasing insight and subsequent behavior changes. Medications are used as needed. In substance abuse treatment the goal is accepting one's dependency, maintaining sobriety, and abstaining from alcohol and drugs. The goal is to eliminate all drugs that affect the central nervous system.

The concept of power differs in the mental health and substance abuse fields. In the mental health view, empowerment is used to enhance self-esteem and to assist clients to better deal with their problems. From the substance abuse perspective, recognizing one's powerlessness is an important step in accepting one's disease. (This is the paradox inherent in the AA philosophy: When one accepts that one is powerless over the disease, it comes under control.)

Clinicians from *both* fields suffer from negative attitudes, some of which are rooted in their own backgrounds or are complicated by their own family histories, use of substances, or psychiatric symptoms (e.g., chronic depression). Clinicians also are hampered by lack of knowledge about one illness or the other. They get stuck trying to determine which illness came first. Some are fearful of trying to address both problems. As a result, the client's treatment may become splintered; clients are referred to other facilities who then also refer, causing a "dumping syndrome" and delaying necessary, coordinated, comprehensive treatment.

The major stumbling blocks to effective treatment are as follows: determining (1) a primary diagnosis, (2) who treats the client, (3) in which facility, and (4) with what approach. As a result, the client might not receive treatment until crises arise and hospitalization or emergency room visits are needed.

A model for treatment

Treatment must address both substance abuse and the psychiatric problem *simultaneously*. As noted, the occurrence of one increases the risk for the other. The synergistic effect of both disorders makes success unlikely if one disorder is treated without addressing the other.

The model used for designing treatment is crucial and is most often based on a combined treatment model that includes the *recovery* model from the substance abuse field and the *biopsychosocial* model from the mental health field. Box 12-1 illustrates the differences as well as the similarities of the two models. Both treatment approaches are active, participative, and encourage continuous care (outpatient support groups, twelve step groups). Both use interdisciplinary teams of health care providers including physicians, nurses, social workers, psychologists, and counselors.

Some areas of difference between the two models must be addressed. These include *medication use, confrontation, abstinence,* the use of *self-help groups,* and how *lapses* and *relapses* are handled.

Use of medications. Two rules guide the use of medications for clients with

Box 12-1
Selected Comparisons of Recovery and Mental Health Models

Recovery model (chemical dependency)	Biopsychosocial model (mental health)
Disease process	Syndrome concept
Biopsychosocial/spiritual factors	Biopsychosocial factors
	Some attention to philosophical issues
Chronic condition	Chronic condition to many major disorders
Relapse issues	Relapse issues
Genetic/physiological component	Genetic/physiological component in many disorders
Chemical use primary	Psychiatric disorder primary
Loss of control	Ineffective coping
Denial	Poor insight
Despair	Demoralization
Family issues	Family issues
Social stigma	Social stigma
Abstinence an early goal	Stability an early goal
Recovery a long-term goal	Rehabilitation a long-term goal
Powerlessness	Empowerment
No use of mood-altering chemicals	Psychotropic medications used
Education about illness	Education about illness
Halfway houses, ALANO clubs	Group homes, day treatment
Sponsors	Case manager/therapist
AA, Al-Anon, self-help groups	Support groups
Concrete action	Behavior change
Self-examination and acceptance	Awareness and insight
Labeling of self as alcoholic/addict	Seeing self as whole person with a disorder
Practice of communication and social skills	Practice of communication and social skills
Slogans, stories, affirmations	Positive self-talk, imagery
"Step-work"	Psychotherapy
Use of spiritual concepts	Use of existential, transpersonal concepts
Family therapy	Family therapy
Group and individual work	Group and individual work
Continuum of care	Continuum of care
Nutrition, exercise, growth as value	Wellness concepts

From Evans, K. & Sullivan, J.M. (1990). *Dual diagnoses: Counseling the mentally ill substance abuser.* New York: Guilford Press.

coexisting conditions. They are: (1) addictive medications should not be prescribed for regular use after detoxification; and (2) if a psychiatric examination indicates the need for medication, nonaddicting psychotropic medications should be used. Antidepressants, antipsychotics, and lithium are among medications commonly prescribed.

Confrontation.   Confrontation is commonly used in substance abuse treatment to break through denial. For clients with psychiatric disorders (especially schizophrenia), a supportive approach is more conducive to responsiveness and, in fact, confrontation can precipitate a psychotic episode (Evans & Sullivan, 1990). Gentle confrontation in a supportive environment can help the client with a dual diagnosis recognize unhealthy thinking. It also is important to make clients accountable for their actions; the disability is not an excuse to be irresponsible. Direct confrontation is indicated, however, for one group of psychiatric clients—those with antisocial personality disorders.

Abstinence.   Abstinence from alcohol and addictive drugs is the goal for clients with a dual diagnosis. Explaining the illness nature of substance abuse helps these clients and their families understand the need for abstinence. Mental health professionals generally discourage the use of labels, such as "alcoholic," because of concern about a threat to self-esteem. For these clients, however, accepting their substance abuse diagnosis can be positive and help them understand that they have two problems, both of which can be treated.

Self-help groups.   For many clients an essential part of substance abuse recovery is a twelve step group. Attendance at self-help groups is encouraged for the person with a dual diagnosis. In addition to helping maintain abstinence, the groups provide models for appropriate behavior in an accepting environment, which can help improve social skills. Distorted thinking and unproductive behavior also are addressed in these groups.

In the last few years Alcoholics Anonymous has recognized the problems of the mentally ill alcoholic. Although AA states that it has no position regarding medications for mentally ill people (AA, 1976), some AA or NA members continue to believe that a recovering individual should take no mind-altering chemicals, and may discourage people from taking needed medications. Developing relationships with local AA members, arranging meetings in treatment facilities, and attending meetings in person all help the practitioner facilitate the involvement of mentally ill clients with AA or NA. In some areas of the country, "double trouble" meetings have been established. These meetings are geared toward the needs of psychiatric clients and help them feel less out of place and more accepted. A new book has recently been published, modeled on the "Big Book," that tells stories of AA members who also have psychiatric diagnoses (Cleveland & Cleveland, 1992).

Another self-help group useful to the client with a dual diagnosis is Rational Recovery. These groups focus more on thought and behavior change and less on spirituality (AA, 1993). Al-Anon and Adult Children of Alcoholics are self-help groups that also might be recommended after a period of recovery (see Chapter 4). Practitioners should screen meetings carefully before recommending them to the more disturbed clients, because of the intense feelings and detailed personal histories that may be discussed.

Lapses and relapses.   One of the most problematic issues in treating coexisting diagnoses is how lapses and relapses (a return to regular use) are viewed and handled. Using the more classic mental health model, a "slip" or lapse (a return to drinking or using drugs) can be seen as coping, as a form of self-medication, as an acting-out of unresolved conflicts, or simply as misbehavior. Using a mental health approach, a slip would be discussed with the client, asking why it happened, the feelings involved, and how to prevent its reoccurrence. A substance abuse clinician might see a slip as a result of not following ("working") the program (usually twelve step). With this model, only a small number of lapses are tolerated, as opposed to the mental health model in which any number might be accepted.

While the program's ideology is important in treating clients with a dual diagnosis, slips and relapses have highly individualized meaning for each client and need to be handled based on the individual's ego strength and level of psychiatric impairment. With a psychiatric client who has poor judgment, poor impulse control, and few coping skills, slips may be viewed by the client as socially acceptable self-medication. A relapse because the client returns to substance abuse or discontinues psychiatric medications so that psychiatric symptoms reappear also reflects the client's denial of one or both problems. In contrast, a client with significant psychiatric pathology who has repeated slips or who has not been attending twelve step meetings or therapy would be treated differently than a chronic schizophrenic who smokes marijuana on a weekend after an increase in auditory hallucinations.

Developing a set of principles and clearly identifying one's belief system and frames of reference becomes a major issue in treating both problems effectively. Some clinicians may decide that while the use of alcohol and drugs is problematic, sporadic use does not jeopardize the client's capacity for treatment. Others believe that any use of nonprescribed mind-altering substances interferes with recovery.

CHARACTERISTICS OF TREATMENT FOR THE CLIENT WITH DUAL DIAGNOSIS

Several important components of treatment for the client with a dual diagnosis address these clients' special needs. Contingency contracts, family treatment, and group techniques are all used.

Contingency contracts

Clear expectations and goals for clients are reflected not only in staff philosophy and approaches but in agreements made with clients. These agreements are called contingency contracts because they spell out expected behaviors and consequences contingent upon those behaviors. They can either be formal—written and signed—or primarily verbal. Contracts often include expectations about attending the treatment program on a regular basis, taking only prescribed medications, abstaining from alcohol and other drugs, and attending AA or NA meetings with a set frequency. Contracts also may spell out guidelines for preventing and responding to relapse. Agreements should be clear regarding behaviors that will precipitate discharge. This is especially important for personality-disordered or unmotivated clients. Staff must have a unified approach or clients will use one illness to manipulate the other (i.e., "splitting"). This will impede the client's treatment and promote havoc with the staff. Because substance abusers feel that they must use substances to feel normal, relapse is possible.

Family treatment

Dysfunctional family systems often are found in families of clients with a dual diagnosis. These families may be chaotic or rigid. Chaotic families offer little structure or consistency. Rigid families, on the other hand, are inflexible and respond in fixed ways regardless of the circumstances. Dysfunctional families also may vary from enmeshment to disengagement. Enmeshed family members have few boundaries and are overly responsive to each other, whereas disengaged families seldom interact and are emotionally distant (Evans & Sullivan, 1990).

There is wide variation in family involvement by the time a client has been dually diagnosed. Clients may have no family involvement, yet others have supportive families. The family should be assessed early in treatment. This helps the clinician involve the family in treatment.

Often families and clients can accept one illness but find it difficult to acknowledge the other. On the other hand, family members often are relieved to learn that both problems are finally identified and addressed. Sometimes parents of schizophrenic clients are surprised to learn about the possible impact a beer has on behavior and the potential for relapse that drinking poses. When family members become informed, they can reinforce appropriate behaviors and discourage others. An additional resource is the local National Alliance for the Mentally Ill chapter, which often sponsors educational or support programs for relatives.

Group treatment

Group treatment, a major emphasis in treatment of clients with a dual diagnosis, is structured, supportive, and educational. Groups may be didactic or they may use a more process-oriented approach. Skills such as relapse prevention, assertiveness, and relaxation techniques are taught. Basic information on substance abuse is given, including the medical and physiological aspects of the disease and concepts from twelve step programs. The nurse also might teach characteristics of mental health and illness as well as the disease concept of addictions. The fact that the client has a dual problem is clearly recognized and openly discussed in a structured manner. Working toward a shared identity and offering a reservoir of support are goals of group treatment.

An increasingly common form of group treatment that nurses often conduct is client education groups. These have been a standard component of most substance abuse treatment programs. These groups need to be planned with the client's level of comprehension considered. This may have little to do with the client's intelligence but more with the degree of psychiatric impairment and frequency and severity of drug or alcohol use. The amount of material covered, and over what period of time, depends on the type of treatment program. On a short-stay acute unit, for example, clients may be exposed to: (1) the concept of dual diagnosis, (2) the disease concept of addiction, (3) where to obtain help, (4) principles of twelve step programs, and (5) relapse prevention techniques. Through education, dual diagnosis problems can be addressed simultaneously. For example, when discussing depression, the practitioner can explain how drugs and alcohol use might accentuate psychiatric symptoms and precipitate relapse. Many appropriate educational materials exist, including films, pamphlets, and instructional manuals.

As clients become more stable, both psychiatrically and in substance abuse recovery, they can engage in more intensive and process-oriented groups, which are structured so that dual problems are addressed. Learning to trust, sharing with others, and being open with the group are possible, as well as essential, for recovery. The group can help clients learn how to deal with feelings without alcohol or drugs. Even very ill clients can discuss topics such as loss and grief, anger, loss of control, what it is like to be both "crazy" and "stoned" on substances. Over time, these groups can develop to the extent that clients confront and support each other.

Discussion, support, and therapy groups are essential during all phases of treatment. Although it is helpful to have clients at somewhat the same level of sobriety as well as recovery from mental illness, this is not always possible. In fact, a mixed group utilizes the progress of those who are further into recovery to encourage those who are early in recovery or who are still in denial.

Educating the staff

To successfully serve clients with a dual diagnosis, the first step is to educate the staff and to identify attitudes, potential difficulties, stereotypes, and biases. The education of health care professionals has been limited regarding substance abuse. Even when the professional is educated to care for clients with mental illness, substance abuse content is inadequate. Conversely, substance abuse training includes little information about psychopathology. These differences result in parallel rather than integrated treatment (Clement et al, 1993). Staff members trained in either discipline need additional information. Whether the program is located in a primary psychiatric or primary alcoholism setting, staff members need to examine their own attitudes of ignorance, chauvinism, fears, and stereotypes. Philosophies about medications, sobriety, and twelve step programs, as well as beliefs about mental illness and substance abuse, must be openly discussed.

Staff members also need ongoing training and consultation on a case-by-case basis. Psychiatric staff need to become familiar with twelve step and recovery models, the meaning of denial, and the process of recovery. Addictions staff need to learn theories of and approaches to clients with various forms of mental illness (e.g., suicide potential, hallucinations) and to grapple with the realization that these substance abusing clients may need a more individualized form of treatment. Addictions staff need to understand the action of medications on brain chemistry and their importance in managing schizophrenia, obsessive compulsive disorder, and bipolar and other mood disorders. The staff in both specialties must become intellectually and attitudinally sophisticated.

THE NURSE'S ROLE IN TREATMENT

Treatment of the client with a dual diagnosis occurs in inpatient settings, day treatment or partial hospitalization, residential settings, and in outpatient, vocational, rehabilitative, and other community-based programs. Ideally, treatment is designed to meet the needs of a specific population. More often, acutely ill and/or severely disabled clients are mixed in with those who are less impaired and more responsive to treatment. Since treatment is usually short-term, staff can use admissions to deepen the therapeutic relationship and view them as steps on the road to recovery. Each type of treatment has a role for the nurse who works with the interdisciplinary team.

The nurse's role in inpatient treatment

Most psychiatric inpatient units and substance abuse treatment units are struggling with the limitations and pressures of reimbursement resulting from widespread use of managed care. Length of inpatient stays has now decreased dramatically. The 28-day substance abuse treatment program is passé, and psychiatric admission longer than 2 weeks has become obsolete. Treatment in both settings, therefore, is more intensive.

Assessment.   The client who has both a psychiatric disorder and a substance abuse disorder requires comprehensive assessment. A complete history and physical assessment is performed. The intrapersonal domain is explored for the client's present feelings, thoughts, and behaviors. Assessment of the intrapersonal domain involves the quality and quantity of relationships with significant others and the adequacy of functioning in school or job, parental or child responsibilities, and leisure and recreational activities. It is important to include past history as well as the present. Then a comprehensive assessment to determine that two disorders coexist is essential because the effects of substance abuse can mimic psychiatric symptomatology. Clement and associates (1993) adapted criteria for substance abuse (Hoffman et al, 1991) to include psychopathology; they suggest that assessment of at least six areas is required. These are: (1) acuity of intoxication or withdrawal and/or the positive symptoms of mental illness, (2) biological comorbidity, (3) psychological comorbidity, (4) acceptance or rejection of treatment, (5) relapse potential/residual negative signs of mental illness, and (6) the recovery environment.

Assessments follow a systematic process; standardized tools exist for mental status, psychiatric history, and substance abuse. Elements particular to the client with a dual diagnosis are:

Psychiatric elements
1. Presenting problem, reason for admission; description of client at admission; vital signs on admission
2. Mental status, especially mood and affect lability; cognitive ability and orientation
3. Psychiatric history, past hospitalizations and reasons; suicide attempts and reasons; history of mental, physical, sexual abuse; trauma
4. Family history of mental illness
5. Medical history, current medical problems

Substance abuse/dependency elements
1. Occasion for admission, client's level of intoxication; last use of alcohol or drug; withdrawal risk assessment
2. Pattern of use of alcohol, illicit drugs, caffeine, nicotine, prescription medications, and over-the-counter drugs
3. Past treatments for substance abuse/dependency; experiences with detox-

ification; rehabilitation; outpatient treatment; attendance at AA/NA, Al-Anon, or ACOA self-help groups

4. Family history of alcoholism/substance abuse, including teetotalism and use by less-close relatives, including in-laws

Assessments must be completed quickly, obtaining the most information possible in the least amount of time. (Chapter 3 includes several assessment tools.) Family and significant others often provide information, particularly when the client is either too psychotic or too impaired to give an adequate history. The nurse plays a vital role in completing an extensive nursing history that includes both psychiatric and substance-abuse information. Despite the need for speed, both psychiatric and substance abuse assessments may have to take place over time, because of the client's attention span and/or stress tolerance. Simply doing both assessments and naming them as mental health and substance abuse assessments helps counter denial in the client and family and makes clear that both aspects of an individual's history are important.

Since distinguishing psychiatric symptoms from substance abuse symptoms is sometimes difficult, it is important for the nurse to document descriptions of these symptoms, both qualitatively and quantitatively, in detail. Additionally, because some symptoms abate with detoxification and time, it is important to document the progress of symptoms over time. The nurse relates incidents and important elements of the history to other caregivers and plans needed care. For example, the nurse might note that the client has been admitted to a psychiatric hospital three times in the last two years and that each admission was the result of a suicide attempt with an overdose of prescribed benzodiazepines and alcohol. The nurse might glean from the history that a client was admitted for a substance abuse relapse following 8 months of sobriety, attendance in an outpatient program, and regular AA/NA involvement. The client's course may have been complicated by a profound sense of hopelessness and helplessness that has become progressively more demoralizing and paralyzing. At some point during the client's stays on the unit, it is useful to describe the relationship of events and findings to the client, other caregivers, and to the family. Such a description interferes with denial, provides education, and emphasizes that there are two problems, both of which need attention and treatment.

The standard monitoring of physical functions (e.g., vital signs, lab tests, physical complaints) and the continuous, 24-hour availability of the nursing staff provide opportunities to observe more subtle signs of substance abuse. A slight rise in vital signs may be the first indication of impending withdrawal in a client who denied heavy alcohol use. Elevated liver enzymes can indicate liver damage from alcohol; nontherapeutic levels of lithium or other psychotropic medications also may portend a relapse. The nurse is in an ideal position to track these medically related phenomena and describe them to the client, family, and other caregivers. (See Care Plans 12-1, 12-2, and 12-3.)

The nurse's role in partial hospitalization

Most partial-hospitalization programs are designed for clients whose illness is more severe. These clients have a poor prognosis without a structured, long-term reha-

Text continued on p. 364.

Care Plan 12-1

Depression and Alcoholism

Carl, a 60-year-old married male, was admitted to the psychiatric unit by his wife of 35 years, severely depressed and suicidal. Both say their marriage is happy and they know of no reason why he is depressed. Assessment revealed long-term, six-pack-a-day alcohol use. They both considered his alcohol use irrelevant. He is employed as an assistant manager of a motor vehicle repair service. He says his job is going fine.

ASSESSMENT

Complete history and physical revealed liver enlargement, elevated AST and SGOT, anemia, and gastric ulcer. Client cried frequently during interview, facial expression was sad. Movements and speech were slowed. He complains that it has become increasingly hard to get out of bed and go to work each day and he has difficulty remembering and concentrating. He and his wife have had increasingly infrequent sexual relations "because I feel so down." The last time was six weeks ago. His children are now grown, but "they are busy and don't have time to come see me anymore." He doesn't "do much in the evenings anymore but just sit and watch TV with his wife." He denies being depressed in his younger years and "just doesn't understand why I am now." He began drinking alcohol when he was in high school, enjoys drinking, and has drunk a six-pack of beer every day for thirty years. "It's never hurt me." He states, "It's not worth living anymore feeling like this." He has a plan to take the car and drive at a high rate of speed into a bridge abutment.

NURSING DIAGNOSES

High risk for violence toward self related to verbalization of suicidal ideation
Denial related to long-term alcohol use
Hopelessness related to ineffective management of his life and excessive alcohol use

Outcome identification	Nursing interventions	Rationale	Evaluation
Nursing diagnosis: High risk for violence toward self related to verbalization of suicidal ideation			
1. Client will remain safe with no self-harm by discharge.	1a. Contract with the client that he will not harm himself for a specific period of time.	1a. The client's commitment to refrain from self-harm for a specific period dramatically reduces the possibility of suicide.	1. Carl contracted with the nurse while in the hospital on a day-to-day basis. By day seven, he declared he would not hurt himself. By discharge, he said he no longer felt like harming himself. Goal met.
	1b. Mobilize family and friends to contract with the client also and to monitor the client's actions and self-statements.	1b. The enlistment of assistance from family and friends reinforces the nurse's actions to keep the client safe.	

Outcome identification	Nursing interventions	Rationale	Evaluation

Nursing diagnosis: High risk for violence toward self related to verbalization of suicidal ideation—cont'd

	1c. Assess client's environment for any object that could be used for self-harm.	1c. Removing objects that could be used for self-harm reduces the possibility of impulsive self-harm.	
	1d. Contract with the client that he will contact the nurse if feelings of self-harm become too strong.	1d. This gives the client a source of social support when feelings overwhelm him.	
	1e. Give medication as ordered or request medication for assistance from the physician.	1e. In case the client continues to talk of self-harm, medication can be used to calm him.	

Nursing diagnosis: Denial related to long-term alcohol use

1. Client will state that alcohol is a problem in his life within 2 weeks.	1a. Teach about AODA and the disease concept.	1a. Knowledge about the disease will convince the client that he has the disease.	1. By 2 weeks, Carl acknowledged that his alcohol use had caused problems in his life. Goal met.
	1b. Teach the client about the relationship between alcohol use and depression.	1b. Heavy alcohol use can precipitate depression in those predisposed, exacerbate depression, and cause symptoms of depression.	
	1c. Have him list ways his life has become unmanageable through his alcohol use.	1c. This is AA Step 1.	

Continued.

Care Plan 12-1

Depression and Alcoholism—cont'd

Outcome identification	Nursing interventions	Rationale	Evaluation
Nursing diagnosis: Denial related to long-term alcohol use—cont'd			
2. Client will make a commitment to complete treatment for both the depression and the alcoholism within 2 weeks.	2a. If depression is not severe, don't be too quick to assist the client in his depression.	2a. Depression can be a window through denial for these clients.	2. After 2 weeks, Carl agreed to complete treatment for both disorders. Goal met.
	2b. Gently point out ways in which alcohol has exacerbated his depression.	2b. Confrontation should be done gently with the depressed client.	
	2c. Point out hope for feeling better and successes he may expect from treatment.	2c. A ray of hope may be the strongest impetus for treatment.	
Nursing diagnosis: Hopelessness related to ineffective management of his life and excessive alcohol use			
1. Client will state hopes for the future and make plans to fulfill them by discharge.	1a. Point out to the client that he will feel better as he increases his activity. If he refuses, ask him if he feels good now, not being active.	1a. Client may want to wait until he feels better to increase activity.	1. By discharge, Carl had been stabilized on an antidepressant and had completed treatment for his alcoholism. He was attending AA meetings and agreed to continue. He stated that he felt better than he had for years. He and his wife decided to complete marital therapy and were making plans for vacation the following summer. Goal met.
	1b. Point out client's negative thoughts.	1b. Depression is sustained by persistent negative thoughts.	
	1c. Place strong emphasis on client's strengths.	1c. The depressed client has very low self-esteem; this helps to raise self-esteem.	
	1d. Help him find pleasant activities with other people.	1d. Clients begin to feel better when engaged in pleasant activities. Association with other people also enhances mood.	

Outcome identification	Nursing interventions	Rationale	Evaluation

Nursing diagnosis: Hopelessness related to ineffective management of his life and excessive alcohol use—cont'd

Outcome identification	Nursing interventions	Rationale	Evaluation
	1e. Use kind, gentle approach.	1e. This client feels very bad about himself and needs gentleness and kindness.	
	1f. Do not allow the client to castigate himself over past behaviors.	1f. Ruminating over past behaviors lowers his self-esteem and deepens his depression.	
	1g. Set time limits, such as 5 minutes, for him to talk about "poor me."	1g. Limits negative thoughts.	
	1h. When teaching, use auditory input and ask for feedback, then be prepared to repeat.	1h. Persons who are depressed have difficulty with memory and concentration and require repetition.	
	1i. Teach necessity of taking medication as ordered if it is prescribed.	1i. Often AA groups discourage clients from taking psychiatric medications, teaching that all chemical use is bad.	
	1j. Monitor and document lifting of depression with passage of time.	1j. Depression may have been caused by the alcohol and may lift as the system returns to normal.	

Care Plan 12-2

Bipolar Disorder and Marijuana Abuse

Mike is a 22-year-old male who was recently readmitted to the psychiatric unit. He is diagnosed with bipolar disorder, manic phase, and was psychotic both at his original admission and the new admission. The second admission occurred 2 weeks after discharge from a 3-week inpatient stay. A review of all of the activities during Mike's 2 weeks at home disclosed that he had resumed his job on the night shift. In addition, he smoked marijuana several times a day each day. He had been taking his lithium regularly as prescribed, however.

ASSESSMENT

Complete history and physical revealed that Mike was slightly overweight and had a slightly elevated SGOT; everything else appeared within normal limits. He stated that he felt really good. His affect was bright and his face flushed. He moved constantly and exhibited push of speech. Thought was tangential and difficult to follow. The interview had to be extremely brief because he could not stay in the room. He currently takes lithium, 1500 mg/d. He was diagnosed with bipolar disorder three years ago at the age of 19, his sophomore year in college. At that time, he was staying up all night and instigating a campus revolution plan. He has been unable to complete his college education and has taken a job as a night watchman. The current hospitalization is the fifth for this disorder. He said that he first began trying marijuana at age 15. Initially, he used with friends only about once a month at parties, but his use increased to daily by age 18. After that time, use increased to the current 3 joints per day.

NURSING DIAGNOSES

Knowledge deficit: Bipolar disorder, medication and substance use related to need for
   repeated hospitalizations
Altered health maintenance related to need for repeated hospitalizations
Ineffective individual coping related to overactive behavior and substance abuse

Outcome identification	Nursing interventions	Rationale	Evaluation
Nursing diagnosis: Knowledge deficit: Bipolar disorder, medication and substance use related to need for repeated hospitalizations			
1. Client will describe process of bipolar disorder within 2 weeks.	1a. Use only simple explanations until the client is stabilized and mania is under control. 1b. When client is stabilized, explain how bipolar disorder is related to disruption of the biological rhythms.	1a. Client's thought processes are too disorganized to follow complex thought. 1b. This will give the client rationale for some lifestyle interventions.	1. After one week, Mike could explain the process of bipolar disorder. He hadn't heard about the biological rhythm disruption before and thanked the nurse for the information. Goal met.

Outcome identification	Nursing interventions	Rationale	Evaluation
Nursing diagnosis: Knowledge deficit: Bipolar disorder, medication and substance use related to need for repeated hospitalizations—cont'd			
	1c. Explain how lithium modulates the highs and the lows in bipolar disorder and must be taken for life.	1c. Client needs explanation for need for continued medication.	
	1d. Teach about lithium, signs of toxicity, need for periodic blood levels, need to continue to take medication.	1d. Knowledge will motivate client to continue taking medication.	
2. Client will list critical elements for controlling bipolar disorder within 2 weeks.	2a. Help client lead a balanced lifestyle.	2a. Balance in work, nutrition, and play reduces stress.	2. Client complained about how difficult it would be for him to eat and sleep regular hours because of his dating and work hours. Client listed critical elements to control bipolar disease, but expressed doubt that he could live up to the elements. Goal partially met. *Revision:* Help client understand the problems with working nights. Help him find a way to date and keep somewhat regular hours.
	2b. Help client reduce stress.	2b. The stress response may precipitate imbalance and trigger mania or depression.	
	2c. Teach importance of regular medication.	2c. Medication modulates the highs and lows of bipolar disorder.	
	2d. Teach value of eating, sleeping, and working regular hours.	2d. Regular eating, sleeping, and working assists the body in regulating biological rhythms.	
	2e. Make clear to client that he must avoid substances that stimulate or depress the CNS.	2e. Mind-altering drugs cause imbalance in the CNS.	

Continued.

Care Plan 12-2

Bipolar Disorder and Marijuana Abuse—cont'd

Outcome identification	Nursing interventions	Rationale	Evaluation
Nursing diagnosis: Knowledge deficit: Bipolar disorder, medication and substance use related to need for repeated hospitalizations—cont'd			
	2f. Make client know he must notify caregiver when body electrolytes may be disrupted, e.g., very hot weather, vomiting, or diarrhea.	2f. Anything which disrupts electrolytes has the potential to precipitate a manic or depressive episode.	
3. Client will discuss the relationship between substance use and bipolar disorder within 2 weeks.	3a. Explain how mind-altering substances either stimulate or depress the nervous system and exacerbate the bipolar disorder.	3a. The client needs this information to have a rationale for not using the drugs.	3. Client could discuss this relationship but stated that when he becomes too stressed it really helps him relax to use the marijuana. Goal partially met. *Revision:* Help him find more ways to reduce stress.
Nursing diagnosis: Altered health maintenance related to need for repeated hospitalizations			
1. Client will describe a balanced lifestyle within 2 weeks.	1a. Help the client plan a reasonable mixture of work, play, and love.	1a. The manic client often engages in excesses and needs to know how to plan for a reasonable balance.	1. Client can describe a balanced lifestyle and is motivated to try one. Goal met.
	1b. Help client plan nutrition and exercise that is acceptable to him and plausible.	1b. The manic client may be malnourished because he forgot to eat, and exercise may be nonexistent or it may be excessive.	
	1c. Teach him to use stress management.	1c. The manic client generally overestimates his capacities and gets himself into many scrapes. He	

Outcome identification	Nursing interventions	Rationale	Evaluation
Nursing diagnosis: Altered health maintenance related to need for repeated hospitalizations—cont'd			
	1d. Teach him time management.	needs to know how to manage stress and plan more realistically. 1d. The manic client overestimates his ability to accomplish something and needs help to plan his time realistically.	
2. Client will demonstrate at least two elements of a balanced lifestyle within 1 month.	2a. Give client a checklist to list activities undertaken during free time while in the hospital.	2a. A checklist may help a manic client manage time.	2. Client could work on and succeed in time management while in the hospital and was eager to set up an exercise plan. He exercised while in the hospital but found it problematic with a job on the night shift. Goal partially met.
	2b. Ask client what he would like to do while in the hospital.	2b. Enlisting the client's input will make success more likely.	
	2c. Help him make a plan to do two activities that he would like.	2c. Client's self-esteem is raised by a simple plan he has made.	
	2d. Help client develop a reasonable exercise program while in the hospital.	2d. An exercise program can help the client dissipate excess energy and will be fairly easy to do while in the hospital.	
Nursing diagnosis: Ineffective individual coping related to overactive behavior and substance abuse			
1. Client will be able to sit in a group situation for 1 hour without disruption of the group within 2 weeks.	1a. Work with client for only short periods while he is still manic.	1a. The manic client has only a short attention span.	1. After 2 weeks, the client could sit and participate in a group. Goal met.
	1b. Avoid any attempt to stop manic behavior.	1b. Any attempt to stop the behavior is nontherapeutic and the client is likely to become highly agitated.	

Continued.

Outcome identification	Nursing interventions	Rationale	Evaluation
Nursing diagnosis: Ineffective individual coping related to overactive behavior and substance abuse—cont'd			
	1c. Redirect the excess energy.	1c. Client's behavior is better controlled when he is allowed to channel his excess energy by constructive means.	
	1d. Keep stimulation at a low level.	1d. The client is already over-stimulated so it is important to reduce this as much as possible.	
	1e. Set limits gently, but firmly.	1e. The client needs to have help to control his behavior. Consistent limit setting lets the client know when to stop.	
2. Client will participate in treatment within 1 week.	2a. When mania is under control, engage client in standard AODA treatment.	2a. The client with bipolar disorder, when mania or depression is under control, can handle standard treatment as well as anyone.	2. Client agreed to participate in AODA treatment. Goal met.
	2b. Teach him about special affinities he may have for stimulants and the dangers of this.	2b. Manic clients may want to seek a hyperactive state because they find this pleasant.	

bilitative program. Programs can be either day or evening. Day treatment is used most often with psychiatric clients and evening treatment often is used for clients with substance abuse who are able to work or attend school during the daytime hours. Nurses can participate in group and individual counseling and educational groups.

Educating both clients and families about medications also is a role for the nurse. Medications are and will continue to be a part of these clients' lives. They

Outcome identification	Nursing interventions	Rationale	Evaluation

Nursing diagnosis: Ineffective individual coping related to overactive behavior and substance abuse—cont'd

	2c. Ask him to keep his responses in group sessions clear, concise, and reality-based.	2c. This client may dominate groups or ramble excessively, but can control this when limits are set.	
	2d. Use gentle but firm limit setting.	2d. The excessive activity is biologically based but will respond to kind, gentle limits.	
	2e. Use the recovery approach for both AODA and bipolar disorder.	2e. Both disorders are chronic and need lifelong recovery responses.	
	2f. Help him learn boundaries for his behavior.	2f. Often the exuberance of the person with bipolar disorder will overwhelm others. He needs to learn boundaries so as to participate in AA appropriately.	

need accurate information. In educational groups, nurses can expand the focus from traditional psychotropic medications to street drugs, alcohol, and over-the-counter drugs, particularly those containing alcohol or caffeine. Learning why addicting drugs are "bad" even though they make you "feel good" and why "good" drugs (e.g., antipsychotics) make you feel bad is valuable information. Dosages, also, are important. Clients may think if one pill is good, three are better.

Educating and supporting the family in both a formal and informal manner is

Text continued on p. 370.

Care Plan 12-3

Schizophrenia and Alcohol Abuse

Gerald is a 43-year-old man who was diagnosed with paranoid schizophrenia, chronic type, 23 years ago. He averages about three hospitalizations per year. The current hospitalization is the third this year. He was brought to the hospital by his parents, who said he was brought to their home by the police after he was found incoherent and wandering through the streets. He has been living in a halfway house but periodically is kicked out for being drunk. At those times, he comes home to his old room at his parents' home.

ASSESSMENT

History and physical exam were done. Physical revealed normal adult male. His affect is flat, any emotion shown was inappropriate to the content discussed. He had to be asked repeatedly to remain seated throughout the brief interview. Thoughts were incoherent. History was completed with information from parents. He had been an average student during high school, a quiet boy that had a few friends but mainly was a loner. He began college and at first made average grades. His sophomore year, he failed several courses and stated that he couldn't complete assignments. He said that "voices told me not to write the papers." He lived at home with his parents for five years after the first psychotic break, but they stated they couldn't handle him anymore. He was placed in a group home, then later began living in a halfway house. They reported that his hospitalizations increased after placement in the halfway house. They thought that his heavy alcohol use began at that time and has increased a great deal since. They were aware of only infrequent social drinking before that time.

NURSING DIAGNOSES

Alteration in thought processes related to acute psychotic episode and substance abuse
Ineffective individual coping related to his inability to function on his own and to substance abuse
Impaired social interaction related to altered thought processes

Outcome identification	Nursing interventions	Rationale	Evaluation
Nursing diagnosis: Alteration in thought processes related to acute psychotic episode and substance abuse			
1. Client will do own ADLs, take medication consistently, and attend clinic appointments, social activities, and skills training within 2 weeks.	1a. Assist the client in self-care while medication is taking effect.	1a. The psychotic and disoriented client may not be able to care for himself.	1. After one week Gerald was able to resume his own ADLs in the hospital. He began attending groups at this time. Goal met.
	1b. Reduce stimulation for the psychotic client; may need to stay in room.	1b. Excess stimulation increases anxiety in the psychotic client.	

Outcome identification	Nursing interventions	Rationale	Evaluation
Nursing diagnosis: Alteration in thought processes related to acute psychotic episode and substance abuse—cont'd			
	1c. Protect the client from intense affect.	1c. The client diagnosed with schizophrenia cannot handle intense affect.	
	1d. Provide the client with schizophrenia with plenty of structure, e.g., hour-by-hour schedule, or checklist for ADLs.	1d. The client's thought processes may be too disorganized to plan and carry through even simple activities.	
	1e. Provide supervision with a passive, friendly, low-key approach.	1e. This client needs supervision and support, but closeness will increase anxiety.	
Nursing diagnosis: Ineffective individual coping related to his inability to function on his own and to substance abuse			
1. Client will state three reasons why he needs to take his medication and three reasons why he needs to stay away from drugs and alcohol by discharge.	1a. Teach about substance abuse in a simple, concrete way and repeat material frequently.	1a. This client thinks in a concrete manner and will need material repeated many times to comprehend and retain information.	1. Gerald stated that he needed to take his medication so the voices weren't so loud, because the doctors wanted him to, and because he could live at the halfway house. He said he needed to quit drinking and using marijuana because he couldn't stay at the halfway house if he continued, it cost him too much money, and it made his parents mad. Goal met.
	1b. Use visual aids and attention-getting devices. Avoid videotapes used for other clients.	1b. This client will learn readily if material is broken down into simple pieces. Concrete visual aids make the concepts easier to understand.	

Continued.

Care Plan 12-3

Schizophrenia and Alcohol Abuse—cont'd

Outcome identification	Nursing interventions	Rationale	Evaluation
Nursing diagnosis: Ineffective individual coping related to his inability to function on his own and to substance abuse—cont'd			
	1c. Help client apply new material to each specific situation.	1c. Client will have difficulty applying new knowledge appropriately and will need much assistance.	
	1d. Use modeling and role-playing to practice new behavior.	1d. Watching someone else and practicing new behaviors will assist the client to integrate new material.	
	1e. Assess client for abuse of anticholinergic medication by determining whether he frequently "runs out" of this medication.	1e. Clients who abuse other substances sometimes use anticholinergic medications for a "buzz."	
	1f. Avoid giving the substance abusing client antianxiety medications.	1f. Antianxiety medications do not relieve psychotic symptoms and are addictive, whereas the antipsychotic medications also relieve anxiety.	
	1g. Use cue cards to illustrate: (1) why the client needs to take medication, (2) three reasons why he needs to stay away from alcohol and drugs, and (3) the consequences of failure to comply.	1g. Concrete visual aids will assist the client to comprehend and remember the new information.	

Outcome identification	Nursing interventions	Rationale	Evaluation
Nursing diagnosis: Ineffective individual coping related to his inability to function on his own and to substance abuse—cont'd			
	1h. Teach the family about substance abuse and about schizophrenia.	1h. The family's knowledge about the two disease processes will reinforce the client's learning. It will also assist the family to respond therapeutically to the client's behavior.	
	1i. Help the family set realistic expectations of the client.	1i. With increased knowledge, the family's expectations more likely will be realistic and appropriate for this client.	
	1j. Help the family set contingency plans for possible behaviors of the client.	1j. With plans in place, the family will have tools to respond therapeutically to relapses into either disease and/or inappropriate behavior.	
Nursing diagnosis: Impaired social interaction related to altered thought processes			
1. Client will attend classes on AODA within 2 weeks.	1a. Give feedback to client in a matter-of-fact style.	1a. This client cannot handle intense affect.	1. Client began attending classes at the hospital. He said they helped him learn about drugs. Goal met.
	1b. Keep levels of confrontation, challenge, and criticism at a minimum.	1b. Confrontation, challenge, and criticism will cause extreme anxiety in this client.	

Continued.

Care Plan 12-3

Schizophrenia and Alcohol Abuse—cont'd

Outcome identification	Nursing interventions	Rationale	Evaluation
Nursing diagnosis: Impaired social interaction related to altered thought processes—cont'd			
	1c. Slowly and methodically build into the client's world the knowledge that he cannot use alcohol and drugs.	1c. This client's ability to integrate new information and make changes is extremely limited and occurs very slowly.	
	1d. Assess client's ability to handle classes on AODA.	1d. Classes may need to be leveled for him and other clients whose thought processes are impaired.	
2. Client will participate in an AA group by discharge.	2a. Avoid the concept of powerlessness in stepwork with client.	2a. This client is already too powerless. He needs to be empowered.	2. Gerald went to an AA meeting but declared that he wasn't going back because they laughed at him. Goal not met. *Revision:* Find another recovering person who un-
	2b. Teach group about the disease of schizophrenia.	2b. This knowledge prepares them to accept client into the group.	

an essential role for the nurse. Discussion of how the outside world affects the individual's recovery is emphasized.

The nurse's role in residential treatment

Both mental health and substance abuse treatment are offered in residential centers for clients who are more impaired and in need of longer-term maintenance, structure, and monitoring. Nurses' roles in these settings are similar to those in inpatient and partial hospitalizations. Nurses here, however, often coordinate the various components of a client's treatment. Many clients are involved in other kinds of treatment and have other medical problems in addition to social and financial problems. Nurses can monitor random drug screens and can provide other general health maintenance and care such as checking blood pressure, monitoring chronic conditions, providing nutrition information, and offering safe-sex coun-

Outcome identification	Nursing interventions	Rationale	Evaluation
Nursing diagnosis: Impaired social interaction related to altered thought processes—cont'd			
	2c. Teach the group to tolerate unusual behavior, to set limits on this behavior, and to keep stimulation low.	2c. If the group can tolerate the occasional unusual behavior, set limits for disruptive behavior, and keep the stimulation low, this client may be able to tolerate an AA group.	derstands schizophrenia to help Gerald find an appropriate AA group and go with him at least until he feels comfortable attending.
	2d. Prepare the client in how to respond if group members confront his use of medication to control the schizophrenia.	2d. Many AA group members believe that conquering substance abuse means avoiding *all* mind-altering substances.	
	2e. Help the client find an AA group that will be helpful for him.	2e. Many clients with schizophrenia can function in an AA group but will need one that operates on a simple level and tolerates differentness.	

seling. In these settings nurses have a unique opportunity to help individuals adapt to a structured living situation, as well as to the demands of interacting with society.

The nurse's role in outpatient, vocational, and rehabilitation settings

Nurses provide various functions in these settings. The nurse may serve as a primary group, individual, or family therapist or counselor. In these roles, nurses are most likely to be certified clinical nurse specialists, certified as addictions nurses, or certified alcoholism counselors. Interdisciplinary team work continues to be important. Ongoing assessment of clients' progress, interactions with families, and monitoring recovery of both the mental health and substance abuse problems are essential. Many of these clients are on medications which require monitoring to prevent serious side effects. Close collaboration with the physician is essential.

SUMMARY

Nurses have vital roles in all aspects and components of the care of the client with a dual diagnosis. In assessment, intervention, and coordination of services, the nurse must be alert to subtle changes that could indicate withdrawal, adverse medication reactions, increased relapse, or suicide risk. While not necessarily unique to the nurse's role, these are skills readily performed by nurses. The nurse as a member of the interdisciplinary team has a unique opportunity to provide family support and to help the client reenter the community as soon as possible.

These clients are both difficult *and* rewarding. The difficulty comes from working with clients whose problems need to be prioritized and with whom goals often have to be set at small gains. The rewards come when a client who has a long history of psychiatric illness, hospitalizations, or suicide attempts becomes sober, stays out of the hospital, and stops making suicide attempts. Some clients have progressed through vocational, high school, and college programs. Many count their days of sobriety and their months when they have not been hospitalized. Accepting their dual problem and agreeing to continue taking prescribed psychotropic medications and avoid illicit drugs and alcohol may upgrade their prognosis from poor to good. Many are able to engage to some extent in continued twelve step groups or ongoing treatment. Although these clients present clinical challenges, improvement is possible.

REFERENCES

Alcoholics Anonymous. (1993). *The dual diagnosis recovery book.* New York: World Services, Inc.

Alcoholics Anonymous. (1976). *Alcoholics anonymous* (3rd ed.). New York: World Services, Inc.

American Psychiatric Association. (1994). *Diagnostic and statistical manual of mental disorders.* (4th ed.) Washington, D.C.: The Association.

Clement, J.A., Williams, E.B., & Waters, C. (1993). The client with substance abuse/mental illness: Mandate from collaboration. *Archives of Psychiatric Nursing, 7*(4), 189-196.

Cleveland, M. & Cleveland, A. (1992). *The alternative twelve steps: A secular guide to recovery.* Deerfield Beach, FL: Health Communications, Inc.

Drake, R.E. & Wallach, M.A. (1989). Substance abuse among the chronic mentally ill. *Hospital and Community Psychiatry, 40*, 1041-1046.

Evans, K. & Sullivan, J.M. (1990). *Dual diagnosis: Counseling the mentally ill substance abuser.* New York: Guilford.

Galanter, M., Casteneda, R., & Ferman, J. (1988). Substance abuse among general psychiatric patients: Place of presentation, diagnosis, and treatment. *American Journal of Drug and Alcohol Abuse, 14*, 211-235.

Group for Advancement of Psychiatry Committee on Alcoholism and the Addictions. (1991). Substance abuse disorders: A psychiatric priority. *American Journal of Psychiatry, 148*, 1291-1300.

Hoffman, N.B., Halikas, J.A., Mee-Lee, D., & Weedman, R.D. (1991). *Patient placement criteria for the treatment of psychoactive substance use disorders.* Washington, D.C.: American Society of Addiction Medicine.

Miller, N.S. & Gold, M.S. (1991). Dependence syndrome: A critical analysis of essential features. *Psychiatric Annals, 21*, 282-290.

National Institute on Drug Abuse. (1991). *Third biennial report to Congress: Drug abuse and drug abuse research.* (DHHS Publication No. ADM 91-1704), Washington, D.C.: U.S. Government Printing Office.

Reiger, D.A., Farmer, M.E., Rae, D.S., Locke, B.Z., Keith, S.J., Judd, L.L., & Goodwin, F.K. (1990). Comorbidity of mental disorders with alcohol and other drug abuse: Results for the epidemiologic catchment area study. *JAMA, 264*, 2511-2518.

Wilen, T.E., O'Keefe, J., & O'Connell, J.J. (1993). A public dual diagnosis detoxification unit, part one: Organization and structure. *American Journal of Addictions, 2*, 91-98.

13 Nursing Care of Special Populations

Sensitive nursing strategies related to special populations and substance abuse often are lacking in the areas of prevention, treatment, and education. Most nurses are not adequately prepared to meet the needs of diverse populations with addictive illnesses. Only through an increased awareness of special issues related to alcohol and other drug abuse can nurses provide appropriate care to these differing groups. This chapter addresses nursing issues concerning racial and ethnic minorities, women, homosexuals, clients with HIV and AIDS, the homeless, older adults, and health care professionals.

RACIAL AND ETHNIC MINORITIES

There are four major racial and ethnic minority groups in the United States today: African Americans (12%), Hispanics (7%), Asian Americans (2%), and Native Americans (1%) (USDHHS, 1990a). Although there is great diversity in drinking and other drug use *within* these groups, there are also distinguishing collective cultural patterns *among* them that add to their vulnerabilities. These patterns form a cultural composite of life experiences related to such variables as religion, education, communication, family practice, and health or illness.

Religion plays a primary role in the attitudes and lifestyles of many cultures (Niederhauser, 1989). Health may be attributed to spiritual harmony and illness associated with punishment for religious or moral infractions. Formal education is valued by the more literate cultures that focus on long-range life plans, as opposed to those with informal learning styles absorbed with the "here and now." Communication styles vary widely among cultures (e.g., some groups respect written words more than those spoken, and others place more value on what is said). Public and private communication patterns differ sharply among cultures in that some restrict discussion of personal matters to the confines of intimate associates, while others expose their private selves to peripheral groups (i.e., Japanese vs. Americans). Family practices reflect the roles assigned to individual members according to culturally learned behaviors. Gender expectations, tasks, birth control, child rearing, and discipline are just a few of the issues involved. Finally, the ways in which individuals perceive health give meaning to the illness experience. Many cultures define health in terms of the absence of disease, which leaves no room for preventive interventions (Niederhauser, 1989).

African Americans

African Americans have traditionally believed that health is a state of harmony with nature, whereas illness is a state of disequilibrium between nature and the mind/body (Spector, 1985). Many health practices can be traced back to Africa, but others have merged with beliefs of the Native Americans to whom African Americans were exposed and whites with whom they lived. The old and the young are commonly cared for by all members of the African-American community; however, traditional healers who possess added knowledge of herbs, roots, and/or religion are sometimes summoned. Health is maintained with an appropriate diet, rest, clean environment, and laxative; and the most common form of treating illness is prayer.

In order to understand the problems that alcohol and other drug use creates in the African-American community, one needs to examine the unique history of this racial-ethnic group. In the early 1800s alcohol was used as a method to control slaves in the South (Bell, 1992). It was distributed generously on holidays as an ostensible reward for obedience and hard work. Many slave owners hoped drunkenness would quell insurrection. Ironically, a revolt ensued in 1830 that caused concern about alcohol as a precipitator of rebellion, and several laws were enacted that placed tighter controls on drinking by African Americans. After the Civil War and the granting of citizenship, many African Americans moved to Northern industrial cities. Discrimination met them "head on" and forced most into ghettos without employment. For some, drinking became a means of coping with a continually disruptive environment. This history of slavery, institutionalized racism, and segregation resulted in what African Americans have come to know as "cultural pain" (Bell, 1992). In spite of these historic and current disadvantages, African Americans have maintained a resiliency that enables them to derive positives from insurmountable hardships (Williams, 1982).

In 1984 the first major national survey of drinking patterns among African Americans was conducted by the Institute of Survey Research at Temple University (Herd, 1990). In contrast to earlier sociocultural studies, the more recent survey indicates that rates of heavy alcohol use and related problems are similar between African Americans and whites. A relatively higher proportion of African Americans are abstainers (29% vs. 23%), and there are lower rates of drinking at all levels for African-American men and women (USDHHS, 1990a). Very different relationships between drinking and age are found in African-American men than in their white counterparts. White men are at highest risk for alcohol abuse in the youngest age group (18 to 29) whereas African-American men are at their lowest risk in this age group. White high school students therefore are important targets for programs that warn about problems related to alcohol use after leaving high school (OSAP, 1990a). Problem use declines sharply for whites in their 30s but escalates for African Americans. Problem usage remains higher for African Americans throughout middle and old age.

Overall patterns of use and abuse are reversed among women, with African-American women indicating fewer alcohol-related problems than white women. Although African-American women are more likely than white women to abstain from alcoholic beverages, they are more likely to drink heavily when they do drink

(Clark & Midanik, 1982). However, Herd (1989) did not report higher rates of heavy drinking among African-American women. African-American women do appear more likely than women from any other racial-ethnic group to use crack co-caine (1.5% as compared with 1.3% of Hispanic women and less than 1% of white women) (NIDA, 1990). Although African-American women are arrested more often for drunk driving, five times more white women report driving while intoxicated (USDHHS, 1990a). African-American women suffer disproportionately from alco-hol-related morbidity and mortality compared with white women, and twice as many African-American deaths are caused by cirrhosis of the liver (Lillie-Blanton et al, 1991).

Late onset of heavy drinking, characterized by sustained patterns of high con-sumption, may predispose African Americans to high risk of many acute and chronic alcohol-related diseases such as cirrhosis, hepatitis, fatty liver, heart disease, malnutrition, intestinal disaccharidase, hypertension, birth defects, and cancers of the mouth, larynx, tongue, esophagus, and lung (USDHHS, 1990a; Herd, 1990). Esophageal cancer for African-American males aged 35 to 44, for example, is ten times that of whites.

Because African Americans have more health problems because of drug use, poverty, societal conditions, and oppression, the larger society tends to believe the media portrayal that African Americans and their families support the drug culture (Williams, Richardson, & Watson, 1991). Inaccurate images occur when the media misrepresents the number of African Americans involved in inner-city drug raids and other drug-related activities. National Institute on Drug Abuse (NIDA) statis-tics demonstrate that African Americans have the lowest rates of substance abuse of any group in the country (Williams et al, 1991). African-American families usually work as a team for the good of the individual members and believe that addiction signifies a lack of willpower and religious faith. They often believe that the sub-stance abuse will cease if (1) the family prays hard enough, (2) the substance abuser can get a job, (3) the addicted person can get out of the neighborhood, (4) family members will leave her or him alone, (5) church attendance is more active, (6) the family had more money, (7) the family lived in a better place, and (8) whites were not so indifferent (Lillie-Blanton et al, 1991). Although some of these may be true, they should not be used to deny the powerlessness felt by family members. Sub-stance abuse should be interpreted as a disease that controls a person's life if not treated.

Hispanics

The Hispanic-Latino population in this country is a diverse group that includes Mexican Americans (62%), Puerto Ricans (13%), Cuban Americans (5%), and immi-grants from El Salvador, Nicaragua, the Dominican Republic, and other Central and South American countries (20%) (OSAP, 1990c). This racial-ethnic group is the sec-ond largest minority, representing 8% of the U.S. population, and it is expected to become the largest minority group in the next 20 to 30 years. Hispanic-Latinos are increasing three times faster than non-Hispanics and are the youngest of the mi-nority groups, having a median age of 25 (OSAP, 1990c).

A national survey by the NIAAA (1980) indicated that the rate of alcoholism for

Hispanics is two to three times higher than the national rate. This suggests that 6% to 10% of the Hispanic population (934,000 to 1,386,000) could be considered alcoholic (De La Rosa, 1989). Add the fact that three to four persons' lives are touched by each alcoholic, and the statistics of those adversely affected by alcoholism increases to 18% to 35% of the Hispanic population (or approximately 2,800,000 to 5,544,000 persons). Abuse of other drugs is also a major problem in this community. Cocaine-related deaths among Hispanics tripled between 1982 and 1984 while they doubled among white non-Hispanics. In addition, Hispanics report primary problems with heroin, cocaine, and phencyclidine more often than whites (NIDA, 1986).

The traditional view of health in Hispanic cultures is attributed largely to good luck, a gift from God that should not be taken lightly. It can be maintained by behaving in a proper way, eating good foods, working diligently, wearing religious medals, and keeping relics in the home. Illness is caused by an imbalance in the body caused by wrongdoing. The most popular form of treatment involves folk healers, or *curanderos,* and herbal teas that are believed to maintain harmony between the hot/cold and wet/dry humors (Spector, 1985).

Macho is a culturally expected form of conduct for Hispanic men that requires them to be dominant, strong, protective, brave, and authoritative. Although many of these qualities indicate strengths, the concept also condones drinking large quantities of alcohol and "holding it like a man" (OSAP, 1990c). The irony is that although heavy drinking in men is considered machismo, alcoholism and loss of self-control are considered weaknesses. Hispanic-Latino men demonstrate a higher prevalence of heavy drinking than non-Hispanic American men as a whole and report a higher incidence of certain alcohol-related cancers, such as oral cavity, pharynx, and esophageal. Heavy drinking levels are usually maintained into the late 40s. Hispanic men also have a higher rate of homicides while legally intoxicated than African Americans and non-Hispanic whites.

In contrast to Hispanic-Latino men, women of this cultural group are expected to either abstain from alcohol or drink very little. Virtue, subservience to men, and serving the family are valued highly. Because of the ideals of female purity, discipline, and self-sacrifice, alcoholic women are sources of shame to families. This would suggest that alcohol and other drug use in women is probably under-reported and that there is reluctance to seek outside help for addictive problems. Although most reports agree that the majority of Hispanic women abstain from alcohol, the rate of abstention varies among different Hispanic groups. Caetano (1984) found that the number of Mexican-American women who abstained (71%) was substantially greater than among Puerto Rican (45%) and Cuban (48%) women living in the United States. Although Hispanic women who have immigrated most recently report the lowest levels of drinking, there is a progressive decline in abstention and an increase in moderate drinking in each succeeding generation of women following immigration (Gilbert, 1987).

Not surprisingly, Hispanic men have consistently reported higher levels of alcohol consumption and greater numbers of drinking-related problems than Hispanic women (Corbett et al, 1991). It is interesting to note, however, that there is a positive association between husband and wife drinking patterns. Frequent and heavy drinking is reported three times as often among men with wives who drink than among men whose wives drink less than once a month. Also, abstinence is ten times as high among men with abstinent wives (Corbett, Mora, & Ames, 1991). Acculturation seems to be a strong predictor of heavy drinking for Hispanic women, especially younger women.

Alcohol use among Hispanic-Latino youth is similar to that of Anglo youth, but those who drink, drink more as they get older (OSAP, 1990c). Almost 3.7 million (18.5%) Hispanic youths between the ages of 12 and 17 have used an illicit drug at least once in their life and are more likely than Anglo- or African-American youth to have used cocaine at least once. Boys have higher use rates than girls, but the gender gap is shrinking in this age group.

Hispanic-Latinos place great importance on the family, which may include grandparents, godparents, neighbors, and close friends. All members contribute to family rules and solving problems. This kind of teamwork encourages interdependence rather than independence, and discourages revealing secrets outside the family unit.

Asian Americans

Asian Americans represent a broad racial and ethnic group that includes people from Japan, China, Korea, India, the Philippines, Vietnam, and other Asian countries. They are one of the fastest growing minority populations in the country; there are more than 5 million Asian Americans in the United States (OSAP, 1990b). A recent study (Kitano & Chi, 1987) compared drinking patterns among Asian Americans of Chinese, Japanese, Korean, and Filipino origin and found that almost half of all Korean men are abstainers and one third of Chinese, Japanese, and Filipino men abstain. Four fifths of Korean and Filipino women are abstainers; two thirds of Chinese women abstain; and one third of Japanese women abstain from alcohol. Asian Americans are notably underrepresented in treatment admissions (0.3%) (USDHHS, 1990b).

To understand Asian-American attitudes toward health and illness, it is important to understand the ancient Chinese philosophy of Taoism. There are two basic world principles: yin and yang. Yin symbolizes female negative energy, or the forces of darkness, cold, and emptiness; while Yang represents male positive energy, producing light and warmth (Spector, 1985). The inside and front of the body are yin, and the back and surface are yang. To remain healthy, all actions must conform to the balance of yin and yang and can be facilitated by traditional healers, acupuncture, and herbal remedies.

Patterns of alcohol and other drug use vary widely with this population because of diverse cultural backgrounds. However, Asian Americans in general have the lowest level of alcohol consumption and related problems of all the primary racial and ethnic groups. This may be attributed in part to the "flushing response" found in many Asian people. This classic Oriental reaction to alcohol includes rapid absorption and elimination of ethanol with a corresponding increase in levels of acetaldehyde, facial and body flushing, increased heart rate, decreased blood pressure, sweating, nausea, vomiting, headaches, diarrhea, and general dysphoria. Not all Asians experience these symptoms; 20% to 25% do not (USDHHS, 1990a).

As Asian Americans are assimilated into American society, they often begin using alcohol and other drugs at the same rate as the larger culture. Youth, especially, are under great pressure to "fit in" and succeed; and because of the stress of limited language and social skills, they sometimes turn to alcohol and other drugs as a coping mechanism. Chinese-American youth use methaqualone (Quaaludes), for example, twice as often as their white and Hispanic counterparts and five times as often as African-American youth (OSAP, 1990b). Chinese-American youth do have, however, a lower use rate of heroin, PCP, amphetamines, and benzodiazepines than other similar cultural groups. Alcohol and other drug use for all age groups may be underreported, since Asians tend to deal with problems within the family unit rather than turning to outside treatment sources (OSAP, 1990b).

Although Asian Americans are more likely than other racial-ethnic minorities to be abstainers, their rates of frequency and amount of drinking appear to be increasing. Japanese men are particularly influenced by friends who drink; highly educated Chinese men drink more; and Korean men are strongly influenced by the drinking behaviors of their parents (OSAP, 1990b).

Although insufficient data exist to estimate the proportion of Asian women who drink, it appears that Asian women of all ethnic groups (Japanese, Chinese, Korean, Filipino, and Vietnamese) are more likely than women from the other racial-ethnic groups to abstain (USDHHS, 1990b). However, as with Hispanic women, the amount and frequency of drinking may increase with acculturation.

Native Americans

There are presently 505 federally recognized Native-American tribes in the United States and 304 federal reservations (Moncher, Holden, & Trimble, 1990). The Native-American population has grown to an estimated 1.4 million according to the current census.

Traditional Native-American beliefs about health and illness focus on total harmony with nature. The earth is considered a living organism and is periodically healthy and ill just like humans. When one harms the earth, one harms the self, and vice versa. The reason for all sickness and pain is associated with something in the past; illness is simply something that must "be." Meditation, massage, sweatlodge, roots/herbs, chanting, and religious ceremonies are all important to the healing process (Spector, 1985).

The Native-American predisposition to substance abuse has increased because of many biological, sociological, psychological, and cultural forces (USDHHS, 1990b). Research on these causal influences is complicated, however, by a nature-nurture controversy in which nature phenomena (biological-physiological-biochemical) are contrasted in importance to nurture phenomena (social-psychological-cultural). The question that arises is whether transmission is through genetics and/or values, beliefs, or psychological mindsets (USDHHS, 1990b).

Alcoholism is considered the number 1 health problem of Native Americans and is related to four of the ten leading causes of death. Marijuana is the second most widely used drug, followed by smokeless tobacco. The only drug not used more frequently by Native Americans than other ethnic groups is cocaine. Native Americans lead the country in rates of alcohol-related cirrhoses (5 times higher in 25- to 44-year-olds than the general population); diabetes; fetal abnormalities (33 times higher than for whites); and homicide (80% alcohol-related) (Moncher et al, 1990). Also, use of both smoked and smokeless tobacco is linked to several types of cancers, coronary damage, and cardiovascular disease.

Alcoholism accounts for 35 Native-American deaths per 100,000, as compared to 6 for the general population (Breda, 1989). Because drinking was formerly illegal, many Native Americans learned to consume available alcohol as quickly as possible. The object was to get as drunk as possible as fast as possible (Hagemaster et al, 1992). A major barrier to improving rates of alcoholism in the past has been the practice of not interfering with either individual or tribal decisions. A precedence may have been established, however, with the Alkali Lake Band of Canadian Indians, who addressed alcoholism as a major problem by mobilizing the entire community (Rhoades et al, 1988). The essential component here seems to be the declaration that the community will no longer tolerate alcoholism and alcohol abuse.

Although Native-American women drink much less than men, they are particularly vulnerable to alcohol-related health problems (USDHHS, 1990a). They account for nearly half of all cirrhosis deaths and give birth to infants with fetal alcohol syndrome 33 times more frequently than women in the general population (OSAP, 1991).

Native-American adolescents use alcohol and other drugs more heavily than members of other racial and ethnic groups. The use of inhalants is five times greater than that of non-Native American youth; 12% have used stimulants as compared to 4% of the general population; and 72% have smoked cigarettes in comparison with 42% of non-Native American youth (OSAP, 1991).

Culturally specific treatment interventions

It is important that treatment programs providing services to diverse cultural communities understand the unique cultural, historical, and psychological characteristics of each. Nurses, counselors, and other health care providers must be aware that African Americans, Hispanics, Asian Americans, and Native Americans are not merely four separate cultural groups, but represent peoples with diverse experiences based on their geographical origins. Culturally sensitive programming is not simply matching minority clients with minority counselors, but involves many factors that can shape a client's response to treatment and long-term recovery. Spirituality, for example, includes personal philosophy, religion, and church and is critically important to each of the major racial ethnic groups. Recognizing this, the nurse can tap into the client's inner strengths and important resources. Secondly, health and illness beliefs should be among the first areas of assessment and include beliefs about healing, as well as practices associated with the use of alcohol and other drugs. Finally, it is important to determine the role of family and various family members in the dynamics of addiction. What are their feelings toward substance abuse and how do they see themselves in the recovery process? A review of the literature (OSAP, 1990a, 1990b, 1990c; USDHHS, 1990a; Bell, 1992) reveals considerations specific to each racial-ethnic group that can be summarized as follows:

African Americans

1. Identification of both nuclear and extended family network, including neighbors, church members, and/or friends

2. Tolerance of substance abuse within the family and community
3. Consequences of racism and oppression on treatment
4. African Americans normally enter treatment as adults and at later stages of the disease
5. Defense mechanisms such as "black anger" can allow African-American clients to slide through treatment
6. African Americans' refusal to see substance abuse as a primary problem but rather as secondary to poverty and racism
7. Importance of education (i.e., high school equivalency) on recovery and treatment of African-American females
8. Issues of trust and mistrust intensified by a language barrier between agencies and the African-American community
9. Accessibility of treatment programs with an emphasis on group counseling for African-American clients
10. Socialization of African Americans to handle their own problems without assistance from helping agencies
11. Thinking that people who seek counseling are "sick"

Hispanics/Latinos

When working with this racial and ethnic group, it is important to remember:
1. The necessity to teach "tough love" for Hispanic women and children who are reluctant to "go against" their substance-abusing spouses, partners, or other family members
2. Low level of acculturation
3. Tendency to rely on family members rather than outside agencies
4. Use of traditional healing and spiritualists for treatment
5. Machismo reluctance to discuss personal problems in the presence of other men (preference for individual rather than group therapy)
6. Role of the Hispanic pastor in fundamentalist churches to interpret secular and spiritual needs and encourage family unity
7. Language and cultural barriers can make or break the therapeutic relationship
8. Educational efforts to reduce shame associated with women substance abusers and to encourage asking for outside help

Asian Americans

Some of the most important features to remember in intervening with this group are:
1. Drug use by this specific ethnic group, as influenced by place of birth, generational status, and degree of acculturation
2. Awareness of Asian values, health practices, and social and environmental influences
3. Adherence to spiritual forms of healing
4. Encouragement of trust and interaction by assigning Asian staff as counselors and management
5. Use of traditional Asian norms to keep young people from using and abusing substances
6. Stigma and shame associated with seeking professional help

Native Americans

With this racial and ethnic group it is important to consider:

1. Bicultural interventions to help this group achieve a level of comfort in both worlds
2. Include "story telling" for examples in dealing with substance abuse
3. Value system of sharing, cooperation, patience, respect for elders, and harmony
4. Strong feelings of noninterference
5. Involve cultural components in treatment program, such as pow-wows, arts, and crafts
6. Available resources through the Indian Health Service

Regardless of the racial-ethnic group, nurses need knowledge of the history and impact of alcohol and other drug abuse on its members. Although it is valuable to have staff with the same ethnic backgrounds, treatment professionals should resist "cultural seduction" that implies *you* cannot help if you are the wrong nationality. (See Care Plan 13-1.)

WOMEN

Despite the growing concern about substance abuse in the United States, relatively little is known about the causes and developmental course of substance abuse in women. Much of the existing information has been extrapolated from research on men, and most theoretical perspectives have been developed by male researchers studying men (Hughes, 1990). Studies on women have frequently focused on the impact of women's substance use on their children, spouse, and family life. Particular emphasis has been placed on the health problems of the infant born to a mother who drinks heavily or abuses drugs. In addition, most studies on women's use of substances have explored the use of a single drug or drug class, usually alcohol, heroin or other opiates, or psychotherapeutic drugs (Hughes, 1988, 1989). This limited focus is questionable given that women may be more likely than men to use more than one substance. Another factor limiting our understanding of substance abuse in women is the fact that many researchers have obtained research subjects from psychiatric, or alcohol and drug, treatment facilities. The few population studies have, for the most part, concentrated on alcohol use and abuse and have seldom included representative numbers of racial and ethnic minorities (Hughes & Fox, 1993).

Because of these limitations it is not possible to determine accurately the prevalence of substance abuse among women. However, a number of findings have reported potential patterns and gender differences.

For example, fewer women than men use both alcohol and illicit drugs. Marijuana and cocaine, the most commonly used illicit drugs, are used by significantly greater numbers of men than women. Women more commonly use alcohol and medically prescribed psychotherapeutic drugs (Verbrugge, 1982). Few people of either gender or age who report use of illicit drugs use only one drug. Multiple drug use is increasingly common, especially among the 18- to 25- and 26- to 34-year-old

Care Plan 13-1

African-American Inner City Client with IV Heroin Abuse

Jerod Smith is a 33-year-old African-American client admitted to a medical unit in an inner-city hospital because of a systemic infection that had spread from an abscess in his forearm. He had been living in a vacant building that was known to be inhabited by a number of drug users.

ASSESSMENT

Jerod was emaciated and had a temperature of 104. On his left arm were red streaks ascending from an abscess on the inner surface of the forearm. He complained of chills and lethargy.

NURSING DIAGNOSES

Hyperthermia related to systemic infection
High risk for infection related to injection of drugs
Altered health maintenance related to drug use, poverty, and homelessness

Outcome identification	Nursing interventions	Rationale	Evaluation
Nursing diagnosis: Hyperthermia related to systemic infection			
1. Client's temperature will return to normal within one week without additional complications.	1a. Give medication as ordered. Provide wound care for abscess. Assist with ADLs.	1a. Allows client to heal with good medical-nursing care.	1. Mr. Smith's temperature did not return to normal for four weeks because he developed cardiac valve involvement. Goal not met.
Nursing diagnosis: High risk for infection related to injection of drugs			
1. Client will acknowledge within one week that injection of drugs places him at high risk for infection.	1a. Refer to client as Mr. Smith. 1b. Explain matter-of-factly that he became sick because of the sore on his arm.	1a. Reflects respect in client's culture. 1b. It is important to refrain from implying that he was "bad" or "has a problem." Negative racial implications are inferred from those phrases.	1. Client was too ill to discuss drug use at one week. After two weeks, client acknowledged that injecting drugs might cause infection. Goal met within a longer time frame.

Outcome identification	Nursing interventions	Rationale	Evaluation
Nursing diagnosis: High risk for infection related to injection of drugs—cont'd			
	1c. Ask him if he has been sticking anything into his arm. Then explain that the skin protects and holes in the skin can result in sickness. Use language which the client can understand. Avoid blaming or accusing language.	1c. Client will not be likely to cooperate with the nurse should he feel attacked or threatened.	
2. Client will state measures to take to reduce risk within 2 weeks.	2a. Teach the client to not share needles and to wash them in household bleach after use with attention to washing out all of the blood first. Demonstrate for the client how to draw the bleach into the syringe.	2a. Client may continue to inject drugs and needs instructions on how best to avoid infection.	2. Client could demonstrate how to clean needle and syringe after four weeks. Goal met over longer time frame.
	2b. Explain the risk of acquiring AIDS. Emphasize that he cannot tell if someone is infected and that the disease is always fatal.	2b. Explaining the risk may give him motivation to take precautions.	

Continued.

Care Plan 13-1

African-American Inner City Client with IV Heroin Abuse—cont'd

Outcome identification	Nursing interventions	Rationale	Evaluation
Nursing diagnosis: High risk for infection related to injection of drugs—cont'd			
3. Client will state alternatives to using IV drugs within 2 weeks.	3a. If possible, bring in an African-American person formerly addicted to heroin who now takes methadone to explain about methadone substitution.	3a. A person with whom he can identify who has taken the step can best present the alternative.	3. Client stated that he would consider taking methadone instead of injecting drugs. Goal met, but it took four weeks.
	3b. Have a recovering African American talk to him about obtaining treatment.	3b. Same as above.	
Nursing diagnosis: Altered health maintenance related to drug use, poverty, and homelessness			
1. Client will state sources for assistance within 2 weeks.	1a. Ask client if he has family the nurse can contact.	1a. The extended family provides social support in the African-American culture. Mr. Smith has obviously disconnected from this network, and it would be beneficial if he could reestablish connections.	1. Client stated he wasn't interested in calling his family. He refused to talk to the social worker. Goal not met. *Revision:* Be sure to find an African-American social worker.

groups (NIDA, 1990). Data collected from women in treatment and compiled by the Chemical Abuse-Addiction Treatment Outcome Registry (CATOR) indicate that younger women (those under 35 years) report more regular and varied use of alcohol and drugs, whereas those over 35 are more likely to use only alcohol (Harrison, 1989).

Cocaine use has always been lower among women than men. The use of cocaine rose in the late 1970s and early 1980s but leveled off in the mid-1980s and began to decline in 1987. Among younger adults the decline was sharper for men than women. However, for 23 to 26 year olds, the decline for men and women was approximately equal. In 1987, 19% of men and 13% of women one to ten years after high school reported using cocaine in the previous year. Older men and women

Outcome identification	Nursing interventions	Rationale	Evaluation
Nursing diagnosis: Altered health maintenance related to drug use, poverty, and homelessness—cont'd			
	1b. Refer to social worker for evaluation for public assistance. Determine the conditions for his receiving assistance.	1b. Assistance may not be available for someone who continues to abuse drugs.	
2. Client will agree to go for drug treatment within 2 weeks.	2a. Ask client what he found out from the social worker about assistance.	2a. It is important to obtain the client's involvement.	2. Client would not agree to accept drug treatment. Goal not met.
	2b. Complete a client referral to allow an addictions nurse to interview the client and suggest treatment.	2b. The addictions nurse has the experience and knowledge to better move this client into treatment.	

reported lower rates of use (USDHHS, 1988). Women who do use cocaine appear less likely than men to progress to regular use (Kandel, Murphy, & Darus, 1985).

Adolescents and young women

The fact that the rates of use of most drugs among high school students have declined or leveled off over the past several years (Johnson, O'Malley, & Bachman, 1989) indicates that educational efforts aimed at youth may be having an effect. However, a notable exception to this trend is the increase in numbers of young women who are smoking cigarettes. A primary explanation for young women's initiation of smoking is weight control. For this reason, treatment programs for women, particularly those that include adolescents and young women, should incorporate educational programs on other, more healthy methods of controlling weight.

Influence of employment

Alcohol and other drug-use patterns not only differ with age; they also vary with life roles, employment, and marital status. Some investigators believe that women employed outside the home may be at increased risk for substance use and abuse. Exactly how employment interacts with women's substance abuse is not clear. For example, Armor and associates (1977) and Johnson (1982) found that married women employed full time reported higher rates of heavy drinking than those reported by unmarried or unemployed women. However, a later national survey, conducted by Wilsnack and associates (1984), found that employed women who were divorced, separated, or never married were significantly more likely than were married employed women to be moderate or heavy drinkers. Only 18% of full-time employed, married women reported moderate or heavy drinking, compared with 49% of women employed full-time who never married. Employed women who were cohabitating reported the highest levels of moderate or heavy drinking (53%). Parker and associates (1980) also found employment status to be an important predictor of drinking; however, they found no association with marital status. Finally, Fillmore (1984), in a cohort analysis of data from three national surveys conducted in 1964, 1967, and 1979, found some evidence for heavy drinking among employed women, particularly among the youngest (21 to 29).

Potential explanations for employed women's greater vulnerability to substance use and abuse are the stressors related to multiple roles, wage discrimination, few opportunities for career advancement, pressures to behave like male employees, and sexual harassment (Klitzman et al, 1990). These issues, as well as others that affect employed women, must be addressed when working with addicted women.

Racial and ethnic minority women

Whether racial and ethnic differences in women's substance-related problems are grounded in cultural attitudes or have a significant physiological basis should be ascertained. Are some groups more susceptible than others to the physiological effects of alcohol? Do ethnic and racial minority women who use substances do so to escape the realities of depressed socioeconomy, poor living conditions, or discrimination? More data about the patterns and correlates of substance abuse among various groups of women are needed to better understand the factors that contribute to substance use and to plan more effective outreach, prevention, and treatment programs.

Health consequences of substance abuse in women

Alcohol and other drug use has significant health consequences for both women and men; however, an increasing number of recent studies have documented that women are more susceptible to the physiological effects of alcohol than men (Hasin, Grant, & Weinflash, 1988; Mello, 1988; Van Thiel & Gavaler, 1988). In each study, regardless of design, method, or study population, women who drank less and for shorter periods of time than men suffered greater physiological consequences. In particular, a recent landmark study demonstrated clear gender differences in the metabolism of alcohol. This study is among the first to demonstrate conclusively that under certain conditions, women do not metabolize alcohol as efficiently as men and that this ability is almost completely impaired in alcoholic women (Frezza et al, 1990). Because of diminished activity of the gastric enzyme, alcohol dehydrogenase, even when moderate amounts of alcohol are ingested following a standard meal, women metabolize significantly less alcohol than do men. Thus, more alcohol reaches the circulatory system and must be filtered through the hepatic portal system.

Other explanations for the increased physiological consequences of alcohol in women include higher concentration of alcohol in the blood because of women's smaller blood volume, smaller proportions of body fluid, higher proportions of fat tissue, and fluctuations in hormonal levels during the menstrual cycle.

Other consequences of substance use in women

Increasingly, data support the relationship between substance use and physical or sexual abuse. Miller and associates (1989) point out that most studies exploring the relationship between violence and substance abuse have focused on male perpetrators' use of alcohol and drugs. Only recently has it been acknowledged that addicted women may be at greater risk for physical and sexual abuse than non-addicted women. Use of alcohol or drugs appears to increase women's risk of violence, abuse (Gorney, 1989; Ladwig & Anderson, 1989), and suicide (Blankfield, 1989). Suicide often occurs as a result of accidental overdose following ingestion of alcohol or drugs. Finally, the risk of harm to the fetus in pregnant women who use alcohol or drugs is well documented. (See Chapter 8.)

Implications for treatment

The life context in which excessive drinking or drug use is embedded significantly differs physiologically, psychologically, and socially for women and men. An understanding of these differences is crucial in planning care for women with alcohol, and other drug, problems.

Barriers to treatment.   Women may experience motivators and barriers to treatment that differ from those encountered by men. The fact that there is greater stigma attached to substance abuse among women than among men is widely recognized. While society is more likely to "excuse" a man with alcohol abuse because of his high-pressure job, family responsibilities, demanding wife, etc., little justification is offered for women who drink excessively (Bauer, 1982). When women's problems are viewed as less important than those of men, women who drink excessively are perceived as behaving self-indulgently and irresponsibly. This is particularly true for women with children. Furthermore, women with alcohol and substance abuse are seen as more immoral than their male counterparts. Drinking among women has historically been linked to a loss of sexual inhibitions (Blume, 1991). Only recently has the presumed link between alcoholism and sexual promiscuity among women been seriously questioned.

Women may be more reluctant than men to seek treatment for substance abuse. Women with alcohol or substance abuse are more likely to seek help for marital or family problems, physical complaints, or emotional problems. Because addictions are incongruent with stereotypes of women, physicians, nurses, and other health care professionals are less likely to recognize the underlying problems in female clients.

Women who seek help for alcohol or drug problems do so more often because of family problems, whereas men more often seek help because of work-related problems (Gomberg, 1992). While men are usually encouraged to seek treatment by their wives, women more often are encouraged to seek help by parents or children.

The greater social sanctions against alcoholism and drug addiction in women make them less willing to seek help and others less willing to recognize that they need help. Once they seek help, they often encounter staff who are ill-prepared to deal with women's issues and treatment programs that are unresponsive to women's needs (Marsh & Miller, 1985). The male-as-norm bias has contributed to the myths and misconceptions about treatment of women with addiction. Because women's response to treatment has been measured against male standards, they often have been viewed as sicker and harder to treat (Marsh & Miller, 1985; Reed, 1985).

Just as treatment models based on men's experience are inadequate for women, so too are models based on the experiences of white, middle-class women inadequate for women of other racial and ethnic groups. There continues to be a great need for attention to the diversity of women. However, although having information about minority and other subgroups of women is important, we must be careful when tempted to make generalizations, even within seemingly distinct groups. Rather than generalizing to African-American, Hispanic, Asian, or lesbian groups, we must make clear what subgroups, socioeconomic strata, and age levels the women represent. The inclusion in treatment planning of the unique concerns of these subgroups of women acknowledges the importance of cultural variation and context and will likely increase the effectiveness of treatment.

Finally, because women are less likely to be employed, or more likely to be employed in positions that offer minimal or no health benefits, many cannot afford treatment. Furthermore, a great many treatment programs do not admit pregnant addicts or addicted mothers, even though substantial numbers of women with substance abuse problems are pregnant or have children, and many more women than men have the major caretaking and financial responsibility for their children. In fact, lack of child care is one of the most frequently reported barriers to treatment for women with alcohol and substance abuse.

Other treatment considerations. Women with alcohol and drug addictions frequently have issues and problems other than substance abuse that must be addressed in conjunction with treatment for addictions. For example, women reportedly have poorer self-concepts and lower self-esteem than their male counterparts (Beckman, 1978) and are more likely to be depressed (Turnbull & Gomberg, 1988). Low self-esteem coupled with depression can have an immobilizing effect. Education and other components of treatment should be geared toward helping women gain a greater sense of control in their lives and confidence in their abilities. Assertiveness training and career counseling, as well as skills training in practical aspects of daily life such as child care, financial management, and personal goal setting can be helpful. For many women in treatment, programs and referral services must be geared toward meeting basic survival needs such as food, housing, and health care.

Women in treatment should routinely be given information about HIV and AIDS. In addition to basic information about transmission, risk factors, and safe sex practices, strategies for instituting safe sex practices may be needed. Women with alcohol and other drug addictions may not have the confidence or assertive skills necessary to insist on precautions during sexual contact. Female role models often are most effective in communicating the importance of women taking responsibility for their own bodies. Discussions about safe and unsafe sexual practices should use vocabulary at the client's level. Because nurses and other health care providers are frequently uncomfortable discussing topics related to sex and sexuality, special training is helpful to increase comfort and effectiveness in communicating such information.

Education for women with substance abuse should include issues related to body image, overeating, and eating disorders. Because a disproportionate number of women in treatment may also have a history of physical and sexual abuse, these issues must also be addressed.

Consideration of gender differences must extend to planning for aftercare. Women with substance abuse may have difficulty with some aspects of traditional twelve step programs. For example, the emphasis in Alcoholics Anonymous (AA) on attacking denial is based primarily on a male phenomenon. Women with substance abuse experience more anxiety and depression and less denial of their problems than men (Colten & Marsh, 1984). Women with substance abuse often have low self-esteem and high levels of shame and guilt, feel powerless, and tend to blame themselves for their failures (Colten & Marsh, 1984). Therefore, the emphasis on surrendering to a higher power and renunciation of past failures may in fact impede rather than facilitate women's recovery.

One alternative to AA is Women for Sobriety (WFS). Developed in the 1970s, WFS offers a positive, self-affirming alternative. Rather than dwelling on past problems and behaviors, the thirteen statements of acceptance in WFS help women to focus on the present and to build emotional strength, self-esteem, and a positive approach to life (Kirpatrick, 1986). Unfortunately, there are far fewer WFS groups than AA/NA groups from which women can choose.

Clearly, AA has helped countless alcoholics gain and maintain sobriety, and twelve step groups can provide women with much needed support during recovery. Particularly when no other alternatives are available, women can be helped to "reframe" troubling aspects of traditional twelve step programs. Where available, women's AA or NA groups often provide a safe and supportive forum for exploring addiction difficulties and dealing with other gender-related issues and concerns. (See Care Plan 13-2.)

HOMOSEXUAL MEN AND WOMEN

The prevalence of alcohol and other drug problems among homosexual men and women is unknown but presumed to be high. Although studies have been few and methodologically flawed (Glaus, 1989), most sources report that lesbians and gay

Text continued on p. 394.

Care Plan 13-2

Native American Woman with Alcoholism at an Outpatient Clinic

Winona was a 29-year-old Native American woman, brought in by a neighbor to the outpatient clinic for a broken arm after a fall down a flight of stairs. She was dirty and disheveled and smelled strongly of alcohol. Blood alcohol level was .22. She lived on the outskirts of town with her husband and five children ranging in age from 10 years to 6 months. She had not been seen in the clinic before. Her neighbor reported that the children were often outside late at night without coats or shoes when the weather was cold and that sometimes she saw them outside playing during school hours.

ASSESSMENT

History and physical exam revealed enlarged liver, decayed teeth, fracture of the right humerus. Chest x-ray revealed tubercular lesions on the right upper lobe of her lung. Significant lab results were elevated SGOT and AST, reduced RBC and HCT. Her mood was stoic and she said that she tripped at the top of the stairs. She described her family relationships as "fine." When asked about her alcohol use, she reported approximately one pint of whiskey per day. She did not see that as a problem. She spent her time caring for her home and children and the small acreage upon which they lived.

NURSING DIAGNOSES

High risk for injury to self related to heavy alcohol use
Alteration in parenting related to heavy alcohol use
Ineffective individual coping related to inadequacy of coping skills

Outcome identification	Nursing interventions	Rationale	Evaluation
Nursing diagnosis: High risk for injury to self related to heavy alcohol use			
1. Client will relate how alcohol imbalances her system within 1 week.	1a. Establish therapeutic relationship with the client.	1a. Nurse-client rapport is crucial to recovery.	1. Winona said that she guessed that alcohol did imbalance her system. Goal met.
	1b. Mention something positive about her in feedback.	1b. Focus on the positive aspects of the person helps reduce shame.	
	1c. Gently point out to her objective signs of intoxication.	1c. Objective evidence combats denial.	
	1d. Use "storytelling" to teach how alcohol causes imbalance between animals and nature.	1d. This technique is much used in the Indian culture.	

Outcome identification	Nursing interventions	Rationale	Evaluation
Nursing diagnosis: High risk for injury to self related to heavy alcohol use—cont'd			
	1e. Ask her if she thinks she might be having the same difficulty.	1e. Connects her difficulties to her alcohol use.	
2. Client will relate her injury to her alcohol use within 1 week.	2a. Tell her that her imbalance must have caused her to fall down the stairs.	2a. Connects her fall from drunkenness to cultural terms.	2. Winona stated that she may have been drunk when she fell and broke her arm. Goal met.
	2b. Elicit client's thoughts about her alcohol use.	2b. Client unlikely to discuss feelings with the nurse at this point. Thoughts will assist the nurse in deciding how to proceed.	
3. Client will agree to evaluation for treatment within 1 week.	3a. Determine if the client has access to traditional Indian healers.	3a. Assessment determines connection to her native culture.	3. Winona has not been in touch with traditional healers and didn't know any. She was distrustful of the treatment center. Goal not met. After several weeks, however, she reappeared at the clinic with complications with her arm because of an additional fall while drunk. At this time she agreed to go for evaluation. Goal was then met.
	3b. If so, ask if she has talked to the healer about her alcohol use.	3b. Determines whether client is using native sources for health.	
	3c. Let her know that help is available for healing.	3c. Information needed by client.	
	3d. Request the client go for evaluation. Use terminology that she will accept. Find a treatment center that uses Native Americans for counselors or is sensitive to cultural issues.	3d. Important to find culturally acceptable treatment alternative.	

Continued.

Care Plan 13-2

Native American Woman with Alcoholism at an Outpatient Clinic—cont'd

Outcome identification	Nursing interventions	Rationale	Evaluation
Nursing diagnosis: Alteration in parenting related to heavy alcohol use			
1. Client will agree that she could use help with her parenting within 4 weeks.	1a. Visit the client's home after treatment.	1a. Shows acceptance in her natural setting.	1. At six weeks, after treatment when Winona and the nurse met, she agreed that she would like help with her parenting. Goal met.
	1b. Observe her with her children.	1b. Provides assessment for parenting skills.	
	1c. Elicit her hopes and then her worries for her children.	1c. Shows concern and also assesses expectations and limitations.	
	1d. Ask her if she would like help for the above.	1d. Obtains client's permission for assistance.	
2. Client will participate in a class for parenting within 6 weeks.	2a. Find a parenting class conducted by a non-drinking Native American.	2a. Person from the same culture can assist the client with parenting skills in line with the client's cultural values.	2. Winona was delighted when she discovered the class was conducted by a Native American woman and participated with enthusiasm. Goal met.
	2b. If a class is not available, search out a nurse or other professional of Indian heritage to assist her on a personal basis.	2b. Information will be more acceptable from someone who understands her own culture.	
Nursing diagnosis: Ineffective individual coping related to inadequacy of coping skills			
1. Client will state sources of personal strength within 4 weeks.	1a. Assess client's resources, including financial.	1a. Determines what is available for her.	1. Winona expressed a great deal of powerlessness. She did not state any source of strength until after she began attending the parenting classes. Goal partially met.
	1b. Help her find ways to meet basic needs.	1b. Need to meet basic needs before she can work on higher-order needs.	

Outcome identification	Nursing interventions	Rationale	Evaluation
Nursing diagnosis: Ineffective individual coping related to inadequacy of coping skills—cont'd			
	1c. Help client identify strengths that she has.	1c. Helps her identify her own resources, raises self-esteem.	
	1d. Help client identify sources of strength she has available outside herself, especially using resources within the Indian community.	1d. She will be more likely to use resources from her own value system.	
2. Client will state coping skills that she would like to acquire within 6 weeks.	2a. Assist client to make list of situations with which she has difficulty.	2a. Assesses need for additional coping.	2. Time frame was not met. After three months, however, she could state coping skills she would like to acquire. Goal was then met.
	2b. Ask her what she now does in these situations.	2b. Assesses current coping.	
	2c. Help her find alternative coping methods for each situation. Look at consequences and practice most appropriate solutions.	2c. Teaches coping and problem solving.	
	2d. If needed, refer her to a culturally sensitive counselor to continue to work on coping skills.	2d. Needs different skills to cope. Learning new skills may be a long-term effort.	

men have a greater incidence of substance abuse problems, in part, perhaps, because they are thought to rely on bars more than their heterosexual counterparts for socialization. Prevalence rates are also difficult to estimate because homosexuals frequently do not disclose their sexual orientation and agencies rarely collect information about sexual orientation. Because of the difficulties in defining and measuring substance abuse among homosexuals, as well as the barriers in obtaining representative samples, caution should be used when evaluating current estimates.

In a recent study, McKirnan and Peterson (1989a, 1989b) found that lesbian women and gay men were less likely than women and men in the general population to abstain from alcohol and other drugs and were less likely to be heavy users of these substances. However, gay men and lesbian women who drink or use other drugs reported higher levels of problems associated with that use than members of the general population.

An additional finding of interest is that the lesbian women and gay men in this study were psychologically healthy and socially well integrated. This finding, also reported by Deevey (1990), is particularly important considering that homosexual women and men often experience high levels of harassment and discrimination, factors thought to contribute to both substance abuse and mental health problems.

It is possible that substance use, particularly alcohol abuse, has declined in the gay community over the past several years. Reasons for this assumption include the overall increased awareness and concern for health in American society generally, increased dissemination of information about risk status (in part stimulated by the AIDS epidemic) among gay groups and organizations, some lessening of the social stigma and oppression of gay people, and increased alternatives to gay bars for social interaction.

Implications for treatment

The addicted lesbian woman or gay man carries a double stigma that affects both help-seeking behaviors and treatment. This stigma may be even greater for homosexual women because society would prefer to deny the existence of both lesbianism and addiction in women.

The general prejudice against homosexuals constitutes a formidable deterrent to self-disclosure. Many lesbians and gay men spend a great deal of psychic energy keeping their identities hidden from family, employers, colleagues, and health care professionals, including staff of treatment programs. The changing political climate and increased media attention to issues affecting homosexual women and men may help to eliminate some of the stereotypes and stigma associated with the gay lifestyle and thus facilitate the development of more sensitive treatment alternatives.

Considering that homosexuals account for approximately 10% of the United States population (Lewis & Jordon, 1989), it is important that nurses and other health care professionals learn more about this special population. It is imperative that nurses first explore their own attitudes, stereotypes, and myths about homosexual identity and experience. Homophobia is defined as "the revulsion toward homosexuals and often the desire to inflict punishment as retribution . . ." Weinberg (1972, p. 133). It is difficult, if not impossible, to grow up in our culture without some degree of homophobia; therefore it is important to acknowledge these attitudes or feelings and actively work toward their elimination. Schwartz (cited in Israelstam, 1986) suggests that counselors ask themselves the following questions:

1. Do you believe that being gay is just as good as being straight?
2. Can you conceive of a homosexual living a happy life?
3. Do you conceal from yourself attitudes of pity, condescension, and moral superiority toward gay men and lesbians?

Examining one's responses to questions such as these can help identify homophobic attitudes which, if present, will inevitably be communicated to gay clients. In addition, acquiring accurate information about the gay lifestyle and learning about common issues that confront persons who are gay are essential to the process of coming to terms and dealing with homophobia.

Some of the common issues experienced by lesbians and gay men include "coming out," gender identity, relationship issues, alienation, oppression and discrimination, unique friendship and kinship networks, and general psychological health. For example, the gay woman or man is continually confronted with the decision of whether or not to acknowledge her or his identity. "Passing" involves the burden of a double identity that may lead to a sense of alienation and to unauthentic or deceptive interactions (Lowenstein, 1980). Recognizing that every gay client lives daily with such oppression is essential to understanding the context in which substance abuse problems develop and continue or are eliminated.

There are considerable resources for homosexual women and men in most major cities. In addition to gay twelve step meetings, there are a host of groups (e.g., coming-out groups, couples groups, gay professionals, gay parents) in many cities that serve as important resources for gay women and men. Other resources, such as gay literature, films, and music that portray positive images of the gay lifestyle, also can be helpful.

Although it can be argued that separate services for homosexual clients are ideal, few cities or communities have the resources to offer such arrangements. At present, only one such treatment facility exists. Pride Institute is a freestanding substance abuse–treatment program in Minneapolis that treats gay and bisexual persons exclusively. Unlike many programs that "accept" gay women and men, Pride actively "values" and affirms the homosexual lifestyle as a viable alternative to the heterosexual lifestyle. As Bushway (1991) notes, treatment programs that are accepting and accommodating of differences are to be commended. However, these accommodations are usually special considerations and do not constitute a shift in perspective that would define the status of "special" as the norm.

Although lesbians and gay men have common issues and problems, it is also important to recognize that life experiences, personality types, and needs of homosexuals are as diverse as those of heterosexuals. Of particular importance is the recognition of differences between bisexual women and men and those who identify themselves as lesbian or gay. In general, bisexual women and men have a relatively undefined subculture and few organized political resources or support systems. Some bisexual women and men may be confused and conflicted about their sexual identity and may lack acceptance from both homosexuals and heterosexuals. In addition to these difficulties, female and male bisexuals also experience discrimination and oppression. A recent commentary written by bisexual female and male coauthors emphasizes the "double dose" of discrimination experienced by bisexuals: "As bisexuals, we do not get half-bashed or only partly discriminated against, we don't lose half our children or half our jobs" (Raymond & Perez, 1993).

Therefore for every client, the sociopolitical and environmental influences, as well as potential psychological conflicts and stresses, should be considered when attempting to understand factors influencing use of alcohol and drugs and when planning treatment and aftercare.

CLIENTS WITH HIV AND AIDS

Use of alcohol and drugs is associated with HIV and AIDS in several important ways. The best-known connection is HIV transmission through exchange of infected blood or blood products, most frequently among intravenous drug users. A second connection is that alcohol and other drugs can impair normal immune responses that protect the body from disease. Finally, substance abuse is associated with other high-risk behaviors, including unprotected sexual activity with an HIV-infected person (Bagnall, 1990). Sexual activity that places a person at high risk for acquiring HIV includes vaginal or anal intercourse without a condom and any sexual practices that allow exchange of blood, semen, or other body fluids. Both the number of sexual partners and the frequency of engaging in the defined sexual behaviors increase the risk of exposure to HIV.

More than 1 million persons in the United States are believed to be infected with HIV. The most rapid growth in incidence is among heterosexuals who have sexual contact with a person who has HIV.

Current research indicates that minorities are disproportionately affected. Although African Americans and Hispanics make up only 21% of the total U.S. population, they account for 43% of AIDS cases reported to the CDC (U.S. Bureau of the Census, 1989; Centers for Disease Control, 1990). Approximately 80% of IV drug users with HIV infection in the United States are African American or Hispanic (Shilling et al, cited in Singer, 1991).

The racial distribution of HIV positive female IV drug users also reflects the disproportionate number of minority women who are affected by HIV. A study of methadone clients in New York found that almost 75% of the female clients were African American or Hispanic and that nonwhite men and women had a higher antibody prevalence rate than white men and women (Schoenbaum et al, cited in Cohen, Hauer, & Wofsy, 1989). Further, Mondanaro (1989) cites a Centers for Disease Control (CDC) spokesperson as stating that the cumulative incidence of AIDS in African-American and Hispanic women is more than ten times that found in white women.

Most women who are HIV-positive or have AIDS acquire the infection through intravenous drug use or sexual contact with men who are intravenous drug users. Although the dual problem of addiction and AIDS besets a comparatively small number of women in the United States, those who do suffer from this combination have a catastrophic illness. The women themselves have a terminal illness and often are the sole caretakers of children. The children also may have acquired AIDS in utero. Education and treatment are limited by lack of funding; and, unfortunately, this population of women is particularly lacking in the political force to demand federal funding for prevention and treatment programs.

Implications for treatment

It is impossible to provide care for addicted clients without encountering HIV- and AIDS-related issues and concerns. Inextricably linked to HIV/AIDS are a myriad of issues and concerns that must be addressed. Some of these include "coming out," sexual behaviors and sexual identity, alternative lifestyles, family and relationship disruption, alienation and isolation, homelessness, poverty, lack of access to care, guilt, embarrassment, sickness and disease, death and dying, and, often, the most difficult to deal with—tremendous stigma.

Those who work with addicted clients have an important responsibility to provide them with adequate and accurate information about HIV/AIDS. Such information is important in decreasing fear as well as encouraging changes in behavior. Providing this information is important for all clients in treatment but particularly important for those in high-risk groups (gay men, IV drug users, partners of IV drug users, prostitutes).

For a client to change behavior the following must occur: (1) recognition that the behavior is in fact high risk, (2) personalization of the risk so that the client identifies with the risk, and (3) acquisition of skills for beginning as well as sustaining the required changes (Pohl, 1988). For these reasons, it is important that lay persons or staff who are viewed as legitimate by particular client groups be included whenever possible in educational programs.

Because of the high dropout rate from drug treatment programs, information should be presented at both intake and orientation (Mondanaro, 1989). Material should be presented in small, safe, homogenous groups. To avoid stigmatizing certain groups, sessions should be mandatory for all clients.

For treatment programs that have several HIV-positive clients, support groups can serve the important functions of answering questions, recommending resources, and providing emotional support. This is particularly important for women and other clients who do not have strong support networks already.

THE HOMELESS

The "new homeless" of the 1980s and 1990s include significant numbers of young women, children, veterans, elderly men and women, and large numbers of racial and ethnic minorities. Although the prevalence of homelessness is difficult to assess, estimates range from 250 to 350 thousand in 1984 to 2 to 3 million today (Lindsey, 1989). A disproportionate number of this population are minorities, 30% are families, and 85% of families are headed by single women (Berne et al, 1990).

The homeless have been categorized into three groups: (1) street people who live regularly on the street, (2) episodic homeless, and (3) situational homeless made so by crises (Kinzel, 1991). The two most significant precipitants to homelessness are family conflict and loss of job, discharge from a living facility, loss of welfare benefits, conflicts with a friend, and eviction because of behavior.

Alcohol abuse and dependence is greatest among the homeless in the middle years in direct contrast to the general population, in which abuse is highest among the young. Chronic health problems, primarily diabetes and hypertension, are reported by 57% of homeless alcohol abusers as compared with 43% of homeless nonabusers (USDHHS, 1990a; Lindsey, 1989). Risk for other health problems includes tuberculosis, scabies, lice, AIDS, peripheral vascular disease, hypothermia, malnutrition, dental problems, drug abuse, and trauma.

Alcoholic homeless women are predominately African American (66%), in their early 40s, have never been married, and were thrown into homelessness by crisis. Women in this population report more chronic health problems (63%) than men (32%) and are particularly vulnerable to high blood pressure, mental illness, injuries, infections, physical and sexual abuse, and sexually transmitted diseases (Francis, 1991).

Families with children comprise the fastest-growing subgroup. Approximately 16% of homeless children (double the rate of the general population) demonstrate chronic physical problems, including asthma, anemia, malnutrition, upper respiratory infections, skin ailments, gastrointestinal problems, ear infections, eye disorders, immunization delays, and dental problems.

Concurrence of alcohol and other drug abuse with mental illness is of particular significance among the homeless. Mental illness has been diagnosed in more than half of all female abusers as compared to one fourth of male abusers. The most common diagnoses are affective disorders, schizophrenia, generalized anxiety, and panic disorder (USDHHS, 1990a). Children are especially at risk for depression, anxiety, sleep problems, shyness, withdrawal, aggression, and suicidal ideations (Berne et al, 1990). Because homelessness, mental illness, and substance abuse each reinforce the other problems, it is often difficult to identify the original problem. (See Chapter 12 for more about clients with both mental health and substance abuse problems.)

One approach to coping with the many problems of this special population is to devise strategies to mitigate the effects of the poverty that underlies homelessness. But in addition to housing and job opportunities, there must be increased availability of drug and alcohol treatment programs, health care, and mental health–treatment facilities.

OLDER ADULTS

The elderly constitute the fastest-growing segment of the general population (11%) (Glantz & Backenheimer, 1988; Gomberg, 1987). Percentages of older persons vary in the different cultures, with 8% in the African-American population, 4% in the Hispanic-Latino community, 6% in the Asian-American, and 5% in the Native American groups (Kail, 1989).

There is some empirical evidence that older adults do not usually engage in illicit drug use (Glantz & Backenheimer, 1988; Gomberg, 1987). Marijuana smoking, cocaine use, and heroin addiction are rare among the elderly, but misuse and abuse of prescription drugs is common. Community health nurses learn quickly to ask to see all medications when they visit a home, often finding dozens of bottles of prescription medications, many outdated.

Prescription and polydrug use

Older adults receive 25% of all medication prescriptions, and 20% of those written for nonbarbiturate sedative-hypnotics. It is interesting to note that of the ten drugs most commonly prescribed, four are psychoactive sedative-hypnotics (Gomberg, 1987).

Although younger persons normally take prescription drugs for short-term infections, older people take multiple prescription drugs for treatment of chronic conditions, often prescribed by more than one physician. To further complicate the pattern, many older clients have a tendency to self-administer over-the-counter drugs that can have hazardous synergistic effects with other medications. Aspirin and antacids, for example, may retard or intensify the actions of some prescribed drugs. "Swapping" medications adds to the problem when an elderly person with good intentions shares his or her medication with someone else. All these factors, combined with age-related changes in drug metabolism, contribute to the fact that older adults have adverse drug reactions two to three times more often than younger patients and are twice as likely to develop iatrogenic disease (Glantz & Backenheimer, 1988). These are all issues of incorrect dosage, overmedication, drug combinations, self-prescription, and noncompliance, rather than problems of addiction (Gomberg, 1987).

The elderly often are not treated for psychiatric diagnoses, insomnia, and depression the same way their younger counterparts are treated. Instead they are prescribed psychoactive medications, as evidenced by the fact that 32% of women and 21% of men 60 to 74 years of age reported using psychoactive drugs within the past year (Gomberg, 1987; Kail, 1989). Anxiety is often manifested as hypochondriasis, which intensifies depression and insomnia. Minor tranquilizers are then prescribed. Many older adults state without hesitation that they have come to depend on their medications and they would not be able to get along without them. Is this a problem with addiction or a problem with health care delivery?

Problems with alcoholism

It is difficult to assess the prevalence of alcoholism in the geriatric population because older people tend to drink less in both quantity and frequency and also have physical problems common to alcoholism. For example, repeated falls, incontinence, hallucinations, malnutrition, social isolation, self-neglect, myopathy, and accidental hypothermia are red flags for identifying substance abuse in younger clients but are common among the elderly (Gomberg, 1987). Assessment is further complicated by inaccurate self-reporting, confounding symptoms of other conditions, and effects of prescription medications. More importantly, the criteria for measuring abuse is standardized for the younger population and often is inappropriate for the elderly.

Although the overall prevalence of alcohol abuse or dependence is lower in the later years (2% to 10%), those who do abuse alcohol may be early onset or late onset. Early-onset alcoholics are those older adults who developed a drinking problem before the age of 40 and now demonstrate personality characteristics similar to younger alcoholics. They are more likely to have legal problems, a family history of alcoholism, severe medical problems associated with abusive drinking, and greater psychopathology. In contrast, late onset heavy drinking may start in response to stressful life experiences such as loss of a loved one, poor general health, economic adjustments, and/or retirement (Glantz & Backenheimer, 1988; USDHHS, 1990a). These individuals generally had stable early lives, are more likely to be divorced, and have health problems that existed before abusive drinking (Bennett & Woolf, 1991). Early-onset drinkers comprise approximately two thirds of elderly alcoholics, and late-onset drinkers represent the remaining one third.

Psychosocial and physical complications

The social, psychological, spiritual, and physiological stressors of aging contribute to a connection between alcoholism, depression, and suicide in late life. The many losses faced by older adults, coupled with the complexities of old insecurities and lack of dependable social resources, may result in feelings of emptiness and meaninglessness that can lead to depression. This depression, along with an accompanying sense of loss of control over significant life events, can then lead to alcohol and/or other drug use and abuse (Bennett & Woolf, 1991).

The process of aging causes alterations in human physiology that influence absorption, tissue distribution, metabolism, and excretion of drugs and alcohol. Generally speaking, aging slows down the processing of drugs by the body and can lead to neurotoxic effects such as a change in mental functioning, altered gait, insomnia, visual disturbances, slurred speech, ototoxicity, seizures, tremors, irritability, and anticholinergic effects including dry mouth, constipation, urinary retention, headache, and restlessness (Gomberg, 1987; Stolley et al, 1991).

Because of the high incidence of dementia among the elderly and its association with alcoholism, organic mental syndromes deserve special attention. One example is alcohol amnestic disorder, or Wernicke-Korsakoff syndrome. This is a severe form of encephalopathy manifested by confusion, ataxia, eye-movement disorders, severe amnesia, confabulation, personality alterations, difficulty learning new information, and difficulty recalling events from the recent past (Bennett & Woolf, 1991). Early assessment and treatment with large doses of thiamine can avert a full-blown syndrome.

Alcohol serves as an irritant to the gastrointestinal tract and can result in esophagitis and gastritis with poor absorption, utilization, and storage of nutrients. Chronic abuse of alcohol also can cause irreparable damage to the liver and pancreas. In normal aging, there is a decrease in liver mass, a reduction in hepatic blood flow, impairment in microsomal enzymatic activity, and a reduction in plasma protein synthesis (Bennett & Woolf, 1991). Alcohol abuse further impairs functioning.

With aging come a decrease in the size of the kidney and a reduction in functional capacity of glomeruli and tubular systems (Bennett & Woolf, 1991). The resulting impairment in excretory and reabsorbative functions leads to impairment of drug clearance and increased drug toxicities.

Intervention with the older adult

Treatment groups for the elderly are necessary to address issues such as normal physical changes that occur with aging, loss, grief therapy, and assertiveness training. Group therapy is recommended so that clients can receive positive reinforcement from peers and engage in social interaction. This is critical when considering the loneliness and social isolation. A unified and informed intervention team should include a psychiatrist, nurse, and paraprofessional who are knowledgeable about aging and alcoholism (Lindblom et al, 1992). Finally, in order to reach the elderly who are not enrolled in traditional treatment facilities, group programs should be located in geriatric health care facilities such as senior citizen programs, outpatient geriatric, medical, or psychiatric programs, nursing homes, and home care programs.

HEALTH CARE PROFESSIONALS

Substance-abusing health care professionals not only suffer the personal consequences of substance abuse but also may jeopardize public health and safety because of impaired clinical judgment and skills. As a result of their impaired practice, health care professionals often lose their license to practice their profession, a prolonged or even permanent consequence that few others experience. Health care agencies also experience increased financial burden and legal liability related to impaired professional practice.

Because the prevalence of substance abuse among health care professionals is not known, estimates of incidence and prevalence of substance abuse have varied greatly. The proposed figures have usually been above the level in the general population. Until recently, information regarding the number of substance-abusing health care professionals and the patterns of their use included primarily those receiving formal disciplinary action or those in a particular treatment program. More recently a population-based study of nurses' substance use showed that use of alcohol and specific drugs was no different for currently employed nurse and non-nurse subjects (Trinkoff et al, 1991). Although further study is needed, the prevalence of substance abuse among health care professionals may not differ from that in the general population. Differences have been found, however, in the choice of substances and use patterns.

Although alcohol is the most commonly abused substance for health care professionals, as it is for the general population, health care professionals have unique access to and special knowledge about drugs that may contribute to the use of substances other than alcohol. Because of their special knowledge, they may idealize the efficacy of drugs and minimize the potential of tolerance or other side effects. Therefore, they may be more likely to use drugs for self-treatment of physical or emotional pain, a phenomenon sometimes called "pharmaceutical coping" (Sullivan, 1991). Unique job stresses and the belief that one has earned the right to relaxation after long hours of caring for others also are described as contributing to substance abuse (Haack & Hughes, 1989).

Identification of the health care professional with substance abuse is especially difficult because of a reluctance to censure one's colleagues. Also, health care professionals may still believe that alcoholics and drug addicts are "skid-row bums," or unable to function professionally. However, when worksite behavioral and personal indicators are evaluated carefully, a substance abuse problem may become apparent (Sullivan, Bissell, & Williams, 1988).

Worksite intervention is an effective technique to get the substance-abusing health care professional to accept treatment, even though the conventional wisdom has been that the alcoholic must "hit bottom" before being responsive to treatment (Williams, 1989). Preparation for the intervention includes gathering and documenting specific data and evidence of inappropriate behavior in the workplace, employee complaints, and suspicions of substance abuse. The goal is to get the professional to agree to evaluation by an expert in substance abuse and into treatment if indicated. Those who enter treatment as a result of intervention can be expected to do just as well, if not better, than those who come into treatment voluntarily (Hester, 1989). This may be especially true for health care professionals because of the added power the professional organization or regulatory board has over a professional's license.

Mandatory reporting of a substance-abusing professional is legislated in some states, but only a few of those states include a diversion program as a part of the regulation. A few states have established comprehensive assistance programs. Most peer assistance programs are sponsored by professional organizations and offer support and referral services, monitoring of recovery, and educational programs to the health care community. Services offered vary widely, however. Many programs rely on volunteer help and may be chronically underfunded.

Hester (1989) identifies the unique characteristics of health care professionals that may affect the treatment process: caregivers' difficulty in receiving care, strong tendency to intellectualize feelings, severe guilt, highly entrenched denial, rationalizations of self-medication due to worksite availability, licensure issues, and stigma. Extended treatment is best provided to health care professionals by an interdisciplinary team that includes at least one member with specialized knowledge of the patient's professional discipline. Some providers favor a separate and special treatment program (Valentine, 1988), whereas others believe that "special treatment" may contribute to the denial system of the health care professional and interfere with an effective treatment outcome. Most treatment professionals would agree that a support group for health care professionals provides a confidential place where issues related to licensure or situations that may have endangered clients can be discussed. Monitoring for continued abstinence may include a return to work contract that specifies consistent attendance at mutual health groups, documentation of continued treatment, and random drug screens. Contingency contracting specifies the consequences in case of relapse.

Although recovery rates have not been reported for all health professionals, and outcome criteria and methodology of existing studies differ substantially, there are some indications that health professionals experience a better incidence of recovery and have fewer relapses than the general population of substance abusers. For example, Morse and others (1984) compared data on 73 physicians with that of 185 middle-class patients treated similarly for alcoholism and other drug dependence. The prognosis was better for the physicians (83% improved) than for the general patients (62%). The threat of licensure sanction and the close monitoring of recovery by a peer assistance program or employee assistance program (EAP) may contribute to improved recovery rates (Morse et al, 1984; Handley, Plumlee, & Thompson, 1991).

SUMMARY

There is no question that alcohol and other drug problems produce major challenges for today's nurse. The disturbing consequences of substance abuse are evident in each of the special populations discussed in this chapter, including racial and ethnic minorities, women, homosexuals, clients with HIV/AIDS, homeless, older adults, and health care professionals. In order to be sensitive to the needs of each, nurses need to develop an awareness of the multicultural perspectives, gender issues, economic barriers, and access to treatment for all special populations. The client's frame of reference should be the cornerstone for development of therapeutic strategies as both practitioner and client engage in a mutual acceptance of one another as human beings.

REFERENCES

Armor, D.J., Polich, J.M., & Stambul, H.B. (1977). *Alcoholism and treatment.* (R-1739-NIAAA.) Santa Monica, CA: Rand Corporation.

Bagnall, G., Plant, M., & Warwick, W. (1990). Alcohol, drugs, and AIDS related risks. Results from a prospective study. *AIDS Care, 2*(4), 309-317.

Bauer, J. (1982). *Alcoholism and women. The background and the psychology.* Toronto: Inner City Books.

Beckman, L.J. (1978). The self-esteem of women alcoholics. *Journal of Studies on Alcohol, 36*(70), 797-824.

Bell, P. (1992). *Cultural pain and African Americans.* Center City, MN: Hazelden Educational Materials.

Bennett, G. & Woolf, D. (Eds.) (1991). *Substance abuse* (2nd ed.). New York: Delmar Publishers.

Berne, A., Dato, C., Mason, D., & Rafferty, M. (1990). A nursing model for addressing the health needs of homeless families. *IMAGE, 22*(1), 8.

Blankfield, A. (1989). Female alcoholics. Alcohol dependence and problems associated with prescribed psychotropic drug use. *Acta Psychiatrica Scandinavica, 79,* 355-362.

Blume, S.B. (1991). Sexuality and stigma: The alcoholic woman. *Alcohol Health & Research World, 15*(2), 139-146.

Breda, A. (1989). Health issues facing Native American children. *Pediatric Nursing, 15*(6), 575-577.

Bushway, D.J. (1991). Chemical dependency treatment for lesbians and their families: The feminist challenge. In C. Bepko (Ed.) *Feminism and addiction.* (pp 161-172). New York: The Haworth Press Inc.

Caetano, R. (1984). Drinking patterns and alcohol problems in a national sample of U.S. Hispanics. In *Alcohol use among U.S. ethnic minorities.* (DHHS Publication No. ADM 87-1435.) Washington, D.C.: National Institute on Drug Abuse.

Centers for Disease Control. (1990). *HIV/AIDS surveillance: U.S. AIDS cases reported through July, 1990.* Atlanta, GA: The Centers.

Clark, W.B. & Midanik, L. (1982). *Alcohol use and alcohol problems among U.S. adults: Results of the 1979 national survey, Alcohol consumption and related problems. Alcohol and Health Monograph 1.* (DHHS Publication No. ADM 82-1190.) Washington, D.C.: U.S. Government Printing Office.

Cohen, J.B., Hauer, L.B., & Wofsy, C.B. (1989). Women and IV drugs: Parenteral and heterosexual transmission of human immunodeficiency virus. *Journal of Drug Issues, 19*(1), 39-56.

Colton, M.E. & Marsh, J.C. (1984). A sex-role perspective on drug and alcohol use by women. In N.C.S. Widom (Ed.) *Sex roles and psychopathology.* (pp 219-248). New York: Plenum Press.

Corbett, K., Mora, J., & Ames, G. (1991). Drinking patterns and drinking-related problems of Mexican-American husbands and wives. *Journal of Studies on Alcohol, 52*(3), 215-223.

Deevey, S. (1990). Older lesbian women: An invisible minority. *Journal of Gerontological Nursing, 16*(5), 35-39.

De La Rosa, M. (1989). Health care needs of Hispanic Americans and the responsiveness of the health care system. *Health and Social Work, 14*(2), 104-113.

Fillmore, K.M. (1984). When angels fall: Women's drinking as a cultural preoccupation and as reality. In S.C. Wilsnack & L.J. Beckman (Eds.) *Alcohol problems in women: Antecedents, consequences, and interventions.* New York: Guilford Press.

Francis, M. (1991). Homeless families: Rebuilding connections. *Public Health Nursing, 8*(2), 90-96.

Frezza, M., DiPadova, C., Pozzato, G., Terpin, M., Baraona, E., & Lieber, C.S. (1990). High blood alcohol levels in women: The role of decreased gastric alcohol dehydrogenase activity and first-pass metabolism. *The New England Journal of Medicine, 322*(22), 95-100.

Gilbert, M.J. (1987). Alcohol consumption patterns of immigrant and later generation Mexican American women. *Hispanic Journal of Behavioral Sciences, 9*(3), 299-313.

Glantz, M. & Backenheimer, M. (1988). Substance abuse among elderly women. *Clinical Gerontologist, 8*(1), 3-26.

Glaus, K.O. (1989). Alcoholism, chemical dependency, and the lesbian client. *Women and Therapy, 8*(1/2), 131-145.

Gomberg, E. (1987). Drug and alcohol problems of elderly persons. In T. Nirenberg & S. Maistro (Eds.) *The assessment and treatment of addictive behaviors.* Ablex.

Gomberg, E.S.L. (1992, September). Overview of women, substance abuse and violence. Presented at conference on issues related to women, substance abuse, and violence. University of Illinois at Chicago.

Gorney, B. (1989). Domestic violence and chemical dependency: Dual problems, dual interventions. *Journal of Psychoactive Drugs, 21*(2), 229-238.

Haack, M.R. & Hughes, T.L. (1989). *Addiction in the nursing profession: Approaches to intervention and recovery.* New York: Springer.

Hagemaster, J., Allen, K., Bailey, M., Cross, P., & Medina, M. (1992). Models of addiction: Relevance for minorities. *Addictions Nursing Network, 4*(2), 61-66.

Handley, S.M., Plumlee, A.A., & Thompson, N.C. (1991). The impaired nurse: Organizational and professional models of response. *AAOHN, 39*(10), 478-482.

Hasin, D., Grant, B., & Weinflash, J. (1988). Male/female differences in alcohol-related problems: Alcohol rehabilitation patients. *The International Journal of the Addictions, 23*(5), 437-448.

Herd, D. (1989). Drinking by black and white women: Results from a national survey. *Social Problems, 35*(5), 493-505.

Herd, D. (1990). Subgroup differences in drinking patterns among black and white men: Results from a national survey. *Journal of Studies on Alcohol, 51*(3), 221-232.

Hester, T.W. (1989). State-of-the-art treatment programs. In T.W. Hester (Ed.) *Professionals and their addictions.* Macon, GA: Charter Medical Corporation.

Hughes, T.L. (1988). Women, alcohol, and drugs. In C. Leppa and C. Miller (Eds.) *Women's health perspectives: An annual review,* Vol. 1, (pp 54-70). Phoenix, AZ: Oryx Press.

Hughes, T.L. (1989). Women and substance use. In C. Leppa (Ed.) *Women's health perspectives: An annual review,* Vol. 2, (pp 17-35). Phoenix, AZ: Oryx Press.

Hughes, T.L. (1990). Evaluating research on chemical dependency among women: A women's health perspective. *Family and Community Health, 13*(3), 35-46.

Hughes, T.L. & Fox, M.L. (1993). Patterns of alcohol and drug use among women: Focus on special populations. *Clinical Issues in Perinatal and Women's Health Nursing, 4*(2), 203-212.

Israelstam, S. (1986). Alcohol and drug problems of gay males and lesbians: Therapy, counseling and prevention issues. *The Journal of Drug Issues, 15*(3), 443-461.

Johnson, L.D., O'Malley, P.M., & Bachman, J.G. (1989). *Illicit drug use, smoking and drinking by America's high school students, college students, and young adults: 1975-1987.* (National Institute on Drug Abuse. Publication No. ADM 89-1602.) Washington, D.C.: U.S. Government Printing Office.

Johnson, P.B. (1982). Sex differences, women's roles and alcohol use: Preliminary national data. *Journal of Social Issues, 38,* 93-116.

Kail, B. (1989). Drugs, gender and ethnicity: Is the older minority woman at risk? *The Journal of Drug Issues, 19*(2), 171-189.

Kandel, D.B., Murphy, D., & Darus, D. (1985). Cocaine use in America: Epidemiologic and clinical perspectives. In *National Institute on Drug Abuse Research Monograph Series,* No. 61. (Publication No. ADM 87-1414.) Washington, D.C.: U.S. Government Printing Office.

Kinzel, D. (1991). Self-identified health concerns of two homeless groups. *Western Journal of Nursing Research, 13*(2), 181-194.

Kirkpatrick, J. (1986). *Turnabout: New help for the woman alcoholic.* Seattle, WA: Madrona.

Kitano, H. & Chi, I. (1987). Asian-Americans and alcohol use. *Alcohol Health and Research World, 11*(2), 42-47.

Klitzman, S., Silverstein, B., Punnet, L., & Mock, A. (1990). A women's occupational health agenda for the 1990s. *New Solutions, 1*(1), 7-17.

Ladwig, G.B. & Anderson, M.D. (1989). Substance abuse in women: Relationship between chemical dependency of women and past reports of physical and/or sexual abuse. *International Journal of Addictions, 24*(8), 739-754.

Lewis, G.R. & Jordon, S.M. (1989). Treatment of the gay or lesbian alcoholic. In G. Lawson & A.W. Lawson (Eds.) *Alcoholism and substance abuse in special populations.* Rockville, MD: Aspen.

Lillie-Blanton, M., MacKenzie, E., & Anthony, J. (1991). Black-white differences in alcohol use by women: Baltimore survey findings. *Public Health Reports, 106*(2), 124-133.

Lindblom, L., Kostyk, D., Tabisz, E., Jacyk, W., & Fuchs, D. (1992). Chemical abuse: An intervention program for the elderly. *Journal of Gerontological Nursing,* April, 6-14.

Lindsey, A. (1989). Health care for the homeless. *Nursing Outlook, 37*(2), 78-81.

Lowenstein, S.F. (1980). Understanding lesbian women. *Social Casework, 64,* 29-38.

Marsh, J.C. & Miller, N.A. (1985). Female clients in substance abuse treatment. *The International Journal of the Addictions, 20,* 995-1019.

McKirnan, D.J. & Peterson, P.L. (1989a). Alcohol and drug use among homosexual men and women: Epidemiology and population characteristics. *Addictive Behaviors, 14,* 545-553.

McKirnan, D.J. & Peterson, P.L. (1989b). Psychosocial and cultural factors in alcohol and drug abuse: An analysis of a homosexual community. *Addictive Behaviors, 14,* 555-563.

Mello, N. (1988). Effects of alcohol abuse on reproductive function in women. In M. Galanter (Ed.) *Recent developments in alcoholism,* Vol. 6, (pp 253-276). New York: Plenum Press.

Miller, B.A., Downs, W.R., & Gondoli, D.M. (1989). Spousal violence among alcoholic women as compared to a random household sample of women. *Journal of Studies on Alcohol, 50*(6), 533-540.

Moncher, M., Holden, G., & Trimble, J. (1990). Substance abuse among Native-American youth. *Journal of Consulting and Clinical Psychology, 58*(4), 408-415.

Mondanaro, J. (1989). Chemically dependent women: Assessment and treatment. Lexington, MA: Lexington Books.

Morse, R., Martin, M., Swenson, W., & Niven, R. (1984). Prognosis of physicians treated for alcoholism and drug dependence. *MANA, 251*(6), 743-746.

National Institute on Alcohol Abuse and Alcoholism. (1980). *Facts in brief: Alcohol and Hispanics.* Rockville, MD: National Clearinghouse for Alcohol Information.

National Institute on Drug Abuse. (1986). *Drug abuse warning network (DAWN).* (DHHS Publication No. ADM 86-1530, Series 1, No. 6.) Washington, D.C.: U.S. Government Printing Office.

National Institute on Drug Abuse. (1990). *National household survey on drug abuse: Main findings.* (DHHS Publication No. ADM 90-1682). Washington, D.C.: U.S. Government Printing Office.

Niederhauser, V. (1989). Health care of immigrant children: Incorporating culture into practice. *Pediatric Nursing, 15*(6), 569-574.

Office for Substance Abuse Prevention. (1990a). Alcohol and other drug use is a special concern for African American families and communities. *The Fact Is . . . ,* August, 1-15.

Office for Substance Abuse Prevention. (1990b). *Asian and Pacific Islander Americans.* Rockville, MD: National Clearinghouse for Alcohol and Drug Information.

Office for Substance Abuse Prevention. (1990c). Reaching Hispanic/Latino audiences requires cultural sensitivity. *The Fact Is . . . ,* September, 1-12.

Office for Substance Abuse Prevention. (1991). *American Indians and Native Alaskans.* Rockville, MD: National Clearinghouse for Alcohol and Drug Information.

Pohl, M.L. (1988). Counseling patients in chemical dependence treatment programs about AIDS. *Journal of Psychoactive Drugs, 20*(2).

Raymond, V. & Perez, L.M. (1993, February). *March on Washington for lesbian, gay and bisexual rights and liberation.* Washington, D.C.: Committee for the 1993 March on Washington, Inc.

Reed, B.G. (1985). Drug misuse and dependency in women: The meaning and implications of being considered a special population or minority group. *International Journal of the Addictions, 20,* 13-62.

Singer, M. (1991). Confronting the AIDS epidemic among IV drug users: Does ethnic culture matter? *AIDS Education and Prevention, 3*(3), 258-283.

Spector, R. (1985). *Cultural diversity in health and illness.* Norwalk, CT: Appleton-Century-Crofts.

Stolley, J., Buckwalter, K., Fjordbak, B., & Bush, S. (1991). Iatrogenesis in the elderly: Drug-related problems. *Journal of Gerontological Nursing, 17*(9), 12-17.

Sullivan, E.J. (1991). Impaired health care professionals. In G. Bennett & D.S. Woolf (Eds.) *Substance abuse: Pharmacologic, developmental, and clinical perspectives* (2nd. ed., pp 293-304). Albany, NY: Delmar Publishers.

Sullivan, E.J., Bissell, L., & Williams, E. (1988). *Chemical dependency in nursing: The deadly diversion.* Menlo Park, CA: Prentice-Hall.

Trinkhoff, A.M., Eaton, W.W., & Anthony, J.C. (1991). The prevalence of substance abuse among registered nurses. *Nursing Research, 40*(3), 172-175.

Turnbull, J.E. & Gomberg, E.S.L. (1988). Impact of depressive symptomatology on alcohol problems in women. *Alcoholism: Clinical and experimental research, 12*(3), 374-381.

U.S. Bureau of the Census. (1989). *Statistical abstract of the United States* (109th ed.). Washington, D.C.: U.S. Government Printing Office.

U.S. Department of Health and Human Services. (1988). *National household survey on drug abuse: Main findings 1985.* (National Institute on Drug Abuse Publication No. ADM 88-1586.) Washington, D.C.: U.S. Government Printing Office.

U.S. Department of Health and Human Services. (1990a). *Alcohol and Health Monograph No. 4. Special population issues.* Rockville, MD: National Clearinghouse for Alcohol Information.

U.S. Department of Health and Human Services. (1990b). *Seventh special report to the U.S. Congress on alcohol and health.* (DHHS Publication No. ADM 281-88-0002.) Rockville, MD: The Department.

Valentine, N.M. (1988). The genesis of Nightingale: Alternative treatment for female health care providers. *Holistic Nursing Practice, 2*(4), 45-55.

Van Thiel, D. & Gavaler, J. (1988). Ethanol metabolism and hepatotoxicity. Does sex make a difference? In M. Galanter (Ed.) *Recent Developments in Alcoholism,* Vol. 6, (pp 291-304). New York: Plenum Press.

Verbrugge, L.M. (1982). Sex differences in legal drug use. *Journal of Social Issues, 38*(2), 59-76.

Weinberg, G. (1972). *Society and the healthy homosexual.* New York: St. Martin's Press.

Williams, B., Richardson, T., & Watson, D. (1991). *Recovery for the African American family.* Center City, MN: Hazelden Educational Materials.

Williams, E. (1989). Strategies for intervention. *Nursing Clinics of North America, 24*(1), 95-107.

Williams, M. (1982). Blacks and alcoholism: Issues in the 1980s. *Alcohol Health and Research World,* Summer, 31-37.

Wilsnack, R.W., Wilsnack, S.C., & Klassen, A.D. (1984). Women's drinking and drinking problems: Patterns from a 1981 national survey. *American Journal of Public Health, 74,* 1231-1238.

OPPORTUNITIES AND CHALLENGES IN SUBSTANCE ABUSE

14 Education, Research, and Theory Development

15 Financing, Legal Issues, and Public Policy

16 Drug Testing

17 Challenging Practice Opportunities in Substance Abuse Nursing

14

Education, Research, and Theory Development

Although nursing combines both art and science, the recent growth of scientifically based nursing knowledge strengthens nursing theory and practice. For the first time in the history of the profession, knowledge grounded in the nursing discipline and appropriate to guiding practice is emerging from research. This chapter describes the evolution of nursing knowledge in the substance abuse field and focuses on a theoretical framework to guide nursing practice in substance abuse care. Theory development and knowledge building are discussed, with emphasis on recent contributions of nurse researchers to the knowledge base. Indications for curricular change in the education of nurses about substance abuse and its treatment are delineated.

Nurse researchers, in an evolutionary way, have sought to identify theories that evolve out of nursing practice, as well as to evaluate conceptual models of the phenomenon that is nursing and the phenomena that are the focus of the profession. Nurses delivering care to clients and families with alcohol, tobacco, and/or other drug problems use a variety of nursing theories to organize care and identify outcomes. The knowledge base from which they have traditionally drawn understanding of the addictions and treatment approaches, however, has been largely developed by researchers in other disciplines: the basic sciences, medicine, and psychology in particular. Before the 1960s, biomedical and psychosocial knowledge about addiction and the physical and psychological ways in which it compromises health was very limited. Nursing knowledge then, as now, derived largely from experience.

Florence Nightingale recognized and actively addressed alcohol dependence. Since her time, nurses have cared for individuals with alcohol and other drug problems, and their associated ills, most frequently in medical-surgical settings, in psychiatric treatment, and often in the community. Nursing assessment and care traditionally have been performed systematically and in relation to general health criteria, making use of basic nursing and interpersonal skills. General nursing care of addicted individuals has evolved from nursing's paradigm, that is, an overall perspective of human, environmental, and nursing interaction. Nursing interventions with clients with substance abuse, however, have often lacked a scientific relevance to clients' health and autonomy because most nurses have been limited by an insufficient knowledge base.

Nursing theorists, educators, and researchers frequently identify health as nursing's central paradigm; and, for purposes of this discussion, nursing's knowledge about, interventions with, and manifestations of addiction are assessed from that perspective. By defining health as the process of expanding consciousness, we observe that all manifestations of life as it is evolving, including disease and disability, reflect this pattern. Consciousness is defined as the capacity of the system (person) to interact with the environment (Newman, 1990). This perspective allows nursing to conceptualize addictive patterns and processes and formulate nursing interventions derived from nursing assessments of the uniquely individual patterns which characterize clients and families. As nursing and the drug and alcohol research and treatment fields have advanced, the absence of a discrete body of nursing knowledge about the nature, processes, and treatment of various addictions has become apparent. While many individuals working in the field were aware of the gaps in knowledge, these were graphically highlighted in the late 1970s when specialty nursing organizations became more visible and the American Nurses Association acknowledged drug- and alcohol-related problems in nurses as contributing to impaired practice. The question of impaired practice was explored and answers were sought within the profession and its traditional educational models. How, educators and administrators asked, could practitioners be expected to deal with addiction in themselves and others when they knew nothing about the process through which one becomes addicted and only recognized the end results in the forms of medical illness and long-term organic deficits?

CURRICULAR CHANGE FOR ALCOHOL AND OTHER DRUG EDUCATION

The need to expand education and incorporate new knowledge, to update assessment skills, and to define nurses' roles in addiction treatment was noted by Hoffman and Heinemann in the mid-1970s and in a later survey noting the lack of progress in this area (Hoffman & Heinemann, 1987). While nursing care of clients with long-term medical consequences of alcohol and opiate abuse had long been part of nursing curricula, newer views of alcoholism and other addictions, including the *disease* model, were not taught. In addition, psychiatric nursing theories on addiction often were limited to analytic hypotheses about the origins of alcoholism. Newer approaches such as behaviorism, learning theory, and dysfunctional family systems theories were not included as models for understanding addictive behavior.

The need for education was partially addressed in 1988, when three federal agencies—the National Institute of Drug Abuse, the National Institute of Alcohol Abuse and Alcoholism, and the Office for Substance Abuse Prevention (now known as the Center for Substance Abuse Prevention)—granted funds to selected nursing schools to identify models for curricular change and develop learning strategies which could readily be incorporated into nursing education. The curricula developed at the New York University, the Ohio State University, and the University of Connecticut are constituted of learning modules of common content for basic nursing preparation and additional modules with specific goals, such as master's level courses and faculty inservice education. All three curricula use the conceptual framework of developmental phases of the life process for organizing content about alcohol and other drug use, abuse, and dependence. Content and learning resources form a matrix that connects skills, related problems that occur at all ages, and concepts central to health-professional intervention generally and nursing intervention in particular.

Models for curricular change

Generalist nursing practice.   Nursing curricula are designed to achieve learning and performance objectives for generalist- and specialist-practitioners of nursing. Basic nursing education prepares the graduate for *generalist practice* at minimum professional standards for the safe delivery of nursing care in wellness states and for major illnesses. Expectations for knowledge and skills to identify and address alcohol, tobacco, and other drug problems parallel desired learning-outcomes in other content areas. They should reflect primary, secondary, and tertiary levels of intervention with these problems. General learning outcomes for the nurse with basic preparation in the addictions field are reflected in the following objectives (Naegle, 1993). On completion of the baccalaureate degree in nursing the graduate will be able to:

1. Develop an awareness of personal attitudes and values about alcohol, tobacco, and other drugs
2. Formulate understanding of patterns of use for nicotine, caffeine, alcohol, and over-the-counter, prescription, and illicit drugs by self, clients, peers, and coworkers
3. Identify patterns of alcohol and other drug use and abuse by clients and families and in communities
4. Assess manifestations of alcohol, tobacco, and other drug use, abuse, and dependence (history taking, examination, community assessments, and use of screening tools)
5. Identify human and environmental factors which place individuals and families at risk for the development of alcohol, tobacco, and other drug problems
6. Describe modalities implemented for the prevention, treatment, and long-term care of human responses in relation to alcohol, tobacco, and other drug problems
7. Describe societal, cultural, ethical, and legal factors related to alcohol, tobacco, and other drug use and their impact on clients and the delivery of health care
8. Formulate nursing diagnoses and strategies in response to drug-using patterns, including co-occurring illnesses and conditions secondary to alcohol, tobacco, and other drug abuse, specifically dual diagnoses and HIV-spectrum illness
9. Assess the effectiveness of nursing strategies implemented with patterns of alcohol, tobacco, and other drug use
10. Demonstrate skills in interdisciplinary planning and collaboration for the development of comprehensive care approaches and delivery

Options for incorporating this content include formal course offerings, clinical experiences and practica, and the integration of the content into courses which form the core knowledge base for beginning practice of the nurse-generalist. Clinical experiences that include contact with clients with diagnosed addictions, as well as clients who are at risk, are the basis of experiential learning and attitude change. Clinical integration provides the most broadly based opportunities for learning, primarily because health problems related to alcohol and other drug use occur across the life span and because the majority of problems are identified in general care settings, not in facilities treating alcohol and other drug problems. Fewer than one half of the individuals who experience alcohol and/or other psychoactive drug dependence ever seek treatment for these problems. The majority of this group, however, use health care agencies for assessment of psychological and physical complaints and treatment of medical illness. Furthermore, at any given time, 35% to 50% of individuals hospitalized in general health care facilities also meet the criteria for alcohol dependence or abuse (Moore et al, 1989). Because of the prevalence of these problems, nurses in staff, specialist, and supervisory positions will encounter the alcohol- and/or drug-dependent client. Each practitioner should be prepared to assess, intervene, and make the appropriate referrals for existing problems. When problems beyond the scope of practice of the generalist nurse are identified, the nurse should refer the client and/or family to providers and/or practitioners with specialized skills.

Specialization in the care of clients and families with alcohol, and other drug, problems has historically been learned through the nurse's employment in settings specializing in treatment of addicted individuals, rather than through educational preparation or certification. In response to educational and affiliative needs of nurses, three specialty nursing organizations have been formed: the Drug and Alcohol Nursing Association, the National Nurses Society on Addictions, and the National Consortium of Chemical Dependency Nurses. None of these groups differentiates the specialty practice by education. All three organizations develop educational materials and provide continuing education at annual meetings. The National Nurses Society on Addictions has published two volumes on nursing care planning for the addicted individual, as well as a core curriculum for inclusion in formal and informal education. Both the National Nurses Society on Addictions and the National Consortium of Chemical Dependency Nurses offer certification examinations to validate practitioner competence; and both the Consortium and the Drug and Alcohol Nursing Association offer membership to licensed practical nurses as well as professional nurses (see Chapter 17).

Specialist nursing practice.   It is increasingly recognized, however, that educational preparation is an important defining characteristic of role performance. The recent American Nurses Association requirement for master's degree education in a specific content area, or "area of concentration," now defines *specialist* status. Consequently, specialist certification no longer will be available from the American Nurses Credentialing Center for baccalaureate or other basic graduates. At present, debates central to developing the specialty of addictions nursing revolve around identifying components that constitute expert knowledge for advanced practice in this area, the viability of a freestanding specialty in addictions nursing versus a subspecialty in psychiatric-mental or community health nursing, and what constitutes uniquely nursing functions in the care of the addicted client or family.

Murphy and Hoeffer (1987) note that the development of specialization in any field can be attributed to three social forces: (1) new knowledge pertinent to the field, (2) technological advances, and (3) responses to public need or demand. All three apply to the identification and treatment of alcohol- and other drug-related problems; and a growing body of knowledge about the many forms of addiction supports the need to delineate specialty practice. "Expert knowledge" at the master's-degree level in nursing usually is acquired as preparation for nursing roles such as clinical specialist, nurse practitioner, or nurse manager. An example of additional expectations for the master's-degree graduate in addictions nursing is described in the terminal objectives of the master's-degree program at the Division of Nursing, New York University. On completion of the 45-credit master's degree, all students will be able to:

1. Select contemporary theories from nursing and from the basic sciences to develop strategies for use with individuals at risk for the development of alcohol or other drug problems
2. Apply the research process in the identification and critical analysis of alcohol- and other drug-related health problems
3. Use findings derived from alcohol and other drug research to formulate theory-based approaches to nursing practice
4. Synthesize knowledge from research related to alcohol and other drugs for education, management, or clinical practice

Graduates, through the selection of courses using the master's-degree modules, also have the option of choosing courses that prepare them to meet the following additional objectives:

1. Use advanced nursing knowledge about alcohol and other drugs to design and evaluate nursing strategies for individuals or groups and families
2. Demonstrate independent decision making in nursing interventions within an interdisciplinary framework for clients and families experiencing alcohol and other drug problems
3. Use knowledge of sociological trends, ethical and legal factors, and health policy related to alcohol and other drug use in formulating and implementing strategies for prevention or care and rehabilitation

These objectives reflect the distinguishing characteristics of master's-degree education for the formulation of scientifically based strategies whether applied to direct care, nursing management, or research-related activities. As new knowledge on addictions nursing is incorporated into nursing curricula, the development of master's-degree curricula will follow suit and the advanced practice role will become more clearly and consistently defined.

THEORY DEVELOPMENT AND KNOWLEDGE BUILDING

Nurse researchers have only recently focused their attention on substance abuse. Early studies addressed impaired practice by nurses as a special phenomenon and addicted nurses as a special population. A physician, LeClair Bissell, is credited with identifying characteristics of the impaired nurse, inspiring nurse researchers to address this population, and encouraging policy changes to aid nurses' recovery (Bissell & Jones, 1981; Sullivan et al, 1988).

This trend to study nurses and nursing students rather than the phenomena of concern, that is, addiction or a related aspect of health, follows an early pattern of nurse researchers that occurred at a time when conceptual models of the discipline had not yet been developed. These studies, essentially descriptive surveys of recovering nurses, have provided consistent, although selected, information about nurses, primarily women, who develop alcohol and other drug problems. The findings provide information about the disciplinary process, return to employment, and predisposing factors for female nurses who are recovering from addictions (Sullivan, 1987; Farley & Hendrix, 1992). These findings profile nurses who develop and recover from addictions. Implications of the findings cannot be extended to other professional women because of nonrandom sampling procedures and the absence of research on factors that differentiate nurses from other professional women and nursing from other professions/occupations. Additional studies (Trinkoff et al, 1991; Floyd, 1991) that compare alcohol and other drug use by nurses and nursing students with nonnurses and other professional student groups show promise for replication and further investigation. This work may be helpful in identifying profession-specific or workplace-specific factors related to drug abuse and dependence in nurses.

Appraisal of nurse and nursing student attitudes about alcohol and other drug problems is another area of investigation by nurse researchers (Cannon & Brown, 1988; Sullivan & Hale, 1986; Long, 1990). Some descriptive-survey findings date from the 1960s and, although limited in applicability, are important in their emphasis on a key treatment variable: attitudes of care providers as determinants of quality of care. In addition, they demonstrate the need for study of attitudes and provide the rationale for the development of educational offerings for nurses and other health-professional students.

Nurses also have identified substance abuse content in nursing curricula (Hoffman & Heinemann, 1987) and have examined the impact of various educational interventions on nurses' and nursing students' attitudes and behaviors (Jack, 1989; Rowland & Maynard, 1989). The studies of nursing curricula indicate that there has been limited content on substance abuse. These reports, however, are several years old and were done before recent initiatives by NIAAA, NIDA, and CSAP to develop this content in nursing education. The limited studies on the impact of education on attitudes and, especially, nurses' treatment of clients with substance abuse hold promise. If what is needed to improve nurses' abilities to care for addicted clients can be determined, appropriate educational programs can be devised.

Other research pursued by nurses includes studies on prevalence, research on clients with alcohol and drug abuse, studies on substance abuse in specialty clinical areas, and research on education in alcohol and drug abuse (Sullivan & Handley, 1992). Table 14-1 illustrates the variety of research on substance abuse problems conducted by nurses. Although the examination of actual nursing interventions is sparse and the lack of conceptual frameworks a concern, nursing's interest in the topic is increasingly apparent.

Table 14-1

Clinical studies on substance abuse by nurses

Researcher	Year	Content
Arneson, et al.	1983, 1987	School nurses' ability to identify and assist children of alcoholic parents
Banonis	1989	Qualitative study of recovery
Bartek, et al.	1988	Difficulty of care by nursing diagnoses
Bennett		Impact of stress and social support on self-esteem in young alcoholic men
Busch and McBride	1986	Pelvic pain and infertility in alcohol- or drug-dependent women
Byers, et al.	1990	Interventions to improve self-esteem
Colon and Radinsky	1981	Impact of referral procedures on outcomes
Engs	1977, 1985, 1990	Prevalence of alcohol use among college students
Fortin and Evans	1983	Disease progression in alcoholic women
Foy, et al.	1988	Assessment of withdrawal potential in high-risk clients
Hoffman and Estes	1986, 1987	Physiological and psychological withdrawal symptoms
Kus	1988a, 1988b	Qualitative study of addiction and recovery
London	1982	Children's beliefs about intoxication
Reynolds and Ried	1985	Assessment and referral skill of community health nurses
Rosenfield and Stevenson	1988	Eating behaviors and stress in alcoholic women
Scavnicky-Mylant	1986	Emotional and social development of children of alcoholic parents
Shelley and Anderson	1986	Menstrual problems in alcoholic women
Talashek	1987	Ego identity in adolescents with an alcoholic parent
Trinkoff, et al.	1990	Cocaine use in large populations

From Sullivan, E.J. & Handley, S.M. (1993). Alcohol and drug use. In J.J. Fitzpatrick & J.S. Stevenson. (Eds.) *Annual review of nursing research,* Vol. 11. New York: Springer.

In addition to increasing interest among nurse researchers, federal agencies are addressing the absence of nurse involvement. Initiatives from NIAAA, NIDA, and CSAP to fund model curriculum projects and faculty development indicate their interest in including nursing in the education of health care professionals. Funding of nursing research grants by NIAAA and NIDA and the appointment of a nurse to the National Advisory Council of NIAAA illustrate an increasing awareness in federal agencies of nursing's contribution to the addictions field.

Theories about addictions

The profession of nursing has not formulated systematically organized knowledge about addictions, nor has theory emerged to guide nursing care of individuals, families, and communities experiencing substance abuse problems. Furthermore, limitations in the alcohol and drug abuse scientific community are a result of the narrow research focus on basic science and reliance on research findings more biological than psychosocial in nature. The dominance of the biomedical model has resulted in more research findings that address the physiology of addiction to alcohol and other drugs than in findings that evaluate comprehensive treatment approaches using psychosocial modalities, as well as medical treatment. Few studies have examined health or correlates of health—nursing's central focus. Instead, investigators have sought to understand addictive disease and its predisposing factors and correlates, physiological consequences, and medical treatment.

Although specialty organizations of nurses working in the addictions have existed for 20 years, their educational efforts have been clinically oriented rather than research oriented, and knowledge building has not been a focus. Consequently, prevention, health implications, phases of addiction, and appropriate nursing care beyond the biological have rarely been studied in the context of a nursing conceptual model. Neither have nursing strategies been designed and evaluated as derivations of nursing's postulated interpretations and definitions of addiction.

Despite the development of a scope-of-practice statement and standards for addictions nursing, nursing theory rarely serves as the basis for nursing practice. Further, nursing frameworks have not been used to generate new knowledge about addictions and their prevention and/or treatment. Articles and textbook content suggest that the development of nursing theory in the nature and origins of addictions as human responses is slowly progressing toward the development of nursing knowledge (Naegle & Mitchell, 1991). Continued reliance on concepts central to the medical model, as well as a biological focus and epidemiological approaches, are evident in the earliest nursing manuscripts and reference books on alcoholism and other drug dependence. These have influenced practice in such a way that the current nursing role is implemented in a very narrow fashion and restricted to physical care and basic interpersonal interactions.

The latest nursing research, however, indicates that the profession is moving toward a stage of theory building in which clinical interventions are evaluated and human beings are viewed more holistically. As long as nurse investigators borrow theory from other disciplines, particularly the social sciences, to explain the multidimensional nature of abuse and addiction, theory is used in accurate and appropriate ways, although not in a nursing paradigm. An example of this is Hutchinson's use of sociologic theory to describe the phenomena of becoming addicted and recovering from addiction (Hutchinson, 1986; 1987). Nursing, like other disciplines, has a predominant paradigm but uses multiple conceptual models which seek to focus the various concepts of greatest relevance to nursing and nursing practice. The use of models not only helps differentiate the phenomena of specific concern to the profession, but provides direction for questions which explore phenomena and nursing's reaction to them. Although the four concepts central to major nursing models—person, health, environment, and nursing—provide a highly relevant framework for establishing perspectives on the addictions and their associated physiological, psychological, and social attributes, nursing models have not been developed. In addition, nursing lacks concepts and propositions about the addictive process and its predispositions and associated problems for appropriate integration into existing models (Hughes, 1989). Florence Nightingale's model is a particularly apt one because it includes metaphysical attributes and potentialities. It is the only nursing model that alludes to the spirit of a person as vulnerable to, and affected by, diminished levels of health. For those caring for drug-dependent individuals, attention to this human manifestation has particular salience because dependence diminishes one's spirituality, that is, one's sense of purpose and belonging in the universe.

Theoretical frameworks

In the professional nursing community there are differing views and theoretical perspectives on addiction. Furthermore, the lack of consensus about terms and concepts among practitioners and researchers compromises both communication and the initiation of research to build a common scientific knowledge base. Consensus does exist, however, that the addictions are determined by interacting variables that can be influenced by nurses practicing in generalist and specialist roles. But the determination of what constitutes effective nursing actions or interventions requires the evaluation of propositions within a variety of paradigms and conceptual models. The use of models appropriate to one or more selected nursing paradigms would allow for flexibility and innovative propositions which would reflect the evolving knowledge base on addictions and the nature of nursing.

Naegle and Mitchell (1991) suggest that theories grounded in the existential-phenomenological perspective reflect philosophical trends in the profession and move nursing research away from the traditions of logical positivism. Since nursing theory on addictions is in its infancy, and scientific knowledge about its nature and treatment is just beginning to coalesce, it would seem that the use of nursing models which are dynamic and consider multiple variables are particularly desirable.

Rogers' theoretical framework, the "science of unitary human beings," moves away from more rigid medically and socially defined models to a broader, more open model of health (Rogers, 1970). Because the human being is viewed "holistically" as an energy field, the *totality* model of an individual as a sum of his or her parts can be set aside. The "energy field" is dynamic and four-dimensional and is manifested in the individual's personality and behavioral and developmental characteristics. The multidimensional nature and range of manifestations that characterize the addictions is readily understood because addictions are viewed as human-field manifestations, emerging from the interaction of human and environmental fields, rather than as effects of particular causes. To Rogers, the human being is involved in a continuous mutual process with the environment, and this "mutual, simultaneous interaction" is linked with continuous change that is innovative, probabilistic, and characterized by higher frequency field-patterning, i.e., an increasingly complex relationship between human and environmental energy fields (Compton, 1989b).

Rogers' theoretical framework is one of the few that has been used by nurses in efforts to conceptualize addiction from the nursing perspective. Figure 14-1 illustrates the current limitations of theory development and the steps necessary to

Nursing Paradigm: human—environment—health—nursing

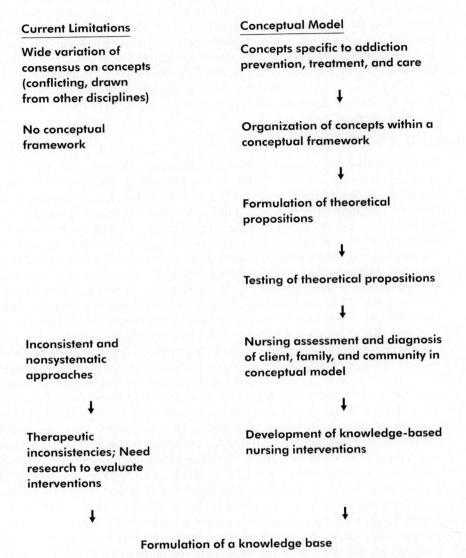

Current Limitations	Conceptual Model
Wide variation of consensus on concepts (conflicting, drawn from other disciplines)	Concepts specific to addiction prevention, treatment, and care
No conceptual framework	Organization of concepts within a conceptual framework
	Formulation of theoretical propositions
	Testing of theoretical propositions
Inconsistent and nonsystematic approaches	Nursing assessment and diagnosis of client, family, and community in conceptual model
Therapeutic inconsistencies; Need research to evaluate interventions	Development of knowledge-based nursing interventions

Formulation of a knowledge base

Fig. 14-1. Developmental status of the addictions nursing knowledge base.

formulate a knowledge base in addictions nursing. Compton (1989a) postulates that drug use represents a mode of seeking alternative ways to participate with the world through an altered sense of perception. Addiction arises out of the mutual process occurring between the drug-using human field and the drug-rejecting environmental field (Compton, 1989b). Different interconnections with the environmental field develop as a function of drug involvement, and these "manifestations" are identified as outcomes of drug-using behaviors. Since addiction arises out of a mutual process of human-environmental interaction, identification of patterns of such interaction can provide opportunities for detection and prevention of addiction by the recognition of, and intervention with, similar patterning. While nurses cannot change the patterning of a drug using/abusing human being, nurses can participate knowingly in helping individuals repattern their interactions and can encourage growth-promoting elements of the environmental field to which the client is integral (Compton, 1989b).

The Rogerian model as a conceptual system has the advantage of providing a value-neutral perspective. Drug use and addiction are viewed not as negative or morally unacceptable behaviors but simply as manifestations which are realities of human-environmental process. The Rogerian model also stresses the unique quality of the individual while acknowledging that field patterns can be similar. Since change is ongoing, the opportunity to increase the integral fit between human and environmental fields is a hopeful probability. The nurse "knowingly participates" with the client to improve his or her well-being to an optimal level, whatever that individual's potential may be.

Anderson and Smereck describe a nursing model for intervention with drug-addicted women, using a blend of the Rogerian theoretical framework and the Aristotelian view of well-being. They describe how "personalized care" and "personalized action" facilitate joint participation by nurse and client in the continuous process of innovative change. In a step-wise fashion the LIGHT (Love, Intent, Giving of Care, Help, and Touch) model is an approach to assisting clients repattern their human-environmental energy fields in creatively individualized ways which promote well-being (Anderson & Smereck, 1989).

The choice of the Rogerian framework is an example of delineating practice approaches from a model congruent with a nursing paradigm or world view. It offers further opportunities to develop guidelines for practice in relation to the phenomena of addictions. Unlike reductionistic or static models, this model incorporates new knowledge as evolutionary and a diverse extension of learning. Most importantly, it provides for "participating with" the client in producing change, rather than acting on the client in accord with standardized approaches that may not be integral with that person's interaction with a larger environmental field.

SUMMARY

Drug abuse and addiction have developed into major health problems. The roles of nurses and nursing have emerged as central potential resources in society's efforts to prevent and treat the medical problems created by use and dependence on alcohol, tobacco, and other drugs. Although standard nursing approaches of assessment and intervention shape nursing action with clients and families, the profession has not placed the range of human responses to addictions within a nursing-conceptual framework. The nursing paradigm of health has been bypassed, for the most part, in favor of the narrow "illness" focus on frank addiction studied and described in the biomedical literature. If nurses are to contribute in a meaningful way to the health care of individuals, families, and communities using drugs and experiencing related health problems, a nursing knowledge base must be developed. This knowledge base must be composed of learning about the phenomena of drug use and addiction gleaned from basic science and psychosocial research by nurse investigators and others.

Components of this knowledge base specific to nursing practice must be identified and interpreted in nursing paradigms that serve as the basis for nursing's perspectives and practice. For a specialty known as *addictions nursing* to advance, a knowledge base specific to the phenomena of the addictions and their nursing care must be established. Necessarily, the thinking of nurse educators and nurse researchers must coalesce to form central concepts and the development of theoretically sound propositions derived from nursing models. These concepts and propositions can be used to generate nursing theory and evaluate principles and guidelines for practice. Of the few nursing models applied to addictions and addictions nursing practice, the Rogerian model of unitary human beings offers a world view conducive to an understanding of addiction, its development, and its illness course, as well as directions for health promoting nursing interventions.

REFERENCES

Anderson, M.D. & Smereck, G.A.D. (1989). Personalized nursing LIGHT model. *Nursing Science Quarterly, 2*(3), 120-130.

Bissell, L. & Jones, R.W. (1981). The alcoholic nurse. *Nursing Outlook, 29*(2), 96-100.

Cannon, B.L. & Brown, J.S. (1988). Nurses' attitudes toward impaired colleagues. *Image: Journal of Nursing Scholarship, 20,* 96-101.

Compton, P. (1989a). Drug abuse: A self-care deficit. *Psychosocial Nursing and Mental Health Services, 27*(2), 22-26.

Compton, M.A. (1989b). A Rogerian view of drug abuse: Implications for nursing. *Nursing Science Quarterly, 2*(2), 98-105.

Farley, P.B. & Hendrix, M.J. (1992). Impaired and non-impaired nurses during childhood and adolescence. *Nursing Outlook, 41*(1), 25-31.

Fawcett, J. (1989). *Analysis and evaluation of conceptual models of nursing* (2nd ed.). Philadelphia: F.A. Davis.

Floyd, J.A. (1991). Nursing students' stress levels, attitudes toward drugs, and drug use. *Archives of Psychiatric Nursing, 1*(1), 46-53.

Hoffman, A. & Heinemann, M.E. (1987). Substance abuse education in schools of nursing: A national survey. *Journal of Nursing Education, 26,* 282-287.

Hughes, T.A. (1989). Models and perspectives of addiction: Implications for treatment. *Nursing Clinics of North America, 24*(1), 1-12.

Hutchinson, S. (1986). Chemically dependent nurses: The trajectory toward self-annihilation. *Nursing Research, 35*(4), 196-201.

Hutchinson, S. (1987). Toward self-integration: The recovery process of chemically dependent nurses. *Nursing Research, 36*(6), 339-343.

Jack, L.W. (1989). The educational impact of a course about addictions. *Journal of Nursing Education, 28*(1), 22-28.

Long, D. (1990). Changing nursing students' attitudes toward alcoholism. *Perspectives on Addictions Nursing,* June 1990, 3-5.

Moore, R., Bone, L., Geller, G., Mamon, J., Stokes, E., & Levine, D. (1989). Prevalence, detection, and treatment of alcoholism in hospitalized patients. *Journal of the American Medical Association, 261,* 403-407.

Murphy, S.A. & Hoeffer, B. (1987). The evolution of subspecialties in psychiatric and mental health nursing. *Archives of Psychiatric Nursing, 1*(3), 145-154.

Naegle, M. (Ed.) (1993). *Substance abuse education in nursing.* New York: National League for Nursing.

Naegle, L.M. & Mitchell, G.J. (1991). Theoretic diversity: Evolving paradigmatic issues in research and practice. *Advances in Nursing Science, 14*(1), 17-25.

Newman, M.A. (1990). Newman's theory of health as praxis. *Nursing Science Quarterly, 3,* 37-41.

Rogers, M. (1970). *An introduction to the theoretical basis of nursing.* Philadelphia: F.A. Davis.

Rowland, N. & Maynard, A.K. (1989). Alcohol education for patients: Some nurses need persuading. *Nurse Education Today, 9,* 100-104.

Sullivan, E. (1987). A descriptive study of nurses recovering from chemical dependency. *Archives of Psychiatric Nursing, 1*(3), 194-200.

Sullivan, E.J., Bissell, L., & Williams, E. (1988). *Chemical dependency in nursing: The deadly diversion.* Menlo Park, CA: Addison-Wesley.

Sullivan, E.J. & Hale, R.E. (1986). Nurses' attitudes toward alcohol abuse: A national survey. Fourth Annual Research Conference, *Proceedings of the Southern Council on Collegiate Education.* (pp 235-236). Dallas, Texas.

Sullivan, E.J. & Handley, S.M. (1992). Alcohol and drug abuse in nurses. In J.J. Fitzpatrick, R.L. Taunton, & J.Q. Benoliel. (Eds.) *Annual review of nursing research,* Vol. 10. New York: Springer.

Sullivan, E.J. & Handley, S.M. (1993). Alcohol and drug abuse. In J.J. Fitzpatrick & J.S. Stevenson, (Eds.) *Annual review of nursing research,* Vol. 11. New York: Springer.

Trinkoff, A.M., Eaton, W.W., & Anthony, J. (1991). The prevalence of substance abuse among registered nurses. *Nursing Research, 40*(3), 172-175.

15

Financing, Legal Issues, and Public Policy

Politics permeates all activities in American life; substance abuse is no exception. Providers, insurers, researchers, and consumers all have questions and answers. Some serve the public good, others serve themselves, and some serve both. Providers are charged with being interested only in increasing their revenues when they argue for treatment. Insurers are accused of caring only for the "bottom line" at the expense of claimants' health. Researchers and treatment staff use different information for decision-making (anecdotal clinical experiences versus research data) and then argue over appropriate treatment.

The question of whether alcohol- and drug-related disorders are indeed diseases or self-inflicted injuries continues to be controversial and fuels the argument against coverage. Also, substance abuse treatment is somewhat unconventional. It occurs in diverse settings: hospital-based units, freestanding facilities, and residential sites. It often uses nonprofessional care providers such as alcohol counselors and recovering persons. In fact, even the name is different. Clients with other health problems receive *health care.* Persons with substance abuse problems receive *treatment.*

This chapter chronicles the evolution of substance abuse financing in this country. Current efforts at cost containment are described. Drug abuse problems in the workplace are discussed, with a focus on the legal issues surrounding drug testing and discrimination. The legal and public policy issues involved in treating individuals with substance abuse problems also are explained.

FINANCING SUBSTANCE ABUSE TREATMENT

Paying for substance abuse treatment is the major concern of those in the field and others who recognize that treatment is effective in reducing substance use and ameliorating its problems (both individual and societal). Compared to compensation for other medical conditions, payment for substance abuse services is not equitably offered (Rogowski, 1992). A number of reasons for this discrepancy are proposed, including negative attitudes of policy makers, lack of public support for such treatment, and a general belief that treatment is ineffective. In addition, determining the optimal length of treatment and thus the appropriate cost has been difficult.

Evolution of financing policy

Until the 1970s, clients with problems related to substance abuse often were admitted to general hospitals with primary diagnoses of associated problems (e.g., trauma, cirrhosis) or to psychiatric hospitals for concomitant diagnoses (e.g., depression, anxiety). Clients with chronic substance abuse received custodial care in state mental hospitals. Few general hospitals had treatment units nor were there specialized hospitals.

With the growing recognition of substance abuse as a primary diagnosis, with more favorable reimbursement for treatment, and with the success of Alcoholics Anonymous (AA) and treatment programs modeled on AA, specialty treatment for substance abuse flourished. By 1986, more than 1000 hospitals and over 50 freestanding facilities provided specialized alcoholism or substance abuse treatment (AHA, 1987). Outpatient and residential facilities expanded similarly. In 1967 only 130 outpatient clinics and 100 halfway homes were in existence, but by 1987 more than 2000 outpatient facilities and 1300 residential facilities such as halfway houses were in operation (NIDA/NIAAA, 1989).

Both voluntary associations (e.g., National Council on Alcoholism, now known as the National Council on Alcoholism and Drug Dependence) and governmental agencies led the efforts to encourage a stable funding base for substance abuse treatment. The Hughes Act (P.L. 91-616) established NIAAA and NIDA in 1970 and is named after Senator Harold Hughes, who led the congressional effort to recognize alcohol and drug abuse as disorders distinct from mental illness. A program of federal funding for substance abuse research, treatment, and prevention was established.

The Hughes Act provided funding mechanisms for treatment services, including formula grants to states, project grants to public agencies and nonprofit organizations, and contracts with private and public organizations. These were combined later into block grants to states. This authority was given to the states to enable them to have maximum flexibility in designing programs to meet unique state needs. States use block grants to provide a variety of substance abuse education, prevention, and treatment programs. In 1992 the block grant program awarded $1.36 billion to states for antidrug activities. Since 1984, there has been a steady increase in funding to the block grant program (Klebe, 1992).

Reorganization of the Alcohol, Drug Abuse, and Mental Health Administration (ADAMHA)

In 1992 the Alcohol, Drug Abuse, and Mental Health Administration Reorganization Act (PL 102-321) moved the research activities of ADAMHA to the National Institutes of Health (NIH). Now there are three new institutes in NIH: the National Institute on Alcohol Abuse and Alcoholism, the National Institute on Drug Abuse, and the National Institute of Mental Health. This move made the addictions' research programs parallel with other components of the United States Public Health Service, in which service activities (e.g., prevention, treatment) are separated from research enterprises. In this regard ADAMHA had been aberrant, and the research component suffered from a lack of prestige.

A new federal agency, the Substance Abuse and Mental Health Services Administration (SAMHSA), was created to house the prevention and treatment components of the former ADAMHA. SAMHSA, which focuses on treatment and services for people who are mentally ill or dependent on alcohol or drugs, is comprised of three agencies: the Center for Substance Abuse Treatment (CSAT) (formerly the Office of Treatment Improvement), the Center for Substance Abuse Prevention (CSAP) (formerly the Office of Substance Abuse Prevention), and a newly created Center for Mental Health Services (CMHS). The purpose of this realignment was twofold: (1) to develop fully the federal government's ability to effectively target substance abuse and mental health services to the people most in need and (2) to translate research in these areas more effectively and more rapidly into the general health care system.

How treatment is financed today

There are two major sources of funding for substance abuse treatment. These are (1) third-party payers, who are either private (insurance companies) or public (Medicare, Medicaid), and (2) direct support, most often federal block grants to states (discussed previously). Third-party payers provide the majority of funding for substance abuse treatment for the employed (through insurance) and the retired (through Medicare). The federal government offers treatment to its employees through the Federal Employees Health Benefits Program (FEHBP). Other federal programs include the Department of Defense and the Veteran's Administration; the Bureau of Prisons; and the Indian Health Service.

Public treatment financing.   *Medicaid.* Medicaid is a joint federal and state financing mechanism that provides health services (including substance abuse treatment) to low-income and indigent state residents. These services are especially inadequate to provide care needed by individuals with multiple complex health and social service problems. Each state devises its own plan for substance abuse treatment and services; these plans vary widely from state to state. Also, Medicaid is tied to the welfare system, whose recipients are primarily female heads of households. The low-income group most likely to abuse drugs—men between the ages of 18 and 64—is the least likely to be included in Medicaid. A recent Institute of Medicine report argues that federal funding should be mainstreamed from block grants into Medicaid to provide more services to those who need them most (Gerstein & Harwood, 1990).

Although Medicaid was not designed specifically to fund alcohol and drug treatment, an increasing number of states are using it for that purpose. The National Drug and Alcoholism Treatment Unit Survey (NDATUS), reports that Medicaid reimbursements for substance abuse treatment doubled between 1982 and 1987 (NIDA/NIAAA, 1989). However, obtaining Medicaid dollars for substance abuse treatment can be a complicated process. The client, the service, and the provider institution are all required to meet a complex set of qualifying criteria. States participate in the Medicaid program on an optional basis and administer it within broad federal requirements and guidelines. This allows considerable discretion in determining eligibility, covered benefits, and provider-payment processes. Therefore, very little uniformity exists from one state to another.

Medicaid eligibility for individuals.   At a minimum, states must cover individuals with a net income less than or equal to 133% of poverty, or 33% above the poverty line ($14,463 for a family of four in 1992). Asset tests (ownership of durable goods), normally required for Medicaid eligibility, have been eliminated for pregnant women in 46 states.

Medicaid eligibility for institutions.   Medicaid covers almost all hospital-based services. Most substance abuse treatment services, however, are provided in nonhospital (freestanding) residential treatment institutions. Services provided within these facilities are the most difficult to have reimbursed under Medicaid because of the IMD (Institution for Mental Disease) exclusion. The IMD exclusion is a provision of the Medicaid statute that prohibits coverage for anyone under 65 who is an inpatient in an institution for mental diseases having more than 16 beds. The Health Care Financing Administration (HCFA), the agency that approves federal reimbursement for health care, has declared residential substance abuse treatment centers to be IMDs; so any person under the age of 65 is excluded from Medicaid coverage for treatment in such institutions.

Medicaid eligibility for services.   Medicaid is designed to finance services that typically fit the medical model. Although most states cover short-term hospital treatment for a three-to-six-day inpatient detoxification stay, as well as a limited number of outpatient counseling visits, there are very few long-term substance abuse treatment options for Medicaid patients. The result is a recurring cycle of relapse and return to the hospital for detoxification (GAO, 1991).

State of Missouri comprehensive plan for substance abuse treatment.   The state of Missouri has addressed the need for comprehensive services for indigent men and women. A shift away from a "provider-driven" to a "client-driven" treatment philosophy in the Missouri Department of Mental Health permitted services to be restructured according to eligibility criteria for Medicaid reimbursement. Missouri's Medicaid plan uses the rehabilitation option so that outpatient services can be delivered by a variety of different professionals and paraprofessionals in settings that can include clients' homes.

C-STAR (Comprehensive Substance Treatment and Rehabilitation Program), one of the most innovative state substance abuse programs in the country, is designed to provide holistic treatment and support to all individuals and families with substance abuse problems in the state of Missouri. It began in June 1991 with 33 C-STAR programs across the state. C-STAR programs are located within 60 miles of each other and serve both rural and urban communities. Built on a community-based model, C-STAR offers a wide range of individualized services organized according to three levels of care: the community-based primary treatment level, community-based rehabilitation level, and the supported-recovery level. All programs are culturally sensitive and some are specialized for pregnant and postpartum women and their children.

A major restructuring of services and a seamless system of electronic processing allows all C-STAR providers to electronically transmit authorization plans, demographic data, and invoices to the Missouri Division of Alcohol and Drug Abuse (ADA), so most services can be reimbursed efficiently through Medicaid funds or other sources. The ADA maximized the potential for Medicaid reimbursement by requiring residential facilities for women and children to provide room, board, and overnight nursing supervision in establishments with 16 beds or less. This precluded the IMD exclusion barrier. Providers are required to be eligible for Medicaid reimbursement in order to be certified as part of the C-STAR network of services. Clients and services not eligible for Medicaid are automatically identified and directed through the unique fiscal and billing system to alternative funding sources such as substance abuse block grant monies from the state department of mental health.

Private health insurance. Treatment for addictive disorders was slow to be included in private health coverage and, in fact, individuals with these problems were often discriminated against in reimbursement policies (Holder & Hallan, 1983). Concentrated efforts to change these policies have been successful to some degree. An analysis of pre- and posttreatment health care claims clearly indicated that substance abuse treatment costs were much less than the higher medical care costs of substance abusers and their family members. Employers also found that a workplace program to intervene with substance abusers, offer treatment, and monitor return to work resulted in cost savings compared to the reduced productivity, absenteeism, and turnover otherwise encountered in employees who abused substances.

Today, basic insurance usually covers physical illnesses and trauma related to substance abuse, as well as detoxification in general hospital settings. Rehabilitation, especially in a specialized treatment unit, continues to be an add-on benefit requiring additional premiums in the form of a rider to the benefit policy. Since few people with substance abuse problems recognize their need for treatment, they are unlikely to choose the extra benefit and expense. Furthermore, stringent restrictions on reimbursable services and length of coverage vary greatly among companies. In spite of these restrictions, the use of substance abuse treatment services has increased with a concomitant increase in costs (Rodriguez & Maher, 1986; Walsh & Egdahl, 1984).

Block grants to states. As a result of the 1992 reorganization law, the ADAMHA block grant was split into two grants: one for mental health services and one for substance abuse treatment and prevention services (Government Information Services, 1992). The 1992 reorganization law established CSAT as the administrator of block grants for substance abuse.

The formula under which each state's block-grant allotment is determined also was modified. Today funds authorized for substance abuse block grants are to be used to implement recommendations of the Institute of Medicine that include comprehensive treatment for pregnant women and intravenous drug users, reduction of waiting lists, improvement of treatment quality, and dedicated efforts to treat expectant mothers and provide on-site child care for parents of young children (Gerstein & Harwood, 1990). Substance abuse block grants are designated for planning, implementing, and evaluating activities to prevent and treat substance abuse. Specifically, 35% of block grants is to be used for alcohol services, 35% for drug abuse services, and 20% for prevention. In addition, the new formula modifies the previous 10% amount set aside for women to 5% targeted specifically to pregnant women and women with dependent children. The remaining 5% of the block grant formula SAMHSA uses for technical assistance, data collection, program evaluation, and for a national prevention database. A portion of this set-aside amount also may be used to assist state prevention efforts. The block grant is one of the most substantial funding sources for public substance abuse services.

Cost containment.   Health care costs have skyrocketed in spite of efforts of the federal government and other third-party payers to contain costs with prospective reimbursement (DRGs) that began in the mid-1980s. The cost of health care is a primary concern of federal and state governments, third-party payers, employers, the health care industry, health care professionals, and the general public. Mental health care in general, and substance abuse care in particular, are often the targets of cost containment, particularly since the move to fund only "medically necessary" care has intensified.

The nature of substance abuse treatment is controversial. Third-party payers have attributed the increase in the use, and thus the costs, of substance abuse treatment to marketing efforts by treatment providers. Conversely, providers suggest that cost containment efforts by insurers reflect persistent negative attitudes toward substance abusers. Regardless, cost containment is a fact of life in health care today, and substance abuse care is no exception. While the impact of health care reform is unknown at this time, several measures have been used to contain health care costs. These are: (1) health maintenance organizations, (2) preferred-provider arrangements, and (3) managed care.

Health maintenance organizations.   HMOs are increasingly used as mechanisms for cost containment. HMOs are prepaid health insurance plans that deliver health care services directly to subscribers at the HMO's expense. Costs are calculated on a per-capita basis and contracts for services negotiated with providers. Therefore, HMOs have an incentive to control costs while still meeting medical, ethical, and legal care requirements. Substance abuse treatment services in most HMO plans include outpatient treatment and follow-up.

Preferred provider arrangements.   Preferred provider arrangements are another method of cost containment. These are arrangements between insurers and health care providers in which costs are contained through incentives (e.g., lower copayments and deductibles) to encourage subscribers to use providers in the preferred-provider network.

Managed care.   Managed care is another cost-cutting strategy of third-party payers. Managed-care firms negotiate contracts with selected providers and institutions. Using a prospective-payment process, managed-care systems establish a standard plan of care for an illness, using preadmission screening, continuous utilization reviews, and discharge planning. As in other cost-containment strategies, managed care emphasizes the least intensive care. In substance abuse, outpatient and residential treatment for both detoxification and rehabilitation are common.

Various combinations of hospitals, physicians, HMOs, and managed-care organizations have formed networks to offer a variety of services on a capitated or fee-for-service basis. These networks can contract with private employers or state governments for comprehensive health care services.

A major concern of substance abuse treatment providers is that cost containment limits access to the range of services needed by patients with substance abuse to achieve and maintain sobriety. Additionally, although outpatient treatment is appropriate and effective for some clients, others need a supportive, therapeutic milieu 24 hours a day. "One size fits all" substance abuse coverage does not allow treatment providers to tailor treatment to the individual needs of clients.

Matching clients to treatment

To date, an adequate database for comparing the cost of treatment with outcomes for specific clients does not exist. Thus, a broad-brush approach is used by both providers and insurers: providers offer essentially the same program to all clients and insurers require that all receive identical coverage. After a lengthy study, the Institute of Medicine (IOM) recommended a comprehensive plan for assessment, referral, and insurance coverage. The underlying premise of their recommendations is that the least intensive program of treatment *that promises to be successful* should be used. The IOM established detailed criteria for assessment so that appropriate treatment modalities could be selected at each stage of treatment.

Another promising endeavor is NIAAA-sponsored research that supports studies to match client characteristics with treatment strategies to produce the most successful outcomes. "Project Match" is a large nationwide study matching clients to various forms of treatment and following their progress for more than a year. Results of this research hold promise for establishing guidelines for better matching clients to treatment.

Recommendations for coverage

In addition to matching clients to appropriate treatment, the IOM study also recommends that ". . . coverage for the treatment of alcohol problems should be subject to the same deductibles, coinsurance, limits, case management, and utilization review as are applied to coverage of treatment for other medical conditions" (IOM, 1990). Gerstein and Harwood (1990) recommend that individuals who have problems with other drugs also should receive this level of care.

Several strategies can be used to encourage implementation of the recommended policy. These range from providing information to employers and subscribers about the cost-effectiveness of treatment, to mandating that insurers provide such coverage. Specifically, the IOM suggests:

1. Increasing and careful use of case-managed coverage, which ideally should perfectly match clients with treatment
2. Reimbursement limits similar to those for other health care problems
3. Public financing through direct service (e.g., the military) and through public insurance (Medicare, Medicaid), again matching the most cost-effective option to specific patient needs

The study also recommends that costs and effectiveness be continually monitored and treatment strategies altered accordingly.

A DRUG-FREE WORKPLACE

To ensure a safe, healthy environment for workers, Congress enacted the Drug-Free Workplace Act of 1988 (41 U.S.C. 701 et seq.). The act requires that any individual or agency who receives a contract or grant from the federal government meet certain standards to ensure a drug-free workplace. Such individuals and agencies must:

1. Establish and publish a drug-free workplace policy, which states that manufacture, distribution, dispensing, possession, or use of controlled substances is prohibited in the workplace
2. Specify actions that will be taken against employees who violate the policy
3. Require adherence to the policy as a condition of employment and require the employee to notify the employer of any criminal drug statute conviction or violation occurring in the workplace, no later than five days after such conviction
4. Provide copies of the policy to all employees
5. Establish a drug-free awareness program
6. Take appropriate personnel action against an employee who is convicted as described above, up to and including termination, or require participation in a drug abuse rehabilitation program for the identified abuser as a condition of continued employment
7. Notify the federal granting or contracting agency within ten days after receiving notice of a criminal drug statute conviction or a violation occurring in the workplace

The law does *not*:

1. Require drug testing as part of the policy
2. Include private companies without government contracts
3. Include the most common addictive problem in the country—alcohol abuse and dependency

Although this law forces selected U.S. employers to address illegal drug use in the workplace—including illegal use of controlled substances—other substance abuse problems, especially alcohol abuse and secondary smoke inhalation from tobacco, are not addressed.

LEGAL ISSUES IN DRUG TESTING

The purpose of drug testing initially was punitive. The objective was to detect employees who were using drugs and dismiss them; treating the problem was not the goal. Today, the more progressive policies aim to arrange treatment for identified employees, provide support during rehabilitation, and encourage their return to work. (See Chapter 16 for information about the drug testing process.)

Drug testing, however benevolent employers' intentions, is fraught with conflict. Both labor and management have strong feelings about testing. Many citizens favor a rigorous approach to testing because of their frustration with escalating drug-related crime and the seeming inability of the legal and social system to contain drug use. The American Civil Liberties Union (ACLU) vigorously opposes testing.

Drug testing may be legally performed any time the agency doing the testing and the individual being tested agree to it. Legal controversies occur when an individual does not agree to testing. These conflicts involve both civil liberty and due-process issues.

Civil liberty issues

The increasing erosion of civil liberties worries many citizens. One's right to privacy is invaded by unauthorized credit reports, check-cashing identification, x-rays of one's person and belongings at airports, and a host of other encroachments. People opposed to drug testing argue that taking body fluids and examining them for illegal drugs is yet another intrusion into citizens' privacy.

The right to privacy is guaranteed by the Fourth Amendment to the Constitution, which states, "The right of the people to be secure in their persons, houses, papers, and effects, against unreasonable searches and seizures, shall not be violated and no Warrants shall issue, but upon probable cause. . . ."

This amendment prohibits an "unreasonable" search and seizure of persons and/or their property by government officials. Drug testing is considered by opponents to constitute an illegal search and seizure (of body fluids). In addition, the process of obtaining specimens for testing is degrading and dehumanizing. Direct observation of voiding, an especially embarrassing procedure, is required for reasonable certainty of an uncontaminated specimen.

Restrictions of the Fourth Amendment apply only to the federal, state, and local governments including public hospitals (i.e., state university hospitals). Private companies, even hospitals that receive government funding (e.g., Medicare, federal grants) are excluded from Fourth Amendment restrictions. Drug testing is common in the private sector and in certain industries. Such testing is governed by state law (see the following section).

Random testing of employees without cause is the most controversial issue, which includes both the reasonableness of searches under the Fourth Amendment by government employers, and the violation of the contract rights of employees by private employers. Cases of preemployment testing, testing for cause (or at least "reasonable suspicion"), and testing in rehabilitation monitoring have withstood legal challenges (*Wilkinson v Times Mirror Corp.*, 1989; *Willner v Thornburgh*, 1990; *Brown v Winkle*, 1989). Suspicionless testing of employees whose work affects public safety generally has been upheld in the courts (*Skinner v Railway Labor Executives' Association*, 1989).

Opponents argue that reliable and accurate results cannot be assured. Today, however, laboratories that adhere to the demanding federal standards (NIDA, 1988) can assure reasonable accuracy. Rigorous standards for collecting, identifying, handling, and transporting specimens also must be followed to ensure reliable results.

The ACLU opposes workplace drug testing because of its potential for abuse by managers. They contend that drug testing presents the opportunity for supervisors to discriminate against employees by harassing them (e.g, requesting frequent specimens). Their arguments are that (1) impaired job performance is not being tested and (2) one positive test does not indicate drug *abuse*, only recent use.

On the other side, employers maintain that they have a legal and moral obligation to ensure a drug-free workplace for all employees, most of whom are not drug users. Employers also have corporate responsibilities (e.g., to protect shareholders' investments). Protecting employees' civil liberties while maintaining a drug-free environment presents a continual challenge to employers (Walsh & Trumble, 1991).

Due process issues

In addition to concern about civil liberties, the Fourteenth Amendment to the Constitution provides protection of due process rights. This amendment states that a citizen may not be deprived of "life, liberty, or property without due process of law. . . ." Employment is a "property" right and cannot be taken away by governmental entities without due process (*Cleveland Board of Education v Loudermill*, 1985). Also, one's employment reputation is a "liberty" interest and any action that poses a threat to that reputation (e.g., a positive drug test) cannot be taken without due process (Scott & Fisher, 1990). Due process rights were violated in a case of mass testing of fire fighters when (1) employees were not given prior notice, (2) standards to guarantee reliability and accuracy of testing were not established, and (3) confidentiality of results was not assured (*Capua v City of Plainfield*, 1986).

Private employers, while not bound by constitutional due process restrictions, must adhere to state regulations regarding drug testing. Some states have "right to privacy" laws as well as legislation governing drug testing. Some state laws forbid disciplinary action following a positive drug test without offering treatment.

Common law liability

In addition to statutory or constitutional law, employees may bring suit against an employer under common-law theories including wrongful discharge, defamation (libel or slander), intentional infliction of emotional distress, or a common-law theory of privacy (Scott & Fisher, 1990). These claims are not yet well tested in the courts. Nevertheless, they demonstrate the importance of clearly delineating policies and procedures for drug testing that respect employees' rights.

PROTECTING CLIENTS' LEGAL RIGHTS

Two federal laws specifically protect the legal rights of substance abuse clients. They provide for (1) confidentiality of records of clients with alcohol and drug abuse problems and (2) protection of individuals with disabilities from discrimination. Since federal laws in these areas supersede state and local laws, including state licensure laws, these statutes ensure adherence for virtually all companies, organizations, and institutions.

Confidentiality of client records

Originally enacted in 1975, the Federal Drug and Alcohol Abuse Act (42 U.S. Code, Sections 290ee-3 and 290dd-3) established guidelines for confidentiality of client identification, information, and records. Regulations specify details of implementation of the law and are commonly cited as 42 CFR Part 2. These laws ensure the right to privacy of all clients receiving substance abuse treatment in a specified unit or in a general hospital if that organization receives any form of government (federal, state, local) assistance, including Medicare or Medicaid. Even clients who receive consultation and referral regarding substance abuse are covered by these regulations. Only clients treated by nonspecialists (e.g., general physicians) are not covered. Since essentially all institutions (public, private, nonprofit, for-profit) providing health care (including substance abuse care) receive some form of outside funding or third-party reimbursement, it would be rare for any institution not to be covered by these regulations.

Exceptions.   There are some specific instances in which confidentiality need not be maintained. These include the following circumstances:
1. When the client has provided prior written consent for release of information, including what information may be released, to whom, and the time limits for release
2. Internal communication within the treatment unit
3. When the client is known or suspected of child abuse
4. When authorized by a court order
5. When the client has a dual diagnosis, leaves the facility (either medically discharged or against medical advice), and is considered dangerous (*Tarasoff v Regents of the University of California*, 1976) (This case is discussed in more detail later in the chapter.)
6. In case of a medical emergency

Implementation.   The regulations require that the treatment program develop policies and procedures for implementing the law. These must include statements about how client privacy and confidentiality of records will be maintained and explanations of situations in which client information might not be protected. These policies and procedures must be widely disseminated and the program must ensure that all clients receive and understand them. *All* personnel (professional, nonprofessional, employees, volunteers) must be educated to follow the procedures for implementing the regulations.

Some examples of areas affected by the regulations include how the telephone is answered, what visitors are admitted, how client and fiscal records are kept (including electronic record-keeping), and how requests from legal authorities regarding other legal problems of clients (e.g., divorce, child custody, crimes, DWIs) are handled. Any person who answers the telephone must not divulge either the presence or absence of a specific client. Often the caller will be told "We cannot confirm nor deny that Mr. X is a client here." The same rules apply when someone appears in person at the facility. Visitors can only be admitted with the client's prior knowledge and approval. These rules regarding information and access apply to legal authorities (e.g., police, probation officers, attorneys). With electronic record-keeping, dual records may need to be kept in order to maintain client confidentiality. Fiscal records and audit information may contain descriptive data without identifying information.

Special populations.   An exceptional challenge to treatment providers are the clients who may endanger others. These populations include health care professionals, persons suspected of child abuse, those who test positive for HIV or AIDS, and dually diagnosed clients with the potential for violence. During treatment, health care professional clients (e.g., physicians, nurses, pharmacists, psychologists, social workers) may reveal prior illegal activities or acts of negligence that potentially endanger people in their care. Unless the state requires licensing board consent before treatment of a health care professional, treatment staff must adhere to the federal regulations regarding disclosure. If the health care professional client has already been reported to the board, he or she may release information that reflects success in the program and thus bolsters a claim of recovery.

In 1987 amendments to the law, staff members are required to meet state regulations for reporting suspected child abuse or neglect. Entire records, however, do not need to be revealed—only information about the abuse or neglect.

Individuals who test positive for HIV or AIDS also are protected by these regulations. Although state laws require reporting of HIV and other infectious diseases, federal law overrules state law, so identifying information may not be revealed.

One 1976 case has had widespread effect on the reporting of dually diagnosed clients with substance abuse and mental illness who are potentially dangerous. In the Tarasoff case (*Tarasoff v Regents of the University of California*, 1976) the psychiatrist, the university, and, ultimately, the Board of Regents were found liable for assaults by a client released from the hospital.

In two subsequent cases involving schizophrenic clients with comorbid substance abuse diagnoses, psychiatric liability was found (*Davis v Lhim*, 1983; *Peterson v Washington*, 1983). Essentially, the courts directed that clinicians with dually diagnosed clients must inform potential victims if the client made threats. Informing the public in general is not required. The clinician also may need to inform the police or initiate civil commitment procedures (Bartels & Drake, 1990).

Protection from discrimination

Public Law 101-336, The Americans with Disabilities Act (ADA) of 1990, protects individuals with physical or mental disabilities from employment discrimination on the basis of the disability. An "individual with a disability" is defined as a person who has a physical impairment (e.g., a vision or hearing deficit, or is confined to a wheelchair) or mental impairment (e.g., a psychiatric diagnosis) or a record of such impairment. People identified as alcohol- or drug-dependent who are no longer using illegal drugs or alcohol are protected. People currently using illegal drugs or alcohol are not protected.

The mandate to employers is clear. Neither the job nor benefits may be denied to a qualified individual because of a disability. As in other antidiscrimination legislation, selection criteria, employment tests, medical histories, and physical examinations may not be used to screen out the disabled. A test to determine the illegal use of drugs is not considered a medical exam and is not precluded. A medical exam may include tests to determine alcohol abuse (e.g., liver function tests) and, therefore, may not be used to disqualify applicants.

The 1990 legislation went much further than previous laws in specifying that employers not only could not discriminate but that they must provide "reasonable accommodation" for an individual with a disability to perform the job. Disabled employees, then, may be held to the same standards for employment, job performance, and behavior as employees without disabilities.

What does this mean to employers of individuals with substance abuse disorders? First, only those who have been identified with substance abuse disorders (either diagnosed or self-reported) are "protected." A person using drugs in the workplace or "under the influence" is not protected from the job-related consequences of that use.

Employees' drug abuse histories must be kept private. The ADA confidentiality provisions require the employer to keep records on an employee's drug abuse (i.e., disability) in separate, locked files with access limited to a need-to-know basis.

"Reasonable accommodation" for identified substance abusers has yet to be determined in the courts but, presumably, it includes modifying an employee's schedule so that counseling and support groups (e.g., Alcoholics Anonymous, Narcotics Anonymous) may be attended. It may include unpaid leave so the employee may enter residential rehabilitation. Often, an employer enters into a return-to-work agreement with a recovering employee regarding responsibilities of both (e.g., random urine screens, disciplinary action). The agreement also may specify restricted access to controlled substances for such employees as pharmacists and nurses.

POLITICS AND POLICY

Political action has influenced national policy, as typified by the Hughes Act in 1970; federal confidentiality laws; protection for substance abusers under the ADA; the move of NIAAA, NIDA, and NIMH to the National Institutes of Health (NIH); and the establishment of the Substance Abuse and Mental Health Services Administration (SAMHSA) in 1992. These policies affect funding, government activities, treatment providers, researchers, and the public.

Scientific data can provide compelling evidence for policy decisions. For example, research evidence about drinking age and traffic fatalities supported successful efforts to raise the drinking age to 21. Scientific data alone is not enough, however. Only political action can transform compelling evidence into policy.

Political activity at the state and federal level determines policies for funding for substance abuse education, prevention, and treatment, as well as drug-testing regulations. Political action in organizations such as the American Hospital Association has resulted in recommended policies for hospital drug testing (AHA, 1992). Finally, institutional or company policy determines how individual employers handle substance abuse problems in their employees. Political activity is especially important in determining policies regarding resource management (e.g., reimbursement policies of third-party payers).

SUMMARY

Identifying individuals with substance abuse problems and providing treatment is a complex and confusing societal problem. Ethical considerations, legal protections, and financing of substance abuse treatment offer public policy challenges. These challenges will escalate as marketplace pressures dominate health care and the debate over health care reform continues. Nurses can play a vital role in influencing policy decisions in their institutions and professional organizations and in local, state, and national governments.

REFERENCES

Alcohol, Drug Abuse, and Mental Health Administration Reorganization Act of 1992, P.L. 102-321 (1992).

American Hospital Association. (1987). *Hospital statistics.* Chicago: American Hospital Publishing.

American Hospital Association. (1992). *Substance abuse policies for health care institutions.* Chicago: The Association.

Americans with Disabilities Act, P.L. 101-336 (1990).

Bartels, S.J. & Drake, R.E. (1990). Tarasoff and the dual-diagnosis patient. In J.C. Beck, (Ed.) *Confidentiality versus the duty to protect: Foreseeable harm in the practice of psychiatry.* (pp 141-156). Washington, D.C.: American Psychiatric Press.

Brown v Winkle, 715 F. Supp. 195, N.D. Ohio (1989).

Capua v City of Plainfield, 643 F. Supp. 1507, D. N.J. (1986).

Cleveland Board of Education v Loudermill, 470 U.S. 532 (1985).

Davis v Lhim, 335 NW 2nd. 481, 124, Mich. App. 291 (1983).

Drug-Free Workplace Act, 41 U.S.C. 701 et seq. (1988).

Federal Drug and Alcohol Abuse Act, 42 U.S.C. Sections 290ee-3 and 290dd-3 (1975).

General Accounting Office. (1991). *Substance abuse treatment: Medicaid allows some services but generally limits coverage.* Report to Congressional Requesters (GAO/HRD-91-92.) Washington, D.C.: General Accounting Office.

Gerstein, D. & Harwood, H. (Eds.) (1990). *Treating drug problems: A study of the evolution, effectiveness, and financing of public and private drug treatment evolution, effectiveness, and financing of public and private drug treatment systems.* Washington, D.C.: National Academy Press.

Government Information Services. (1992). *ADAMHA reorganization act. Federal funding opportunities: An analysis of funding available as a result of the 1992 restructuring of federal anti-drug programs.* Arlington, VA: Government Information Services.

Holder, H.D. & Hallan, J.B. (1983). *Development of cost simulation study of alcoholic insurance benefit packages.* Rockville, MD: National Institute on Alcohol Abuse and Alcoholism.

Hughes Act, P.L. 91-616 (1970).

Institute of Medicine. (1990). *Broadening the base of treatment for alcohol problems.* Washington, D.C.: National Academy Press.

Klebe, E. (1992). *Alcohol, drug abuse, and mental health block grant programs.* Washington, D.C.: Congressional Research Service, The Library of Congress.

National Institute on Drug Abuse. (1988). *Medical review officer manual: A guide to evaluating urine drug analysis.* Washington, D.C.: U.S. Government Printing Office.

National Institute on Drug Abuse/National Institute on Alcohol Abuse and Alcoholism. (1989). *Highlights from the 1987 national drug and alcoholism treatment unit survey (NDATUS).* Rockville, MD: NIDA/NIAAA.

Peterson v Washington, 671 P2d 230, 100, Wash. 421 (1983).

Rodriguez, A.R. & Maher, J.J. (1986). Psychiatric case management offers cost, quality control. *Business and Health, 3*(5), 14-17.

Rogowski, J.A. (1992). Insurance coverage for drug abuse. *Health Affairs, 11*(3), 137-148.

Scott, M. & Fisher, K.S. (1990). The evolving legal context for drug testing programs. *Anesthesiology, 73,* 1022-1027.

Skinner v Railway Labor Executives' Association, 109 S. Ct. 1402 (1989).

Tarasoff v Regents of the University of California, 551 P.2d. 334, 17 Cal.3d. 425, Cal. Sup. Ct. (1976).

Walsh, D.C. & Egdahl, R.H. (1984). Treatment for chemical dependency and mental illness: Can this utilization be managed? *Health Affairs, 3*(3), 130-135.

Walsh, J.M. & Trumble, J.G. (1991). The politics of drug testing. In R.H. Coombs & L.J. West, (Eds.) *Drug testing: Issues and options.* (pp 22-49). New York: Oxford University Press.

Wilkinson v Times Mirror Corporation, 215 Cal. Ap. 3d. 1034, 264 Cal. Rptr. 194, Cal. Ct. App. (1989).

Willner v Thornburgh, 738 F. Supp. 1, D.C.C. (1990).

16 Drug Testing

Drug testing is a relatively recent strategy used in an attempt to control the increasing abuse of drugs and their effect on the workplace. Drug testing has become available because of the technological ability to detect various substances (e.g., alcohol, other drugs) in biological specimens (e.g., urine, blood).

This chapter describes the drug-testing process, the information it yields, and procedures used to collect and test specimens. Considering drug-testing costs, situations for appropriate use of drug testing are explored.

Drug-use costs to American industry result from lost productivity, drug-related accidents, enforcement and treatment expense, drug-related crime, property damage, and increased demands on health care benefits (including AIDS cases related to IV drug use) (White House, 1990). Of the estimated $116.9-billion cost of alcoholism and alcohol abuse for 1983, nearly $71 billion (61%) was attributed to lost employment and reduced productivity, and $15 billion (13%) to health care costs and treatment (USDHHS, 1990). Costs of illicit drug use in 1988 were estimated to be $58.3 billion, which included $7.2 billion for lost productivity and $3 billion for premature death (NIDA, 1991).

WHAT IS DRUG TESTING?

Drug testing is a screening method used to detect the presence of a drug or its metabolite in a body fluid, either urine or blood. Detectability depends on the (1) type of drug; (2) size of the dose, especially the last dose; (3) frequency of use; (4) route of administration; (5) individual variation in drug metabolism; (6) body weight; (7) amount of liquids consumed; (8) sample collection time (first void specimen is the most accurate); and (9) sensitivity of the analytical method used.

Drug testing provides only one piece of information: that the person who provided the specimen used the drug in the immediate past. It is not diagnostic for alcohol or drug dependency nor does it determine the possible severity or extent of that use. In fact, the person may have used the drug only on that one occasion. Unfortunately, policy makers, employers, and others (e.g., malpractice insurance carriers) often view drug testing as the panacea for drug abuse. While drug testing is not such a panacea, it can effectively be used with other methods to identify substance abuse and can assist in monitoring recovery from dependency.

THE DRUG TESTING PROCESS

Definitions

The following definitions will help clarify drug-testing methods (Sullivan et al, 1988).

Sensitivity. The detection limit of the test. The more sensitive the test, the longer the drug can be detected and the smaller the amount that can be measured; also the greater the risk of "false positives."

Specificity. The ability of a test to discriminate between drugs. The more specific the test, the more accurate the determination of specific drug use.

Assay. The analysis of a substance to determine its composition.

Screening assay. An analysis used to screen a sample for the presence of drugs. Samples testing positive with a screening assay should be followed by a confirmation assay to ensure that the result is not a false positive.

Confirmation assay. A follow-up test, more sensitive and more specific than the screening test, to confirm the presence of a drug. When the presence of drugs is not validated by the confirmation assay, the test is reported as negative.

Cross-reactivity. The misidentification of a drug when the reaction of one metabolite mimics the presence of another (e.g., novocaine can be reported as cocaine).

Nanograms and micrograms. Concentrations of metabolites in urine that are reported as amounts per milliliter. The amounts are reported in nanograms (ng) or micrograms (μg). There are 1000 nanograms in one microgram. A microgram is one millionth of one gram. There are 28 million micrograms in one ounce. The presence of marijuana is usually reported in nanograms per milliliter, and cocaine metabolite is reported in micrograms per milliliter.

Quality assurance (QA). The ability of a laboratory to conduct consistently accurate tests. To meet high quality assurance standards, rigorously controlled procedures should be followed in handling, storing, labeling, and testing samples for the presence of drugs. To test a laboratory for QA, a nursing administrator can send a sample of urine containing a known quantity of a drug. The laboratory's ability to produce accurate results can be determined by comparing its report with the known quantity. The known quantity samples are referred to as quality-control samples.

Random drug testing. Random drug testing means that specimens are collected without prior warning to the individual. A random schedule of collection is used. Unannounced testing for drugs provides greater assurance that drug use is not occurring and, conversely, that an individual using drugs will be identified.

Cut-off value. The cut-off value is the point at which the presence of a drug is considered to be present. The cut-off value must be set high enough to avoid a false positive report and possible litigation, but not so high that the presence of the drug is undetected.

Types of drug tests

Thin-layer chromatography (TLC).   TLC is commonly used to detect very high recent doses of drugs or toxic levels of drugs. It is extremely useful in emergency-room admissions for drug-overdose cases in which a patient is unable to report what drug or how much has been taken. However, the test is not sensitive enough to use in drug screens in the workplace because only very large doses are detected. False negatives are common for people using smaller quantities.

Gas chromatography (GC) and gas chromatography mass spectrometry (GC-MS).   Gas chromatography and gas chromatography mass spectrometry is about 100 to 1000 times more sensitive than TLC; it also specifically identifies the drugs present. A urine sample is heated to a vapor inside a gas chromatogram, which measures the amount of time the vaporized drug takes to pass through a column filled with the testing substances. This test can identify extremely small quantities of several drugs in a single analysis. Its sensitivity can be increased with mass spectrometry, which breaks down drug vapor into smaller fragments that are measured for electrical charge. Although these tests are considered the most reliable, they are also expensive, time-consuming, and require complex procedures. With the increased computerization of laboratories, however, these tests are becoming more widely used.

Enzyme immunoassay (EIA) and radioimmunoassay (RIA).   Enzyme immunoassay and radioimmunoassay use the sensitivity and specificity of antibodies to indicate the type and quantity of drug metabolites present in the urine. For EIA, the urine sample is mixed with reagents used to detect specific drugs. The mixture is placed in a spectrometer, which measures the amount of light the mixture absorbs. The degree of absorption indicates the presence or absence of the drug. RIA uses radioactive substances similarly.

Sometimes cross-reaction of compounds can occur, making RIA and EIA less specific than GC or GC-MS. Nevertheless, RIA and EIA are commonly used for screening assays because the laboratory procedure is less complex, more widely available, and less expensive. Table 16-1 compares the various tests for drug screening.

Elimination times

As can be seen by Table 16-2, drugs have varying elimination times. Some drugs have long elimination times (e.g., PCP, marijuana) while others are retained in body fluids for only a short period of time (e.g., cocaine, narcotics). The metabolites of short-acting drugs, however, are retained for longer periods of time (e.g., 98% of cocaine is eliminated from the body in five hours, but its metabolite, benzoylecgonine, is detectable for two to four days). Although alcohol can be measured in urine as well, methodological problems caused by alcohol's prompt excretion and volatility commonly produce false negative results that are not reliable (Pottash et al, 1983).

Accuracy

The accuracy of a drug test is the most common concern of the company or agency testing employees and of the employees themselves. Erroneous results occur because of (1) contamination of the specimen or container, (2) the quality of the laboratory, (3) the type of test(s) used, (4) carelessness in collection, and (5) technician

Table 16-1

Comparison of laboratory tests for drug screening

Name	Type	Sensitivity	Specificity	Availability
TLC	Toxicology screen	Poor	Poor	Inexpensive, fast, can be done in most labs
GC GC-MS	Chemical analysis	Excellent	Excellent	Expensive, requires complex equipment and trained personnel, available in some labs
RIA EIA	Immunoassay	Excellent	Good	Moderate cost, available in many labs, easily automated procedures

From Sullivan, E.J., Bissell, L., & Williams, E. (1988). *Chemical dependency in nursing: The deadly diversion.* Menlo Park, CA: Addison-Wesley.

error in testing. In addition, deliberate sabotage can occur. For example,

- Placing chemical substances under the fingernails to release into the sample
- Puncturing the specimen container with a pin, thus allowing the urine to escape slowly during transport
- Adding soap from rest room dispensers to the specimen
- Releasing fluid from a fluid-filled bulb (placed under the arm with a tube leading to the genitalia) into the container in place of urine
- Procuring urine from drug-free friends or saving urine from non-drug use periods and substituting it for a newly voided specimen
- Scooping water from the commode to dilute the specimen
- Concealing a plastic tube filled with drug-free urine in vagina, unscrewing cap, and "urinating" into container

Table 16-2

Drug detection period

Drug	Type	Detection period
Amphetamine	Stimulant	2 to 4 days
Barbiturate	Sedative	12 hours to 3 weeks
Cocaine	Stimulant	2 to 4 days
Fentanyl	Narcotic	Can be less than an hour
Heroin/morphine/ meperidine (Demerol)	Narcotic	2 to 4 days
Marijuana	Euphoric	3 days to more than one month
Methadone	Analgesic	2 to 4 days
PCP	Anesthetic	1 to 30 days
Benzodiazepine	Tranquilizer	Up to 1 week

Sullivan, E.J., Bissell, L., & Williams, E. (1988). *Chemical dependency in nursing: The deadly diversion.* Menlo Park, CA: Addison-Wesley.

- Sending friend to give specimen
- Catheterizing bladder and substituting urine obtained from a family member, then urinating under careful observation

Both false positive or negative results can occur. A false negative is a much more common occurrence than a false positive. A *false negative* occurs when the drug is actually *present* but the test is reported as negative. A *false positive* occurs when the drug is *not present* but a positive test is reported. A false positive can take place with the ingestion of certain foods, over-the-counter medications, or prescription medicines. For these reasons, and because false positives can be nearly eliminated by the use of confirmatory tests (such as GC-MS), a positive result is likely to be accurate. A negative result may or may not be correct.

PROCEDURES FOR DRUG TESTING

Collecting the specimen

Specimen collection is the first step in testing. Urine is the most common specimen used because there is 1000 times the amount of drug in urine as in the blood, and urine is relatively easy to collect (NIDA, 1988). Obtaining a blood specimen is, of course, a more invasive procedure. Urine collection requires only a clean container, a private area for voiding, and a reliable person to receive custody of the specimen. There are, however, a number of complications to accurate urine specimen collection. If the collection is not witnessed, the possibility of substitution or adulteration is possible. Since it is usually experienced drug users who alter specimens, most employers have opted for employees' privacy rather than witness the collection. In fact, a determined person can find ways to change specimens in plain view of a witness.

Chain of custody

The chain of custody is a method of accountability for the specimen from collection to final disposal. After the specimen is collected, it must remain in sight of assigned personnel at all times or it must be locked in a secure area with restricted access. It must be tightly capped, sealed, and labeled. A logbook should be maintained to designate each person responsible for the specimen and the times that the specimen was in her or his care. Every individual who handles, transports, or receives the specimen should sign the logbook.

The laboratory

The specimen can be collected without contamination, and all who handle it can follow the chain-of-custody requirements, but if the laboratory fails to accurately test the specimen the results are worthless. When selecting a laboratory, accreditation and certification should be required and staff should meet state requirements, at a minimum. The U.S. Department of Health and Human Services has issued standards for laboratories conducting drug testing for the federal government. A laboratory adhering to these standards, "Mandatory Guidelines for Federal Workplace Drug Testing Programs," can virtually assure the user of accuracy and reliability (USDHHS, 1988).

THE COST OF DRUG TESTING

The actual cost of a urinalysis to determine the presence of drugs is about $100, but the total expense to a company and the employee is much more (Strasser, 1990). Added cost factors include establishing a collection site, assigning employee(s) to collect specimens, managing the chain of custody, handling necessary paperwork, and defending legal challenges.

Although a regular rest room can be used for collection, large companies arrange special facilities. They may have the water turned off or add blue coloring to the toilet bowl. Employees may be required to remove coats and jackets, leave purses outside, and empty pockets before providing a specimen. Staff must be assigned to handle the collection process.

The chain of custody must be guaranteed or the results are useless. This involves keeping the specimen in sight at all times and maintaining records and signatures of all responsible parties. Recordkeeping for the entire process, including results, is an additional expense.

Drug testing is a useful tool when used for cause and after accidents, but mass testing is inappropriate and costly. Many argue that the expense involved in drug testing could be better spent in educating employees and providing confidential employee assistance programs.

WHEN IS DRUG TESTING USED?

During treatment and follow-up

Random drug testing during treatment can be a useful adjunct to therapy. It encourages the client to avoid drugs, which is especially important if outpatient treatment is used. It provides assurance to both treatment staff and the client that abstinence is being maintained.

During outpatient treatment or follow-up care, drug testing also helps protect the public if the substance abuser presents a particular danger to society. For clients who have a history of drug use concurrent with criminal activity, or workers whose substance abuse can endanger others (e.g., health care workers, airline pilots), random drug testing offers additional assurance of compliance with treatment. Drug testing, of course, offers little help in determining abstinence from alcohol.

To protect the public

People who have the potential to endanger others (e.g., police officers, railroad engineers, physicians, nurses) have been targeted for drug testing in an attempt to protect the public. In circumstances where injury has already occurred (e.g., railway accident, traffic collision), drug testing may be used to determine culpability. In this situation, the consequences of drug use may be considered a crime rather than merely results of an illness. The argument, however, is a powerful one—no third party should suffer or die at the hands of another, even if the other has an illness.

Public safety concerns have resulted in stringent procedures to identify and either rehabilitate or terminate substance abusers. To maintain integrity of the federal work force, to protect public safety, and to safeguard sensitive information, suspicionless testing is allowed. Challenges to random testing, however, continue in the courts (Angarola, 1990).

In the workplace

In the workplace, drug testing is used (1) to screen potential employees; (2) for cause (e.g., suspicions of use); (3) following a suspicious event; and (4) to monitor returning employees after rehabilitation. Random drug testing of employees who do not present a threat to public safety is not allowed. A multitude of complex legal and ethical issues surrounds drug testing in the workplace. Chapter 15 describes these issues and their impact on public policy.

GUIDELINES FOR TESTING

Drug-testing programs must respect the rights of individuals and, at the same time, fulfill the employer's responsibility to provide a drug-free workplace. While these obligations often are in conflict, there are some guiding principles to protect employees that also help management to meet its goal. Suggested guidelines are:

1. The goals of testing must be to rehabilitate the individual and prevent harm to others.
2. The opportunity for treatment must be made available.
3. All individuals to be tested must be informed.
4. Confidentiality must be maintained.
5. Alternative methods for identifying substance abuse also should be used, including:
   a. testing job performance,
   b. educating employees and supervisors,
   c. providing a mechanism for voluntary treatment without job loss, and
   d. offering an employee assistance program (EAP).
6. Testing must:
   a. be scientifically sound,
   b. adhere to strict standards for specimen collection and handling,
   c. utilize confirmatory test(s) following positive screens,
   d. be performed by a reliable laboratory, and
   e. have quality controls built into procedures (Coombs & West, 1991).

SUMMARY

Drug testing is not a panacea for controlling drug use; rather it is an adjunct technique used to identify substances. The screening techniques available identify the presence of a drug or its metabolite in urine or other body fluids. Enzyme assay techniques are commonly used in initial screening because they are less complex and relatively inexpensive. Gas chromatography and mass spectrometry are more sensitive, although also more time-consuming and expensive; they are generally used as follow-up to a positive screen.

Strict laboratory standards for collection, handling, processing, and reporting must be maintained to ensure accuracy and confidentiality. The cost of a urine drug screen and ethical-legal considerations preclude routine screening in the work-place. Random drug testing is indicated in professions that place the public at risk, in circumstances in which drug use is suspected, or to monitor employees reentering the work force after drug treatment.

REFERENCES

Angarola, R.T. (1990). Substance abuse testing in the workplace: Legal issues and corporate responses. In R.H. Coombs & L.G. West, (Eds.) *Drug testing: Issues and options.* (pp 155-189). New York: Oxford University Press.

Coombs, R.H. & West, L.G. (1991). *Drug testing: Issues and options.* New York: Oxford University Press.

National Institute on Drug Abuse. (1988). *Medical review officer manual: A guide to evaluating urine drug analysis.* (DHHS Publication No. ADM 88-1526.) Washington, D.C.: U.S. Government Printing Office.

National Institute on Drug Abuse. (1991). *Third triennial report to congress: Drug abuse and drug abuse research.* (DHHS Publication No. ADM 91-1704.) Washington, D.C.: U.S. Government Printing Office.

Pottash, A.C., Gold, M.S., & Extein, I. (1983). The use of the clinical laboratory. In L.I. Sederer, (Ed.) *Inpatient psychiatry: Diagnosis and treatment.* (pp 205-207). Baltimore: Williams & Wilkins.

Strasser, A.L. (1990). Drug testing requires examination of methods, reasons and usefulness. *Occupational Health & Safety, 59*(6), 52.

Sullivan, E.J., Bissell, L., & Williams, E. (1988). *Chemical dependency in nursing: The deadly diversion.* Menlo Park, CA: Addison-Wesley.

United States Department of Health and Human Services. (1988). Mandatory guidelines for federal workplace drug testing programs; final guidelines; notice. *Federal Register, 53,* 11970-11989.

White House, The. (1990). *National drug control strategy.* Washington, D.C.: U.S. Government Printing Office.

17 Challenging Practice Opportunities in Substance Abuse Nursing

The reasons why a nurse selects a particular clinical specialty can be as varied as nurses themselves. Determining factors may include inspiring teachers, personal situations in which a specific disease or illness played a central role in the family, or employment opportunities that offered attractive working conditions. Variables such as these, either singly or in combination, frequently influence the direction of a nurse's career. However, there are specialty areas in the field of nursing that initially get overlooked, perhaps until an opportunity presents itself with challenge. Substance abuse nursing is an area of practice that many nurses easily bypass at first glance and might not discover until their careers develop. Only upon reflection, usually, does the choice seem to fit the profile of the variables mentioned.

Today, there are more opportunities than ever before for nurses interested in exploring the challenging practice-opportunities in substance abuse nursing. Researchers, clinicians, and educators from all the health disciplines have responded to society's call for expert assistance in solving one of the most complicated social problems facing our culture in this century.

This chapter provides an overview of progress in the development of addictions nursing practice as a specialty. Highlighting specific populations who are in need of services, it explores roles that exist and can be developed, at both the generalist and advanced practice levels, to meet the needs of clients, families, and communities.

CONTEXT OF SUBSTANCE ABUSE NURSING

The context for exploring practice opportunities in substance abuse nursing begins with creativity and commitment to caring for whole clients and families in any practice setting. In this age of managed care and specialization, we have yet to build an alternative health care system in which holistic care of clients will be viewed as the normative approach to cost-effective care. For now, we continue to function in an era of specialization that we hope soon will be balanced with a renewed emphasis on primary care. What makes the future particularly exciting is the potential for a "level playing field" for nurses to contribute their particular expertise to a new system of care, one which values the added effects of prevention, education, and community-based support (Naylor & Brooten, 1993). As existing barriers to practice are systematically removed, opportunities for development of clinical nurse specialists appear to be unparalleled (Safriet, 1992).

The scope of this book illustrates that one does not have to work in a designated substance abuse treatment unit to encounter clients with addictive disease. Caring for clients in any setting presents opportunities to apply substance abuse nursing. Whether a professional is a recognized expert in the field or a general practitioner of nursing with curiosity and interest in human behavior and addictions, the ground is fertile for integrating skills in addictions management into a day-to-day professional role.

Excerpts of poems from R.D. Laing's collection entitled *Knots* (1970) balance a clinical discussion of professional opportunities. Sensitivity to the humanistic side of the problems that clients, families, and communities face in dealing with addictive disorders must be acknowledged. The emotional entanglements, impasses, and binds that Laing so eloquently addresses in his poetry serve as a literary reference for the problems that nurses recognize and try to remedy. We hope to challenge nurses to find, within their span of practice, new opportunities to explore skill acquisition in substance abuse nursing. These skills will add new areas of professional reward for nurses. (See poems on pp. 453 and 457.)

The addiction field's state of the art is growing. Over the past 25 years a considerable body of knowledge has emerged to describe the etiology, behavior, treatment, and outcomes of the diseases of alcoholism and drug dependency (Mendelson & Mello, 1985; Bratter & Forrest, 1985). Despite the proliferation of books and articles on the topic, there is still ambivalence about how to accurately describe even the diagnosis of alcoholism, the most familiar of the addictions.

Recently, a multidisciplinary committee of the National Council on Alcoholism and Drug Dependence and the American Society of Addiction Medicine conducted a two-year study to determine a definition of alcoholism that would be considered scientifically valid, clinically useful, and understandable to the general public. The committee agreed to the following definition of alcoholism (Morse & Flaven, 1992, p. 1013):

> A primary, chronic disease with genetic, psychosocial, and environmental factors influencing its development and manifestations. The disease is often progressive and fatal. It is characterized by impaired control over drinking, preoccupation with the drug alcohol, use of alcohol despite adverse consequences, and distortions in thinking, most notably denial. Each of these symptoms may be continuous or periodic.

The committee also underscored the need to recognize alcoholism as a primary illness and to integrate this concept throughout existing psychiatric classification systems. (See Chapters 2 and 3 for more detailed descriptions of substance abuse and its diagnosis.) The theory that chemical dependency is a disease has allowed society and clinicians alike to be more comfortable in approaching the substance abuser as an individual who is in need of help, compared to the moral attitude that these individuals are simply weak-willed and undesirable to treat.

Theories about alcohol and drug dependency range from describing substance abuse as a disease primarily genetically determined to a theory that substance abuse is a consequence of negative environmental factors. Theories can be useful for understanding the underlying dynamics of an individual's inability to sustain a healthy state of homeostasis. They are helpful also in understanding how nurses' use of good interpersonal skills can assist a client in choices to regain a state of wellness.

Any nurse interested in working effectively in the addictions field needs to understand its psychological, social, and physiological dimensions. Substance abuse is better understood and treated when viewed as a disease that can respond to properly designed treatment that fosters clients' active participation and responsibility. The nature of the disease of addiction and its prominence as a major health threat has forced members of society and the health care profession alike to recognize that substance abuse demands compassionate and specialized skills.

The opportunities for nurses to work with clients who have substance abuse are limited only by our own lack of skill in recognizing the problems that exist in every population encountered: infants, children, adolescents, women, men, professionals, and people with AIDS. As this book has shown, it is not uncommon for a client with underlying substance abuse to be admitted to the hospital for another diagnosis. What typically results in these cases is a lack of recognition of, or interest in exploring, the true cause of the client's problem. Choosing to treat only the symptoms at the expense of the underlying causes is simply poor (and very expensive) care, in both the short and long run.

THE EMERGENCE OF ADDICTIONS NURSING PRACTICE

Nurses are gaining opportunities in many settings to expand their role and scope of practice. There is no better example than substance abuse and addictions nursing. Whether the nurse's title is "clinical specialist," "nurse-clinician," "clinical nurse," or "nurse-practitioner," he or she can bring a wealth of knowledge and skill to each environment. With specialization in an area of clinical practice, nurses are in positions to work as primary care providers and collaborators with other members of a multidisciplinary team.

The specialty of addictions nursing practiced at basic and advanced levels had little visibility in nursing until the 1980s, when the prevalence of substance abuse problems, the growth of new treatment centers, and a new focus on impairment in health professionals highlighted the specialty. Further progress toward delineating nursing standards and specialization was made in 1983, when representatives of the American Nurses Association (ANA), the Drug and Alcohol Nursing Association (DANA), and the National Nurses Society on Addictions (NNSA) convened to discuss the scope of nursing practice in relation to the prevention, diagnosis, and treatment of alcohol and other drug problems. This was the first time consensus had been reached on various nursing roles and practice concerns in treating persons with alcohol and other drug problems. The resulting publication, *The Care of Clients with Addictions: Dimensions of Nursing Practice,* defines addictions nursing as an area of specialty practice concerned with care related to dysfunctional patterns of human responses.

Continuing collaboration in 1986 among representatives of the NNSA and the ANA produced *Standards of Practice in Addictions Nursing* (ANA, NNSA, 1988). This publication describes professional practice standards for addictions nursing and selected diagnoses from the North American Nursing Diagnosis Association

(NANDA) listing (see Chapter 3 for more on nursing diagnosis). It is intended for generalist-nurses working in various settings. This effort did much toward establishing standard approaches and practice expectations for nurses with basic education who practice in this area and to delineate distinct and relevant nursing behaviors which contribute to the restoration of health for addicted individuals.

Today, several certification programs exist to formally recognize the expertise and self-regulation of nurses practicing in the addictions. The certification process "by which a nongovernmental agency or association validates an individual registered nurse's qualifications, knowledge, and practice in a defined functional or clinical area of nursing, based on predetermined standards of nursing practice has assisted greatly in establishing addictions nursing as a recognized specialty within the profession" (Addictions Nursing Certification Board, 1992; Nelson, 1989).

There are currently three specialty nursing organizations dedicated to addictions nursing: NNSA, NCCDN (National Consortium of Chemical Dependency Nurses), and DANA. These specialty nursing organizations have a vested interest in the role development of the nurse, offer certification, and focus attention on the special problems associated with the impaired nurse (see Appendix for addresses for these organizations).

The ANA also has established other standards documents for specialized practice, which are useful in providing care for addicted clients. The ANA *Standards of Clinical Nursing Practice* provides a framework for the steps involved in the care of clients in any health care setting. The ANA *Standards of Psychiatric and Mental Health Nursing Practice* build on the basic standards; they outline the need to incorporate theory, specific psychosocial interventions, and community health systems. The *Standards of Addictions Nursing Practice* relates both generic and psychiatric mental health nursing standards to the needs of addicted clients and includes attention to the therapeutic alliance and self-help groups.

Table 17-1 compares the three standards of practice statements and orients nurses practicing under the clinical nursing practice standards to additional standards for psychiatric and addictions care nursing. The *Standards of Psychiatric and Mental Health Nursing Practice* and the *Standards of Addictions Nursing Practice* provide focus for clients with a dual diagnosis of mental illness and addiction. For nurses working with primarily addicted clients, the *Standards of Addictions Nursing Practice* are applicable.

PRACTICE OPPORTUNITIES

Generalist roles

The generalist nurse in the addictions is one who has satisfied requirements for certification at the basic level. This means that the nurse has a fundamental understanding of addictions and how the nursing process can be applied to care planning, treatment delivery, and evaluation of services. The generalist uses these skills in a variety of settings and demonstrates in clinical practice the ability to apply knowledge to a broad spectrum of clients. Box 17-1 illustrates creative approaches to acquiring the education and skills needed. There are unique problems with mothers addicted to alcohol and drugs (Gigliotti, 1992), in adolescent drug use (Jack,

Text continued on p. 453.

Table 17-1

Comparison of generic, psychiatric-mental health and addictions nursing practice standards for use by nurses practicing at the generalist or advanced practice levels

ANA Standards of Clinical Nursing Practice*	ANA Standards of Psychiatric and Mental Health Nursing Practice†	ANA and NNSA Standards of Addictions Nursing Practice‡
Standards of care		
Standard I: *Assessment*. The nurse collects client health data.	Standard I: *Assessment*. The psychiatric-mental health nurse collects client health data.	Standard I: *Theory*. The nurse uses appropriate knowledge from nursing theory and related disciplines in the practice of addictions nursing.
Standard II: *Diagnosis*. The nurse analyzes the assessment data in determining diagnoses.	Standard II: *Diagnosis*. The psychiatric-mental health nurse analyzes the assessment data in determining diagnoses.	Standard II: *Data Collection*. Data collection is continual and systematic and is communicated effectively to the treatment team throughout each phase of the nursing process.
Standard III: *Outcome Identification*. The nurse identifies expected outcomes individualized to the client.	Standard III: *Outcome Identification*. The psychiatric-mental health nurse identifies expected outcomes individualized to the client.	Standard III: *Diagnosis*. The nurse uses nursing diagnoses congruent with accepted nursing and interpersonal physiological and psychological disorders to express conclusions supported by data obtained through the nursing process.
Standard IV: *Planning*. The nurse develops a plan of care that prescribes interventions to attain expected outcomes.	Standard IV: *Planning*. The psychiatric-mental health nurse develops a plan of care that prescribes interventions to attain expected outcomes.	Standard IV: *Planning*. The nurse establishes a plan of care for the client that is based upon nursing diagnoses, addresses specific goals, defines expected outcomes, and delineates nursing actions unique to each client's needs.
Standard V: *Implementation*. The nurse implements the interventions identified in the plan of care.	Standard V: *Implementation*. The psychiatric-mental health nurse implements the interventions identified in the plan of care.	Standard V: *Intervention*. The nurse implements actions independently and/or in collaboration with peers, members of other disciplines, and clients for prevention, intervention, and rehabilitation phases of the care of clients with health problems related to patterns of abuse and addiction.

Standard Va: *Counseling.* The psychiatric-mental health nurse uses counseling interventions to assist clients in improving or regaining their previous coping abilities, fostering mental health and preventing mental illness and disability.

Standard Vb: *Milieu Therapy.* The psychiatric-mental health nurse provides, structures, and maintains a therapeutic environment in collaboration with the client and other health care providers.

Standard Vc: *Self-Care Activities.* The psychiatric-mental health nurse structures interventions around the client's activities of daily living to foster self-care and mental and physical well-being.

Standard Vd: *Psychobiological Interventions.* The psychiatric-mental health nurse uses knowledge of psychobiological interventions and applies clinical skills to restore the client's health and prevent further disability.

Standard Ve: *Health Teaching.* The psychiatric-mental health nurse, through health teaching, assists clients in achieving satisfying, productive, and healthy patterns of living.

Standard Va: *Intervention: Therapeutic Alliance.* The nurse uses the "therapeutic self" to establish a relationship with clients and to structure nursing interventions to help clients develop the awareness, coping skills, and behavior changes that promote health.

Standard Vb: *Intervention: Education.* The nurse educates clients and communities to help them prevent and/or correct actual or potential health problems related to patterns of abuse and addiction.

Standard Vc: *Intervention: Self-Help Groups.* The nurse uses the knowledge and philosophy of self-help groups to assist clients in learning new ways to address stress, maintain self-control or sobriety, and integrate healthy coping behaviors into their lifestyle.

Standard Vd: *Intervention: Pharmacological Therapies.* The nurse applies knowledge of pharmacological principles in the nursing process.

Standard Ve: *Intervention: Therapeutic Environment.* The nurse provides, structures, and maintains a therapeutic environment in collaboration with the individual, family, and other professionals.

*From American Nurses Association. (1991). *Standards of clinical nursing practice.* Washington, D.C.: The Association.
†From American Nurses Association. (1994). *A statement on psychiatric-mental health clinical nursing practice and standards of psychiatric and mental health nursing practice.* Washington, D.C.: The Association.
‡From American Nurses Association and National Nurses Society on Addictions. (1988). *Standards of addictions nursing practice with selected diagnosis and criteria.* Washington, D.C.: The Association.

Continued.

Table 17-1

Comparison of generic, psychiatric-mental health and addictions nursing practice standards for use by nurses practicing at the generalist or advanced practice levels—cont'd

ANA Standards of Clinical Nursing Practice*	ANA Standards of Psychiatric and Mental Health Nursing Practice†	ANA and NNSA Standards of Addictions Nursing Practice‡
Standards of care—cont'd		
	Standard Vf: *Case Management.* The psychiatric-mental health nurse provides case management to coordinate comprehensive health services and ensure continuity of care.	Standard Vf: *Intervention: Counseling.* The nurse uses therapeutic communication in interactions with the client to address issues related to patterns of abuse and addiction.
	Standard Vg: *Health Promotion and Health Maintenance.* The psychiatric-mental health nurse employs strategies and interventions to promote and maintain mental health and prevent mental illness.	
Standard VI: *Evaluation.* The nurse evaluates the client's progress toward attainment of outcomes.	Standard VI: *Evaluation.* The psychiatric-mental health nurse evaluates the client's progress in attaining expected outcomes.	Standard VI: *Evaluation.* The nurse evaluates the responses of the client and revises nursing diagnoses, interventions, and the treatment plan accordingly.
		Standard VII: *Ethical Care.* The nurse's decisions and activities on behalf of clients are in keeping with personal and professional codes of ethics and in accord with legal statutes.
Standards of professional performance		
Standard I: *Quality of Care.* The nurse systematically evaluates the quality and effectiveness of nursing practice.	Standard I: *Quality of Care.* The psychiatric-mental health nurse systematically evaluates the quality of care and effectiveness of psychiatric-mental health nursing practice.	Standard VIII: *Quality Assurance.* The nurse participates in peer review and other staff evaluation and quality assurance processes to ensure that clients with abuse and addiction problems receive quality care.

Standard II: *Performance Appraisal.* The nurse evaluates his or her own nursing practice in relation to professional practice standards and relevant statutes and regulations.

Standard III: *Education.* The nurse acquires and maintains current knowledge in nursing practice.

Standard IV: *Collegiality.* The nurse contributes to the professional development of peers, colleagues, and others.

Standard V: *Ethics.* The nurse's decisions and actions on behalf of clients are determined in an ethical manner.

Standard VI: *Collaboration.* The nurse collaborates with the client, significant others, and health care providers in providing client care.

Standard VII: *Research.* The nurse uses research findings in practice.

Standard VIII: *Resource Utilization.* The nurse considers factors related to safety, effectiveness, and cost in planning and delivering client care.

Standard II: *Performance Appraisal.* The psychiatric-mental health nurse evaluates own psychiatric-mental health practice in relation to professional practice standards and relevant statutes and regulations.

Standard III: *Education.* The psychiatric-mental health nurse acquires and maintains current knowledge in nursing practice.

Standard IV: *Collegiality.* The psychiatric-mental health nurse contributes to the professional development of peers, colleagues, and others.

Standard V: *Ethics.* The psychiatric-mental health nurse's decisions and actions on behalf of clients are determined in an ethical manner.

Standard VI: *Collaboration.* The psychiatric-mental health nurse collaborates with the client, significant others, and health care providers in providing care.

Standard VII: *Research.* The psychiatric-mental health nurse contributes to nursing and mental health through the use of research.

Standard VIII: *Resource Utilization.* The psychiatric-mental health nurse considers factors related to safety, effectiveness, and cost in planning and delivering client care.

Standard IX: *Continuing Education.* The nurse assumes responsibility for his or her continuing education and professional development and contributes to the professional growth of others who work with or are learning about persons with abuse and addiction problems.

Standard X: *Interdisciplinary Collaboration.* The nurse collaborates with the interdisciplinary treatment team and consults with other health care providers in assessing, planning, implementing, and evaluating programs and other activities related to addictions nursing.

Standard XI: *Use of Community Health Systems.* The nurse participates with other members of the community in assessing, planning, implementing, and evaluating community health services that attend to primary, secondary, and tertiary prevention of addictions.

Standard XII: *Research.* The nurse contributes to the nursing care of clients with addictions and to the addictions area of practice through innovations in theory and practice and participation in research, and communicates these contributions.

Box 17-1
Routes to Skill Acquisition for Integrating Knowledge of the Addictions into Clinical Practice: A Self-Evaluation Guide

Do you have a knowledge base of substance abuse and the addictions that you can apply to your clinical, educational, and/or administrative practice?

Yes   **No** (Identify resources where you can gain the knowledge base, i.e., reading, audio/video tapes, identification of local experts, professional associations, CE offerings.)

Have you received supervision in the specific applications of this knowledge base in your clinical, educational, and/or administrative practice?

Yes   **No** (Seek out opportunities for such supervision from educators, clinical nurse specialists, or knowledgeable peers.)

Do you conduct a detailed assessment of an individual's or family's use of substances as part of your routine nursing assessment?

Yes   **No** (Consult the literature and substance abuse treatment resources for sample questionnaires devised to elicit information with the necessary details in order to make an accurate assessment.)

For both physical and mental disorders, substance use and abuse are frequently either the underlying cause of the illness or the use of these substances potentiates the disability. Do you routinely consider the connection between one of the major public health problems in our country to the problems you encounter in the patients, families, students, employees, and co-workers with whom you interact?

Yes   **No** (Explore the literature, talk with experts in the field or conduct more detailed patient interviews in order to assess, first hand, the prevalence of substance abuse among patients in your practice setting.)

Do you have ready access to experts in the field of substance abuse?

Yes   **No** (Network within your facility or community to locate an expert willing to provide some consultation to you and your work group. Examples may be recognized experts in clinical/academic settings, an EAP counselor, or a clinician in private practice. Consider volunteering in a substance abuse treatment program that provides access to patients, counselors, and seminars so you can develop your expertise.)

Do you have access to educational and treatment resources for substance abuse treatment (including smoking cessation) as a means of being current on referral sources?

Yes   **No** (Perhaps you and your co-workers could develop a survey project to explore and identify community resources.)

Have you ever suspected a patient, family member, co-worker, or student to be personally involved in the abuse of substances and have you actively participated in devising treatment intervention for that individual?

Yes   **No** (Become educated in the steps to conducting an intervention in order to assume this important responsibility as part of your professional role.)

From Valentine, N.M. (1988). The genesis of Nightingale. Alternative treatment for female health care providers. *Holistic Nursing Practice, 2,* 45-55.

1992; Washburn, 1991), in women's health concerns (Teusch, 1993; Gullman et al, 1990), in the special needs of geriatric populations (Mathwig & D'Arcangelo, 1992; Lindblom et al, 1992), and in impaired health professionals (Farley & Hendrix, 1993; Naegle, 1992). There are endless applications for assessment, intervention, and evaluation by nurses across all settings, at both generic and advanced levels.

> *She has started to drink*
> *as a way to cope*
> *that makes her less able to cope*
>
> *the more she drinks*
> *the more frightened she is of becoming a drunkard*
>
> *the more drunk*
> *the less frightened of being drunk*
>
> *the more frightened of being drunk when not drunk*
> *the more not frightened drunk*
> *the more frightened not drunk*
>
> *the more she destroys herself*
> *the more frightened of being destroyed by him*
>
> *the more frightened of destroying him*
> *the more she destroys herself*
>
> R.D. Laing

Clinical specialists in substance abuse

The clinical specialist has training and experience in mental health and psychiatric nursing and has advanced training in the addictions. This combination of skills permits the nurse to apply the nursing process to the most complex treatment and rehabilitation situations. Specialists can be found in inpatient and outpatient alcohol and drug rehabilitation settings, or they can be available to staff in other practice areas, functioning in a consultative role.

There is no area of general practice—hospital, clinic, or home-care setting—that does not present opportunities for the specialist nurse to use addictions knowledge and skill.

The following clinical examples demonstrate missed opportunities and how the situation could be changed with the additional skills of an advanced practice nurse.

Emergency room setting.

ⅢⅢ➡ Clinical Example

A 24-year-old, single, white female is seen in the emergency room for a migraine headache twenty-four hours after a minor car accident. She is not badly injured but indicates she had been in numerous accidents within the past year. She attributes this to having an "inability to concentrate because of stresses at home and at work." The patient expresses no need to consult a psychiatrist because she feels that she is improving and can "work this out." She is given a physical examination as well as the name of a therapist in case she needs additional assistance. Twenty-four hours later she arrives by ambulance following a head-on car collision caused by extreme intoxication. In the emergency room the previous evening, questions about alcohol or drug consumption had not been asked.

Alternative scenario: The patient is seen in the emergency room as described. When she casually mentions her previous car accidents, the intake nurse begins to explore the circumstances of each. Although the patient evades many details, the nurse is alerted to underlying stress and anxiety and the possibility of an alcohol or drug problem. The nurse suggests to the doctor on call that an alcohol level and drug toxicology screen be drawn. The intake nurse calls the psychiatric unit and requests that the clinical nurse specialist stop by and talk with the patient. A further assessment is conducted and an appointment is made for the patient to come back for an outpatient visit at the substance abuse center.

Community health clinic.

⫸ Clinical Example

The well-baby clinic, held weekly in the community nursing services center, notes the frequency of missed appointments by a 13-year-old mother who had been accompanied to the clinic in previous months by her mother. A series of telephone calls are made to the home and several messages left with an older woman who sounds distracted and whose speech is slurred. Finally, after three months of postcard reminders, the young woman returns with her baby alone, stating that her mother was not able to come because she had the flu and had lost several weeks at work. The baby is inoculated and an appointment made for a return visit.

Alternative scenario: The mother and baby are greeted back to the clinic and treated as described. The clinic nurse explores the problems with the grandmother and notes the sad and lonely expression on the young mother's face. The nurse suggests that a home visit might be useful to discuss the adjustment of the family to the new baby, and an appointment is made. The clinic nurse then follows up with the clinical nurse–case manager for the family, and the issue of the maternal grandmother's potential alcohol problem is explored before the home visit.

Medical inpatient setting.

⫸ Clinical Example

A 40-year-old gentleman with chest pains is admitted to a local general hospital. The change-of-shift staff notice a marked difference in his personality since admission and increased agitation as the shift progresses. The patient ultimately requires four-point restraints, and a psychiatrist is called in for assessment. The patient's wife is consulted about his possible history of psychiatric problems. Eventually the topic of pills and alcohol surfaces, and it is determined that the patient is clearly withdrawing from alcohol and barbiturates. The nurse notes that the patient's history indicates that he only drank socially and occasionally used drugs recreationally. Neither "social drinking" nor recreational use of drugs was explored in any detail.

Alternative scenario: When the patient is first admitted and asked about the use of substances, the admissions nurse recalls her recent in-service class where there was a review of the updated admissions form and role-playing that taught how to query patients for details of their alcohol and drug use. She uses her new knowledge to interview the patient.

Visiting Nurse Association. VNA nurses often request expanded education in drug and alcohol abuse because they see so many cases as they visit clients in their home environments. Abnormal behavior in the aged, in particular, is difficult to diagnose definitively because of the possibility of other causes (e.g., organic brain damage syndrome).

ⵊⵊ➡ Clinical Example

Susan is a 70-year-old female living alone in a housing complex for the elderly in a small community. Her children live in other states but communicate frequently by telephone. The VNA is involved in the case because Susan had been discharged from the hospital eight months earlier with congestive heart failure. The VNA nurse visits twice weekly and notices a dramatic decline in Susan's intellect and organizational activities. What is not noticed or explored is Susan's alcohol consumption. The VNA nurse is aware that she drinks "a little wine at dinner," but the quantity is never questioned. Ironically, in order to explain the change in personality and the decline in her ability to handle activities of daily life, great effort is expended in reviewing Susan's meds with her.

Alternative scenario: Carefully and thoughtfully exploring the patient's use of alcohol, a major variable in the assessment of the patient's health status is identified. The nurse contacts AA and arranges for Susan to attend a meeting.

In each of these examples, the nurse missed the cues that the client or family member needed a substance abuse evaluation. Because of haste to cure, rather than to care, clients received only services that attended to the presenting symptoms. The professionals neglected to explore the more complex picture of declining ability to cope and adapt. It is in the skillful unmasking of the basic issues in a client's health that professional nursing can make a difference in the lives of individuals and families.

The following clinical examples represent total patient care. Hopefully they will be used in establishing standards for nursing assessment, intervention, and evaluation.

ⵊⵊ➡ Clinical Example

A male client scheduled for a day–surgical procedure arrives agitated and confused about the printed directions for preoperative preparation. Although he tolerates the surgical procedure well and is stabilized before discharge, the nurse-anesthetist notes that his smoking history and obesity made him a surgical risk for this intervention as well as for future episodes. The day–surgical center recently had networked with the hospital's smoking cessation and nutrition clinics to coordinate referrals for follow-up care. As part of the nurse's case-finding activities, she counsels the client on the need for intervention in these two areas and makes an appointment for the client to be seen in both clinics as part of the follow-up plan of care.

ⵊⵊ➡ Clinical Example

A female client is referred to an inpatient facility for the treatment of depression. As part of the initial nursing assessment, the nurse inquires about the client's use of alcohol. In a recent in-service education class the nurse had learned that a response such as "social drinking" is not adequate, so the nurse spends extra time on this question—inquiring about the quantity, type, and drinking patterns of the client. This approach yields information that assists in determining that the client might be best placed on the dual-diagnosis unit rather than on the depression unit. The nurse shares this information with the director of admissions, and a decision is made for the client to receive further evaluation for the potential for alcohol abuse *and* depression on the dual-diagnosis unit.

In each of these clinical examples, the nurse views the health care incident as an opportunity to conduct a complete physical and psychosocial assessment and to make the appropriate referrals for follow-up care. These cases illustrate the role of nurses as primary care providers in their respective settings, as contrasted with a specialized role in one exclusive area (Naylor & Brooten, 1993). With basic skills in addictions counseling and referral, all nurses have the potential for making a difference in the overall health status of their clients.

Consultation/liaison roles

Those who are specialists in addictions nursing can play a role as a consultant or liaison, especially in settings where systems are designed to facilitate intervention. At one hospital, nurse practitioners have been decentralized to work on the client care units, rather than in the medical clinic. Working with psychiatric nurses, nurse practitioners have added a substance abuse assessment of the client. In cases where additional consultation is needed to assess or intervene with a patient's suspected addiction, the nurse-manager of the alcohol and drug abuse unit, a clinical specialist, also is available for consultation. In this way, the interdisciplinary skills of all the nurses can be used in client care.

Collaborative roles

Collaborative practice with physicians and other members of the health-care team is also an opportunity for nurses with a specialty in addictions. Peplau (1991) defines professional collaboration as "the authority and direction for designing nursing functions derived from situations in which professional workers collaborate to bring about health improvement."

The contributions of the team combine synergistically to meet the needs of families and clients. This is particularly important at a time when health-care consumers are demanding improved quality and cost-effective care. The benefits of a collaborative approach are twofold: increased satisfaction for clients and professional satisfaction for nurses and other team members.

Team members bring with them a host of characteristics, values, perceptions, assumptions, and skills that greatly influence how they behave, both in task and relationship activities. The field of substance abuse has fewer constraints than most medical fields, in which only certain specialists are recognized as experts. Members of the team tend to view addiction from their own perspective. These different perspectives regarding treatment and management of a client with substance abuse are helpful in expanding the scope of treatment. What the different perspectives reveal is that substance abuse is a complex condition, and the various perspectives are vital in understanding the larger picture.

The very nature of substance abuse mandates that more than a single individual or profession be involved. As Pluckhan (1972, p. 310) states, "The alternative to working together is working alone, which is totally unrealistic in today's society." No health care professional in the addictions field can be as effective working in isolation. The importance of collaboration with physicians, counselors, and other health care professionals cannot be overemphasized.

Opportunities in management and administration

The management of large groups of employees, whether employed in health care or other settings, represents another sector of people in need of services. Many companies have handled employees' substance abuse by developing an employee assistance program (EAP) or by contracting with an established firm. Often these services employ social workers as providers, but the role is congruent with that of a nurse-clinician with addictions training and certification.

In addition to services, policy statements have been developed in many institutions and companies, which specify the employer's position on drug use and rehabilitation. This approach is based on the assumption that the solution to the problem is greater user-accountability, which translates into making employees responsible for their actions—a particularly useful approach because the employer controls the greatest reinforcer for change: the paycheck. Given industry's interest in controlling and eliminating drug use in the workplace, a clinical specialist with skills in the addictions is an ideal candidate on staff, or in a consultation capacity, to develop policies, procedures, and intervention plans that support positive change in the workplace (deBernardo, 1991).

Other examples illustrate how nursing organizations can be more effective in the management of substance use and abuse in the workplace. Every clinical department of nursing in the United States should review its programs annually to ensure increased awareness and active prevention/intervention among the nursing staff. Some agencies have established committees to oversee these reviews. Clinical nurse-specialists can be a creative force for change in bringing relevant issues to the attention of the staff.

Educational considerations

If I don't know I don't know
I think I know
If I don't know I know
I think I don't know

R.D. Laing

Education is the key to changing our attitudes and consequently our practice patterns. Creative instruction (Ellis, 1990; Gee et al, 1990) and commitment to curriculum changes (Valentine, 1983) threaded through all clinical specialties is crucial to the education of nurses who will be able to deliver comprehensive and effective care to substance abuse clients.

SUMMARY

Nurses have both the relationship and the opportunity to influence clients' wellness from a holistic perspective. Knowledge of substance abuse and addictive behavior, and empathy for people with dependency and illness, demands much from a nurse. But the rewards can be very gratifying because behavioral change, although difficult to achieve and maintain, enhances the lives of individuals, families, and entire communities. Except for mass immunizations, there is no other single intervention in health care that has the same far-reaching consequences. Successful contributions to health and well-being are immeasurable. Nurses can use a close alliance with clients and a personalized approach to the health-assessment process to open up discussions on diet, spending, gambling, and alcohol and substance use patterns. It is as important to evaluate how clients cope with stress in their lives as it is to evaluate their cholesterol level. The goal of quality nursing care is to balance the routine concern focused on the functional status of a client's health with an emphasis on the assessment of behavioral health indicators.

We are in an age of reorientation to health and the delivery of health care services. Throughout the health care system, behavioral issues are gaining more attention; they should be explored and creative interventions devised for quality care. As health policies shift to emphasize personal responsibility for self-help and self-care, new partnerships are predicted in which nurses, as primary health care providers, will be expected to address the full spectrum of physical and behavioral health. All nurses will need more experience in these areas. Those with expertise in the addictions will be on the cutting edge of new delivery approaches as they work toward wellness with clients and their families.

REFERENCES

Addictions Nursing Certification Board. (1992). *Certification for addiction nurses.* Skokie, IL: Addictions Nursing Certification Board.

American Nurses Association. (1991). *Standards of clinical nursing practice.* Washington, D.C.: The Association.

American Nurses Association. (1994). *A statement on psychiatric-mental health clinical nursing practice and standards of psychiatric and mental health nursing practice.* Washington, D.C.: The Association.

American Nurses Association and National Nurses Society on Addictions. (1988). *Standards of addictions nursing practice with selected diagnoses and criteria.* Washington, D.C.: ANA, NNSA.

Bratter, T.E. & Forrest, G.G. (1985). *Alcoholism and substance abuse.* New York: MacMillan.

deBernardo, M.A. (1991). Why do your workers abuse drugs? *Institute for a Drug-Free Workplace report, 3,* 73-78. Washington, D.C.: Law Office of Littler, Mendelson, Fastiff, and Tichy.

Ellis, M.A. (1990). Teaching nursing students and clinicians family intervention for substance abuse. *Association For Medical Educational Research in Substance Abuse, 2*(1).

Farley, P.B. & Hendrix, M.J. (1993). Impaired and non-impaired nurses during childhood and adolescence. *Nursing Outlook, 41,* 25-30.

Gee, M.S., Oldham, S.B., Sharpe, K.P., Strohm, M.P., Tittle, L.A., Vaughn, M.P. (1990). Peer teaching: A two year experience of a student-organized alcoholism education workshop. *Association For Medical Educational Research in Substance Abuse, 2*(1).

Gigliotti, E. (1992). Fetal effects of maternal alcohol and drug use. *NLN Publication,* Module 11.1 (15-2463), 1-116.

Gullman, H., Hornung, C.A., Johnson, N.P., & Rabbins, K.H. (1990). *Characteristics of women alcoholics.* Washington, D.C.: Association for Medical Educational Research in Substance Abuse.

Jack, L.W. (1992). Primary prevention of alcohol and other drug use. *Journal School Nurses, 8*(2), 25-33.

Laing, R.D. (1970). *Knots.* New York: Vintage.

Lindblom, L., Kostyk, D., Tabisz, E., Jacyk, W.R., & Fuchs, D. (1992). Chemical abuse—An intervention program for the elderly. *Journal of Gerontological Nursing, 18*(4), 6-14.

Mathwig, G. & D'Arcangelo, J.S. (1992). Drug misuse and dependence in the elderly. *NLN Publication,* Module 11.2 (15-2493), 463-530.

Mendelson, J.H. & Mello, N.K. (1985). *Treatment of alcoholism.* (2nd ed.). New York: McGraw Hill.

Morse, R. & Flavin, D. (1992). Definition of alcoholism. *JAMA, 268*(8), 1012-1014.

Naegle, M.A. (1992). Impaired practice by health professionals. *NLN Publication,* Module 11.2 (15-2463), 117-219.

Naylor, M.D. & Brooten, D. (1993). The roles and functions of clinical nurse specialists. *Image, 25,* 73-78.

Nelson, N. (1989). The certification process. History and significance for addictions nursing practice. *Nursing Clinics of North America, 24*(1), 151-159.

Peplau, H. (1991). *Interpersonal relations in nursing.* New York: Springer.

Pluckhan, M.L. (1972). A problem affecting the delivery of health care. *Nursing Forum, 9,* 310.

Safriet, B.J. (1992). Health care dollars and regulator. *Alcohol, 35,* 210-214.

Teusch, R. (1993). Women and addictions. *Developments, 2,* 1-4.

Valentine, N.M. (1994). Nurses in need of care: Substance abuse and impairment in nurses. In D. Fishman and O. Strickland. (Eds.) *Nursing issues in the '90s.* Delmar.

Valentine, N.M. (1988). The genesis of Nightingale. Alternative treatment for female health care providers. *Holistic Nursing Practice, 2,* 45-55.

Valentine, N.M. (1983). Approaches to educating professional nurses in the field of addiction and treatment. *Toward a coordinated approach: current issues and future directions.* Proceedings of the second Pan Pacific Conference on Drugs and Alcohol. Hong Kong.

Washburn, P. (1991). Identification, assessment and referral of adolescent drug abusers. *Pediatric Nursing, 17*(2), 137-140.

APPENDICES

A   Diagnostic Instruments
   A-1   CAGEAID Questionnaire
   A-2   Michigan Alcoholism Screening Test (MAST)
   A-3   Alcohol Use Disorders Identification Test (AUDIT)
B   Organizational Resources and Services
C   Publications and Periodicals

A-1

CAGEAID
Questionnaire

**CAGE Questions Adapted to Include Drugs
(CAGEAID)**

Have you felt you ought to cut down on your drinking *(or drug use)*?
_____ Yes _____ No

Have people annoyed you by criticizing your drinking *(or drug use)*?
_____ Yes _____ No

Have you felt bad or guilty about your drinking *(or drug use)*?
_____ Yes _____ No

Have you ever had a drink *(or used drugs)* **first thing in the morning to steady your nerves or get rid of a hangover** *(or to get the day started)*?
_____ Yes _____ No

From Fleming, M.F. & Barry, K.L. (1992). *Addictive Disorders.* St. Louis: Mosby; and Ewing, J.A. (1984). Detecting alcoholism: The CAGE questionnaire. *Journal of the AMA, 252:*1905-1907.
NOTE: Boldface text shows the original CAGE questions; boldface italic text shows modifications of the CAGE questions used to screen for drug disorders. In a general population, two or more positive answers indicate a need for more in-depth assessment.

A-2 Michigan Alcoholism Screening Test (MAST)

Points		Yes	No
	0. Do you enjoy a drink now and then?	____	____
(2)	1. Do you feel you are a normal drinker? (By normal we mean you drink less than or as much as most other people.)*	____	____
(2)	2. Have you ever awakened the morning after doing some drinking the night before and found that you could not remember a part of the evening?	____	____
(1)	3. Does your wife, husband, a parent or other near relative ever worry or complain about your drinking?	____	____
(2)	4. Can you stop drinking without a struggle after one or two drinks?*	____	____
(1)	5. Do you ever feel guilty about your drinking?	____	____
(2)	6. Do friends or relatives think you are a normal drinker?*	____	____
(2)	7. Are you able to stop drinking when you want to?*	____	____
(5)	8. Have you ever attended a meeting of Alcoholics Anonymous (AA)?	____	____
(1)	9. Have you gotten into physical fights when drinking?	____	____
(2)	10. Has your drinking ever created problems between you and your wife, husband, a parent, or other relative?	____	____
(2)	11. Has your wife, husband (or other family member) ever gone to anyone for help about your drinking?	____	____
(2)	12. Have you ever lost friends because of your drinking?	____	____
(2)	13. Have you ever gotten into trouble at work or school because of drinking?	____	____
(2)	14. Have you ever lost a job because of drinking?	____	____

*Alcoholic response is negative.

NOTE: *Scoring System:* In general, five points or more would place the subject in an "alcoholic" category. Four points would be suggestive of alcoholism. Three points or less would indicate the subject was not alcoholic.

Programs using the above scoring system find it very sensitive at the five-point level and it tends to find more people alcoholic than anticipated. However, it is a screening test and should be sensitive at its lower levels.

From Selzer, M.L. (1971). The Michigan Alcoholism Screening Test (MAST): The quest for a new diagnostic instrument. *American Journal of Psychiatry*, 3, 176-181.

Points		Yes	No
(2)	15. Have you ever neglected your obligations, your family, or your work for two or more days in a row because you were drinking?	_____	_____
(1)	16. Do you drink before noon fairly often?	_____	_____
(2)	17. Have you ever been told you have liver trouble? Cirrhosis?	_____	_____
(2)	18. After heavy drinking have you ever had delirium tremens (DTs) or severe shaking, or heard voices or seen things that really weren't there?†	_____	_____
(5)	19. Have you ever gone to anyone for help about your drinking?	_____	_____
(5)	20. Have you ever been in a hospital because of drinking?	_____	_____
(2)	21. Have you ever been a patient in a psychiatric hospital or on a psychiatric ward of a general hospital where drinking was part of the problem that resulted in hospitalization?	_____	_____
(2)	22. Have you ever been seen at a psychiatric or mental health clinic or gone to any doctor, social worker, or clergyman for help with any emotional problem, where drinking was part of the problem?	_____	_____
(2)	23. Have you ever been arrested for drunk driving, driving while intoxicated, or driving under the influence of alcoholic beverages?‡ (If YES, how many times _____)	_____	_____
(2)	24. Have you ever been arrested, or taken into custody, even for a few hours, because of other drunk behavior?‡ (If YES, how many times _____)	_____	_____

†5 points for delirium tremens.
‡2 points for *each* arrest.

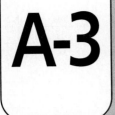

A-3

Alcohol Use Disorders
Identification Test (AUDIT)
(Revised to Include Drugs)*

This questionnaire asks you some questions about your use of alcohol and drugs during the past year. Alcoholic beverages include beer, wine, and liquor (vodka, whiskey, brandy, etc.). Drugs include cocaine, marijuana, narcotics, and tranquilizers.

1. How often do you have a drink containing alcohol or use other drugs (e.g., marijuana, cocaine, narcotics)?

   ☐ Never   (0)   [   ]
   ☐ Less than monthly (1)

   If *more* than once a month:

   Alcohol   ☐ Monthly   (2)   [   ]
                  ☐ Weekly   (3)
                  ☐ Daily or almost daily (4)

   Cocaine   ☐ Monthly   (2)   [   ]
                  ☐ Weekly   (3)
                  ☐ Daily or almost daily (4)

   Marijuana   ☐ Monthly   (2)   [   ]
                  ☐ Weekly   (3)
                  ☐ Daily or almost daily (4)

   Tranquilizers ☐ Monthly   (2)   [   ]
                  ☐ Weekly   (3)
                  ☐ Daily or almost daily (4)

   Other _____ ☐ Monthly   (2)   [   ]
                  ☐ Weekly   (3)
                  ☐ Daily or almost daily (4)

2. On a day when you drink alcohol or use other drugs, how many drinks (alcohol), lines (cocaine), joints (marijuana), or tranquilizer pills do you use?

   Alcohol   ☐ None   (0)   [   ]
                  ☐ 1 or 2   (1)
                  ☐ 3 or 4   (2)
                  ☐ 5 or 6   (3)
                  ☐ 7 to 9   (4)
                  ☐ 10 or more (5)

*Developed by the World Health Organization, AMETHYST project, 1987. Modified by Fleming and Barry, 1990.
From Fleming, M.F. & Barry, K.L. (1992). *Addictive disorders.* St. Louis: Mosby.

Cocaine ☐ None (0) [ ]
☐ 1 or 2 (1)
☐ 3 or 4 (2)
☐ 5 or 6 (3)
☐ 7 to 9 (4)
☐ 10 or more (5)

Marijuana ☐ None (0) [ ]
☐ 1 or 2 (1)
☐ 3 or 4 (2)
☐ 5 or 6 (3)
☐ 7 to 9 (4)
☐ 10 or more (5)

Tranquilizers ☐ None (0) [ ]
☐ 1 or 2 (1)
☐ 3 or 4 (2)
☐ 5 or 6 (3)
☐ 7 to 9 (4)
☐ 10 or more (5)

Other ☐ None (0) [ ]
☐ 1 or 2 (1)
☐ 3 or 4 (2)
☐ 5 or 6 (3)
☐ 7 to 9 (4)
☐ 10 or more (5)

3. How often do you have 6 or more drinks, 1 or more joints, 10 or more lines, or 3 or more tranquilizer pills on one occasion?

Alcohol
☐ Never (0) [ ]
☐ Less than monthly (1)
☐ Monthly (2)
☐ Weekly (3)
☐ Daily or almost daily (4)

Other drugs
☐ Never (0) [ ]
☐ Less than monthly (1)
☐ Monthly (2)
☐ Weekly (3)
☐ Daily or almost daily (4)

4. How often during the last year have you found that you were unable to stop drinking or using other drugs once you had started?

Alcohol
☐ Never (0) [ ]
☐ Less than monthly (1)
☐ Monthly (2)
☐ Weekly (3)
☐ Daily or almost daily (4)

Other drugs
☐ Never (0) [ ]
☐ Less than monthly (1)
☐ Monthly (2)
☐ Weekly (3)
☐ Daily or almost daily (4)

5. How often during the last year have you failed to do what was normally expected from you because of drinking or using other drugs?

Alcohol
☐ Never (0) [ ]
☐ Less than monthly (1)
☐ Monthly (2)
☐ Weekly (3)
☐ Daily or almost daily (4)

Other drugs
☐ Never (0) [ ]
☐ Less than monthly (1)
☐ Monthly (2)
☐ Weekly (3)
☐ Daily or almost daily (4)

6. How often during the last year have you needed a drink or drug in the morning to get yourself going after a heavy drinking or drug-using session?

Alcohol
☐ Never (0) [ ]
☐ Less than monthly (1)
☐ Monthly (2)
☐ Weekly (3)
☐ Daily or almost daily (4)

Other drugs
☐ Never (0) [ ]
☐ Less than monthly (1)
☐ Monthly (2)
☐ Weekly (3)
☐ Daily or almost daily (4)

7. How often during the last year have you had a feeling of guilt or remorse after drinking or using other drugs?

Alcohol
☐ Never (0) [ ]
☐ Less than monthly (1)
☐ Monthly (2)
☐ Weekly (3)
☐ Daily or almost daily (4)

Other drugs
☐ Never (0) [ ]
☐ Less than monthly (1)
☐ Monthly (2)
☐ Weekly (3)
☐ Daily or almost daily (4)

8. How often during the last year have you been unable to remember what happened the night before because you had been drinking or using other drugs?

Alcohol
☐ Never (0) [ ]
☐ Less than monthly (1)
☐ Monthly (2)
☐ Weekly (3)
☐ Daily or almost daily (4)

Other drugs
☐ Never (0) [ ]
☐ Less than monthly (1)
☐ Monthly (2)
☐ Weekly (3)
☐ Daily or almost daily (4)

9. Have you or someone else been injured as a result of your drinking or drug use?

Alcohol
☐ Never (0) [ ]
☐ Less than monthly (1)
☐ Monthly (2)
☐ Weekly (3)
☐ Daily or almost daily (4)

Other drugs
☐ Never (0) [ ]
☐ Less than monthly (1)
☐ Monthly (2)
☐ Weekly (3)
☐ Daily or almost daily (4)

10. Has a relative, friend, or a doctor or other health worker been concerned about your drinking or drug use or suggested you cut down?

Alcohol
☐ Never (0) [ ]
☐ Less than monthly (1)
☐ Monthly (2)
☐ Weekly (3)
☐ Daily or almost daily (4)

Other drugs
☐ Never (0) [ ]
☐ Less than monthly (1)
☐ Monthly (2)
☐ Weekly (3)
☐ Daily or almost daily (4)

Record the total of the specific items. In a general population, a score of 11 or greater may indicate the need for a more in-depth assessment.

B Organizational Resources and Services

Agency or organization	Services
Al-Anon Family Group Headquarters P.O. Box 862 Midtown Station New York, NY 10018-0862	Support group for family members of alcoholics
Alcoholics Anonymous World Services Inc. P.O. Box 459 Grand Central Station New York, NY 10163	Support group for alcoholics; advocacy
Association for Medical Education and Research in Substance Abuse Brown University Center for Alcohol and Addictions Studies Box 6 Providence, RI 02912 (401) 863-7791	Multidisciplinary organization that provides information on substance abuse and offers an annual conference
Children of Alcoholics Foundation 555 Modern Ave., 4th floor New York, NY 10022 (212) 949-1404	Public education; research; information on parent-child relations, development, abuse, and substance abuse in children of alcoholics
Cocaine Anonymous 6125 Washington Boulevard, Suite 202 Culver City, CA 90232	Support group for cocaine users
Drug and Alcohol Nurse Association (DANA) 660 Lonely College Drive Upper Black Eddy, PA 18972-9313	Specialty organization for nurses who work in substance abuse
Narcotics Anonymous P.O. Box 9999 Van Nuys, CA 91409 (818) 780-3951	Self-help group for drug abusers; modeled on AA

National Clearinghouse for Alcohol and Drug Information P.O. Box 2345 Rockville, MD 20847-2345 (800) 729-6686	Information and education on alcohol and other substances of abuse
National Consortium of Chemical Dependency Nurses (NCCDN) 1720 Willow Creek, Suite 519 Eugene, OR 97402	Offers a certification program for RNs and LPNs working in substance abuse, resulting in credentials RNCD
National Council on Alcoholism and Drug Dependence (NCADD) 12 West 21st Street, 8th Floor New York, NY 10010 (212) 206-6770	Information, education, and referral on substance- and abuse-related issues
National Institute on Alcohol Abuse and Alcoholism 5600 Fishers Lane Rockville, MD 20857 (301) 443-3885	Research; information on treatment, rehabilitation training
National Institute on Drug Abuse 5600 Fishers Lane Rockville, MD 20857 (301) 443-6480	Research; information, training
National Nurses Society on Addiction (NNSA) 5700 Old Orchard Road Skokie, IL 60077 (708) 966-5010	Specialty organization for nurses interested in addictions; administers certification program in collaboration with the National League for Nursing (NLN). This exam includes all addictions—eating, gambling, etc.—and awards the credential CARN (Certified Addictions Registered Nurse)
Substance Abuse and Mental Health Services Administration 5600 Fishers Lane Rockville, MD 20857 (301) 443-5407	Supports prevention and treatment services of addictive and mental health problems and disorders
SAMSA Branches: Center for Substance Abuse Prevention Center for Substance Abuse Treatment Center for Mental Health Services	

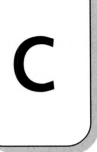

C | Publications and Periodicals

PUBLICATIONS

Eighth Special Report to Congress on Alcohol and Health (1994)

This current report to Congress describes recent progress in the knowledge of alcohol abuse and alcoholism, focusing on research advances made since the Seventh Special Report in 1990. Covers all active areas of research on alcohol-related problems including epidemiology, genetics, neuroscience, medical consequences of alcohol abuse and alcoholism, alcohol use and pregnancy, adverse social consequences of alcohol abuse and dependence, diagnostic criteria and screening instruments.

Fourth Triennial Report to Congress: Drug Abuse and Drug Abuse Research IV (1994)

This report summarizes the extent of drug abuse in the United States, its health implications, and recent advances in the prevention and treatment of drug dependency. This is the fourth in this series, and it emphasizes research developments in the last 3 years.

National Household Survey on Drug Abuse: Main Findings 1988 (1990)

This survey provides data about the prevalence, frequency, and demographic correlates of the use of illicit drugs, alcohol, and tobacco by the household population aged 12 and older.

Diagnostic and Statistical Manual of Mental Disorders

DSM-IV (1994) is the current edition of the manual that defines the American Psychiatric Association–approved diagnoses of mental disorders.

PROJECT NEADA

PROJECT NEADA (Nursing Education in Alcohol and Drug Abuse) is an integrated model program and curriculum prepared under the direction of Dr. Olga M. Church, University of Connecticut, School of Nursing, supported by Contract Number ADM 281-88-0007 from the National Institute on Alcohol Abuse and Alcoholism in cooperation with the National Institute on Drug Abuse. The model curriculum includes 3 undergraduate modules, a post-baccalaureate core module, 3 graduate modules, and 3 faculty development modules. Each module, with instructor's guide, includes the following sections: Introduction, Objectives, Session-specific Outlines, References, and Materials for Module. In addition, 2 training modules and 3 videotapes have been developed to teach alcohol and drug screening and intervention techniques, including use of the AUDIT (Alcohol Use Disorder Identification Test). For further information contact:

Olga Maranjian Church, PhD, FAAN
University of Connecticut
School of Nursing, U-59
175 Auditorium Road
Storrs, CT 06269-3059
(203) 486-0516

PROJECT SAEN—Substance Abuse Education in Nursing

PROJECT SAEN (Substance Abuse Education in Nursing) is a model nursing curriculum prepared under the direction of Dr. Madeline Naegle, supported by Contract Number ADM 281-88-0004 from the National Institute on Alcohol Abuse and Alcoholism in cooperation with the National Institute on Drug Abuse. The model curriculum includes 23 learning modules and instructor's guides designed to develop knowledge and skills at three content levels. The basic undergraduate level includes 7 modules which address the health needs of clients and families across the life-span and the nurse's role in maintaining and restoring health. The advanced undergraduate level includes 8 modules which build on the first level and require comprehension and skill performance at a more complex level. The masters advanced practice level includes 8 modules which can be integrated into the existing structure of the nursing programs which choose to use the modules. Project SAEN materials are published by the National League for Nursing as *Model Curriculum for Substance Abuse Education in Nursing*. The curriculum is available in three volumes through NLN Publications, 350 Hudson Street, New York, NY 10014. For further information contact:

Madeline A. Naegle, PhD, FAAN
New York University
SEHNAP, Division of Nursing
50 West 4th Street
New York, NY 10003
(212) 998-5321

An Addictions Curriculum

AN ADDICTIONS CURRICULUM is a three level–curriculum series prepared under the direction of Dr. Elizabeth M. Burns, Ohio State University, College of Nursing, supported by Contract Number ADM 281-88-0005 from the National Institute on Alcohol Abuse and Alcoholism in cooperation with the National Institute on Drug Abuse. The three levels include the Basic Knowledge and Practice Level (undergraduate), the Advanced Knowledge and Practice Level (graduate and specialized continuing education or inservice), and the Presenter Development Level (faculty development). Each curriculum module includes Module Overview, Module Planning, Guidelines for the Presenter, Visual Aid Masters, Handout Masters, and Evaluation Instruments. It is available in two volumes from Springer Publishing, 536 Broadway, New York, NY 10012. For further information contact:

Elizabeth M. Burns, RSM, RN, PhD, FAAN
Ohio State University
College of Nursing
1585 Neil Avenue
Columbus, OH 43210
(614) 292-4746

Mosby's Nursing Care of Clients with Substance Abuse video series

This video series is a comprehensive set of six videotapes that address the nursing care of clients with substance abuse. Developed in conjunction with this book, the series covers the nursing care of clients in a variety of settings, including the hospital; perinatal care; families, children, and adolescents; the community; chemical dependency treatment programs; and dual diagnosis clients. Each videotape is narrated by Dr. Eleanor Sullivan and comes with an instructor's booklet, a pretest, a posttest, and discussion questions.

PERIODICALS

Addictions Nursing Network

Quarterly journal for nurses treating drug and alcohol problems.
Mary Ann Lubert, Inc.
1651 Third Avenue
New York, NY 10128

Alcohol Alert

Quarterly bulletin that disseminates important research findings to health professionals. Each bulletin addresses a single aspect of alcohol abuse and alcoholism in a succinct, easy-to-read format; issues are free.
NIAAA
ATTN: Alcohol Alert
Office of Scientific Affairs
5600 Fishers Lane, Room 16C-14
Rockville, MD 20857
(301) 443-3860

Alcohol Health and Research World

Quarterly refereed publication of the National Institute on Alcohol Abuse and Alcoholism, which provides current research information in an easily readable magazine format.
Superintendent of Documents
U.S. Government Printing Office
Washington, DC 20402-9371

Alcoholism: Clinical and Experimental Research

Bimonthly official journal of The Research Society on Alcoholism, which reports on current research.

Williams and Wilkins
428 Preston Street
Baltimore, MD 21202-3993

Journal of Substance Abuse

Journal containing reports pertaining to alcohol, drug abuse, smoking, and obesity.

Ablex Publishing Corporation
335 Chestnut Street
Norwood, NJ 07648

Journal of Studies on Alcohol

Journal containing original research reports that contribute to the fundamental knowledge about alcohol, its use, and biomedical and sociocultural effects.

Journal of Studies on Alcohol
Rutgers Center of Alcohol Studies
P.O. Box 969
Piscataway, NJ 08855-0969

NIDA Notes

Information covering the areas of treatment and prevention research, epidemiology, and behavioral pharmacology. The publication is intended to report on advances in the drug abuse field, identify resources, promote an exchange of information, and improve communications among clinicians, researchers, administrators, and policymakers. It is available free through NCADI.

NCADI
P.O. Box 2345
Rockville, MD 20852
(301) 468-2600
(800) 729-6686

Substance Abuse

Official publication of the Association for Medical Education and Research Substance Abuse (AMERSA).

Center for Alcohol and Addiction Studies
Brown University, Box 6
Providence, RI 02912

INDEX

A

AA; *see* Alcoholics Anonymous
Abstinence, 9, 97-98, 106-107, 306, 350
Abstinence syndrome, 136-148
Abuse, 41, 286-288
Acetaminophen (Datril, Tylenol) in pain management, 179
ACLU; *see* American Civil Liberties Union
ACOA; *see* Adult Children of Alcoholic Families
Acquired immunodeficiency syndrome (AIDS), 42, 55,
    109-110, 170-175, 219, 271-272, 389, 396-397
Acute alcohol intoxication, 25
ADA; *see* Americans with Disabilities Act of 1990
ADAMHA; *see* Alcohol, Drug Abuse, and Mental Health
    Administration
ADD; *see* Attention deficit disorder
Addiction Research Foundation Clinical Institute
    Withdrawal Assessment for Alcohol (CIWA-Ar), 315,
    316-318
Addiction Severity Index (ASI), 55, 56
Addictions, 8, 181-182, 418-419, 454
ADDICTIONS CURRICULUM, 474-475
Addictions Nursing Certification Board, 311
Addictions Nursing Network, 475
Addictions nursing practice, 15, 58, 60-61, 119-120, 309,
    448-459
    knowledge base of, 420
Adolescents, substance abuse in, 250-266, 275, 385-386
ADS; *see* Alcohol dependence syndrome
Adult Children of Alcoholic Families (ACOA), 40, 95, 127,
    239, 248, 350
Advil; *see* Ibuprofen
Aerosols, 11
African Americans, 275, 373-375, 379-380, 398
Aftercare, 84, 314
Agency for Health Care Policy and Research (AHCPR), 177
AHA; *see* American Hospital Association
AHCPR; *see* Agency for Health Care Policy and Research
AIDS; *see* Acquired immunodeficiency syndrome
Airway clearance, ineffective, 186-187, 226
Alanine amino transferase (ALT), 56
Al-Anon, 4, 73, 89, 95, 126, 273, 289, 350, 471
Alateen, 95
Alcohol, 4, 6, 8, 10, 12, 24-28, 30-31, 32, 34, 38, 41, 140, 169,
    192-194, 254-255, 278-279, 282-284, 300, 320, 357-358,
    373, 378-379, 390-391, 425-426, 428, 440; *see also*
    Alcoholism
Alcohol abuse, 21, 23-24, 63, 168, 331
Alcohol dependence, 21-22, 63
Alcohol dependence syndrome (ADS), 62
Alcohol Health and Research World, 475
Alcohol teratogenicity, critical period for, 193
Alcohol Use Disorders Identification Test (AUDIT), 48, 49,
    468-470, 474

Alcohol withdrawal, 27, 86, 139-169, 171, 319, 320, 322-324,
    328-329
Alcohol withdrawal syndrome (AWS), 139-140
Alcoholic cardiomyopathy, alcohol abuse and, 167-168
Alcoholic hepatitis, alcohol abuse and, 155
Alcoholics, 276
    adult children of; *see* Adult Children of Alcoholics
Alcoholics Anonymous (AA), 4, 51, 71-72, 73, 91-96, 105, 106,
    107, 126, 134, 273, 306, 313, 346, 389, 425, 436, 471
    twelve step programs and; *see* Twelve step programs
Alcoholism, 2, 19-23, 72-77, 88, 240-241, 399-400; *see also*
    Alcohol
    alteration of nutrition related to, nursing diagnosis of,
    146
    definition of, 8, 62, 447
    depression and, care plan for, 356-359
    harm reduction approach to, 104-106
    hepatic failure and, care plan for, 162-166
Alpha alcoholism, 19-20, 72-73
Alprazolam (Xanax), 11
ALT; *see* Alanine amino transferase
American Academy of Pediatrics, 215
American Civil Liberties Union (ACLU), 214, 431
American Hospital Association (AHA), 436
American Medical Society on Alcoholism and Other Drug
    Dependencies, 312
American Nurses Association (ANA), 15, 118, 307, 414, 415,
    448, 449
American Nurses Credentialing Center, 414
American Society of Addiction Medicine (ASAM), 62, 79-81,
    100, 312, 447
Americans with Disabilities Act (ADA) of 1990, 300-301,
    313
AMERSA; *see* Association for Medical Education and
    Research Substance Abuse
Amphetamine sulfate (Benzedrine), 11, 33
Amphetamines, 4, 11, 25, 31-33, 55, 207, 319-320, 378, 441
Amylase, pancreas and, 167
Amytal, 10-11
ANA; *see* American Nurses Association
ANA Standards of Addictions Nursing Practice, 15, 58,
    119-120, 309, 449, 450-453
ANA Standards of Clinical Nursing Practice, 450-453
ANA Standards of Psychiatric and Mental Health Nursing
    Practice, 450-453
Analgesics, 11-12, 150, 178
    narcotic; *see* Narcotics
Anesthesia, general, sedatives and, 26
"Angel dust," 37
ANS; *see* Autonomic nervous system (ANS)
Antabuse; *see* Disulfiram
Anticholinergics, 184
Antidepressants, 87, 98-99, 329, 349

Antidrug campaigns, 261
Antiemetics in treatment of viral hepatitis, 175
Antihistamines in treatment of viral hepatitis, 175
Antimicrobials for infection control in drug-addicted neonate, 220
Antipsychotics, 329, 349
Anxiety, 160, 181-182, 246-247
AODA; *see* Alcohol and other drug abuse
Appetite suppressants, 11-12
Aromatics, 37
ASAM; *see* American Society of Addictions Medicine
Ascites, alcohol withdrawal and, 155
ASI; *see* Addiction Severity Index
Asian Americans, nursing care of, 275, 373, 377-378, 380
Aspartate amino transferase (AST), 56
Aspirin, 179, 399
Assessment, 55-56, 118-123, 220-222, 296
Asset tests, Medicaid and, 427
Association for Medical Education and Research Substance Abuse (AMERSA), 476
AST; *see* Aspartate amino transferase
Ativan; *see* Lorazepam
Atresia, ileal, cocaine and, 202
Atrial fibrillation in binge drinkers, 168
Attention deficit disorder (ADD), fetal alcohol syndrome and, 199
AUDIT; *see* Alcohol Use Disorders Identification Test
Autonomic nervous system (ANS) activity, increased, alcohol withdrawal syndrome and, 140
AWS; *see* Alcohol withdrawal syndrome
Azene; *see* Chlorazepate

B

BAC; *see* Blood alcohol concentration
Barbital, 33
Barbiturates, 10-11, 25, 32-34, 148, 319-320, 328, 441
Battered women, 286
Bayley Scales of Infant Development, 220
Behavior, 133, 260
Behavioral contracting, substance abuse treatment and, 87-88
Behavioral manifestations, fetal alcohol syndrome and fetal alcohol effects and, 199-200
Behavioral problems, 127-134, 250
Benzedrine; *see* Amphetamine sulfate
Benzodiazepines, 4, 11, 25, 26, 32, 34, 41, 87, 176-177, 180-183, 319, 328, 441
  use of, 109, 140, 141, 378
  withdrawal from, 148, 319, 320, 328, 330
Benzoylecgonine, elimination time of, 440
Beta alcoholism, 20, 72-73
Betty Ford Center, 17
Big Book in Alcoholics Anonymous, 73, 94, 96
Biochemical markers in assessment of substance abuse, 56-57
Biological factors in substance abuse, 255
Biopsychosocial perspective in medical models of substance abuse treatment, 73
Bipolar disorder, 360-365
Birth weight, fetal effects of tobacco on, 205-206
Bissell, L., 415-416
Block grant program, 425, 428-429
Blood alcohol concentration (BAC) in assessment of substance abuse, 25, 57
Breast milk, alcohol consumption and, 194
Brief intervention, 50-51, 288
Brief MAST, 49
Broadening the Base of Treatment for Alcohol Problems, 97
Bromide, sedative-hypnotics and, 33
Bromocriptine, 86, 329
Brown v Winkle, 432
Buprenorphine (Buprenex), 86, 178

Burns, E.M., 474-475
Butisol, 11
Butorphanol (Stadol) in pain management, 178

C

Cadmium, substance abuse in perinatal care and, 205
Caffeine, 4, 11, 28, 38
CAGE questionnaire in assessment of substance abuse, 48, 49
CAGE Questions Adapted to Include Drugs (CAGEAID), 48, 465
Cancer, alcohol and, 169
Candidiasis, 175-176
Cannabinoids, 25
Cannabinols, 36, 151
Cannabis, 11
Capua v City of Plainfield, 433
Carbamazepine, 86
Cardiovascular system, alcohol withdrawal and, 167-169
Care of Clients with Addictions: Dimensions of Nursing Practice, The, 448
Care plan
  for adolescent abusing alcohol and marijuana, 262-265
  for African-American inner city client with IV heroin abuse, 382-385
  for alcohol dependence and withdrawal, 144-147
  for bipolar disorder and marijuana abuse, 360-365
  for bulimia and cocaine abuse, 332-339
  for child with stress-related symptoms, 256-259
  for chronic pain/narcotic and benzodiazepine addiction/ interstitial pulmonary disease, 180-183
  for depression and alcoholism, 356-359
  for early pregnancy, uncertain drug or alcohol use and, 210-212
  for elderly man, alcoholism and, 278-283
  for hepatic failure, alcoholism and, 162-166
  for infective endocarditis/IV drug abuse, 172-174
  for monitoring program in work setting for client recovering from alcoholism, 298-299
  for multidrug withdrawal, 156-160
  for Native American woman with alcoholism at outpatient clinic, 390-393
  for neonate born with crack cocaine in system, 224-227
  for nursing care of the client with alcohol dependence in a social detoxification setting, 322-327
  for overdose of unknown chemicals, 186-187
  for schizophrenia and alcohol abuse, 366-371
  for spouse of husband with substance abuse, 240-247
CARN; *see* Certified Addiction Registered Nurse
CAST; *see* Children of Alcoholics Screen Test
Catecholamines, 31
CATOR; *see* Chemical Abuse/Addiction Treatment Outcome Registry
CCDN; *see* Certified Chemical Dependency Nurse
CEAP; *see* Certified Employee Assistance Program Counselor
Cellulitis as sequela of substance abuse, 170
Center
  for Mental Health Services (CMHS), 426
  for Substance Abuse Prevention (CSAP), 17, 307, 412, 426, 471
  for Substance Abuse Treatment (CSAT), 426, 428, 471
Central nervous system (CNS) depressants, 25, 28, 33-34, 86, 136-137, 149, 154-155, 319-320
Central nervous system (CNS) dysfunction, fetal alcohol syndrome and fetal alcohol effects and, 198-200
Central nervous system (CNS) stimulants, 25, 28, 31, 86, 137, 150
Certification of nurses in substance abuse practice, 307
Chancroid, 42, 175-176
Chemical Abuse/Addiction Treatment Outcome Registry (CATOR), 96, 98, 384

Chemical dependency, 8, 447-448
Chemical dependency treatment settings, nursing care in, 305-344
Chief enabler, dysfunctional family patterns and, 237
Child abuse, 41-42, 251-252, 286-287
Children, 236, 238, 250-259, 292, 398; *see also* Neonate
"China white," 38
Chinese, nursing care of, 377-378
Chlamydia, 175-176
Chloral hydrate, 11, 33
Chlorazepate (Azene, Tranxene), 11
Chlordiazepoxide (Librium), 11, 141, 161, 176-177
Chromatography, 439-441
Chronic illness paradigm, substance abuse and, 22-23
Church, O.M., 473, 474
CIWA; *see* Clinical Institute Withdrawal Assessment
CIWA-Ar; *see* Addiction Research Foundation Clinical Institute Withdrawal Assessment for Alcohol
Cleveland Board of Education v Loudermill, 433
Client, 78, 315-318, 342
Clinical Institute Withdrawal Assessment (CIWA), 143, 315, 316-318
Clinical nurse specialists, role of, with substance abuse patients, 13
Clinical specialists in substance abuse, addictions nursing practice and, 455-456
Clinics, prenatal and well-baby, nursing care in, 302
Clonidine, 86, 329
CMHS; *see* Center for Mental Health Services
Coca leaves, 4
Cocaine, 4, 11, 25, 28, 31-33, 35-36, 38, 42, 87, 227, 320, 439-441
    abuse of, and bulimia, care plan for, 332-339
    lactation and, 202-203
    snorting of, nasal septum damage as sequela of, 170
    substance abuse in perinatal care and, 201-203
    use of, 260-261, 334-337, 376, 378, 381, 384-385
    withdrawal from, 27, 86, 319, 329
Cocaine Anonymous, 4, 73, 471
"Cocaine bugs," 36
Cocaine hydrochloride ("coke"), 35-36
Cocanon, 73
CODA; *see* Codependents Anonymous
Codeine, 11, 34, 320
Codependency, 239-249
Codependents Anonymous (CODA), 95, 127, 239
Cognitive impairment, 199, 282-283
Cognitive-behavioral approach to substance abuse treatment, 74
"Coke"; *see* Cocaine hydrochloride
Comfort, alteration in, 157-158, 181-182, 329
Common law liability, financing substance abuse treatment and, 433
Communication, nursing care in occupational settings and, 301-302
Community, 40-44, 83-84
Community education in substance abuse in perinatal care, 228
Comorbid disorders, substance abuse treatment and, 86
Comprehensive Substance Treatment and Rehabilitation Program (C-STAR), 427
Confidentiality, 300, 433-435
Confirmation assay in drug testing, 439
Confrontation, 128-129, 349-350
Consciousness, 187, 412
Contemplation in substance abuse treatment, 79, 103
Contingency contracts in treatment of client with dual diagnosis, 351
Continuity of care, 79-81, 126-127
Controlled drinking as alternative recovery goal, 108-109
Cost, 42-43, 300, 442-443

Cost containment, financing substance abuse treatment and, 429-430
Cotinine, tobacco and, 206-207
Cough and cold medicines, 11-12
Counseling, 90, 95-96, 273, 296-297, 307, 311-313, 341
Crack cocaine, 35-36, 41, 224-227, 277, 320, 375
Craving, 28, 86-87, 112, 329
Cross tolerance, 11-12, 26, 55, 140, 176, 321-329
CSAP; *see* Center for Substance Abuse Prevention
CSAT; *see* Center for Substance Abuse Treatment
C-STAR; *see* Comprehensive Substance Treatment and Rehabilitation Program
Cuban Americans, nursing care of, 375-377
Curanderos, Hispanic cultures and, 376
Cyanide, substance abuse in perinatal care and, 205

D

DA; *see* Dopamine
Dalgan; *see* Dezocin
Dalmane; *see* Flurazepam
DANA; *see* Drug and Alcohol Nursing Association
Darvon; *see* Propoxyphene
DAST; *see* Drug Abuse Screening Test
Datril; *see* Acetaminophen
Davis v Lhim, 435
Dederick, C., 83
Deep sleep state of drug-addicted neonate, 222
Defense mechanisms, common, in substance abuse, 29-30
Delayed withdrawal syndrome, 320-321
Delirium tremens (DTs), 15, 140, 141, 315, 319
Delta alcoholism, 20, 72-73
Delta-9-tetrahydrocannabinol (THC), 36, 203
Demerol; *see* Meperidine
Denial, 5, 29, 118, 127-129, 236-237, 357-358
Dependence, 9, 26-27, 345
    alcohol; *see* Alcohol dependence
Dependency, 8, 19-46
Depression, 98-99, 218, 277, 329
Designer drugs, 38
Desipramine (Norpramin), 87
Destructive confrontation in substance abuse treatment, 128
Detoxification, 15, 85-86, 273, 306-307, 314-330
Detoxification setting, social, alcohol dependence in, care plan for, 322-327
Developmental care of drug-addicted neonate, 222-227
Dexedrine, 11
Dezocin (Dalgan) in pain management, 178
Diabetes, blood sugar stabilization and, withdrawal and, 330-340
Diagnosis, 47-70, 347
Diagnostic and Statistical Manual of Mental Disorders (DSM), 57-58, 62-64, 74, 473
Diagnostic and Statistical Manual of Mental Disorders, ed. 2 (DSM-II), 63
Diagnostic and Statistical Manual of Mental Disorders, ed. 3 (DSM-III), 63-64, 66
Diagnostic and Statistical Manual of Mental Disorders, ed. 4 (DSM-IV), 8, 20, 63, 64, 66, 68
Diagnostic instruments for clinical practice and research in assessment of substance abuse, 64-67
Diagnostic Interview Schedule (DIS) in assessment of substance abuse, 55, 56, 65, 66
Diazepam (Valium), 11, 141, 321, 328, 330
Digitalis in treatment of alcoholic cardiomyopathy, 168
Dilantin; *see* Phenytoin
Dilaudid; *see* Hydromorphone
Dipsomania, 21
DIS; *see* Diagnostic Interview Schedule
Discussion meetings in Alcoholics Anonymous, 92
Disease, 9, 42, 72-74, 88, 183, 447-448
Disease model versus illness model, 306

Disulfiram (Antabuse), 87, 284-285
Diuretics in treatment of alcoholic cardiomyopathy, 168
Doctoral programs in nursing education, 16-17
Domestic violence, substance abuse and, 41
Dopamine (DA), 28, 31-33
Dopamine receptors, D2, alcohol abuse and, 24
Doriden; *see* Glutethimide
"Double trouble" meetings, dual diagnosis and, 350
"Downers," 33
Drinking, 8, 20, 21, 108-109
Driving under the influence (DUI), 8, 40, 43
Drowsy state of drug-addicted neonate, 222
Drug Abuse Resistance Education (Project DARE), 291
Drug Abuse Screening Test (DAST), 49
Drug and Alcohol Nursing Association (DANA), 414, 448, 449, 471
Drug and alcohol screening, preemployment; *see* Drug testing
Drug overdose, emergency care for, 184-187
Drug seeking behavior, management of, 133
Drug testing, 42-43, 294, 300, 431-445
Drug-addicted neonate, 215-227
Drug-Free Schools and Community Act of 1986, 290
Drug-Free Workplace Act of 1988, 431
Drugs, 38, 86-87, 210-212, 382-385; *see also* Medications
DSM; *see* Diagnostic and Statistical Manual of Mental Disorders
DTs; *see* Delirium tremens
Dual diagnosis, 64, 67, 345-372, 390-391
DUI; *see* Driving under the influence of alcohol
Duodenitis, alcohol abuse and, 161
Dysmorphic characteristics of fetal alcohol syndrome and fetal alcohol effects, 197-198
Dysrhythmias, cardiac, alcohol abuse and, 168-169

E

EAP; *see* Employee assistance program
ECA; *see* Epidemiological Catchment Area
"Ecstasy," 38
Education, 15-17, 88, 290-291, 353, 364-370, 425, 459
    affective, antidrug campaigns and, 261
    community, in substance abuse in perinatal care, 228
    nursing, 311-312, 342, 414, 415
Effectiveness, 96-99
EIA; *see* Enzyme immunoassay
Eighth Special Report to Congress on Alcohol and Health, 473
ELISA test for human immunodeficiency virus, 219
Emergency care, 179-188, 292-293
Emergency room settings, 14, 455-456
Emotional abuse, 251-252, 286-287
Emotional consequences of substance abuse, 38-39, 236, 250
Employee assistance program (EAP), 20, 40, 43, 108, 294-295, 297, 402, 459
Employment, 386, 433
Encephalopathy, portal-systemic, alcohol withdrawal and, 161, 162-166
Endocarditis, 170, 172-174
Environmental support, 137, 141-147, 329-330
Enzyme immunoassay (EIA), 440, 441
Epidemiological Catchment Area (ECA), 7
Epidemiological Catchment Area Survey of National Institute of Mental Health, 234, 346
Epinephrine, 31
Epsilon alcoholism, 20-21, 72-73
Equanil; *see* Meprobamate
Esophageal varices, alcohol withdrawal and, 155-161
Ethanol, 50, 194
Ethchlorvynol (Placidyl), 11
Ethnic and racial minorities, nursing care of, 373-381, 386
Evaluation in nursing care, 126-127
Ewing's 4 *P*'s screening tool, 208, 209

Experimental use by adolescents, 254-255
Explosive drinking, 21

F

Faculty development grants, nursing education and, 307
FAE; *see* Fetal alcohol effects
Fagan Infatest, 220
Failure to thrive (FTT), fetal alcohol syndrome and, 197-199
False negatives in drug testing, 442
False positives in drug testing, 439, 442
Families, 89, 234-239, 248-249, 352, 398
    assessment of, nursing care in home setting and, 285
    effects of substance abuse on, 124-125
    experiences of, interpretations of, children of families with substance abuse and, 252
    nursing care in community settings and, 276-277
    support of, nursing care in community settings and, 288-289
Family counseling, 341
Family hero, dysfunctional family patterns and, 237
Family substance abuse treatment, 89
FAS; *see* Fetal alcohol syndrome
Federal Drug and Alcohol Abuse Act, 433
Federal Employees Health Benefits Program (FEHBP), 426
FEHBP; *see* Federal Employees Health Benefits Program
Fentanyl, 34, 38, 441
Fetal alcohol effects (FAE), 193, 194-200
Fetal alcohol syndrome (FAS), 192-200, 228
Fetal tobacco syndrome, 205
Fetor hepaticus, portal-systemic encephalopathy and, 161
FHR; *see* Fetal heart rate
"Fight or flight" response, amphetamines and, 31
Financial problems in families of substance abusers, 286
Financing substance abuse treatment, 273, 424-430
"Flash," 33
Fluoxetine, 86
Flurazepam (Dalmane), 11
"Flushing response" in Asian people, 377
Fourteenth Amendment to Constitution, 433
Fourth Amendment to Constitution, 432-433
Fourth Triennial Report to Congress: Drug Abuse and Drug Abuse Research IV, 473
Framingham study, substance abuse and, 21
FTT; *see* Failure to thrive
Fuels, 11

G

GABA; *see* Gamma-aminobutyric acid
Gamma alcoholism, 19-20, 72-73
Gamma-aminobutyric acid (GABA), 24, 33-34
GAMMA-glutamyl transferase (GGT), 56
Gas chromatography mass spectrometry (GC-MS), 440, 441
Gas exchange, impaired, related to lung failure, nursing diagnosis of, 163-164, 180-181
Gastrointestinal tract, alcohol withdrawal and, 161-167
Gateway drugs, use of, by adolescents, 254-255
Gateway Foundation, 83-84
Gay men, 389-396
GC; *see* Gas chromatography
GC-MS; *see* Gas chromatography mass spectrometry
General anesthesia, sedatives and, 26
Generalist nursing practice, curricular change for alcohol and other drug education and, 311, 413-414, 449-455
Genetics, alcohol abuse and, 23-24
Genital herpes infection, 175-176
Genital warts, 175-176
Genogram in social assessment of client, 123
GGT; *see* GAMMA-glutamyl transferase
Glutamate, alcohol and, 24
Glutethimide (Doriden), 11
Gonorrhea, 175-176, 213
Graduate programs in nursing education, 311-312

Grants, 307, 428-429
Granuloma inguinale, 175-176
"Grass," 36
Grieving, anticipatory, 166, 183
Group therapy, 88-89, 273, 352-353
Growth deficiency, fetal alcohol syndrome and fetal
    alcohol effects and, 198

H

Habilitation, detoxification versus, 306
Halcion; *see* Triazolam
Halfway houses, substance abuse treatment and, 43, 83,
    273, 425
Hallucinations, alcohol withdrawal syndrome and,
    140
Hallucinogens, 11, 25, 37, 151
Halogenated hydrocarbons, 37
Harm reduction approach to recovery, 104-106, 109
Harrison Narcotic Act of 1914, 5
Hashish, 25, 36, 203
Hazelden Foundation, 17, 73
HCFA; *see* Health Care Financing Administration
Head and neck cancer, alcohol abuse and, 169
Health, 137, 284, 373-378, 412
Health Care Financing Administration (HCFA), 427
Health care professionals, nursing care of, 401-402, 415-416,
    417
Health care versus substance abuse treatment, 424
Health insurance, private, financing substance abuse
    treatment and, 428
Health maintenance, alteration of, 362-363, 384-385
Health maintenance organizations (HMOs), financing
    substance abuse treatment and, 429
Healthy People 2000, 290-291
Heavy users, 8
Hepatitis, 155, 175, 213
Hero, family, dysfunctional family patterns and, 237,
    238
Heroin, 4, 11, 34, 36, 86, 87, 207, 441
    substance abuse in perinatal care and, 200-201
    use of, 376, 378
Heroin dependence, methadone maintenance for, 109
Herpes, HIV transmission and, 42
Hispanics, nursing care of, 275, 373, 375-377, 380
"Hitting bottom," recovery and, 103-104, 288
HMOs; *see* Health maintenance organizations
"Holiday heart syndrome," 168
Home settings, nursing care in; *see* Nursing care in home
    setting
Homelessness, 271, 384-385, 397-398
Homophobia, 394-395
Homosexual men and women, nursing care of, 389-396
"Hookahs," 36
Hospital, nursing care of clients with substance abuse in,
    13-14, 135-190
Hospitalization, 183
    partial, 82, 83, 355-370
    repeated, 360-363
Hostility, 128, 130-132, 174
Hughes Act, 425, 436
Human immunodeficiency virus (HIV), 42, 109-110, 174-175,
    219, 389, 435
    nursing care and, 271-272, 396-397
Hydrocarbons, halogenated, 37
Hydromorphone (Dilaudid), 11
Hyperlipidemia, alcoholic-induced bone necrosis and, 169
Hypertension, 155, 168, 200
Hyperthermia related to systemic infection, nursing
    diagnosis of, 382
Hypnotics, 10-11, 26
Hypoglycemia, blood sugar stabilization and, withdrawal
    and, 330-340

I

Ibuprofen (Advil, Motrin, Nuprin) in pain management,
    179
"Ice," 33, 320
IGR; *see* Intrauterine growth retardation
Ileal atresia, cocaine and, 202
Illness, 9, 374-378
    models of, substance abuse and, 19-23
Illness model versus disease model, 306
IMD; *see* Institution for Mental Disease
Immobilization, 165, 183
Impaired nurse, characteristics of, 401-402, 415-416, 417
Incest, nursing care in home setting and, 288
Indian Health Service, 228, 426
Indians, nursing care of, 377-378
Individual coping, ineffective, 182, 263-264, 298-299,
    324-326, 334-337, 363-369, 392-393
Individual therapy, substance abuse treatment and, 87, 273
Individuals, 285, 427
Infant; *see* Children; Neonate
Infection, 173, 183, 206, 382-384
Infection control in drug-addicted neonate, 219-220
Infective endocarditis, 170, 172-174
Informed consent form for inpatient detoxification, 137, 138
INH; *see* Isoniazid
Inhalants, 11, 37, 153
In-house employee assistance program, 295
Injury, 145, 158, 187, 278-279, 329, 390-391
Inpatient substance abuse treatment, 81, 82, 306, 354-355
Institute
    of Medicine (IOM), 97, 430
    of Survey Research at Temple University, 374
Institution, 427
Insurance, 300, 428
Interdisciplinary aspects of substance abuse treatment,
    309-313
International Classification of Diseases, 20
Intervention, 75-76, 124-126
    brief, 50-51, 288
    nursing care in community settings, 288-290
    nursing care in occupational settings and, 296-297
Intervention team, nursing care in community settings
    and, 289
Interview, 51-55, 64-65
Intoxication, 25, 139-140
Intraoperative care, 176
Intrauterine growth retardation (IGR), tobacco and, 206
IOM; *see* Institute of Medicine
Isoniazid (INH) in treatment of tuberculosis, 175

J

Japanese, nursing care of, 377-378
JCAHO; *see* Joint Committee on the Accreditation of
    Health Care Organizations
Jellinek, E.M., 72
Jellinek model of substance abuse, 19-21, 62
Joint Commission on the Accreditation of Health Care
    Organizations (JCAHO), 67, 310-311
Journal of Substance Abuse, 476

K

"Kinship" foster care placement of infants, 277
Knots, 447
Knowledge building, substance abuse and, 415-421
Knowledge deficit, 240-241, 279-280, 360-362
Koreans, nursing care of, 377-378

L

Labor and delivery, substance abuse in perinatal care and,
    209-213
Laboratory, drug testing in, 444
Lactation, 194, 202-207

Laing, R.D., 447
Lapse, 9, 111, 350-351
Larynx, cancer of, alcohol abuse and, 169
Latinos, nursing care of, 373, 375-377, 380
Legal issues, substance abuse treatment and, 431-436
Lesbians, 389-396
Liability, common law, financing substance abuse
     treatment and, 433
Librium; *see* Chlordiazepoxide
Lifestyle change as goal of recovery, 107-108
Light users, 8
Liminal, 11
Lipase, pancreas and, 167
Lithium, 74, 349
Liver, 155-161
Liver cancer, alcohol abuse and, 169
Liver flap, portal-systemic encephalopathy and, 161
Liver function tests in assessment of substance abuse,
     56-57
Long-term aftercare, substance abuse treatment and, 84
Long-term care versus step-down program, 306
Lorazepam (Ativan), 11, 141
Los Angeles Police Department, Project DARE and, 291
Lost child, dysfunctional family patterns and, 238
Lung failure, impaired gas exchange related to, nursing
     diagnosis of, 163-164, 180-181
Lymphogranuloma venereum, 175-176
Lysergic acid diethylamide (LSD), 11, 73

M

MacAndrew Scale in assessment of substance abuse, 55, 56
Macrocytosis, alcohol abuse and, 57
Magnesium sulfate, alcohol withdrawal and, 141
Maintenance, 79, 103, 306
Managed care, financing substance abuse treatment and,
     429-430
Management opportunities, addictions nursing practice
     and, 458-459
"Mandatory Guidelines for Federal Workplace Drug
     Testing Programs," 444
Manipulation, 129-130, 174
March of Dimes, 228
Marijuana, 4, 11, 25, 36, 262-265, 360-365, 440-441
     chronic effects of, 32
     substance abuse in perinatal care and, 203-204
     use of, 254-255, 260-261, 378, 381
Mascot, dysfunctional family patterns and, 238
MAST; *see* Michigan Alcoholism Screening Test
Master's degree in area of concentration in nursing
     education, 311-312, 414, 415
Mazindol, 86
MCV; *see* Mean corpuscular values
MDMA; *see* Methylenedioxymethamphetamine
Mean corpuscular values (MCV) in assessment of
     substance abuse, 57
Meconium, possible inhalation of, ineffective airway
     clearance related to, nursing diagnosis of, 226
Medicaid, 427, 434
Medical format for detoxification, 321
Medical inpatient setting, addictions nursing practice and,
     456
Medical models of substance abuse treatment, 47, 57-58,
     62-67, 73, 305, 308-309
Medical practitioners in substance abuse treatment, 289,
     312
Medical/surgical units, general, nursing care in, 148-176
Medicare, 434
Medications, 284-285, 348-349; *see also* Drugs
Men, 376-377, 389-398
Mental health model of substance abuse treatment versus
     recovery model, 348-351
Mental status examination, baseline, withdrawal and, 315

Mentally Ill Chemical Abusers (MICA), 95
Mentally ill persons, nursing care in community settings
     and, 276
Meperidine (Demerol), 4, 11, 34, 38, 178-179, 441
Meprobamate (Equanil, Miltown), 11
Mescaline, 4, 11, 38
Mesolimbic system, reinforcement and, 28
Methadone, 11, 34, 87, 179, 201, 284, 329, 441
Methadone maintenance, 104, 109
Methadone maintenance program (MMP), substance
     abuse treatment and, 84-85
Methadone withdrawal, alteration in comfort related to,
     nursing diagnosis of, 157-158
Methamphetamine, 33, 38, 207, 320
Methaqualone (Quaaludes), 378
Methylenedioxymethamphetamine (MDMA), 38
Methylxanthines, 28
Methyprylon (Noludar), 11
Mexican Americans, nursing care of, 375-377
MICA; *see* Mentally Ill Chemical Abusers
Michigan Alcoholism Screening Test (MAST), 48-49, 51,
     466-467
Microcephaly, fetal alcohol syndrome and fetal alcohol
     effects and, 198-199
Mini-Mental Status, withdrawal and, 315
Minnesota model of substance abuse treatment, 72, 73,
     99
Minnesota Multiple Personality Inventory (MMPI), 56
Minor tranquilizers, 11, 55
Minorities, 275, 373-381, 386
Miscarriage, alcohol consumption and, 193
Missouri comprehensive plan for substance abuse
     treatment, 427-428
Mixed Personality Disorder, 239
MMP; *see* Methadone maintenance program
MMPI; *see* Minnesota Multiple Personality Inventory
Model Curriculum for Substance Abuse Education in Nursing,
     474
Model curriculum grants in schools of nursing, 307
Models of illness, substance abuse and, 19-23
Moderate users, definition of, 8
Modified Selective Severity Assessment (MSSA), 142-143
Molluscum contagiosum, 175-176
Mood-altering drugs, 10
Moral defect concept of alcoholism, 72
Moralistic approach to substance abuse, 5-6
Morbidity, fetal effects of tobacco on, 206
Morphine, 4, 11, 26, 34, 178, 441
Mortality, fetal effects of tobacco on, 206
Motrin; *see* Ibuprofen
Mowrer, O.H., 84
MSSA; *see* Modified Selective Severity Assessment
Multidisciplinary interactions in substance abuse
     treatment, 309
Multidrug use; *see* Polydrug use
Muscle relaxants, prescription, abuse of, 55
Musculoskeletal system, alcohol withdrawal and, 169
Myopathies, alcohol abuse and, 169

N

NA; *see* Narcotics Anonymous
NAACOG, 228
Naegle, M.A., 474
Nalbuphine (Nubain) in pain management, 178
Naloxone (Narcan), 184, 218
Naltrexone hydrochloride (Trexan), 86, 285
NANDA; *see* North American Nursing Diagnosis
     Association
Narcan; *see* Naloxone
Narcanon, 73
Narcotics, 11, 34-35, 86, 150, 161, 176-177, 179, 180-183, 207,
     440

Narcotics Anonymous (NA), 4, 73, 107, 134, 273, 313, 389, 436, 471
Nasal septum damage as sequela of snorting of cocaine, 170
NASS; *see* Neonatal Abstinence Syndrome Score
National Alliance for the Mentally Ill, 352
National Certified Addictions Counselor (NCAC), 307
National Clearinghouse for Alcohol and Drug Information, 472
National Commission to Prevent Infant Mortality, 191
National Consortium of Chemical Dependency Nurses (NCCDN), 414, 449, 472
National Council on Alcohol (NCA), 63, 425
National Council on Alcoholism and Drug Dependence (NCADD), 5-6, 51, 62, 125, 126, 191, 254, 425, 447, 472
National Drug and Alcoholism Treatment Unit Survey (NDATUS), 426
National Household Survey on Drug Abuse: Main Findings 1988, 473
National Institute
    on Alcohol Abuse and Alcoholism (NIAAA), 16-17, 24, 87, 294, 307, 412, 425, 430, 472
    on Drug Abuse (NIDA), 16-17, 86-87, 290-291, 307, 375, 412, 425, 472
    of Mental Health, 346, 425
National Institutes of Health (NIH), 425
National Nurses Society on Addictions (NNSA), 58, 311, 414, 448, 449, 472
Nationally Certified Addictions Counselor, 312
Native Americans, 275, 373, 378-379, 381, 390-393
NBRS; *see* Neurobiological Risk Score
NCA; *see* National Council on Alcoholism
NCAC; *see* National Certified Addictions Counselor
NCADD; *see* National Council on Alcoholism and Drug Dependence
NCCDN; *see* National Consortium of Chemical Dependency Nurses
NDATUS; *see* National Drug and Alcoholism Treatment Unit Survey
"Nembies," 33
Nembutal; *see* Pentobarbital
Neonatal Abstinence Syndrome Score (NASS), 215, 216-217, 218
Neonate, 224-227; *see also* Children
    drug-addicted; *see* Drug-addicted neonate
Neuroadaptation, physical dependence and, 26-27
Neurobiological Risk Score (NBRS), 221
Neuroscience model of substance abuse treatment, 73
Neurotransmitters, 24, 73
NIAAA; *see* National Institute on Alcohol Abuse and Alcoholism
Nicotine, 11, 28, 38, 86, 204
NIDA; *see* National Institute on Drug Abuse
NIDA Notes, 476
Nightingale, F., 411, 419
NIH; *see* National Institutes of Health
Nitrites, 37
Nitrosamine, substance abuse in perinatal care and, 204
Nitrous oxide, 11, 37
NNSA; *see* National Nurses Society on Addictions
Noludar; *see* Methyprylon
Nonopioids in pain management, 178, 179, 180-183
Nonpharmacological strategies in pain management, 179, 180-183
Nonspecific urethritis, 175-176
Norepinephrine, 25, 31
Norpramin; *see* Desipramine
North American Nursing Diagnosis Association (NANDA), 59, 68, 123, 448-449
Novocaine, drug testing and, 439
Nubain; *see* Nalbuphine
Nucleus accumbens, dopamine and, 28

Nuprin; *see* Ibuprofen
Nurse, 13-15, 307, 353-371, 401-402, 415-417
Nurse generalists in substance abuse treatment, 311, 413-414, 449-455
Nurse researchers, 411-423
Nurse specialists, 13, 16, 311-312, 414-415
Nursing assessment and diagnosis of substance abuse, 57-61
Nursing care, 115-407
Nursing care plan; *see* Care plan
Nursing diagnosis, 60-61, 123
    of alteration
        in cardiac output, decreased related to recurrent right and left ventricular failure, 173
        in comfort, 157-158, 181-182, 329
        in family processes, related to father's divorce and changed living arrangements, 264-265
        in health maintenance, 362-363, 384-385
        in nutrition, 146, 164, 183, 227
        in parenting related to heavy alcohol use, 392
        in role performance related to substance abuse, 262
        in thought processes related to acute psychotic episode and substance abuse, 366-367
    of anticipatory grieving, 166, 183
    of anxiety, 160, 245
    of denial related to long-term alcohol use, 357-358
    of high risk, 173, 227, 278-279, 356-357, 382-384, 390-391
    of hopelessness related to ineffective management of client's life and excessive alcohol use, 358-359
    of hyperthermia related to systemic infection, 382
    of impaired gas exchange, 163-164, 180-181
    of impaired home maintenance management related to drinking alcohol and cognitive impairment, 282-283
    of impaired skin integrity related to altered nutritional status and immobility, 165
    of impaired social interactions, 174, 369-371
    of ineffective airway clearance, 186-187, 226
    of ineffective family coping compromised related to changes made in response to husband and father's drinking patterns, 241-245
    of ineffective individual coping, 182, 263-264, 324-326, 334-337, 363-369, 392-393
    of knowledge deficit, 210-212, 240-241, 279-281, 360-362
    of personal identity disturbance related to childhood dysfunctional family and history of sexual abuse, 337-339
    of potential, 183, 256-258
        for ineffective individual coping related to recent cessation of substance use, 298-299
        for injury, 145, 158, 187, 329
    of self-esteem disturbance related to dysfunctional home situation, 259
    of sensory-perceptual alteration, 329
        related to withdrawal, 147, 159, 165, 224-225, 322-324
    of sleep pattern disturbance, 226-227, 246-247
    of social isolation related to husband's drinking and wife's role overload, 247
    of spiritual distress related to change in value system contrary to that established in childhood, 326-327
Nursing education; *see* Education, nursing
Nursing Education in Alcohol and Drug Abuse (PROJECT NEADA), 473-474
Nursing model of substance abuse assessment, 47, 57-61
Nursing practice, 311, 413-414, 449-455
    addictions; *see* Addictions nursing practice specialist; *see* Nurse specialists
Nursing practice standards, generic, psychiatric-mental health and addictions, comparison of, 450-453
Nutrition, 146, 164-165, 183, 227, 329

O

Occupational health nurse, substance abuse treatment and, 14
Office
of Substance Abuse Prevention, 17, 307, 412, 426
of Treatment Improvement, 426
Ohio State University, curricula for alcohol and other drug education developed at, 412
Older adults, 276, 278-283, 398-401
Opiates, 11, 25, 73, 86, 137, 154-155, 184, 319-320, 329
Opioids, 26-28, 32, 34-35, 177-179
Opium, 4, 218
Organizational resources and services, substance abuse and, 471-472
Osteonecrosis, alcohol-induced, 169
OTC drugs; *see* Over-the-counter drugs
Otitis media in infants, tobacco and, 206
Outpatient substance abuse treatment, 83, 99, 306
Overeaters Anonymous, 73, 127
Over-the-counter (OTC) drugs, 11-12, 207, 284, 399
Oxazepam (Serax), 11
Oxycodone, 11

P

Pain, 177-183
Pancreas, alcohol abuse and, 161-167
Paraldehyde, 33
Paregoric in drug withdrawal in drug-addicted neonate, 218, 219
Parental substance abuse, recognizing, nursing care in school settings and, 293
Partial hospitalization, 82, 83, 355-370
Passive smoking, effects of, 206
PAW symptoms; *see* Post-acute withdrawal syndrome symptoms
PCP; *see* Phencyclidine
Pediculosis pubic, 175-176
Peer assistance programs for substance-abusing health care professionals, 402
Peer group influences on substance abuse in adolescents, 255
Pentazocine (Talwin), 11, 178, 207, 320
Pentobarbital (Nembutal), 11, 33, 328
Percodan, 11
Perinatal care, substance abuse in, 191-233
Perioperative care, substance abuse and, 176-177
Peterson v Washington, 435
Peyote, 11
Pharmacologic tolerance, 25
Pharmacologic treatment, 85-87, 141, 321-329
Pharmacological support in management of acute withdrawal in hospital, 137-139
Phencyclidine (PCP), 11, 28, 32, 37, 152, 184, 207, 376, 378, 440-441
Phencyclidine-induced psychosis, 293
Phenobarbital, 33, 215, 218, 219, 328, 330
Phenytoin (Dilantin), alcohol withdrawal and, 141
Philosophy of nursing care in substance abuse treatment, 305-307
Physical abuse, nursing care in home setting and, 286, 287
Physical assessment of client in nursing process, 121-122
Physical dependence, 9, 26-27
Physician, 289, 312
Physiological dependence, 9, 27
Physiological factors in relapse, 110-111
Physiological tolerance, 25
PIH; *see* Pregnancy-induced hypertension
Placaters, dysfunctional family patterns and, 238
Placenta previa, tobacco and, 206
Placental transfer of alcohol, substance abuse in perinatal care and, 194
Polydrug use, 38, 54, 156-160, 185, 320, 381-384, 399

POMR; *see* Problem-oriented medical record
Portal hypertension, alcohol withdrawal and, 155
Portal-systemic encephalopathy, alcohol withdrawal and, 161, 162-166
Positive screens, responding to, in assessment of substance abuse, 49-51
Post traumatic stress disorder (PTSD) in adult children of alcoholics, 248
Post-acute withdrawal syndrome (PAW) symptoms, 110-111
Postnatal care, substance abuse in perinatal care and, 213-214
Postoperative care, 176-177
Poverty, 271, 384-385
Preemployment drug and alcohol screening, nursing care in occupational settings and, 300
Preferred provider arrangements, financing substance abuse treatment and, 429
Pregnancy, 191-233, 271, 275; *see also* Perinatal care, substance abuse in
Pregnancy tests, 192, 208
Pregnancy-induced hypertension (PIH), heroin and, 200
Prenatal care, 207-208, 210-212
Prenatal clinics, nursing care in, 302
Preoperative care, 176
Prescription drugs, 54-55, 207, 398, 399
Prevention, 15-17, 228, 261-266
Pride Institute, 395
Primary diagnosis, dual diagnosis and, 347
Primary prevention, 274, 290-291, 294-296
Privacy, right to, drug testing and, 432
Private health insurance, financing substance abuse treatment and, 428
Problem-oriented medical record (POMR), nursing diagnosis and, 67
Professional staff, education of, nursing care in school settings and, 291
Project DARE; *see* Drug Abuse Resistance Education
"Project Match," 430
PROJECT NEADA; *see* Nursing Education in Alcohol and Drug Abuse
PROJECT SAEN; *see* Substance Abuse Education in Nursing
Propoxyphene (Darvon), 11, 320
Proteases, pancreas and, 167
Prune belly syndrome, cocaine and, 202
Pseudoaddiction, pain management and, 177
Psychiatric model of substance abuse treatment, 74
Psychiatric-mental health nursing practice standards for use by nurses practicing at generalist or advanced practice levels, 450-453
Psychiatrists in substance abuse treatment, 312
Psychoactive medications, 178, 399
Psychoactive substances, clinical manifestations and interventions for major classifications of, 149-153
Psychological assessment of client in nursing process, 122-123
Psychological consequences of substance abuse, 38-39
Psychological dependence, 9, 26-27
Psychological support in management of acute withdrawal in hospital, 137
Psychologists in substance abuse treatment, 312
Psychosis, phencyclidine-induced, 293
Psychosocial dimension of nursing care in substance abuse treatment, 340-341
Psychosocial health, monitoring of, nursing care in community settings and, 284
Psychotropic medications in withdrawal from stimulants, 329
PTSD; *see* Post traumatic stress disorder
Public health nurse, substance abuse treatment and, 14
Public Health Service, 290-291
Public laws, 425, 435

Public policy, substance abuse treatment and, 436
Puerto Ricans, nursing care of, 375-377
Punitive approach to substance abuse, 5-6
Pure Food and Drug Act of 1906, 5
Pyrazinamide (PZA) in treatment of tuberculosis, 175

Q

QA; *see* Quality assurance
Quaaludes; *see* Methaqualone
Quality assurance (QA) in drug testing, 439
Quiet alert and sleep states of drug-addicted neonate, 222-223

R

Racial and ethnic minorities, nursing care of, 373-381
Radioimmunoassay (RIA), 440, 441
"Raising the bottom," recovery and, 288
Rational Recovery, 350
Rationalization as defense mechanism in substance abuse, 30, 128
RDC; *see* Research Diagnostic Criteria
Rebound phenomenon, 27, 314
Receptors, substance abuse treatment and, 73
Recovering clients, 9, 248-249, 277-285
Recovering personnel in substance abuse treatment, 313
Recovery, 9, 102-110, 288
    and relapse; *see* Relapse
    twelve step approach to; *see* Twelve step programs
Recovery model of substance abuse treatment versus mental health model, 348-351
Recovery prone clients, 111
"Reds," 33
"Reefer," 36
Referral, 124-126, 200, 288-290, 297
Rehabilitation, 15, 306, 314
Reimbursement for substance abuse treatment, 99-100, 429
Reinforcer, 28
Relapse, 9, 22, 110-112, 350-351
    and recovery; *see* Recovery
Relapse prevention, substance abuse treatment and, 91
Relapse prone clients, 111
Reliability, 48, 65
Religion, 273, 373
Remission, 9, 103-104
Research Diagnostic Criteria (RDC), 65
Residential settings, long-term, substance abuse treatment and, 83-84
Residential treatment of client with dual diagnosis, nurse's role in, 370-371
Respiratory depression, 186-187, 218
Responsible children, dysfunctional family patterns and, 238, 252
Restoril; *see* Tenazepam
Retrospective reimbursement in substance abuse treatment, 99
RIA; *see* Radioimmunoassay
Rifampin in treatment of tuberculosis, 175
Right to privacy, drug testing and, 432
Risk reduction approach to recovery, 104-106
Ritalin, 11
"Rock," 35-36
Rogerian model, 419-421
Role behaviors, dysfunctional family patterns and, 237-239
Role conflict in substance abuse treatment, 310
Rural populations, nursing care in, 272
"Rush," 36
Rush, B., 4, 72

S

SAAST; *see* Self-Administered Alcoholism Screening Test
SADS; *see* Schedule for Affective Disorders and Schizophrenia

SAMHSA; *see* Substance Abuse and Mental Health Services Administration
San Diego Suicide Study, 42
Scapegoat, dysfunctional family patterns and, 238
Schedule for Affective Disorders and Schizophrenia (SADS) in assessment of substance abuse, 65-66
School settings, nursing care in; *see* Nursing care in school settings
SCID; *see* Structural Clinical Interview for DSM-III-R
Screening instruments for general settings in assessment of substance abuse, 47-49
Screens in assessment of substance abuse, 49-51, 57
Secobarbital (Seconal), 11, 33
Secondary diagnosis, dual diagnosis and, 347
Secondary prevention, 275-277, 291-293, 296-297
Secondary withdrawal syndrome, 320-321
Sedative-hypnotics, 33
Sedatives, 10, 11-12, 26-27, 55, 161, 320
Seizures, 215, 315, 330
Self-Administered Alcoholism Screening Test (SAAST), 49
Semistructured interview, 64-65
Sensitivity, 48, 439
Sensory-perceptual alteration, 147, 159, 165, 224-225, 322-324, 329
Serax; *see* Oxazepam
Serotonin, alcohol and, 24, 25
Sexual abuse, 41, 42, 251, 286, 288
Sexually transmitted diseases (STDs) as sequelae of substance abuse, 42, 175-176, 213
Short MAST (SMAST), 49
Short-acting barbiturates, 33
SIDS; *see* Sudden infant death syndrome
Skin integrity, impaired, 165, 183
Skinner v Railway Labor Executives' Association, 432
SMAST; *see* Short MAST
Smokeless tobacco, use of, by Native Americans, 378
Smoking, 28, 206, 254-255, 385-386; *see also* Tobacco
"Snow lights," 36
Social format for detoxification, 321
Social interactions, impaired, 174, 369-371
Social isolation, 236, 247
Social learning theory of substance abuse treatment, 74
Social model versus medical model of substance abuse treatment, 305, 308-309
Social workers in substance abuse treatment, 312
Societal approaches to substance abuse, 5-6
Societal consequences of substance abuse, 40-44
Sociocultural perspective of substance abuse treatment, 74-75
Sociopathic personality syndrome, addictions as part of, 74
Solvents, 11
"Speed," 33
Spiritual assessment of client in nursing process, 123
Spiritual counseling, substance abuse treatment and, 95-96
"Splitting," contingency contracts and, 351
Spontaneous abortion, alcohol consumption and, 193
Spontaneous remission, recovery and, 103-104
Spouse abuse, 41, 286
Staff, professional, education of, 291, 353
Standards
    of Addictions Nursing Practice, 15, 58, 119-120, 309, 449, 450-453
    of Clinical Nursing Practice, 449
    of Psychiatric and Mental Health Nursing Practice, 449
Staphylococcus aureus, cellulitis and, 170
States, block grants to, financing substance abuse treatment and, 428-429
STDs; *see* Sexually transmitted diseases
Step-down program versus long-term care, 306
Steroids, 37
Stimulants, 11, 320, 329

Stress, coping with, in primary prevention of substance abuse, 274
Stroke, alcohol abuse and, 168
Structural Clinical Interview for DSM-III-R (SCID) in assessment of substance abuse, 65, 66-67
Structured intervention, nursing care in community settings and, 288-289
Structured interview, 64-65
Students, 290, 293
Substance Abuse and Mental Health Services Administration, 472
Substance Abuse Education in Nursing (PROJECT SAEN), 474
Substance abuse treatment, 71-101, 314
  availability of, 214, 273
  confrontation in, 128-129
  costs of, 42-43
  emergency, 179-188
  versus health care, 424
  legal issues and, 431-436
  medical models of, 62-67, 73
  Missouri comprehensive plan for, 427-428
  pain management in, 177-179
  public policy and, 436
  in women, 387-389
  workplace effects of, 40, 43
Sudden infant death syndrome (SIDS), heroin and, 201
Suicide, 42, 185, 356-357
Sullivan, E., 475
Surgi-centers, nursing care in, 302
"Swapping" medications by elderly, 399
Symptomatic substance abuse treatment, 87
Synanon, 74-75, 83-84
Syphilis, 42, 175-176, 213

T

T-ACE questionnaire, 208, 209
Talwin; *see* Pentazocine
Taoism, Asian Americans attitudes toward health and, 377
Tarasoff v Regents of the University of California, 434, 435
Taxonomy I, 59
Tegaderm for infection control in drug-addicted neonate, 220
Tegretol in withdrawal from barbiturates, 328
Tenazepam (Restoril), 11
TENS; *see* Transcutaneous electrical nerve stimulation
Teratogens, 192, 193
Tertiary prevention, 277-285, 293-294, 297
Thalidomide, pregnancy and, 207
THC; *see* Delta-9-tetrahydrocannabinol
Therapeutic approach to substance abuse, 6
Therapeutic communities, substance abuse treatment and, 83-84
Therapeutic milieu, substance abuse treatment and, 89-90
Therapy, 87-91, 252-253
Thiamine, 184, 400
Thin-layer chromatography (TLC), 439-440, 441
Three-quarter house, substance abuse treatment and, 273
Tincture of opium in drug withdrawal in drug-addicted neonate, 218
Tissue-building steroids, 37
TLC; *see* Thin-layer chromatography
Tobacco, 87, 204-207, 378; *see also* Smoking
Tobacco-related neoplasms, alcohol and, 169
Tolerance, 25-26, 181-182; *see also* Cross tolerance
Tolerance test in withdrawal from barbiturates, 328
Tranquilizers, minor, 11, 55
Transcutaneous electrical nerve stimulation (TENS), 179
Transitionally relapse prone clients, 111

Tranxene; *see* Chlorazepate
Treatment, 89
Tremors, alcohol withdrawal syndrome and, 139-140
Trexan; *see* Naltrexone hydrochloride
Triazolam (Halcion), 11
Trichomoniasis, 175-176
Tricyclic antidepressants in cocaine withdrawal, 329
Tuberculosis as sequela of substance abuse, 175
Tuinal, 11
Twelve step programs, 43, 71-72, 73, 74, 81, 82, 88, 91-95, 106, 273, 306, 313, 389
Twelve Traditions of Alcoholics Anonymous, 92, 93, 94

U

Unstructured interview, 64-65
Urban populations, special needs in, nursing care in community settings and, 270-272
Urethritis, nonspecific, 175-176
Urogenital anomalies, cocaine and, 202
U.S. Chamber of Commerce, 294
U.S. Department of Defense, 300, 426
U.S. Department of Health and Human Services, 444
U.S. Department of Transportation, 300
Use, 8

V

Vagal response in infants of mothers with substance abuse, 215
Vaillant's study, substance abuse and, 21-22
Validity, 48, 65
Valium; *see* Diazepam
Vancomycin hydrochloride (Vancocin) in treatment of cellulitis, 170
Varices, esophageal, alcohol withdrawal and, 155-161
Vasodilators in treatment of alcoholic cardiomyopathy, 168
Vasopressin in treatment of esophageal varices, 161
Venereal warts, 175-176
Vietnamese, nursing care of, 377-378
Violence, 41, 132, 272, 356-357
Viral hepatitis as sequela of substance abuse, 175
Visiting Nurse Association (VNA), addictions nursing practice and, 456-458
Volatile agents, inhalation of, 37

W

Warts, genital, 175-176
"Weed," 36
Well-baby clinics, nursing care in, 302
Wellness programs, nursing care in occupational settings and, 295-296
Wernicke-Korsakoff syndrome, 184, 400
WFS; *see* Women for Sobriety
WHO; *see* World Health Organization
Wilkerson v Times Mirror Corp., 432
Willner v Thornburgh, 432
Withdrawal, 136-148, 158, 160, 213, 218, 226-227; *see also* Detoxification
Withdrawal assessment scale, 315
Withdrawal seizures, 330
Women, 286, 376-377, 381-398
Workers' compensation, nursing care in occupational settings and, 300
Workplace, 401-402, 431, 443
World Health Organization (WHO), 49

X

Xanax; *see* Alprazolam

Y

"Yellows," 33